Cobert's Manual of Drug Safety and Pharmacovigilance

Fourth Edition

Cobert's Manual of Drug Safety and Pharmacovigilance

Fourth Edition

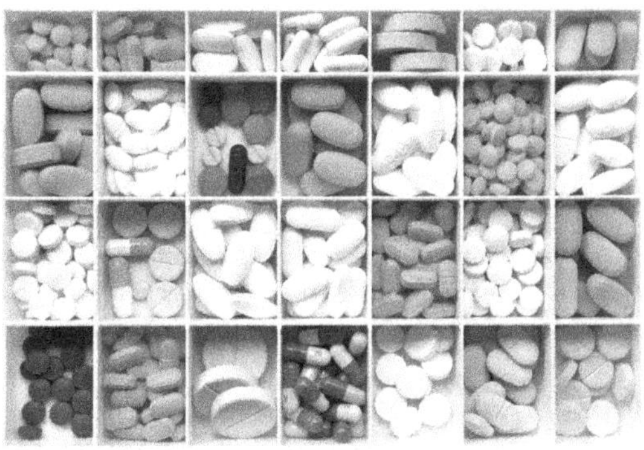

Barton Cobert
BLCMD Associates USA

William W Gregory
USA

Jean-Loup Thomas
Hospices Civils de Lyon, France

Catherine Baldridge
Essential Pharmacovigilance, LLC, USA

World Scientific

NEW JERSEY • LONDON • SINGAPORE • BEIJING • SHANGHAI • HONG KONG • TAIPEI • CHENNAI

Published by

World Scientific Publishing Co. Pte. Ltd.
5 Toh Tuck Link, Singapore 596224
USA office: 27 Warren Street, Suite 401-402, Hackensack, NJ 07601
UK office: 57 Shelton Street, Covent Garden, London WC2H 9HE

British Library Cataloguing-in-Publication Data
A catalogue record for this book is available from the British Library.

COBERT'S MANUAL OF DRUG SAFETY AND PHARMACOVIGILANCE
Fourth Edition

ISBN 978-981-12-9771-7 (hardcover)
ISBN 978-981-98-0021-6 (paperback)
ISBN 978-981-12-9772-4 (ebook for institutions)
ISBN 978-981-12-9773-1 (ebook for individuals)

For any available supplementary material, please visit
https://www.worldscientific.com/worldscibooks/10.1142/13970#t=suppl

Typeset by Stallion Press
Email: enquiries@stallionpress.com

Thank You

Barton Cobert: Thanks to Chris Davis who saw enough merit in the earlier editions to publish a fourth edition. And thank you to the team at World Publishing. Great to work with all of you!

Thanks to our many colleagues in the drug safety world for their advice and clarification.

And again, thanks to my loving and lovely wife Josiane and our children Julien Cobert, MD and Emilie Murray, MD, JD, MPH for their advice and contributions.

Thanks to Catherine, Bill and Jean-Loup for taking much of the work and pressure off my retired shoulders!

Jean-Loup Thomas: Thanks to all my colleagues and ex-colleagues who have been so professional and nice to work with.

William Gregory: To Lauren and Carly for their incredible love and understanding, for giving me a sharper appreciation of lawyers and veterinarians, and for making my soul blossom every day. To my co-authors for being so smart and easy to work alongside, chapter by chapter.

Catherine Baldridge: To my patient husband and three beautiful children for giving me love, support, and encouragement; To my late brother, Philip, for fueling my fire to fight for ethical product development and safety; To my sister for her constant "you can do this" and daily reminder that I have something important to say, and to my parents for providing me with an education & skills that have allowed me to succeed. Lastly, thank you to Bart, Bill, and Jean-Loup for allowing me to contribute to the text and learn from their illustrious careers and valuable experience!

Contents

Manual 4 Introductions

This is now the fourth edition of the Manual.

Edition 1 was published in 2007 which now seems like it was a century ago. This was when the internet was in its "infancy" and the use of information technology was largely unknown in pharmacovigilance which was also younger — perhaps a toddler. Edition 2 was published in 2012 and edition 3 in 2019. Things were clearly changing between 2007 and 2019. We had anticipated another 5 to 7 years for the fourth edition but clearly the changes that have occurred since 2019 were major. Similarly in the four years since edition 3 major changes have occurred in the pharmaceutical world not the least of which has been Covid. There were many causes for these changes. Perhaps the biggest was the rapidly evolving field of information technology, artificial intelligence, new and powerful databases, social media and fake news, instantaneous communication as well as new duties and functions in the FDA, EMA and other health agencies, Brexit (with the MHRA moving from London to Amsterdam), multi-polar global pharmacovigilance rather than dominance by the US, the EU and Japan (the original ICH partners), changes in the pharmaceutical industry, more generics, pharmacoepidemiology, signaling, marijuana "approval", opioid abuses and many others you could name. The first two editions were single author books. At that time, this was reasonable and possible. Now the field has become so large and complicated that expertise is needed from multiple authors. We have still tried to keep this Manual simple and readable. We've tried to minimize jargon and long compound and complex sentences.

We are delighted that Catherine Baldridge has joined the team! She has provided wonderful insight into what is happening in the world of drug safety as well as functioning as Chief Operating Officer of this endeavor! Thank you, Catherine.

The numerous reasons mentioned above pushed us to update this Manual somewhat sooner than we had anticipated. By necessity, we have made some changes to the contents compared to previous editions. There is more on signaling and pharmacoepidemiology but those fields now seem to merit a manual or textbook of their own. We have cut back on looking at global

PV as there are now far too many countries involved in PV with rapidly changing rules, laws, regulations and procedures. Practically speaking, because of language issues and local "unwritten" practices keeping up with PV in over 100 countries is nearly impossible.

Finally, any thought that we might get some breathing room after this edition is probably not going to happen. The next changes on the horizon will be in the field of AI (artificial intelligence). AI will make major changes in the way the whole world works, communicates and analyzes data. There may also be some significant changes in drug approval by regulators. This has been spurred on by the "waivers", shorter review times and other exceptions to the usual rules to allow drugs and vaccines to be used against Covid. We expect new pathways to emerge to get products to the patients faster but with less data. To put it another way, if efficacy can be shown quickly the product can get provisional approval with the proviso that more efficacy and safety data will be collected. This means that we will collect more and more safety data after marketing. This is now being seen with Covid medications and marijuana.

In any case, some of the observations from the introductions in previous editions still apply and are worth looking at:

- We now have four authors not just one. The field has become so complex, diverse, global and messy that it is impossible for one person to be fully versed in the field to do a single author textbook.
- Given the extraordinary changes in IT and data collection, it is now presumed by the health agencies that global data can and will be accurately and completely collected and processed both in clinical trials and in the post-marketing setting. With changes in approval procedures for marketing we are now seeing drugs reach the market with fewer patients studied and less known about the safety profile. The potential to mine safety data from electronic health records is promising and could supplement and, perhaps, reduce some duplication of pharmacovigilanties' efforts. We are also seeing more post-marketing requirements. This may or may not be a good thing.
- Other major changes include the divergences in many areas that were more or less harmonized by ICH. Harmonization seems to have peaked in the early 2000s. We now see divergences in the US and EU and in many other areas, particularly as technology has evolved.
- ISO has entered the picture and many more countries and outside organizations are now involved in the pharmaceutical world. Hopefully these are good things.
- On the disheartening side, we see corporatization, digitalization, depersonalization, politicization, commoditization, and other "-izations" in drug safety and medicine in general. Medicine is now a mass-market commodity, and drug safety is following that path too. We see laxity and bad behavior on the part of industry, healthcare practitioners, patients, consumers, government, universities, and nongovernmental organizations. We see politics and money continue to play a big role in the world of pharmacology. We also see the downside of globalization, with enormous fragmentation and duplication of efforts, and little upside.
- This manual is a practical instruction book on drug safety. It is aimed at newcomers, old-timers, and outsiders to the field who would like a demystification and explanation of what adverse events are and how drug safety departments work. Hopefully, readers, especially those not in the field, will understand that drug safety, like all other areas of medicine, is as much an art as it is a science.
- For newcomers, this is a "Drug Safety 101" course giving a broad overview of how adverse events are handled from start to finish. For old-timers, this book will fill in gaps in knowledge on drug safety. For outsiders not working directly in this field, this book will explain how "side effects" are handled by the industry and by health authorities. This book is not meant to be an encyclopedia. There are other such books already available.
- It is expected that, after carefully reading and absorbing the contents, the reader will be able to begin work in a drug safety department, or, if an outsider, understand what happens in such a department and where listings or adverse events come from.
- We have attempted to avoid excess jargon ("This spontaneous SAE is expeditable since it is unlisted") and make the book approachable for those with limited or no knowledge of medicine or pharmacology.

There it is. We hope you find the book useful, accurate, and easy to read and absorb. Best of luck. You'll need it.

Authors

The original text, and "founding father" of this textbook series, Dr. Barton Cobert, has worked tirelessly over the years to share his knowledge, experience and insight in this scientific field. His contributions to the industry are well known and he was one of the first to set forth and publish a text regarding the basic principles and theory of drug safety and pharmacovigilance. Throughout his illustrious career, he has forged relationships with other key opinion leaders and graciously invited others to contribute their knowledge to the text Each contributor has provided a summary of their background to showcase their experience and for the readers to have a better understanding of who has contributed to the text. Collectively, we as contributing authors are grateful to have been included in this endeavor and hope that our readers will find just as much value in our advice as we have had in providing it.

— Catherine Baldridge

Barton Cobert, MD, FACP, FACG
United States

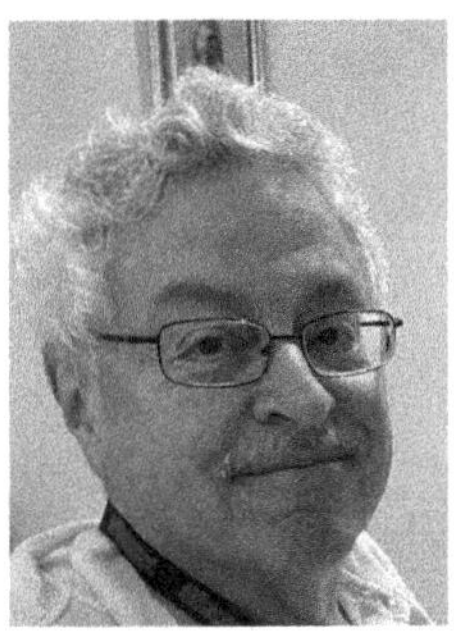

Dr. Cobert is an expert on Drug Safety and medication side effects, and author of several textbooks and multiple journal articles on these topics. He has extensive experience in Drug Safety, Clinical Drug Research, Regulatory Affairs, Risk Management, and Computer Informatics in pharmaceuticals. He was previously in practice doing gastroenterology before entering the pharmaceutical world as Global Head of Drug Safety at Schering Plough and Novartis OTC. He has worked for several pharmaceutical companies and consulted to FDA and other regulatory agencies. He created his own consulting group BLCMD Associates in 2008. Dr Cobert is a 1974 graduate of the New York University School of Medicine where he also did his training in Internal Medicine and Gastroenterology. He also did a post-doctoral fellowship in liver disease in France. He is board certified in Internal Medicine and Gastroenterology.

Dr. Jean-Loup Thomas, MD
France

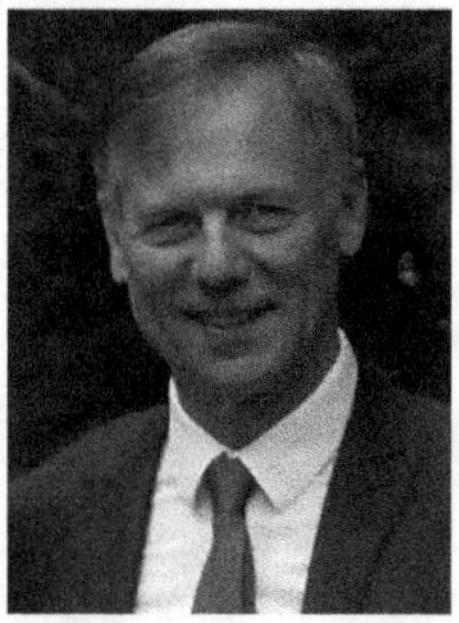

Dr. Jean-Loup Thomas is M.D. graduate of the Paris (France) Medical School (La Pitié Salpétrière), specialized in clinical Pharmaco-Toxicology. He started his medical career at the Paris Poison Control and Pharmacovigilance Center. He then moved to the pharmaceutical industry within Pharmacovigilance for several companies (Lilly, Novartis, Merck-Serono, Sanofi-Pasteur, Sanofi Pharma), at both affiliate and corporate levels. He is an expert in Clinical Pharmacology, Clinical Safety/Pharmacovigilance, Safety Signals and Risk Management, Drug Safety Crisis, Data Monitoring Committees/Data Safety Monitoring Boards, Labelling/ Product Information and Clinical Development. He has been EU QPPV within the Sanofi group and also led the Sanofi Global Labelling team. He is now Senior Consultant for the clinical pharmaco-toxicology department at the Hospices Civils de Lyon (France).

Dr. William W. Gregory
United States

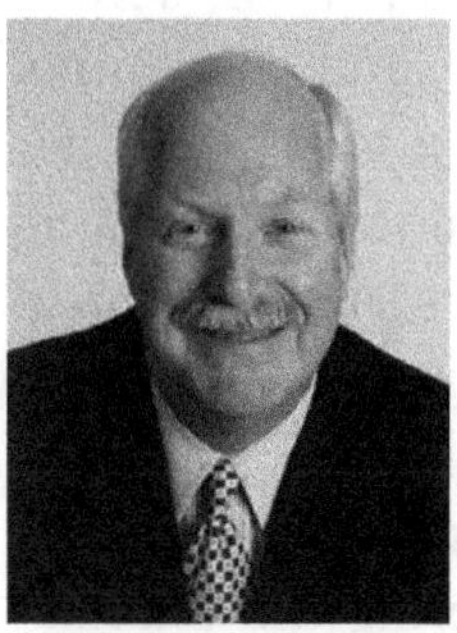

Dr. Gregory received formal training in infectious diseases and molecular mechanisms of pathogenesis at Davidson College, the University of St Andrews (Dundee), and the University of North Carolina Medical School (Chapel Hill) followed by postgraduate fellowships at The University of Chicago Hospitals and Clinics and the University of Rochester Medical Center. He has practical experience in diagnostic methodology/ techniques, product in/out licensing due diligence, pharmacovigilance, benefit-risk assessment, drug safety operations, clinical trial design, pre- and post-registration protocol development and execution, regulatory phases I-IV of medicinals and large molecule development for successful product registration. He also held positions at the US Army Institute for Infectious Diseases (Fort Detrick), the Veterans Administration (consultant in laboratory medicine), the US Army Combat Engineers (Captain), the University of Virginia Medical School (pathology professor), the University of Virginia Hospitals and Clinics, the Blue Ridge Hospital, and a 40-year career at Pfizer Inc. in positions of increasing responsibility and influence in R & D, including Team Leader for several commercially-successful products launched around the world. He was awarded the prestigious Excellence in Research and Development Award by Pfizer for innovation in clinical research and efficiencies in global product development and registration. He has served on many consensus panels, including ICH, CIOMS, ISO, Eu2P, DIA, NCCLS, and HL7 as well as trade groups. He is an accomplished jazz trombonist, dog breeder, and is credited with more than 50 scientific publications as an author or co-author.

Mrs. Catherine Baldridge, MS
United States

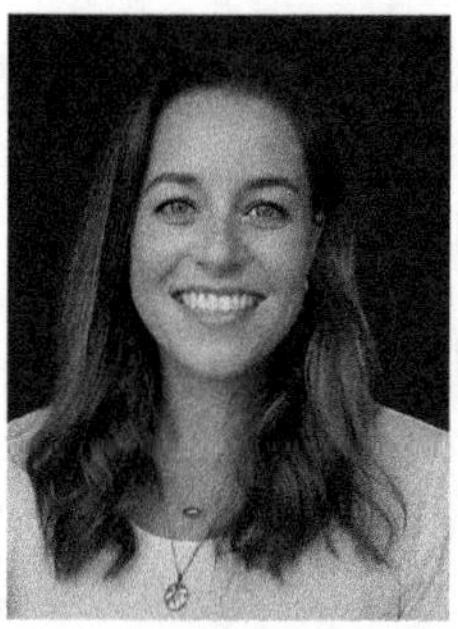

Mrs. Catherine Baldridge is a recognized leader in product safety & pharmacovigilance operations. She is a graduate of Hollins University with a degree in Psychology, with a concentration in both neuro and clinical psychology, and later received her Masters of Science degree from the University of Virginia in Clinical Investigations and Patient Oriented Research. Mrs. Baldridge has worked for several CROs and Pharmaceutical and biotech companies, and has held positions as an Adjunct Faculty at Temple University, teaching several courses in Clinical Trial Safety and Good Pharmacovigilance Operations. She has been a leader within the DIA organization, serving as the Chair of the Clinical Safety and Pharmacovigilance community as well as leading several discussions in the field and providing expert peer review of published articles in therapeutic journals. Mrs. Baldridge has also served as an industry consultant, helping many companies develop safety operations and remediate inspection findings and outcomes.

Chapter Contributions

"You don't know what you don't know"

To acknowledge when you are not the expert, when are still educating yourself, and to realize the power of seeking guidance and advice from others, is really one of the only ways to grow and succeed in life as well as in this industry. We understand our limitations as professionals in the medical and scientific field of drug safety and pharmacovigilance and have sought thoughtful insights and educational wisdom from several other experts within the field, who are listed below.

The authors would like to acknowledge and thank our contributors, without whom some of these chapters could not be realized.

We thank them for their time, dedication, and expert advice and opinion towards the industry and their contribution to this text.

Lisa Beth Ferstenberg, MD
United States

Lisa Beth has worked in the pharmaceutical industry for over 40 years during which she has assisted in the development of multiple biopharmaceutical, monoclonal antibody, cell therapy and vaccine products. Her experience spans four epidemics, the evolution of biotechnology, the remarkable advances in organ and cellular transplantation and the use of gene therapies for rare diseases.

Her global engagement has given her experience in the most sophisticated research centers and the most basic community care outposts. She has had the opportunity to learn the impact of cultural beliefs, economics, social requirements and political influences on the availability and delivery of healthcare.

Currently, Lisa Beth is Executive Director of Pharmacovigilance for the Biopharmaceutical Division of AstraZeneca where she recently oversaw safety management for the deployment of the COVID vaccine.

Chapter Contributions: Author of Chapter 41, Vaccinovigilance

Gretchen S. Dieck, MPhil, PhD

Epidemiologist and safety & risk management consultant
United States

Gretchen Dieck, PhD, is currently an epidemiology, safety, and risk management consultant to the pharmaceutical industry. Previously, she was Vice President, Safety, Epidemiology, and Risk Management at UBC where she was responsible for a group that develops, validates, and supports automated tools for safety, risk management, and cost and utilization. Before working at UBC, Dr. Dieck was 23 years at Pfizer where she was Senior Vice President, Safety and Risk Management. She has over 35 years of experience in the pharmaceutical industry. She was a Founding Board Member of the International Society for Pharmacoepidemiology and is the past Chair of the Pharmacovigilance and Epidemiology Technical Group of PhRMA. She represented PhRMA during PDUFA III and PDUFA IV discussions and co-led the PostMarket Safety Group. Dr. Dieck received an AB in Biological Sciences from Smith College and has obtained M. Phil. and Ph.D. in epidemiology and also completed a Postdoctoral Fellowship in cardiovascular disease epidemiology at Yale University.

Chapter Contributions: Chapter 5, Mathematics of AEs; Chapter 6, Pharmacoepidemiology

Aurore GOURAUD PharmD

Pharmacovigilance Specialist, Clinical Pharmaco Toxicology Department, Lyon, France

Aurore Gouraud, PharmD, is currently a hospital practitioner in the pharmaco-toxicology department of the Hospices Civils de Lyon, where she works as a toxicologist at the poison control center. Formerly, she was Deputy Director of the Lyon Pharmacovigilance Center, where she managed all post-marketing pharmacovigilance activities; her interest is focused on benefit-risk assessment and drug exposure for pregnant and breast-feeding women. She is responsible for the Dynamic Meta-analysis Unit, which deals with the evaluation of the benefits and risks of medicines (http://metaevidence.org/). She has been an expert in pharmacovigilance for the French national agency (ANSM) for over 10 years. She holds a doctorate in pharmacy and a Master of Science in medical engineering, and led a Pharmacovigilance Certificate over ten years (University of Lyon).

Chapter Contributions: Chapter 16: Vulnerable populations, Chapter 17: Pregnancy & Lactation, Chapter 18: Acute & chronic AEs, Chapter 19: Drug-Drug Interactions

Isabelle BRUYERE, PharmD

Therapeutic Area Head — Pneumo, Meninge and Endemic vaccines, Patient Safety & Pharmacovigilance Department, Sanofi-Pasteur

Dr. Isabelle Bruyère is Therapeutic Area Head (TAH) at Sanofi Patient Safety & Pharmacovigilance, dedicated to meninge, pneumo and traveler vaccines. In this role, Isabelle is responsible for a wide range of functions including, management of Global Safety Officers (GSO), providing strategic guidance to ensure best in class evaluation and communication of safety signals, benefit risk assessment and answers to Health Authorities, interactions with external committees and partners.

Isabelle obtained her PharmD with honors, Master of Biological and Medical Sciences and an Inter-University Diploma in Toxicology and Drug Safety from Claude Bernard University, Lyon France. She has also further training in signal substantiation and quantification from the Erasmus University in Rotterdam/European program for Pharmacovigilance and Pharmacoepidemiology. She is involved as a lecturer in various training programs on pharmacovigilance, notably the Master of Vaccinology in Siena, Italy, the Inter-University Diploma curriculum from the Regional PV center and the Eudipharm master from the University in Lyon, France.

She started her career in Pharmacovigilance more than 15 years ago at the Public Regional PV center of Lyon in 2006 in the framework of her Pharmacy Internship. After working in the hospital setting supporting clinical trials, Isabelle joined the industry and served as a Global Safety Officer at Sanofi for 11 years. During this period, she developed expertise in signal management, benefit-risk assessment, and risk management planning.

Chapter Contributions:

Chapter 10: EU Qualified Person for Pharmacovigilance; Chapter 30: Pharma Companies; Chapter 36: Pharmacovigilance System Master File

Magnus Ysander, MD

Executive Director, EU QPPV

Chapter Contributions: Co-author Chapter 41, Vaccinovigilance

Notice

This manual is meant to be a guide to those new to, or those who already have experience with, the history, theory, and basic principles of drug safety and pharmacovigilance. We acknowledge the ever-changing regulatory, legal and "medical culture" environment with regards to the principles and topics outlined within, which makes it an ongoing challenge to keep this text up to date. However, we hope that our insights will help further the understanding of these topics in order to promote best practice when it comes to product development in regard to safety and pharmacovigilance.

This book is not meant to be used in the practice of medicine or for the prescription of medicines, drugs, biologics, over-the-counter medications, health foods, supplements, and so forth. The medications described do not necessarily have specific approval by the U.S. Food and Drug Administration, European Medicines Agency, Health Canada, or any other regulatory or health agency for use in the diseases, patients, or dosages discussed. The approved labeling in the United States and other countries and regions must be consulted for that jurisdiction before any product is used or prescribed. Because standards for usage change, it is advisable to keep abreast of revised recommendations, precautions, safety warnings, and adverse events, particularly those concerning new products.

This book is not intended to express opinions about the value of specific products or their comparative value within a drug class, even when a specific product is used to provide examples of adverse reactions. The content of this book is not meant to be used in choosing therapies in medical practice by healthcare practitioners or consumers. As with all medications and therapies, the official approved product labeling should be consulted before prescribing or using.

And finally, this manual is not meant to be a comprehensive drug development guide.

We have given our opinions on many areas of safety in drug development and marketing, but things change daily. *Therefore, we urge you to investigate further what we have written as reference and realize that this is a science that is ever developing.* Check many sources. Trust but verify.

A brief note on spelling. Just as pharmacovigilance is not totally harmonized (harmonised), the English language suffers similarly. We have used both US and UK spelling inconsistently throughout this book. In particular, we did not change spelling in URLs which, of course, would not allow you to reach the website.

A note on URLS: We learned in the past editions of this Manual, that URLs may have very short half-lives! Organizations merge, reorganize, get new or updated databases, etc. Thus, URLs which were correct at the time of writing often change or disappear by the time the book is published. When we do list URLs, try them. With luck, they'll still work. Otherwise, a Google search should be done.

Good luck!

CHAPTER

1

The History and Theory of Drug Safety and Pharmacovigilance

Why does a biopharmaceutical or device company need a drug/device safety group? What is the mission of such a drug safety group and how is it organized?

■ The Why

This is a question often asked and then taught in programs around the world. Why does a company need a drug/device/product safety group? National laws in many countries require manufacturers, biopharmaceutical companies, and others to comply with certain requirements that are designed to ultimately protect the human patient and recipient of products developed to improve or mitigate a known health outcome. Why do you need a safety group? Because the law requires it, and our ethical obligations to the public and patients lend to the necessity of such a group. Additionally, as a result of inspection findings, outcomes of poor planning, manufacturing, labeling/communication, and other unsavory events, it is in a company's best interest to accurately and diligently study, monitor, and evaluate a product's effect in humans and its safe use in order to avoid legal and financial penalties and burdens.... and to best protect the public health. Put simply, if you don't "do safety" right, you'll pay for it later, quite literally.

In this chapter we review the background and purpose of some of the regulatory agencies as well as notable historical events that led to the development of key principles that make up what we now call good "safety and pharmacovigilance" practices, or GVP.

■ A Brief History, Focusing on the US FDA

The history of balancing benefits and risks of pharmacologically active substances has a very extensive history. Some of the earliest work can be traced back many centuries to Chinese and other Asian herbalists. Written documentation exists to support the preparation and safe and effective use of herbal preparations and herbal combinations to improve human health. However, up until a century or two ago, the requirements for the safety and efficacy of drug products were either non-existent or poorly defined at best. And unregulated. In the US, the Pure Food and Drugs Act (FDA), adopted into law in 1906, prohibited interstate commerce of mislabeled and adulterated drugs and food within the United States. This covered some safety aspects of drugs but not efficacy. The FDA had, at that time, no jurisdiction or control of efficacy claims made for drugs. In 1912, the law was changed to cover false and fraudulent claims made for drugs. However, the law did not mandate safety and, in effect, unsafe products could be and were marketed. The FDA could not seize unsafe drugs and was limited only to issuing public warnings.

Much of FDA's oversight and enforcement authority have emerged because of misbehavior and disasters. In 1937, a company in the United States marketed elixir of sulfanilamide, which contained diethylene glycol (similar to antifreeze) as a solvent. More than 100 people (including many children) died from this product due to kidney failure caused by the solvent. Because the law did not require safety testing for drugs, the company had done none. As a result of this, the Federal Food, Drug and Cosmetic Act was passed into law in 1938. This law required safety testing to be performed and submitted to the FDA in a New Drug Application (NDA). Additional laws were passed in the 1940s requiring testing for purity, strength, and quality of many drugs.

The next major event was the thalidomide disaster of the early 1960s, when the NDA for thalidomide was valiantly opposed by Dr. Frances Kelsey at the FDA because of insufficient safety information despite strong pressure to approve it. The product was intended for use in pregnant women to prevent morning sickness and was widely available for this use in Europe and was even sold OTC in Germany. Though never marketed in the US, thalidomide was used in the investigational setting in the US. By 1962, the terrible teratogenic (birth defect) aspect of the drug became known as babies were born, mostly in Europe, with severely deformed arms and legs (phocomelia).

In 1962, the Kefauver-Harris Amendment became law and introduced the modern era of drug regulation. Drug manufacturers now had to demonstrate to the FDA both safety and efficacy before marketing a new drug. In 1971, the National Drug Experience Reporting System was begun as was the publication of "The FDA Drug Bulletin" to alert physicians and pharmacists to drug issues. In 1985, the regulations on AE reporting for marketed drugs were strengthened, and new requirements for Investigational New Drug Applications (INDs) were introduced. Over the years, the FDA has had multiple reorganizations and alterations in its structure and function as the overseer of drug safety and efficacy in the US. The result is the complex system of AE collection, analysis, and reporting that we know today.

Regulations, Laws, and Guidances

The regulations, laws, guidances, guidelines, and other relevant documents covering drug safety and pharmacovigilance are scattered throughout multiple places in the Code of Federal Regulations (CFR) for the US, in various venues for European Union (EU) and member state documents, and now in many other regions such as Canada, India, Australia, the Asian Pacific and other regions worldwide.

Their ultimate goal remains the same in all countries: ensure the best use of medicines in the interest of any subject/patient.

The EU PV requirements are designed at the EMA level (Regulations, Directives, and Guidances) and then implemented in each EU country; nevertheless, some countries can be more (but never less) demanding. Most of the EU documents are updated fairly frequently. Most other countries in the world have their own set of local laws, regulations, and guidances (often available only in the local language).

Requirements in most countries are fairly similar in their intent of protecting patient safety (including subjects in clinical trials). Some countries, such as Australia, even refer back to EU GVP guidelines. Most local regulations require nearly all SAEs and some non-serious AEs to be reported quickly if there appears to be a potential impact on public health. The definitions of "serious" and "non-serious" AEs are more or less standardized, although there are nuances that apply in various jurisdictions.

More "routine" individual AEs are analyzed and reported at periodic intervals. Most countries also require some form of aggregate reporting of serious and non-serious AEs at periodic intervals (e.g., every 3 months, 6 months, yearly, every 3 years), depending upon whether the drug is in clinical trials or on the market and whether it is new or old. Although the rules are similar throughout the world, they are sufficiently different in detail ("the devil is in the details") they can be very difficult to track and keep up to date. The major documents for the US and the EU are listed below. These should be read and digested by anyone doing drug safety for a living. The contents of these documents are topics of this book. In the US, FDA's regulation-making authority derives from legislation passed by the US Congress and signed into law by the US President. Most of the FDA-directed legislation gives FDA broad ability to introduce regulations and to enforce the related requirements. The FDA regulations do not explicitly state that a department or group must exist to deal with drug safety. Rather, sponsor/applicant obligations are spelled out. A "sponsor" is responsible for clinical trials and an "applicant" is responsible for meeting requirements associated with a marketing application and in the post-marketing phase. To do this adequately, an organized system or department is necessary.

The EU PV requirements are designed at the EMA level (Regulations, Directives, and Guidances) and then implemented in each EU country, with some countries being more (but never less) demanding. The EU regulations are more specific and require that a formal pharmacovigilance (PV) system be put in place and that it is fit-for-purpose: Good Pharmacovigilance Practices (GVPs) Module I — Pharmacovigilance systems and their quality systems. In addition, the EU regulations require an EU Qualified Person for Pharmacovigilance" (EU QPPV) be nominated by the pharmaceutical company: this EU QPPV is legally responsible for ensuring a company meets its legal obligations for the safety monitoring of all registered products and is a significant role within any company.

The United States and EU Laws, Regulations, Guidances, Guidelines, Directives and Practices

Drug safety in the US is covered under several sections of the Code of Federal Regulations (CFR). FDA regulations are consolidated in Title 21 of the CFR or 21 CFR (a searchable version of 21CFR is available at www.regulations.gov).

21CFR312 covers INDs: 21CFR312.32 covers IND safety reports, including expedited 7- and 15-day reports. 21CFR33 covers IND annual reports. The NDA regulations for drugs are found in 21CFR314.80. Updates to regulations are published in the *Federal Register* on a daily basis and are viewable (www.regulations.gov). Note that the consolidated CFR is only updated with the final FDA regulations from the daily Federal Register only once a year, on April 1st.

A summary of safety documents for the EU can be found at the EudraVigilance website (www.eudravigilance.eu), the European Commission website (www.ec.europa.eu), and the EMA website (www.ema.europa.eu).

There are several major documents covering drug safety: EudraLex Volume 10 is for clinical trials (amended in 2019 with the implementation of Regulation (EU) No 536/2014). For post-marketing, the regulations have been completely reviewed in 2010–2012; the main documents are as follows:

- Regulations (EU) Nos. 1235/2010 and 1027/2012.
- Directives 2010/84/EU and 2012/26/EU.
- Good Vigilance Practices (GVP); there is a series of 12 Good Pharmacovigilance Practice (GVP) modules, numbered I to XVI (planned Modules XI, XII, XIII, and XIV are void, as the content has been integrated into other modules). The GVP modules provide guidance to marketing authorization holders (MAHs), the EMA, and national competent authorities in EU member states. They cover medicines authorized in the EEA, regardless of the route of authorization.

There are several subsections devoted to drug safety also available at this website. "Volume 10 — Clinical Trials Guidelines" includes the following:

- Detailed guidance on the collection, verification, and presentation of adverse reaction reports arising from clinical trials on medicinal products for human use;
- Detailed guidance on the European database of suspected unexpected serious adverse reactions (EudraVigilance — Clinical Trial Module);
- Questions and answers specific to adverse reaction reporting in clinical trials.

Pharmaceutical companies are obliged to capture AEs, analyze them, and report them to their health agency locally and to other health authorities, or to companies abroad for submission to their HAs if there are formal corporate arrangements for sales and trials outside the home country. Thus, a company needs to create or have full-time (24/7) access to a safety team or department equipped to handle spontaneous and clinical trial AEs (as required) or to outsource this function. If the company is based solely in one country, the department may be relatively small and uncomplicated. In the simple setting, AEs are reported only to the HA in that country. If, however, AEs can come from (or need to go to) subsidiaries or affiliates in other countries or from business partners with which the company has contractual relationships, the complexity of the needs and requirements grows enormously. If a single-country company is doing clinical trials outside its borders, it must be able to report AEs and handle all other safety and regulatory matters with other countries' health agencies.

Safety & PV Operational Considerations

Different languages, time zones, ever-changing government requirements, reporting due dates, documents and formats, electronic transmission, and so forth must be taken into account. Standard operating procedures, Medical Dictionary for Regulatory Activities (MedDRA®), and training systems must be in place. An electronic safety database must be built (an enormous task) or purchased or leased (still a complex and costly endeavor). Risk evaluation and management/mitigation systems must be in place.

Healthcare personnel, including physicians, nurses, pharmacists, and support staff, must be hired. The business relationships with other concerned departments within the company, such as regulatory affairs, sales and marketing, legal, clinical research, and others, must be established. In other words, creating a safety department is a complex and expensive endeavor that must be done absolutely correctly.

After an AE report is received by the safety department, it must be entered or uploaded into the safety database, which is used for storage, retrieval, analysis, and reporting data. Although such transactional databases may start out in small companies as spreadsheets with the data typed onto paper forms, most companies respond to this need by purchasing an expensive (up to hundreds of thousands or millions of dollars, depending on the number and location of users and information technology, IT, maintenance staff) dedicated safety database. In addition to a transactional database, some large organizations have developed data warehouses to organize and store large amounts of safety data. Much of this is now out-sourced and stored in the cloud. They create complex departments with tight standard operating procedures to ensure that the company remains in full compliance with all laws, regulations, and guidelines and will withstand inspections and audits from the FDA, EMA, and other HAs, business partners, outside auditing companies and others.

There is usually a senior executive (typically a vice president for drug safety) to oversee the entire group. Within the drug safety group, there are multiple functions to handle. Depending on the size of the company, separate people or groups may handle each of the categories below. In small companies, all functions may fall on one or two people or are outsourced.

- Case receipt, triage, and processing by data entry personnel;
- Case evaluation by medical professionals;
- Coding of AEs in MedDRA (sometimes this group is separate from drug safety);

- Coding of drugs in WHO-Drug or another drug dictionary;
- Quality review;
- Medical review by physicians;
- Submission to HAs, subsidiaries, business partners, and so on.

To support the drug safety group, there is often a dedicated informatics (IT/computer) group, a signaling/pharmacovigilance group, a training group, a standard operating procedure (quality) group, an epidemiology group, a risk management group, a quality group and more. These groups may be within or separate from the drug safety department. Sometimes a medical report writing group also falls under drug safety to prepare aggregate reports, such as Periodic Safety Update Reports (PSURs, PBRERs), annual reports, NDA periodic reports, IND annual reports, and so on.

Similar groups often exist within HAs. Some authorities (FDA, MHRA, Health Canada, ANSM, TGA, EMA, and others) receive reports directly from healthcare professionals and consumers. The agencies may form departments similar to those in companies to receive, enter, and evaluate data and make medical judgments on the cases. The volumes in companies may run to tens or even hundreds of thousands of cases per year. The FDA received over 2.3 million post-marketing ICSRs in 2022, of which 1.3 million (57%) were expedited. There were 78,000 (2%) received directly from the healthcare community or consumers (refer to the FDA website, www.fda.gov). These reports (redacted) are available over the Internet using a public dashboard.

This is a large task and is performed by most health agencies throughout the world. Because serious cases tend to be reported to all health agencies, there is enormous duplication of effort in creating databases in each agency and company. In practice, only HAs in large countries with advanced pharmacovigilance practices are able to maintain relatively complete databases and conduct meaningful signal analyses.

There are four major databases with large but not total overlap for post-marketing AEs: the FDA in the United States, the EudraVigilance database in the EMA (Amsterdam), the MHRA database (UK), and the Vigibase at the Uppsala Monitoring Centre in Sweden. There are others as well.

Clinical trial AEs tend to be more scattered and far less transparent than AEs for marketed products because most of the information on drugs not yet on the market is proprietary and guarded as secret information by both companies and HAs. In many countries, clinical trials by pharmaceutical companies, universities, consortia, health agencies, and others must be entered into web-based registries. The largest is the clinical trial website maintained by the US National Library of Medicine at the National Institutes of Health (www.clinicaltrials.gov), with more than 460,000 trials from all over the world registered as of the middle of 2023. The data, however, are variable, and often there is little or no safety data and the data are not always up to date. Various countries, including the US, have mandated regular posting and updating of "Basic Results" for safety (and efficacy) data. When the database first went into production in 2000, trial listings and data were incomplete, but this has gradually improved over the ensuing years.

The Mission of a Safety Group

The mission of the safety group must be clearly defined and made known to all employees of the company, in particular to senior management, marketing and sales. It is also good policy to let the general public know of the company's or health agency's commitment to patient safety. For example, see FDA's Sentinel Initiative Mission Statement. Companies also explain their safety functions to the public, see for example, Pfizer (www.pfizer.com), Merck (www.merck.com), and Novartis (www.novartis.com).

The mission of the drug safety group, whether in a company or a health agency, is first and foremost to protect the public health by maintaining accurate, up-to-date, and complete safety information. Medical analyses must be done with patient safety in mind, not "product and sales protection". It is argued that the best product and sales protection comes from ensuring that full, unbiased, scientific, and complete safety information is available to all stakeholders: patients, medical professionals, health agencies, and the company in a form that can be understood by the particular target audience. Secondary goals within a company's safety department relate to such corporate functions as consultation within the company on safety issues, legal matters including litigation, response to patient and healthcare professional queries, training, and supporting the sales force.

There is often enormous pressure on the safety group to minimize or wait on safety issues until they are proved beyond a shadow of a doubt. The attitude that the "drug is innocent until proven guilty" and those safety warnings should not be issued to the health agency or the public until this point is reached is not at all appropriate in the world of safety. Rather, each safety issue must be evaluated and acted on because of its own merit and criticality in a timely fashion to evaluate and minimize risk. This can become quite challenging because risk must be considered in the context of benefit and alternatives. Some problems must be addressed on Friday at 5 p.m. and over the weekend.

In the corporate world, this attitude runs contrary to the prevailing fiduciary obligation of a corporation ("to increase stockholder value by making more profit"). The personnel in the drug safety department need a fairly thick skin to work in this non-glorious field, unlike the world of clinical research or sales where there are congratulations (and monetary rewards and bonuses) for completing a study, getting drugs approved, or selling more product. Rather, drug safety personnel need strong backbones to be able to say to management that a product has a safety problem that must be acted on immediately or tracked until more data are in. Sometimes expensive studies are required and the outcome may merely strengthen the evidence of a problem. Good and wise corporate management understands this and welcomes "straight talk" from the safety unit. Bad management buries or delays. This is becoming more dangerous as the penalties (commercial, regulatory, and legal) are becoming more severe and bad behavior goes viral on the internet overnight.

It should be noted that the concept of drug safety is often less well understood and less well developed in small start-up companies with only a small number of employees. Their primary task is to develop one or a few drugs and their goal is to complete trials rapidly and either sell the product to another company for further development (e.g., large phase III trials) or get rapid FDA approval with the goal of getting positive cash flow. These companies usually do not have a safety department and sometimes do not even have anyone specifically handling safety or tracking regulations and new requirements. They usually rely on their partners or CROs. They often do not handle safety well and when safety issues or crises occur, they have significant problems often requiring external "emergency" assistance to help resolve the issues.

It is hoped that corporate executives will realize that a safety problem hidden in the short run may, in the long run, appear on the front page of the *New York Times*, on TV or go viral on the Internet, or the six o'clock news. They may need to explain their actions to governmental investigation panels and to the multiple lawsuits — class action, civil, and criminal — that are frequent in the US and, increasingly, now pop up elsewhere in the world on any safety-related issue.

Similarly, the role of drug safety in the health agency is difficult. The primary mission is similar to the corporate safety role: to protect the public health. However, the profit-making motive is not present. Instead, there are always intense budget pressures to save money as well as the need to answer to multiple demanding constituencies: in the US, the FDA answers in one way or another to the Secretary of Health and Human Services, the US Congress, the public, the press, patient advocacy groups, the Internet blogosphere, the health professions, and the companies (and lobbies) the HAregulates. Similar political pressures exist for other agencies around the world.

■ Frequently Asked Questions

Q: Why would anyone want to work in drug safety?

A: Good question. Some of us "stumbled" into research during post-collegiate years, and then further "stumbled" into drug safety, found their passion and stayed. Some of us who decided not to be HCPs, but still wanted to serve in the public health sector, found drug safety to be a way of ensuring compliance by companies and feel it provides a service to the public by constantly monitoring for changes to the safety and efficacy of the product.

Some healthcare professionals decide to move out of direct clinical care, either due to stress, hours, or a combination of both, and find industrial/pharmaceutical medicine. Unlike the "glamor" of clinical research, where new and exciting drugs are tested, drug safety tends to have a different atmosphere, dealing with the problems of the new and exciting (and old and dull) drugs.

There is much more detective work and medical analysis in working hard to obtain all the clinical facts available, perform a defensible medical analysis, and come to a medically sound conclusion often based on incomplete (or even misleading) data. The work can be quite academic when one is working up a complex signal or risk evaluation/mitigation plan. And as always in medicine, one never has enough information. There is always one more test or examination one could do to get closer to the truth. Like the clinician, the drug safety worker is usually dealing with uncertainty and must still make rapid and often irreversible decisions. Yet given the data available, one must come to the medically proper and defensible conclusion and convey this in a cogent way to both medical and non-medical people. The work is challenging and fulfilling when done well.

The ethical issues come up when clear, compelling safety arguments calling for action are made and no action is forthcoming from management. This puts drug safety personnel in awkward and sometimes legally risky positions.

There is also much drama and excitement. Much can be routine, but the next e-mail or Tweet may bring a disaster with widespread consequences if the signal bears out. The adrenaline level rises and the "crisis" team mobilizes. The drug safety department is the emergency room of the company. Those who perform drug safety as a career are often passionate about it. Few decide at the outset of a pharmaceutical career that they want to "do side effects". Rather, they want to discover new drugs or do clinical research or study the pharmacology of drugs. Many come into drug safety after trying other areas in the industry and discover they love it.

There are a few downsides that should be noted. If one wants to move high up in a company's hierarchy this is not a good path for advancement. Of course, one can move up within the safety area with the top job usually being the Vice President of Drug Safety and Pharmacovigilance. However, the people who move up to the executive levels and other high positions almost never come from safety. These positions usually go to marketers, sales, research, legal and other non-safety positions. On the other hand, few people from these areas are clamoring for your job in safety!

Within the company, some people will be wary when they talk or interact with safety people fearing that they might say something that can get them into a delicate position. "Water cooler conversation" usually stops when the PV person approaches.

There is a lot of interaction with legal and regulatory. Sometimes these interactions are fine, sometimes adversarial and sometimes very guarded. People in other sections of the company may have (unstated) agendas that differ from what you might expect.

Finally, sometimes they do "kill the messenger"!

Q: Is there not an inherent conflict of interest in asking a company to police itself?

A: In a sense yes, especially when money is involved. Most regulated professions have some level of self-policing, including aviation, banking and finance, the food industry, medicine, and law. The results of self-policing have not always been happy. Thus, there must be some level of outside oversight to ensure that self-policing is done correctly. Finding the right balance is always the trick. In practice, there is far too much to do and oversee in the pharmaceutical industry to have total outside oversight from health agencies. Rather, practicalities force the system to police itself with regulations, periodic reports, monitoring, reviews, audits, and other mechanisms looking over the industry's shoulder to "keep it honest". In recent times, following terrible banking and investment scandals, there is a strong tendency toward risk aversion and the demand that there be more regulation and control "to prevent another (fill in your own crisis: Oxycontin,Vioxx, AIG, Madoff, earthquake, Covid etc.)". Thus, we are likely to see more regulation and perhaps less risk-taking. Whether or not more regulation will lead to better outcomes (i.e., "safer" drugs) remains to be seen.

CHAPTER 2

Primary definitions relevant to Safety & Pharmacovigilance

What is an adverse event (AE)? A serious AE (SAE)? An adverse drug reaction (ADR)? A suspected, unexpected, serious adverse reaction (SUSAR)? A suspected, expected, serious adverse reaction? What do expected, unexpected, listed and unlisted mean?

Note: Unless otherwise noted, the words "drug" or "drug product" or "medicinal product" should be taken in this book to include "biologics", "Combination products", and "vaccines", too.

■ Introduction

Clinical research and the product development industry contain too many terms to fully outline in this text. This chapter intends to focus on only the primary definitions and terms relevant to safety and pharmacovigilance that deserve clarification and must be understood to achieve the goals of this science. It is hard enough to explain to "outsiders" what "clinical safety and pharmacovigilance" means, so it is even more important for those of us within this profession have a unified understanding of the primary terms relevant to this science to function properly. An exhaustive Glossary can be downloaded from the EMA website. (https://www.ema.europa.eu/en/about-us/glossaries)

■ The Theory

To operate consistently in any area, be it construction, law enforcement, education, and including product development of any kind, one must fully understand and abide by definitions and standards to ensure unity and understanding from person to person. Definitions and standards guide individuals with a universal understanding of any given task or function and are crucial to harmonization, especially when conducting research and activities on a global scale.

Pharmaceutical and biotechnology companies, medical device manufacturers, research and development organizations, etc. would ideally all follow one set of standardized definitions as it pertains to product development and research. However, what we have found is that there are slight variations in definitions of specific terms, documents, and procedures based on region, product type, or as simple as someone's past experience.

For example, the internal document that outlines the roles and responsibilities of a given CRO, Vendor, supplier, manufacturer, sponsor, etc., during a clinical trial can be named a multitude of things, when in reality they have the same goal and are the same document. This document has been referred to as a Safety Management Plan (SMP), Safety and Medical Monitoring Plan (SMMP), Safety Reporting Plan (SRP), Safety Operating Guidelines (SOG), Joint Operating Guidelines (JOG), and on and on. It is our wish to standardize some of these definitions amongst the industry as outlined in this chapter.

Pharmacovigilance terminology and related initialisms can be confusing, especially when comparing the terms between CROs and big/small pharma. Table 1 contains a list of associated initialisms for reference, but this is certainly not a comprehensive list and will unfortunately differ company to company.

The "official" and accepted definitions in most countries are based on the International Conference on Harmonization (ICH) E2A Guideline and are given in the following sections.

Some agencies, such as the EMA, have also gone so far as to develop their own lexicon and dictionary of terms to help close communication gaps due to differing opinions, language nuances, and definitions globally. The European Medicines Agency (EMA) has developed a "Medical terms simplifer," or a plain language description of medical terms related to medicine use and is available on their website. For pharmacovigilance terms in the EU, and for other countries that have adopted EU Good Pharmacovigilance Practices (GVPs), one should refer to the EMA, Guideline on GVP, Annex I — Definitions. This document is complete, simple to read, accessible, and truly should not be regarded as for use only in postmarketing scenarios, but in all aspects of product development, and is a good reference point of terms that are *relevant* to pharmacovigilance, including Off-Label Use, Product Quality Complaints, and Medication errors — terms that are often neglected by

Table 1. Selected Initialisms and Acronyms Used in this Manual

Initialism	Interpretation
AE	Adverse Event, sometimes Adverse Drug Event (ADE) or, for FDA, also means Adverse Experience
AESI	Adverse event of special interest
API	Active Pharmaceutical Ingredient (also application programming interface)
AR/ADR	Adverse Reaction, sometimes Adverse Drug Reaction (ADR)
CCSI	Company Core Safety Information
CFR	Code of Federal Regulations, for US
DCSI	Development Core Safety Information
GVP	Good Pharmacovigilance Practice, for Post-marketing in the EU
ICH	International Council for Harmonization of Technical Requirements for Pharmaceuticals for Human Use (formerly International Conference on Harmonization)
IME	Important Medical Event
SAE	Serious Adverse Event
SAR	Suspected Adverse Reaction, sometimes Serious Adverse Reaction
SADR	Serious Adverse Drug Reaction, sometimes Suspected Adverse Drug Reaction, neither of which is currently in common use
SESAR	Serious Expected Suspected Adverse Reaction
SUSAR	Serious Unexpected Suspected Adverse Reaction, used in the EU trials and outside the US; similar in concept to FDA's Suspected Unexpected Serious Adverse Reaction (no initialism for FDA)
NSAE	Non-serious Adverse Event
NSAR	Non-serious Adverse Reaction

other areas as being relevant to the pharmacovigilance system.

Now let's get down to basics. Each of the terms outlined in this chapter are the basic terms one needs to fully comprehend to survive and operate in this industry. As noted numerous times, however, one will find a difference in language and points of clarification depending on the source and region of the definition, even though ultimately, the intent of the concepts captured in the definitions is basically the same.

Adverse Event (AE)

The "adverse event", its seriousness, classification, and relationship to the product, is what we as researchers tend to look for in product development, and could be considered one of the most critical data points that will be collected and studied for the life of the product. There are varying definitions by region as noted below:

1. Any untoward medical occurrence in a patient or clinical investigation subject administered a pharmaceutical product and which does not necessarily have to have a causal relationship with this treatment (ICH E2A).
2. Any unfavorable and unintended sign (including an abnormal laboratory finding, for example), symptom, or disease temporally associated with the use of any dose of a medicinal product, whether or not considered related to the medicinal product (ICH E2A). Any untoward medical occurrence in a patient or clinical trial subject administered a medicinal product and which does not necessarily have to have a causal relationship with this treatment (Article 2(m) of Directive 2001/20/EC). An AE can therefore be any unfavorable and unintended sign (e.g., an abnormal laboratory finding), symptom, or disease temporally associated with the use of a medicinal product, whether or not considered related to the medicinal product (EMA, Good Pharmacovigilance Practices Annex I Definitions).

In the context of pharmacovigilance and outside a clinical trial, any untoward medical occurrence in a patient to whom a medicinal product is administered and which does not necessarily have a causal relationship with this treatment.

Adverse Event/Experience (AE) — FDA

In practice, most people use the term "AE" to refer to any "bad thing" that occurs during the use of a drug without implying that the bad thing is due to the drug. The bad thing may be due to the drug substance, excipients, packaging, storage issues or other problems and may or may not be due to the active ingredient. Therefore, AEs are events that coincide with the use of a product but may not necessarily be caused by the product.

The FDA uses the term ***adverse event/experience*** and defines it as follows:

For post-marketing cases: Any AE associated with the use of a drug in humans, whether or not considered drug-related, including the following: An AE occurring in the case of the use of a drug product in professional practice; an AE occurring from drug overdose whether accidental or intentional; an AE occurring from drug abuse; an AE occurring from drug withdrawal; and any failure of expected pharmacological action (21CFR314.80(a)).

For clinical trial cases: Any untoward medical occurrence associated with the use of a drug in humans, whether or not considered drug-related.

Adverse Reaction (AR)

A key difference between an "AE" and an "AR" is the **concept of causality**. An "event" is merely something "bad" that occurs, but a "reaction" captures the concept of a relationship between the event and drug exposure.

An Adverse Reaction (AR) refers to an AE that has occurred during the use of a product AND has an associated relationship, or causal relationship with the use of that product. These events would be classified as having at least a possible causal relationship with a product according to most definitions, and these types of events should be clearly defined in protocols and company definitions for clarification amongst team members.

Synonyms: Adverse drug reaction (ADR), Suspected adverse (drug) reaction or serious adverse reaction (SAR), Adverse effect, Undesirable effect (see EMA GVP Module Annex 1 Definitions).

1. For *pre-approval* (i.e., not yet marketed, experimental) products, the definition is as follows:

   "All noxious and unintended responses to a medicinal product related to any dose should be considered adverse drug reactions." This means "that a causal relationship between a medicinal product and an adverse event is at least a reasonable possibility, i.e., the relationship cannot be ruled out." (ICH E2A)

2. For *post-approval* (i.e., marketed) products, the definition is as follows:

   "A response to a drug which is noxious and unintended and which occurs at doses normally used in man for prophylaxis, diagnosis, or therapy of disease or for modification of physiological function." (ICH E2A)

3. **EMA (GVP Module Annex I Definitions):** A response to a medicinal product which is noxious and unintended. Response in this context means that a causal relationship between a medicinal product and an AE is at least a reasonable possibility (see GVP Annex I). An adverse reaction, in contrast to an AE, is characterized by the fact that a causal relationship between a medicinal product and an occurrence is suspected.
4. For regulatory reporting purposes, if an event is **spontaneously reported** (such as in post-marketing reports from patients), even if the relationship is unknown or unstated by the healthcare professional or consumer as the primary source, **it meets the definition of an adverse reaction**.

Therefore, all spontaneous reports notified by healthcare professionals or consumers are considered suspected adverse reactions, since they convey the suspicions of the primary source, unless the primary source specifically states that they believe the event to be unrelated or that a causal relationship can be excluded.

Serious Adverse Event and Serious Adverse Reaction (SAE/SAR)

A key difference between an "AE" and an "AR" is the **concept of causality**. An "event" is merely something "bad" that occurs, but a "reaction" captures the concept of a relationship between the event and drug exposure.

A serious AE or AR are events that meet a specific set of requirements based on definitions echoed globally, and only varying slightly between devices and drugs. SAEs/SARs are additional classifications of events that are heavily scrutinized, reviewed by the sponsors, and reported to the agencies at varying frequencies due to their nature of severity and impact to public health. SAEs and SARs, like other critical events, should be clearly defined in the protocol and procedures at sponsor companies. The definitions should match the local regulations and internal procedures or be a unified definition that encompasses the varying regional definitions (see... this isn't as easy as Websters Dictionary!)

A *serious* AE (experience) or *serious* AR is any untoward medical occurrence that, at any dose, meets one, or more, of the following criteria:

1. Results in death,
2. Is life-threatening,
   a. *Note*: The term *life-threatening* in the definition of *serious* refers to an event in which the patient was at risk of death at the time of the event; it does not refer to an event that hypothetically might have caused death if it were more severe.
3. Requires inpatient hospitalization *or prolongation of existing hospitalization*,
4. Results in persistent or significant disability/incapacity,

5. Is a congenital anomaly/birth defect,
6. Is an Important Medical Event. (See below)

Medical and scientific judgment should be exercised in deciding whether expedited reporting is appropriate in other situations, such as important medical events (IMEs) that may not be immediately life-threatening or result in death or hospitalization but may jeopardize the patient or may require intervention to prevent one of the other outcomes listed in the definition above. These should also usually be considered serious. The EMA has developed a companion document called the "MedDRA Important Medical Events Term List" that is readily available to the public (can be found by a simple search) and should be referenced and used by sponsors as a guideline for what events are automatically considered IMEs, and therefore automatically considered serious.

Examples of such events are intensive treatment in an emergency room or at home for allergic bronchospasm; blood dyscrasias or convulsions that do not result in hospitalization; or development of drug dependency or drug abuse (ICH E2A).

The EMA considers any suspected transmission via a medicinal product of an infection agent to be a serious adverse reaction.

Note that an event or reaction may meet one or more of the criteria for seriousness simultaneously. Only one is needed, however, to consider the event or reaction to be serious. For an individual case safety report (ICSR) to be serious, it takes only one serious AE out of all the AEs present. To be a non-serious ICSR, all the AEs must be non-serious.

A. FDA's definition of a *serious* event or reaction for clinical trials (21CFR312.32(a)) is as follows:

An AE or suspected adverse reaction is considered "serious" if, in the view of either the investigator or sponsor, it results in any of the following outcomes: Death, a life-threatening AE, inpatient hospitalization or prolongation of existing hospitalization, a persistent or significant incapacity or substantial disruption of the ability to conduct normal life functions, or a congenital anomaly/birth defect. Important medical events that may not result in death, be life-threatening, or require hospitalization may be considered serious when, based upon appropriate medical judgment, they may jeopardize the patient or subject and may require medical or surgical intervention to prevent one of the outcomes listed in this definition. Examples of such medical events include allergic bronchospasm requiring intensive treatment in an emergency room or at home, blood dyscrasias or convulsions that do not result in inpatient hospitalization, or the development of drug dependency or drug abuse.

B. FDA's definition of a *suspected* adverse reaction for clinical trials is as follows:

Any adverse event for which there is a reasonable possibility that the drug caused the adverse event. For the purposes of IND safety reporting, "reasonable possibility" means there is evidence to suggest a causal relationship between the drug and the adverse event. Suspected adverse reaction implies a lesser degree of certainty about causality than adverse reaction, which means any adverse event caused by a drug.

Suspected Adverse (Drug) Reaction (SADR) — FDA

This includes any AE for which there is a reasonable possibility that the drug caused the AE. For the purposes of IND safety reporting, "reasonable possibility" means there is evidence to suggest a causal relationship between the drug and the AE. Suspected adverse reaction implies a lesser degree of certainty about causality than adverse reaction, which means any AE caused by a drug.

The point here is the word *suspected*, which means some level of causality with the drug in question, is present. It may be serious or non-serious.

Serious, Unexpected, Suspected Adverse Reaction (SUSAR)

Serious, Unexpected, Suspected Adverse Reactions (SUSARs) are events that are serious (meet one of the 6 main criteria), are unexpected (meaning not listed in the current labeling or known to have previously occurred in nature or severity), suspected (meaning there is a suspected or known causal association with the product), adverse reaction. SUSARs are therefore considered one of the most critical types of events in research as they typically garner the most attention and require a more expeditious reporting timeframe than any other.

EMA uses this phrase for an SAR in a clinical trial that is serious, not listed (i.e., unexpected) in the reference safety information, e.g., investigator brochure, and suspected to be due to the drug in question. See the definitions for serious and unexpected. The FDA does not use this definition or initialism formally for cases, though the concept is similar to SUSAR; FDA wording for this concept is "Suspected, Unexpected, Serious Adverse Reaction". Such an SAR will ordinarily trigger an expedited report in the EU and consideration of expedited reporting to FDA (see below). The acronym "SUSAR" is only applied to clinical trial data, i.e., it does not apply to spontaneous reports in the post-marketing phase.

Serious, Expected, Suspected Adverse Reaction (SESAR)

Serious, Expected, Suspected, Adverse Reactions (SESARs) are events that are serious (meet one of the 6 main criteria), are expected (meaning already listed in current labeling or investigator brochure, or known to have previously occurred in nature or severity), suspected (meaning there is a suspected or known causal association with the product), adverse reactions.

EMA uses this phrase for an SAR in a clinical trial that is serious, listed (i.e., expected) in the reference safety information, e.g., investigator brochure, and suspected to be due to the drug in question. See the definitions for serious and expected.

The FDA does not explicitly define or use this terminology however in 21CFR312.32(c(1)(iv) companies are required to report an "*increased rate of occurrence of serious suspected adverse reactions. The sponsor must report any clinically important increase in the rate of a serious suspected adverse reaction over that listed in the protocol or investigator brochure*." Therefore, if there are known reactions listed in the protocol or investigator brochure (aka "expected" events), and their rate of occurrence increases, sponsors are responsible for reporting on such increases. We have found that this is often a forgotten or missed concept within the industry, however this requirement plays a crucial role in the scientific monitoring and analysis of previously known data. Processes should also exist that outline how these types of events will be identified as it will take an aggregate review of cumulative data in order to determine if there is a clinically significant increase in the previously observed rate.

A few questions come to mind regarding this process; 1) Are there already established rates of occurrence? 2) At what point is the cumulative rate of event occurrence considered "Clinical important"? Does it have to be a statistically significant increase (i.e. p value >.05?) 3) Who makes this determination? Is it a committee or an individual? 4) What is the day 0 when it is identified? Processes for ICSR processing and reporting should include language that addresses the above questions. These questions are only sometimes answered and, when answered, may vary from place to place.

Unexpected Adverse Event — FDA

Pre-marketing: "Unexpected" as applied to clinical trials is defined by FDA in 21CFR312.32(a): An AE or suspected adverse reaction is considered "unexpected" if it is not listed in the investigator brochure or is not listed at the specificity or severity that has been observed, or if an investigator brochure is not required or available, is not consistent with the risk information described in the general investigational plan or elsewhere in the current application, as amended. For example, under this definition, hepatic necrosis would be unexpected (by virtue of greater severity) if the investigator brochure referred only to elevated hepatic enzymes or hepatitis. Similarly, cerebral thromboembolism and cerebral vasculitis would be unexpected (by virtue of greater specificity) if the investigator brochure listed only cerebral vascular accidents. "Unexpected", as used in this definition, also refers to AEs or suspected adverse reactions that are mentioned in the investigator brochure as occurring with a class of drugs or as anticipated from the pharmacological properties of the drug but are not specifically mentioned as occurring with the particular drug under investigation.

Post-approval (Marketed) Products: This takes account of any adverse drug experience that is not included in the current labeling (Package Insert or Summary of Product Characteristics (SmPC)) for the drug product. This includes events that may be symptomatically and pathophysiologically related to an event listed in the labeling but differ from the event because of greater severity or specificity. FDA provides an example in 21CFR314.80(a): Hepatic necrosis would be unexpected (by virtue of greater severity) if the labeling only referred to elevated hepatic enzymes or hepatitis.

AEs that are considered "class-related" (i.e., allegedly seen with all products in this class of drugs) and are mentioned in the labeling (Package Insert or SmPC) or investigator brochure but are not specifically described as occurring with this product are considered unexpected.

Unexpected Adverse Reaction — EMA

An adverse reaction, the nature, severity or outcome of which is not consistent with the Summary of Product Characteristics (SmPC) (Article 1(13) of Directive 2001/83/EC67). This includes class-related reactions which are mentioned in the SmPC but which are not specifically described as occurring with this product. For products authorized nationally, the relevant SmPC is that approved by the Competent Authority in the Member State to whom the reaction is being reported (often in the local language). For centrally authorized products, the relevant SmPC is the SmPC authorized by the European Commission. During the time period between a CHMP Opinion in favor of granting a marketing authorization and the Commission Decision to grant a marketing authorization, the relevant SmPC is the SmPC annexed to the CHMP Opinion (EMA GVP Module Annex I definitions).

These adverse reactions, when the SmPC is used as the reference document, are referred to as *unlabeled*. This is quite different from *unlisted* (see below).

Note: For products registered in the EU, the EU SmPC is the single document to consider, even for clinical trial ICSRs; the investigator brochure is the reference document for clinical trial ICSRs, but only if the product is not registered.

Unlisted Adverse Reaction — EMA

An adverse reaction that is not specifically included as a suspected adverse effect in the Company Core Safety Information (CCSI). This includes an adverse reaction whose nature, severity, specificity or outcome is not consistent with the information in the CCSI. It also includes class-related reactions which are mentioned in the CCSI but which are not specifically described as occurring with this product (GVP Annex IV, ICH-E2C(R2).

Expected (Listed versus Labeled)

As opposed to "unexpected", "expected" refers to an event that is noted in the investigator brochure or labeling (Package Insert or SmPC). One complication is that two different reference documents (labels) are available for marketed drugs for expectedness. One is the regulator-approved prescribing information (e.g., Package Insert or SmPC, etc.), which may vary from jurisdiction to jurisdiction, and the other is the company's core safety information (CCSI). The latter is provided to regulators, but it is a company-driven document that does not ordinarily need approval by regulators. Usually, these are quite similar if not identical, but not always. The CCSI contains the company position on the minimum safety information that should be in every regulator-approved label wherever the product is authorized for marketing. An event/reaction not found in the CCSI may be included in the regular-approved label, but not vice-versa. If the event/reaction is not found in the SmPC, it is considered unlabeled. If it is not found in the core labeling, i.e., the product's CCSI, it is *unlisted*. If it is not found in the PI or SmPC, etc. it is *unlabeled*. The CCSI is used to determine "listedness" for periodic aggregate reports in the post-marketing phase.

Thus, an event in the United States is expected or unexpected depending on whether it is found in the reference safety information (RSI): the investigator's brochure for unapproved products or the FDA-approved labeling for marketed products. In the European Union, it is the same for unapproved products, but for marketed products, an unexpected event/reaction may be unlabeled (not in the SmPC) or unlisted (not in the CCSI).

This is confusing terminology. To summarize "listed" refers to the CCSI; "labeled" refers to the PI or SmPC.

The Practice

For a good summary of post-marketing pharmacovigilance definitions used in the EU (and often elsewhere), see the GVP Annex I Definitions, referenced above. This is a comprehensive document with definitions from the EMA. They are very similar to the FDA definitions.

AEs are unintended events that occur when taking a drug (or biologic or vaccine, etc.). They may or may not be due to the drug itself (the "active moiety", or "active pharmacological ingredient" (API)), the formulation, excipients in the product (e.g., the inactive ingredients, fillers), the packaging (e.g., leaching of products from a container into the liquid drug product), a contaminant, manufacturing problems, the underlying disease, or some other unknown cause or causes. Thus, an AE does not imply that the drug (i.e., the active component) necessarily caused the bad thing to occur.

An AR is an AE in which there is "reasonable possibility" of a causal relationship between the drug and the AE. Some interpret this to mean that the relationship cannot be ruled out. This is probably too extreme as it implies that unless causality can be absolutely, positively ruled out, it is "possibly related" or that there is a "reasonable possibility" of causality. FDA in its guidance on IND Safety Reporting discussed this at length and indicated that they do not want to see cases reported as expedited IND reports if there is "not enough evidence to suggest that there was a reasonable possibility that the drug caused the AE". This is done to increase the likelihood that the information sent to FDA will be "interpretable and will meaningfully contribute to the developing safety profile of the investigational drug and improve the overall quality of safety reporting". The notion of causality is discussed in much greater detail later in this Manual. Thus, an AE possibly or probably due to the drug is an ADR or AR.

These terms are being replaced in practice by SAR, which emphasizes the suspicion that the drug is *a* possible cause of the bad thing or is *the* possible cause of the bad thing. Following logically from this, we now have the phrase *suspected, unexpected, serious adverse reaction*. The addition of the words "serious" and "unexpected" to the SAR term represents the criteria for submission as expedited reports to government health agencies in many countries of serious reactions from clinical trials. This phrase is very similar in meaning to the acronym SUSAR that is used for expedited clinical trial reports in the EU.

Suspected, expected, serious adverse reactions usually do not have to be submitted as expedited reports to governmental agencies. They are usually submitted periodically (e.g., yearly) or at the end of the study in the final study report. However, some regulatory jurisdictions require submission of all "serious" SARs, regardless of expectedness, if there is a reasonable possibility of a causal relationship with the product.

Expectedness represents an often highly subjective area. An event or reaction is expected if it is found in the product reference document (IB for clinical trials or the post-marketing labeling for approved drugs). More specific or more severe events or reactions, however, are considered to be unexpected. Thus, if "pneumonia" is in the brochure or product labeling and the patient has "streptococcal pneumonia", this is considered unexpected because the "streptococcal" designation is more specific. Similarly, "fatal pneumonia" is considered unexpected if only pneumonia is labeled (see Chapter 22).

The bottom line here is that there are multiple definitions and variants floating around. They all more or less add up to the same cases being "expeditable" in the United States, European Union, and elsewhere in many, but not in all situations. There are nuanced differences in the definitions of related/unrelated, but fundamentally what they come down to is that cases that are serious (death, life-threatening, hospitalization, disability/incapacity, birth defect) and related ("reasonable possibility" that the AE is due to the drug) and unexpected (not in the IB or only included in the class labeling section) are expeditable in the clinical trial setting.

Another nuance is the responsibility for the causality determination for clinical trial reports: FDA has assigned this responsibility to the sponsor (only), whereas elsewhere, either the sponsor or the investigator judgment applies. A good rule of thumb: In general, one should be conservative in applying the definitions, and if one has to discuss or debate whether something is serious and/or related and/or unexpected, then it is. That is, if there is any doubt about any of these three definitions, choose the more conservative approach (serious, related, unexpected).

Q&A

Q: What can be done to simplify this process?

A: Companies must adopt a uniform dictionary and process and stick with them. Ideally, all companies would define which dictionary they will use to operate and define events from a safety and pharmacovigilance perspective. Would you start a game a Scrabble without confirming which dictionary would be used to challenge words? No, so then why would you accept a varying degree of understanding of terms when it comes to the evaluation of safety data in order to protect and monitor human health and outcomes?

Q: How can companies achieve this?

A: Create a policy, SOP, or lexicon, that will be referenced throughout all procedures and training for definitions. Train your employees on these definitions; if your employees do not have a uniformed understanding of what it is they are evaluating, what they are looking for, and what they are monitoring and reporting on, we will continue to see discrepancies in data analysis and review.

CHAPTER

3

Regulations, Directives, Guidance, Laws and Consensus Documents

Pharmacovigilance (PV) is governed by a large body of requirements. Some are written and rigid, i.e., legally enforceable. Others are written but are far less rigid. Others are not requirements but only guidances or guidelines, and still others are unwritten customs and (best or optimal) practices. Obviously, laws and regulations, as well as their enforcement, vary from country to country and are subject to change over time. Difficulty in effecting change is roughly in this rank order (beginning with most difficult and time-consuming): Laws, Regulations, Regulatory Guidance, and Consensus Guidelines. The sections that follow concisely summarize the obligations in the US and the EU for drugs and over-the-counter (OTC) products, but also provide selected references to assist with remaining "up to date" on PV requirements.

■ United States

Legal requirements for drug safety come from multiple areas. There are laws, regulations, and guidances issued by the United States' federal government. These are the predominant formal requirements governing drug safety. In the US, a "law" is a written statute, requirement, or ordinance that has been passed by a legislature and then signed into law (where required) by the executive. That is, a federal law is passed by Congress in Washington, D.C., and signed by the president. Laws may be created at multiple levels of government (federal, state, and local). Regulation of interstate commerce is the FDA's main enforcement authority.

The law governing investigational drugs ("New Drugs") is found in Section 505(i) [21 U.S.C. 355], and the law governing marketed drugs is found in Section 505(k) of the Food Drug and Cosmetic Act.

In addition to laws, the US Food and Drug Administration (FDA) is empowered by Congress to create regulations. Regulations are rules issued by government authorities under the power of laws. Regulations thus have the force of law. To create a regulation, the FDA publishes the proposed version of the new or amended regulation in the *Federal Register* (https://www.federalregister.gov/). A period is defined during which time the public may send written comments on the proposal to the FDA. After review, a final regulation is published in the *Federal Register* and in the *Code of Federal Regulations* (https://www.ecfr.gov). A long period may elapse between publishing the draft and the final regulation (e.g., 6 months or more) and FDA is under no obligation to finalize a draft regulation or guidance. Also, a draft regulation or guidance may be withdrawn. While a proposed or final regulation may be published and put into force anytime, the Code of Federal Regulations is updated with final regulations once a year, on April 1st.

Finally, the FDA issues guidances that contain FDA's preferences on how to comply with the agency's interpretation of laws and regulations. Regulatory guidances are often offshoots of guidelines that are developed by consensus organizations, e.g., the International Council for Harmonization (ICH) or the Council of International Organizations of Medical Sciences (CIOMS).

As the FDA states on its Center for Drug Evaluation and Research (CDER) Guidance page: "Guidance documents represent the Agency's current thinking on a particular subject. They do not create or confer any rights for or on any person and do not operate to bind FDA or the public. An alternative approach may be used if such approach satisfies the requirements of the applicable statute, regulations, or both." However, it is generally held in practice in the industry to be a wise course of action to follow FDA guidances as they outline what the FDA currently expects. Some of the applicable pharmacovigilance (PV) guidances can be found by simply looking through www.fda.gov.

■ European Union

The EU situation is different from that in the US, because the EU is composed of 27 separate Member States (formerly 28 before the UK left the EU — Brexit) plus three affiliated states that are organized differently from the 50 United States. The EU member states are sovereign countries, whereas the states that make up the US are not. The EU member states are Austria, Belgium, Bulgaria, Cyprus, the Czech Republic, Denmark, Estonia, Finland, France, Germany, Greece, Hungary, Ireland, Italy, Latvia, Lithuania, Luxembourg, Malta, the Netherlands, Poland, Portugal, Romania, Slovakia, Slovenia, Spain, and Sweden. Additional countries have indicated a desire to become part of the EU: Albania, Bosnia and Herzegovina, Moldova, Montenegro, North Macedonia, Serbia, Turkey, and Ukraine. These countries are working to adopt laws and values of the EU, albeit often with local nuances. How this will affect PV is unclear at this time.

The European legislation often refers to and applies to the European Economic Area (EEA), which consists of the 27 EU member states plus Iceland, Liechtenstein, and Norway. These latter three countries are not EU member states but participate in much of the EU single market and adopt the EU PV legislation. To complicate matters further, one sometimes sees reference to the European Free Trade Association (EFTA), which was set up originally for countries not in the European Union. The EFTA now includes only Iceland, Norway, Switzerland, and Liechtenstein. (Note that Switzerland is not part of the EU.) The Committee for Medicinal Products for Human Use (CHMP)) which facilitates scientific evaluation of medicinal products in the EEA, using resources from the 27 EU countries and Iceland and Norway.

EU "primary legislation" derives from treaties and agreements among the Member States. This includes the Single European Act (1987), the Maastricht Treaty (1992), the Treaty of Amsterdam (1997), and the Lisbon Treaty (2007). "Secondary legislation" derives from the treaties. There are several types. The ones that touch most on PV are as follows:

- **Regulations:** Directly applicable and binding in all EU Member States without the need for any additional national implementation legislation. That is, the regulation as it is published is, word for word, becomes the law in each of the Member States. Note that this is different from the use of the word *regulation* in the United States.
- **Directives:** This legislation binds member states to the objectives of the legislation within a certain timeframe but allows each Member State to create its own form of national law to achieve it. That is, each member state may modify the wording and requirements of the directive as long as the objectives of the directive are met.
- **Recommendations, guidelines, and opinions:** Similar to FDA guidances, though EU guidelines usually hold the force of law and are obligatory.

If Regulations and Directives are in effect for several years while recommendations, guidelines and opinions are frequently updated.

When translated into local law, each EU country can include additional requirements which are then country-specific. Thus, this can lead to somewhat different detailed requirements in various Member States.

The main EU website is, and the website covering legislation can be found at https://europa.eu/european-union/law_en.

The key EU regulatory and procedural documents relating to PV can be found at on the EU EMA website.

Guidelines can be found at www.ema.europa.eu This site contains "Good Pharmacovigilance Practices (GVPs)", which consist of over a dozen "guidelines" for post-marketing PV, which are referred to as "modules", as well as multiple other documents and "annexes". These annexes include other documents and templates. These "guidelines" are soft law in the EU and are obligatory, unlike the FDA "guidances", as noted above, which are not obligatory (although still within your best interest to follow and implement). The modules are discussed in the individual chapters ((in this manual covering each module's topics. Each module has requirements for regulators as well as for applicants (companies).

The EU situation regarding drug safety is, in many ways, far more complex than the US situation. In the US, the requirements for drug safety come primarily from the FDA. Some state and local requirements apply to PV for companies, but in practice, these do not touch on drug safety as much as reimbursement, formularies, health insurance, dispensing, and other non-PV areas. There are, occasionally, requirements for registries or other safety obligations imposed by other governmental entities, such as the National Institutes of Health (NIH) and the National Cancer Institute (NCI) for clinical trials, as well as Risk Evaluation and Mitigation Strategies (REMS) and other post-marketing obligations on NDA or BLA holders. The US regulations are relatively concise and far less detailed than the EU requirements. Many of the US requirements actually fall under guidances which, although strictly non-obligatory, have in fact become standard practices and are de facto obligatory. For example, Data Monitoring Committees (DMCs) are described in a guidance but have become more or less standard in most phase III clinical trials and are expected by FDA.

In contrast, the EU requirements are highly detailed and run to thousands of pages. Many people have said that the US requirements are not detailed enough ("Show me exactly where the regulations say that I have to do this, some say the level of detail in the US affords interpretive flexibility for different organizations while others are of the opinion that the EU regulations are too highly detailed. Another complaint is that many of the EU modules have been revised several times since their creation in 2012 whereas US regulations are revised far less frequently.

The EU has the supra-national body of directives, regulations, and such from the European Medicines Agency (EMA) (empowered by the European Commission, Parliament, Council of Ministers in Brussels), as well as legal requirements in each Member State, which may differ from or add onto the European Union-level requirements. EU documents are generally available in many of the EU languages (of which there are 24 official ones: Bulgarian, Croatian, Czech, Danish, Dutch, English, Estonian, Finnish, French, German, Greek, Hungarian, Irish, Italian, Latvian, Lithuanian, Maltese, Polish, Portuguese, Romanian, Slovak, Slovene, Spanish and Swedish.) Interestingly, the working language of the EU has largely been English. Translation has had a few challenges. Now that the UK has left the EU, there are only two small English-speaking countries (Malta and Ireland), one wonders if English will be used less frequently though so far English still predominates.

Member State documents are published in the official language(s) of the Member State but are not consistently published in other languages. Local documents are often not available in English. Most, if not all, EU-level documents are available in English. Summaries of Product Characteristics (SmPCs), for example, are usually available in the official language of each country where the product is approved. National documents may only be available in that country's The base SmPC language for centrally-authorized products is English language.

Any company dealing in the EU must obtain expertise at the European and Member State level to stay in compliance with all safety obligations. In practice, this usually means the creation of affiliates or subsidiaries or the hiring of local companies or agents in the European countries where the drug is sold or studied.

In particular, the EU requires the presence of a Qualified Person for Pharmacovigilance (EU QPPV). Directive 2010/84/EU: "The qualified person (…) shall reside and operate in the Union and shall be responsible for the establishment and maintenance of the PV system" and GVP Module 1: the EU QPPV "shall have sufficient authority to influence the performance of the quality system and the PV activities and to promote, maintain and improve compliance with the legal requirements". The QPPV is the first EMA contact person for PV activities as well as for preparing reports and responding to questions on safety matters, including the continuous, ongoing risk–benefit analyses of authorized products.

■ Consensus Documents

These are reviewed elsewhere in this manual. Most of the consensus documents that have been developed have been done by international organizations, such as CIOMS, ICH, or ISO. These documents represent the agreed-on consensus for best/optimal practices by governments and pharmaceutical companies and others involved in pharmaceutical research, development, and sales. Many countries and governments do indeed adopt these documents as the laws or regulations in their countries. Others adopt them with changes.

The key point here is that these documents themselves do not hold the force of law and do not have to be followed unless a particular country or health agency implements them into law or regulations. Thus, one must examine the PV requirements in each country or jurisdiction where one is working.

The Practice

In practice, the laws and regulations often leave areas of ambiguity. No law or regulation is ever able to predict or account for every conceivable circumstance that may arise. Where feasible, a "guidance" or some other agency document is issued to clarify issues and intent. However, it is a complex, time-consuming, and difficult bureaucratic process to create laws, guidances, and regulations, and there is always a time lag between the need for a clarification and the publication of such.

For example, the definition of *serious* would seem fairly clear:

> *Any adverse drug experience occurring at any dose that results in … death, a life-threatening adverse drug experience, inpatient hospitalization or prolongation of existing hospitalization, a persistent or significant disability/incapacity or congenital anomaly/birth defect. Important medical events that may not result in death, be life-threatening, or require hospitalization may be considered a serious adverse drug experience when, based upon appropriate medical judgment, they may jeopardize the patient or subject and may require medical or surgical intervention to prevent one of the outcomes listed in this definition.*

In fact, several areas are unclear, and there have been a long series of dialogues, publications, and meetings to address such ambiguities:

1. Is staying in a hospital emergency room overnight considered inpatient hospitalization (and

thus a serious adverse event, SAE)? The consensus: No. It is highly recommended to address the definition of "hospitalization" in the protocol and to clarify if a <24 hr stay constitutes "hospitalization" or not.

2. Is a preplanned inpatient hospitalization that occurs after an adverse event (AE) but perhaps for a totally separate condition considered inpatient hospitalization (and thus a SAE)? The consensus: No.
3. Is a pre-planned inpatient hospitalization for a cosmetic or elective procedure considered "hospitlization" and an AE? The consensus: No.
4. What is an "important medical event"? Is thrombocytopenia, if the count is 5,000 platelets per microliter? Yes. 50,000? Probably yes. 350,000 (where the normal is up to 400,000)? Probably no.
5. Is pulmonary embolism an important medical event? Is the event considered to be clinically significant enough to warrent further investigation as the ultimate outcome of the event could adversely affect the patient?
6. What is "medically important" or "significant"? There is no clear consensus on this. It is left to individual reviewers' and reporters' judgments.

Thus, in circumstances where there is no clear answer, the best approach is to take the most conservative course of action and "overcall":

- If the question is between serious and non-serious, prefer serious.
- If the question is between reporting and not reporting a case to the health authority, prefer reporting.

Calls to the agencies are possible to ask such questions, but it is not always possible to reach the right person to have a policy question answered. Most agencies discourage this practice as it would be burdensome to them. If one does succeed in getting an opinion from an agency on a tricky issue, try to get a written confirmation. If that is not possible, write detailed minutes of the telephone call and file them with the case. For cases submitted to multiple health authorities around the world, it is not practical to call each authority to get an answer, and it is possible the answers would be contradictory. Again, the best course of action is the most conservative and, thus, defensible course.

Over-the-Counter Drugs

Reporting requirements vary from country to country.

United States

In the United States, an over-the-counter (OTC) product is sold based on whether it got to market via (1) an approved New Drug Application (NDA) (Rx to OTC switch) or an Abbreviated New Drug Application (ANDA), or (2) the OTC drug monograph process. The Time and Extent Application (TEA) is another method to get a product onto the market via the monograph process, but this is rarely used.

The safety obligations depend on which method is used to get the product to market. If an OTC product has an approved NDA, the requirements are the same as for a prescription product (expedited reports, periodic reports, etc.). For monograph products, the situation is different. Until 2007, there were no obligatory safety reporting requirements, though many manufacturers voluntarily reported SAEs to the FDA.

The regulations and guidances changed when the federal government put forth the following:

1. Dietary Supplement and Nonprescription Drug Consumer Protection Act, December 2006.
2. Guidance for Industry Postmarketing Adverse Event Reporting for Nonprescription Human Drug Products Marketed Without an Approved Application, July 2009.

These documents changed the reporting requirements for the monograph products:

1. A manufacturer, packer, or distributor whose name is on the label (called the "responsible

person") must submit to FDA all SAEs with a copy of the label within 15 business days.

2. All follow-up information received within 1 year of the initial report must be submitted within 15 business days.
   - The requirements say one year, but FDA expects reports with no time limit. That is, report all follow-ups forever.
3. Report electronically, using E2B according to FDA's specifications (MedWatch forms are not accepted from manufacturers, but can be used by consumers and the healthcare community).
4. Use NDA definitions for minimum criteria, reportability, and so forth.
   - For brand families need to know the active ingredient to have a reportable drug.
   - If multiple suspect drugs, submit Individual Case Safety Report (ICSR) to FDA and to other manufacturers.
5. No aggregate reporting requirements, but FDA has occasionally requested *ad hoc* compilations or reports to address safety concerns.
6. Reporting requirements for NDA/ANDA products were unchanged because of the changed OTC requirements.

European Union

In the EU, all marketed drugs (OTC or Rx) have a Marketing Authorization (MA). Thus, all OTC drug products have the PV requirements for prescription requirements (expedited reporting, PSURs, signals and risk management, labelling etc.) Local requirements should be checked for products, such as neutraceutical and herbal preparations, etc. Agencies collect AEs on OTC products (e.g., the Medicines and Healthcare Products Regulatory Agency, MHRA, collects them under its Yellow Card Scheme). In other words, PV requirements for an OTC drug in the EU are the same as for Rx drugs.

If a product is sold in both the US and the EU, in practice, the product is handled as a drug with expedited reporting, PSURs, and so forth, for global use, although some documents (e.g., aggregate reports) would not be submitted to FDA if not required.

■ Staying Up to Date

As noted in multiple places throughout this manual, the world of drug safety is changing almost daily. Personnel handling drug safety and PV must stay up to date with changes that occur both in the scientific and medical world (new SAEs, new interactions, etc.) for drugs they handle and in the regulatory–operational world. The best way to do both is through journals, meetings, conferences, networking, and the Internet. There are also vendors who will survey the landscape and provide updates to subscribers.

Scientific/Medical Literature

New and important medical information on areas that involve drug safety are found in many medical journals throughout the world, including major pharmacology and medical publications, such as the *New England Journal of Medicine*, the *Lancet*, the *Annals of Internal Medicine*, and specialized drug safety journals, including:

1. *Drug Safety* is published by Springer/Adis.
2. *AdisInsight Safety* is a worldwide resource for PV literature monitoring. It provides access to published adverse drug reaction case reports, drug safety studies and regulatory news covering all drugs and therapeutic areas, updated daily
3. *Expert Opinion on Drug Safety*) covers medical issues on particular drugs.
4. *Pharmacoepidemiology and Drug Safety* is the official journal of the International Society for Pharmacoepidemiology.
5. *Therapeutic Innovation and Regulatory Science*, formerly known as the *Drug Information Journal*, published by the Drug Information Association. This journal carries articles on the whole field of pharmaceuticals, including sections on drug safety.
6. There is an expectation (and a requirement in some jurisdictions) that relevant "local" journals (in the local language) will be identified and periodically reviewed as part of an ongoing comprehensive literature survey.

There are online and open access journals published now that cover many medical areas including PV. Some claim to be refereed.

There are also multiple blogs that cover PV news. They vary in reliability. There are also many PV groups on various websites, such as LinkedIn. They are generally not curated and also vary in terms of reliability.

It is likely AI will play a larger and larger role in tracking PV sources, journals, courses, etc. As of now, however, many of the AI sites do not yet connect to the Internet and thus, the many of the large postmarketing databases contain data that are incomplete as of one to three years ago. This will likely improve over time. Watch this space.

Meetings and Conferences

Many conferences cover drug safety only or have sections dedicated to drug safety.

1. Drug Information Association (DIA) holds many conferences in the United States, Canada, Europe, and Asia, as well as sessions before and during annual meetings held in several regions. Each year, conferences on drug safety are held in the US and there are annual conferences in the EU, Asia, and elsewhere.
2. Other private (non-profit) organizations offer training, including the Pharmaceutical Education and Research Institute (PERI) (www.peri.org), the Uppsala Monitoring Centre (https://www.who-umc.org/) and the Drug Safety Research Unit (http://www.dsru.org/courses/).
3. The FDA, Health Canada, EMA and MHRA often conduct PV training sessions or hold virtual meetings to address relevant topics.
4. The International Society for Pharmacovigilance (ISoP) holds meetings and training courses (http://isoponline.org/).
5. The International Society for Pharmacoepidemiology (ISPE) has conferences, meetings, and training courses (https://www.pharmacoepi.org/).
6. The FDA and certain other agencies hold advisory committee meetings and hearings that are open to the public. Some are also transmitted online or are available as podcasts or webinars on the respective websites.
7. The Regulatory Affairs Professionals Society (www.raps.org) has training sessions and conferences on the general field of regulatory affairs and sometimes addresses drug safety.
8. Many private, for-profit organizations train in drug safety on all continents. They are best found by doing a Google search on drug safety conferences. They vary in quality. Caveat emptor. Various companies, institutions, individuals etc. now claim to offer certification in PV, and some entities in Europe offer graduate degrees in Pharmacovigilance (Eu2P for example), however there is no "official" or "global" recognized body doing this.

The Internet

There are many resources on the internet. They are ever-changing, with new ones appearing, old ones disappearing, and current ones changing:

1. **Government e-mail alerts, e-newsletters, Facebook, X (formerly known as Twitter) and others:** The FDA, EMA, MHRA, Health Canada, TGA, and many other governmental agencies issue periodic alerts in various fora.
2. ***Fierce Pharma*** (https://www.fiercepharma.com/): This is a set of daily publications on various areas of the industry.
3. **Blogs:** There are many blogs on the pharma industry, some serious, some outrageous, some outraged, all opinionated. They change frequently and their credibility varies. Best found by a periodic Google search. Caveat emptor.
4. **Google Alerts:** An excellent Google function is called Google Alerts. This is an automated mechanism that can be set up on Google to deliver, as news becomes available, daily or weekly

information found on the net. The use of keywords such as "PV" and "drug safety" will bring interesting news, press releases, blog addresses, and sites (https://www.google.com/alerts).

It is easy to spend one's entire day just reading blogs and news on the Internet. A good compromise would be to find one or two sources that provide the updates the reader needs for his or her work. Attending (whether live or on virtual media) a conference on drug safety once or twice a year is also valuable for both updates and networking.

CHAPTER

4

The United States Food and Drug Administration

The "granddaddy" of drug safety "regulatory agencies" dates back to 18th century Japan, when the eighth shogun, Yoshimune Tokugawa (1716–1745), upon recovering from an illness, awarded 124 medicinal traders in Osaka special privileges to examine medicines throughout the country. However, the safety of the medicines was difficult to guarantee despite these efforts. A shrine in Osaka, called Shinno-san, was created and dedicated to Shinno, the guardian of the pharmaceutical industry and the divine founder of medicine from China. This information was found at the Osaka tourism website.

Introduction

Very often governments have responded to misbehavior or tragedies by strengthening laws intended to address perceived shortcomings in protecting patient safety. In the past 30 or so years, the number of organizations devoted to drug safety has increased markedly outside the United States. This chapter is focused on key activities of the US Food and Drug Administration (FDA), which regulates biopharmaceutical products and medical devices for human use. FDA also regulates certain foods and veterinary products, for a total of more than US $2.4 trillion worth of products each year. The latter topics are outside the scope of this chapter.

The FDA is a complex organization with over 15,000 employees strategically posted at US domestic locations and overseas stations. Several distinct parts of FDA handle safety matters. The largest areas touching drug safety reside within the Center for Drug Evaluation and Research (CDER) and the Center for Biologics Evaluation and Research (CBER). In addition, within CDER and CBER, functions are generally split between pre- and post-marketing regulatory activities.

The FDA has undergone, and continues to undergo, major changes following various scientific, public, and political controversies, drug withdrawals, investigations, and changes in the law. This chapter will summarize the key functions that deal with medical product safety and will outline some of the initiatives that will undoubtedly lead to further advances in "regulatory science" in the coming years. The current organization of the agency is posted on the FDA website and the information is regularly updated with any changes.

■ Center for Drug Evaluation and Research

This is the prime (and largest) center in the FDA for handling the safety of biopharmaceutical products in the US. The Center for Drug Evaluation and Research (CDER) handles new drugs from the IND stage (when a product first moves into human study) to the evaluation of the NDA/ANDA or BLA for approval or rejection of the request to market the product in the United States. A separate group within CDER then evaluates the post-marketing safety of the product continuously. Although simple in theory, the actual practice is complex and has evolved over time. It continues to change, often in response to Congressional mandate, and should be viewed as a work in progress.

The FDA organization chart is posted online and is quite useful. It gives names, addresses, and contact information on the FDA organization and key personnel (www.fda.gov). The chart is updated regularly with changes (see below). When this chapter was written, there were 45 "offices" in CDER covering many areas, including biotechnology, new medical product evaluation, counterterrorism, pediatric drug development, generic drugs (including biosimilars), compliance, biostatistics, prescription drug promotion, translational sciences, and, of course, product safety.

See CDER's website (www.fda.gov/cder). In 2017, there were 33 advisory committees made up of external members, who provide consultation and give expert and consumer advice to the FDA. The FDA generally follows an advisory committee's recommendation, but is not bound to do so. There is an advisory committee on Drug Safety and Risk Management that evaluates new products and safety concerns across the product lifecycle continuum.

The FDA reorganizes periodically. As of 2024, the structure was as follows (this content is easily accessible via fda.gov): the Office of the CDER Center Director has under it approximately 13 offices and each office has several further divisions and offices including the Office of Surveillance and Epidemiology (OSE). OSE is considered a safety "Super Office", available for consultation on safety concerns across all of FDA, not only CDER-regulated products. In 2024, were two Offices and eight divisions in OSE:

- **Office of Pharmacovigilance and Epidemiology**

  Division of Pharmacovigilance I & II (two divisions): The staff includes safety evaluators whose primary role is to detect and assess safety signals for all marketed drug products. They work closely with medical reviewers in the Office of New Drugs so that potential safety signals are placed in the context of existing preclinical, clinical, or pharmacologic knowledge of the drug(s) being evaluated.

  Division of Epidemiology I & II (two divisions): The staff conducts active surveillance using the Sentinel System and also conducts epidemiologic studies using observational data sources. An increasingly important activity is the review of epidemiologic study protocols, which are conducted by applicants as post-marketing commitments or post-marketing requirements. The Division evaluates various post-marketing surveillance tools that may be incorporated into non-routine risk minimization strategies, such as patient registries and restricted distribution systems. They estimate the public health impact of safety signals by evaluating digital claims databases, healthcare datasets, and the published literature, etc.

- **Office of Medication Error Prevention and Risk Management**

  Division of Medication Error Prevention and Analysis (I and II) (DMEPA I & DMEPA II): The staff provides pre-marketing reviews of all proprietary names, labels, and labeling for CDER-regulated products to reduce the potential for medication errors of a proposed product. The division also provides post-marketing review and analysis of all medication errors received by the Agency.

  Division of Risk Management (DRM): DRM serves as the focal point for risk management activities in CDER. DRM provides risk management expertise on design, development, and implementation of programs and initiatives to support the Center's policies related to Risk Evaluation and Mitigation Strategies (REMS) authorities under the Food and Drug Administration Amendments Act (FDAAA) of 2007. DRM provides input on the need for a REMS for all new molecular entities (NMEs), original BLAs, and post approval for serious risks that warrant consideration of a REMS. Additionally, DRM reviews sponsor-proposed REMS and REMS modifications for all products with an approved REMS for conformance with current FDA standards. REMS decision-making is a joint decision between the Office of Surveillance and Epidemiology (OSE) and the Office of New Drugs. DRM serves as the REMS experts within OSE and the scientific lead for CDER on all new REMS and REMS modifications. In conjunction with the Division of Mitigation Assessment and Medication Error Surveillance (DMAMES) and Office of New Drugs, DRM participates in the review of REMS assessment reports. DRM consists of healthcare professionals with varied backgrounds, including: pharmacists, physicians, nurses, and health communication specialists.[1]
  Division of Mitigation Assessment and Medication Error Surveillance: (DMAMES)

  "DMAMES provides expertise to evaluate risk mitigation strategies and recommend regulatory actions to ensure safe and effective use of drug products. Our focus is on identifying and mitigating medication errors and assessing Risk Mitigation and Evaluation Strategies (REMS) for marketed products. We are the lead for medication error pharmacovigilance, and collaboratively work on safety signal detection, assessment, understanding, and prevention of medication errors. We also collaboratively review proposed new REMS and REMS modifications, REMS assessment methodologies, and REMS assessment reports. We develop standards, policies, and approaches related to health informatics and data management tools and techniques to support REMS standardization and integration initiatives, medication error prevention and analysis, use of structured product labeling, and electronic health record interoperability. We also work closely with other entities, including the Institute for Safe Medication Practices (ISMP), to support research and innovation to advance the science of risk assessment and mitigation and protect public health."

FDA's SOP list is available (www.fda.gov). In fact, almost all of FDA's policies and procedures are available on their website. The FDA has an extensive, useful website, although the information tends to be scattered and difficult to find. There is a search engine that is somewhat useful. The website has extensive information on how the FDA works, its history, drug availability, counterfeits, Internet purchases of drugs, labeling and medication guides for drugs on the market, signals, REMS, guidance, laws and regulations covering pharmaceuticals (as well as devices, biologics, radiologic agents, over-the-counter (OTC) products, nutraceuticals, and more). The main CDER website lists late news and provides a jumping off point to other CDER information, including:

1. **FDA Basics:** This provides fundamental information on the various divisions, functions, and leaders at FDA.
2. **Drug-Specific Information**: This is an alphabetical list of drugs that have an information sheet, Early Communication about an Ongoing Safety Review, or other important information.

[1] Office of Surveillance and Epidemiology (OSE) — Divisions | FDA

3. **Development and Approval Process for Drugs:** This provides information on how drugs are developed and approved.
4. **Guidance, Compliance, and Regulatory Information:** For industry, this key page for pharmacovigilance (PV) professionals has links to information on laws, acts, rules, good review practices, enforcement activities, surveillance, post-marketing commitments requirements, warning letters, enforcement actions, new guidance documents, cyber letters, and the CDER manual of policies and procedures.
5. **Information for Industry:** This is a page for the pharmaceutical industry with links to guidance, post-marketing information, the Prescription Drug User Fee Act (PDUFA, which is renewed every 5 years), industry fees, warning letters, electronic submissions, the Orange Book (approved drug products with therapeutic equivalence evaluations), abbreviations, and types of applications.
6. **JumpStart:** This is a tool for FDA reviewers to gain insights on data fitness in an application and which analytical tools might be appropriate for use in the review. This was spawned by CDER's 21st Century Review Process, which is an integrated review process that partitions work into IT functions and scientific analysis. JumpStart is intended to be applied to electronic data between submission of a marketing application by industry and filing of the application by CDER.
7. **MedWatch:** See below for more detailed information.
8. **Drugs at FDA:** This is a link to the page that has an alphabetical list and search engine to find approved drugs by name, active ingredient, or application number.
9. **openFDA:** This is a software tool designed to facilitate public access and use of public FDA data.
10. **Recalls, Market Withdrawals and Safety Alerts.**

■ The Safety Reporting Portal

FDA has launched a "one-stop shopping" safety portal in which electronic case safety reports for nearly all products regulated by FDA (and NIH) can be submitted. Food (human or animal), drugs, biologics, blood products, gene-transfer research issues, and more can be reported by sponsors/applicants/manufacturers/distributors, healthcare professionals, researchers, public health officials, and "concerned citizens". The features and functionalities of this portal evolve as experience is gained. It allows for initial and follow-up reports. One can enter a case as a "guest" or one can establish an account and use it repeatedly. It is not meant for emergency reporting when a company's safety system is down. See the Safety Reporting Portal FAQ page. Other pages of interest include the following:

1. **Potential Signals of Serious Risks/New Safety Information Identified from the FDA Adverse Event Reporting System (FAERS):** This page contains information about ongoing signals. Along the same lines, the 2007 legislation generally required FDA to perform extensive safety analyses of new drugs at 18-months following approval or after 10,000 individuals had been exposed to the drug, whichever was later. However, the 21st Century Cures Act abolished this requirement because a study showed that these assessments had little value and the requirement was redundant to other FDA safety activities. Results were largely the same as those from established safety surveillance practices and they did not reveal important safety issues any sooner. These activities were not a good use of FDA resources so they were curtailed by the 2016 legislation. In January 2024, FDA published a final document titled, "Best Practices for Food and Drug Administration Staff in the Postmarketing Safety Surveillance of Human Drug and Biological Products." This document segregates products into three categories for safety screening

and gives FDA staff general guidance on the recommended cadence of ICSR reviews for each category. The document updates an earlier version (2019) and, among other things, provides reference to CDER's "Manual of Policies and Procedures for Collaborative Identification, Evaluation, and Resolution of Newly Identified Safety Signals."

2. **Post-market Drug Safety Information for Patients and Providers:** This site contains information on post-market study requirements and commitments, a link to the clinical trials registry, and other safety-related information.
3. **Approved Risk Evaluation and Mitigation Strategies (REMS):** This site contains summary information and links to REMS summaries that are in place and dates of modifications or release. There is a separate link to a repository of released (previously approved, but inactive) REMS.
4. **Guidances:** This site contains FDA's new, current, revised, and withdrawn guidance in all areas, including Drug Safety, ICH, OTCs, Good Review Practices, the FDAAA Food and Drug Administration Amendments Act (2007), the FDA Safety and Innovation Act (2012), the 21st Century Cures Act (2016), and the FDA Reauthorization Act of 2017.
5. **Post-market Drug Safety Information for Patients and Providers: Selected Safety Regulations:** This page has links to the relevant sections of the Code of Federal Regulations covering safety matters for drugs and biologics, as well as INDs, NDAs, BLAs, STNs (submission tracking numbers), and labeling.
6. **Warning Letters:** A site with many years of warning and untitled letters for all matters, not just safety, that are searchable by company (or investigator, etc.), issuing office, and so forth.
7. **Pregnancy and Lactation Labeling**.
8. **Prescription Drug User Fee Act (PDUFA):** The main web page for information on PDUFA, including the current version, with several links.
9. **Office of Surveillance and Epidemiology (OSE)**.
10. **Guidance, Compliance, and Regulatory Information:** This page has links to the various laws, acts, guidance, and so forth.
11. **Surveillance: Post-drug Approval Activities:** Links to the staff guide, regulations and policies, advertising, and promotional information.
12. **FDA Adverse Event Reporting System (FAERS):** This site has the description of the main FDA drug safety database, with post-marketing data files and statistics for chemical drugs and therapeutic biologics, including data migrated from predecessor databases. There is a fairly user-friendly "Public Dashboard" that supports navigation of redacted FAERS data (additional details at www.fda.gov).
13. **Vaccine Adverse Events Reporting System (VAERS):** This site contains post-marketing reports for vaccines regulated by CBER. The database is housed by a vendor and scientific access is shared by CBER and the Centers for Disease Control.
14. **Electronic Medical Device Reporting (eMDR) System:** This site has post-marketing safety ("incident") data for medical devices regulated by Center for Devices and Radiologic Health (CDRH) and reported by manufacturers and user facilities.
15. **MedWatch to Manufacturer Program:** The system whereby FDA informs applicants of SAEs that are received directly by FDA for the first 3 years after a new product is marketed. This is activated only on request of the applicant (see "MedWatch" below). *Note*: The MHRA in the United Kingdom has a similar program.
16. **DailyMed:** This is actually an NIH website that provides "high quality information about marketed drugs". It is not a complete listing but does have information on more than 7,000 drugs. See the Drugs@FDA site.

17. **Medication Guides**.
18. **Medication Errors**.
19. **Safe Use Initiative:** FDA's program to reduce preventable harm from medications. This FDA website is extensive, and almost everything that one wants to find relating to the FDA, drugs, and drug safety are present, though often not easy to find. In addition, FDA changes its websites frequently, and pages may jump or be moved, or URLs may be dead links. It may be necessary to search for the new URL using the FDA search engine on the home page. Note that most, but not all, of the drug safety information is in the CDER section of the website.

■ Risk Management

On the FDA website there is extensive information on risk management initiatives. Other FDA activities are covered elsewhere in this chapter and in other chapters of this manual.

In 1997, the federal government put forth a global framework for federal risk management of drug products. The fundamental concepts include the following:

Risk assessment is the estimation and evaluation of a risk in the pre- and post-marketing areas.

Risk confrontation determines the acceptable level of risk in the large context, including social and community values and the technical judgments of professionals. This includes the use of advisory committees, which get input from various concerned independent experts and stakeholders. In addition, the FDA has relationships with various groups of health professionals, consumer and patient advocacy groups, industry organizations, and other governmental agencies to gather information and advice.

Risk intervention is the evaluation of alternative risk control actions, selection among them, and their implementation. After the risks are identified and assessed, they must be managed or minimized. The FDA can refuse to allow the product to be marketed if the Agency concludes that the product's risk outweighs its benefits. If the product is permitted on the market, the FDA minimizes risk by various mechanisms, including the review and approval of the original labeling and any subsequent changes. FDA also regulates the advertising and promotion of marketed products. Promotional materials must not be false (i.e., they must conform to the label and be substantiated), and they must not be misleading (i.e., they must be balanced and include the material facts). FDA also tracks medication errors and can act on issues there. FDA also can require other risk minimization or mitigation measures, including mandating education for product users, limiting product distribution (e.g., to specific hospitals or specialists), requiring prescriber qualifications, training, or informed consent, etc. The FDA may also require post-approval clinical or epidemiologic studies after marketing. In urgent situations, there are various mechanisms to remove products from the market. In January 2024, FDA issued a final guidance document Titled, "Best Practices for Food and Drug Administration Staff in the Post-marketing Safety Surveillance of Human Drug and Biological Products

Risk communication is aimed at conveying the needed information to the public. There are ongoing and rapidly changing risk communication mechanisms using traditional and social media mechanisms to convey information to consumers and healthcare practitioners. The Internet and various new means of wireless communication challenge all parties to get the correct message out and make it visible in the large sea of available information. The product labeling (Package Insert) has been the classic mechanism of communication. The FDA has redone and revised how labels are made and how the information is communicated both to patients and practitioners. This is a controversial area as some feel the changes make labeling more complete but less useful and more ponderous. Medication guides for patients are also provided for some products in lay language to communicate how consumers should use products. Whether these changes lead to lowering risks for particular products remains to be seen.

Another controversial area is ***Direct-to-Consumer advertising***, which is allowed in the United States but not in many other developed countries. Whether this promotes product use that is safer or more dangerous is a much-debated topic, with no clear answer.

MedWatch

The MedWatch program is the FDA's national pharmacovigilance program for marketed products. It collects safety information and provides clinical information about safety issues involving prescription and OTC drugs, biologics, medical and radiation-emitting devices, and special nutritional products (e.g., medical foods, dietary supplements, and infant formulas). See the MedWatch site at www.fda.gov.

The website provides "one-stop shopping" for information or links to information on medical product safety alerts, recalls, withdrawals, current new and hot topics, educational materials, and a glossary, the NIH Daily Med site (hosted by the National Library of Medicine with up-to-date drug labeling information), Medication Guides, drug-specific information (more labeling), drug shortages, and more.

There is also a set of links to receive periodic e-mail notifications and RSS feeds (which you can have automatically sent to your Internet home page, if it accepts such feeds). There are also social media broadcasts produced by FDA on Facebook, Twitter, etc.

Another little-known MedWatch function is the MedWatch to Manufacturer Program (see above), which allows drug and biologics manufacturers to receive certain serious AEs submitted directly to FDA that would not otherwise be known to the manufacturer. An applicant can subscribe at any time within 3 years after product approval; FDA will send reports for a period of about 3 years after approval.

The other key part of the MedWatch site is information on reporting serious AEs to the FDA using the MedWatch form, which comes in three very similar variations — the 3500-form for the public to voluntarily submit AEs, the 3500B-form that is more consumer-friendly than the 3500-form, and the 3500A-form for mandatory reporting. Manufacturers usually use the 3500A-form only for expedited reporting from clinical trials; structured electronic reporting is required for marketed products.

An information page for health professionals and the public describes the systems used for safety reporting, which then has links to the other pages giving further information. There are links to downloadable PDF versions of the MedWatch forms. There is also a link to an online reporting form for the public.

There is a page with information for industry on the three key serious AE reporting areas. Information and links to the appropriate regulations and forms are included:

- OTC Products and Dietary Supplements;
- Drug/Biologic/Human Cell, Tissues and Cellular and Tissue-Based Product Manufacturers, Distributors, and Packers;
- Human Cell & Tissue Products (HCT/P) Adverse Reaction Reporting.

Safety Databases

The FDA maintains several databases that contain safety information:

- **FDA Adverse Event Reporting System (FAERS):** This is a computerized information system for FDA's post-marketing safety surveillance program for drugs and biologics. It is compliant with the data elements specified in the ICH E2B guideline. This database is one of the largest of its kind and contained over 15-million ICSRs as of mid-2024. More than half of these are classified as serious. Quarterly (non-cumulative) data files since January 2004 are available for downloading as zipped SGML or ASCII files. The data in these files are not cumulative and not searchable online. However, there is a "Public Dashboard" that supports searches of FAERS data. It is also possible to request FAERS cases (redacted) using Freedom of Information (FOI) requests.
- Data freely available for querying via the "Public Dashboard" include patient demographics, the suspect drug(s) reported, the adverse reaction(s),

patient outcome, and the source of the reports. It is possible to stratify and organize data by product, patient age, type of adverse event, the timeframe in which the event occurred, etc.

- **Post-marketing Requirements (PMRs) and Commitments (PMCs):** This database contains information on studies and trials that applicants have committed to carrying out after drug approval.
- **Vaccine Adverse Event Reporting System (VAERS):** VAERS is a cooperative database run by the CDC and the FDA. VAERS collects information about AEs that occur after the use of licensed vaccines, or adverse events following immunization (AEFI). See below under CBER.
- **Manufacturer and User Facility Device Experience Database (MAUDE):** This database contains selected safety information for medical device reports since 1991 and is updated weekly. See below under CDRH.
- **Clinical Trials Database:** This is not a safety database but has information about governmental and private clinical trials under way in the United States and globally. There are tens of thousands of trials in more than 170 countries on file. Some contain safety information. The PDUFA/FDAAA laws require safety information to be put online and this has been a gradual process. See: www.clinicaltrials.gov.
- Other databases include such topics as poisonous plants.

Other Useful FDA Web Pages

- Post-market Drug Safety Information for Patients and Providers: A one-stop shopping page for just about everything you want to know about safety.
- FDA guidance for FDA-regulated products.
- Office of Non-prescription Drugs (OTCs).
- Potential Signals of Serious Risks New Safety Information Identified from the FDA Adverse Event Reporting System (FAERS).
- Prescription Drug User Fee Acts (PDUFA), which are on 5-year cycles. PDUFA legislation specifies deadlines for the FDA to review new drug applications (normally 10-months for new drugs or 6-months for priority review, beginning on the date that FDA accepts the application).
- Food and Drug Administration Amendments Act (FDAAA) of 2007.
- Warning Letters.
- Summaries of approved Risk Evaluation and Mitigation Strategies (REMS).
- Global Health Agencies (links).
- Dietary Supplements.
- Code of Federal Regulations.
- Drugs@FDA — the US labeling for most approved drugs.

Finally, there is a very useful page that covers mandatory post-marketing reporting by drug and biologic manufacturers, distributors, and packers. There are hyperlinks to the applicable federal regulations:

- Labeling
  - 201.56 — Requirements on content and format of labeling for human prescription drug and biological product
  - Other labeling regulations
  - 208 — Medication Guides for Prescription Drug Products
  - 310.501 — Patient package inserts for oral contraceptives
  - 310.515 — Patient package inserts for estrogens
  - 312 — Investigational New Drug (IND) Application
  - 312.32 — IND safety reports
  - 312.33 — Annual reports
  - 312.88 — Safeguards for patient safety
  - 314 — Applications for FDA Approval to market a New Drug (NDAs)
  - 314.80 — Post-marketing reporting of adverse drug experiences
  - 314.81 — Other post-marketing reports
  - 314.97 — Supplements and other changes to an approved abbreviated application (ANDA)
  - 314.98 — Post-marketing reports
  - 314.520 — Approval with restrictions to assure safety use
  - 314.540 — Post-marketing safety reporting
  - 314.630 — Post-marketing safety reporting
  - 601 — Biological Licenses

- 601.12 — Changes to an approved application
- 601.32 — General factors relevant to safety and effectiveness
- 601.35 — Evaluation of safety
- 601.93 — Post-marketing safety reporting
- 610 — General Biological Products Standards
- 610.11 — General safety

In addition, other key documents such as FDA instructions for field staff, E2B ICSR submission information, ICH documents, and others are available.

Center for Biologics Evaluation and Research

The CBER website contains less information regarding product safety than the CDER site because the regulatory responsibility for approval and post-marketing evaluation of many CBER products was transferred to CDER in 2003. The products remaining in CBER include cellular products (e.g., pancreatic islet cells for transplantation, whole cells, cell fragments, or other components intended for use as preventative or therapeutic vaccines); allergenic extracts used for diagnosing and treating allergic diseases and allergen patch tests; antitoxins; antivenins/antivenoms; venoms; blood; blood components; plasma-derived products (e.g., albumin, immunoglobulins, clotting factors, fibrin sealants, proteinase inhibitors), including recombinant and transgenic versions of plasma derivatives (e.g., clotting factors); blood substitutes; plasma volume expanders; human or animal polyclonal antibody preparations, including radiolabeled or conjugated forms; certain fibrinolytics, such as plasma-derived plasmin; and red cell reagents.

More extensive information on this subject can be found at the CBER website. In regard to safety, there is information covering recalls, shortages, biological product deviation reporting (i.e., errors and accidents in manufacturing), AE reporting, and specific information about safety issues on various products, such as flu vaccines, HIV test kits, tissue products, and blood products. As noted, most AEs are reported via MedWatch using the 3500-voluntary reporting form. One exception is vaccine AEs (e.g., Adverse Events Following Immunization (AEFI)). These are reported to the Vaccine Adverse Event Reporting System (VAERS), which is sponsored by the FDA and the CDC. As with drugs, the goal is to collect and analyze safety signals and vaccine AEs. In particular, compared with drug products, vaccines are given to large numbers of children (FDA notes on its website that more than 10 million vaccinations are given yearly to children younger than 1 year old). As with all other products, the full safety picture is not known at the time of vaccine approval. Most of the VAERS reports are mild and include fever and injection site reactions, but some 15% are more severe AEs.

The VAERS website has sections for consumer and healthcare professional reporting of AEs online, by fax, or by mail.

The VAERS database, unlike the drug database, FAERS, has a system called CDC WONDER for obtaining data and producing tables, maps, charts, and various extracts regarding the incidence of vaccine AEs. For example, one can produce a report grouped by symptoms or medical problems (e.g., gastroenteritis) and various other criteria, such as age, gender, manufacturer, US location, date vaccinated, onset interval, seriousness, and outcome. The data are immediately available and are largely up to date. Data downloads are also available. This is a very useful tool. However, many discrepancies have been introduced by the application of SMQs to add an extrapolated diagnosis to the database when a diagnosis was not provided by the reporter. SMQs were not designed or tested for this and, e.g., sometimes age-inappropriate diagnoses are added. Use caution.

Center for Devices and Radiologic Health

Device regulation became much more formalized starting in 1976 with amendments to the Food, Drug and Cosmetics Act, in 1982 when the CDRH was formed and in 1990 when the Safe Medical Devices Act was passed. This is the center that deals with medical devices and radiologic agents. There are three sections in the CDRH website that are worth examining.

The first is the Medical Device Safety section, which covers alerts and notices, recalls, and emergencies. There is a large section on Medical Device Reporting (MDR) of adverse events from manufacturers, importers, and user facilities (e.g., hospitals, nursing homes). Consumer and healthcare professionals report via MedWatch (as with biologics and drugs) using either the 3500- or 3500B-voluntary reporting form. With the introduction of electronic reporting, eMDR was launched and mandatory reports must be sent to eMDR according to CDRH technical specifications.

The second is the Device Advice: Regulations & Guidance section. This is a very useful section that explains the regulations on marketing, standards, guidance, compliance, and post-market requirements. Note that the entire process of approval, marketing, and safety for devices is markedly different from the processes for drugs and biologics.

The third is the section on medical device databases. There are several, but the key one for safety is MAUDE (Manufacturer and User Facility Device Experience). This database contains AE reports involving medical devices. It contains data submitted by mandatory reporters (manufacturers, importers, and device user facilities) and voluntary reporters (healthcare professional, patients, and consumers). Data goes back to 1991 for device user facilities, to 1993 for distributor reports, and to 1996 for manufacturer reports. It is online and searchable by product problem, product, class, manufacturer, event type (death, injury, malfunction, other), brand name, registration number, and time frame. The focus is on medical devices which may have malfunctioned or caused a death or serious injury.

Some of the MAUDE data are downloadable. These files consist of voluntary reports since mid-1993, user facility reports since 1991, distributor reports since 1993, and manufacturer reports since mid-1996. The searchable portion of the data contains records for the most recent 10 years and is refreshed weekly. Note that MAUDE may not include reports made under waivers, exemptions, variances, or alternative reporting requirements. There also is a separate database for pre-1996 reports from manufacturers. A detailed review of medical device safety or drug-device combination products is not in the scope of this manual.

■ Over-the-Counter Products

OTC products are regulated by CDER's Office of Non-prescription Drugs and are drug products that can be sold in the United States without a prescription and, thus, without any medical professional intervention. That is, they are sold without a clear medical diagnosis being made by a medical professional and, thus, are purchased largely for symptoms as self-diagnosed by the lay public. Some products are not truly over the counter and are held by the pharmacist "behind the counter" such that the consumer must speak with the pharmacist, who will/should assess the need and appropriateness of the patient and product. OTC products have benefits that outweigh their risks, have low potential for misuse and abuse, can be adequately labeled, and do not require a health practitioner for their safe and effective use.

Drugs can enter the OTC market in several ways. A drug may be approved via the usual NDA process and then may be moved to OTC status through various routes. One is the "Rx to OTC switch". Other drugs that are "generally recognized as safe and effective (GRAS/E)" are listed in the FDA's "OTC monograph(s)" that specify which drugs may be marketed without further studies, FDA review, or approval. There are also so-called negative monographs that limit specific indications for certain drug ingredients. The monographs are very detailed specifications in the Code of Federal Regulations that specify ingredients, doses, formulations, indications, and labeling.

The FDA can act quickly to restrict marketing or remove a product from sale if there is significant risk or lack of evidence for effectiveness, or if the FDA finds that the usual notice and public procedure method are impracticable, unnecessary, or contrary to the public interest. The FDA can, thus, issue a rule requiring immediate label changes and marketing restrictions. In non-urgent situations, the FDA can use the notice and comment rulemaking mechanism to change marketing status.

Regarding safety reporting, OTC reporting by industry was not required until December 2007 for OTCs that did not have NDAs. That is, there was no requirement for AEs to be collected, analyzed, or submitted by manufacturers. This changed in 2007 when FDA issued a guidance that required reporting of serious AEs for OTC products found to be "associated with the drug". These were to be reported via MedWatch by manufacturers, packers, and distributors, using the 3500A-form. This essentially required that all serious AEs (whether in the label or not) must be reported to FDA within 15 calendar days. Requirements for minimal validity criteria are essentially the same as for drugs. Manufacturers are now required to submit reports electronically, but others are not yet required to use electronic means to make OTC case reports.

■ Drug Safety Oversight Board

The FDA created an internal Drug Safety Oversight Board (DSB) in 2005. The DSB was subsequently mandated by the FDA Amendments Act of 2007 and advises CDER Center Director on handling and communicating important and emerging drug safety issues, especially regarding how such issues impact federal healthcare delivery and payment systems. The DSB is composed of representatives from two FDA Centers and eight other federal government agencies, the Agency for Healthcare Research and Quality (AHRQ), Centers for Disease Control and Prevention (CDC), Centers for Medicare and Medicaid Services (CMS), Department of Defense (DOD), Health Resources and Services Administration (HRSA), Indian Health Service (IHS), National Institutes of Health (NIH), and Department of Veterans Affairs (VA). An important role of the DSB is to help FDA assess the impact of their safety decisions on the healthcare systems of its Federal Partners. The Board, with its broad representation from federal healthcare organizations, can provide valuable input and allows FDA to hear varied perspectives on drug safety issues.

Monthly meeting minutes and outcome reports are available online.

■ Prescription Drug User Fee Act

In 1992, the Prescription Drug User Fee Act (PUFA) was passed and then renewed 5 years later in 1997 (PDUFA II), and again in 2002 (PDUFA III), 2007 (PDUFA IV), 2012 (PDUFA V), and 2017 (PDUFA VI). This Act allows the FDA to collect a fee from an applicant whenever the applicant submits an NDA or BLA. In addition, companies pay annual fees for each manufacturing establishment and for each prescription drug product approved for marketing. Previously, taxpayers alone paid for product reviews for regulatory action by the FDA, through congressional appropriations.

In the program authorized under PDUFA, industry provides the funding in exchange for FDA agreement to meet drug-review performance goals, which emphasize timeliness without a loss of scientific quality of the review. As examples, the PDUFA fee rate for FY 2018 was $2,421,495 for an application requiring review of clinical data and was $1,210,748 for an application not requiring review of clinical data. The fees are adjusted on an annual basis. The typical allowed review time for an NDA under PDUFA is 10-months (or 6-months for priority reviews). Questions have been raised about the appropriateness of what is, in effect, industry funding of the government process for approving a medical product for entry into the commercial marketplace. In reality, user fees are for application review, not approval. Approval is not guaranteed.

■ Prescription Drug User Fee Act: Five-Year Plan

The FDA created multiple action plans to address the requirements of the law. In particular, FDA issued a "Prescription Drug User Fee Act Five-Year Plan" with each sequential renewal of PDUFA. Each plan includes steps to address the requirements in the legislation. Details and milestones are posted on the FDA website.

Other FDA initiatives under way are briefly mentioned below. The landscape changes frequently and

FDA's website should be checked periodically for updates and new initiatives.

Food and Drug Administration Act (FDAAA) of 2007

In 2007, PDUFA was actually a part of major new legislation known as the Food and Drug Administration Amendments Act (FDAAA) of 2007.

The FDAAA has multiple parts. The ones that deal with post-marketing safety are known as Title IX and give enhanced authority to the FDA regarding safety. In particular, it created the concept of Risk Evaluation and Mitigation Strategies (REMS), which are briefly outlined in this chapter and described in more detail elsewhere.

Another section strengthened the FDA's authority to unilaterally modify product labeling. Before 2007, the FDA did not clearly have the power to force labeling changes and most changes were done on a "voluntary" basis, though the FDA, in practice, could force most changes they desired. FDAAA formally empowered FDA to "notify" the applicant of new safety information that the agency "believes should be included in the labeling". The applicant then has 30 days to submit an amendment proposing new labeling that reflects FDA's communication or to notify the FDA that it disagrees and why. FDA may then have discussions with the applicant that usually last no more than 30 days, after which time the FDA may force the applicant to make labeling changes that the agency "deems appropriate". The FDA has used this new authority on several occasions, including the addition of a black box regarding an increased risk of death in elderly patients treated with antipsychotics for dementia, the addition of a black box regarding an increased risk of tendon injury with fluoroquinolone antibiotics, and the addition of a black box regarding the risk of histoplasmosis and other fungal infections with TNF alpha-blockers.

Other sections deal with the following:

1. Pre-approval review of proprietary names;
2. Modernization of information technology;
3. Medical devices, including enhancements in the device review program, inspections by third parties, new requirements for certain single-use devices, and user fees;
4. More studies in the pediatric population;
5. Development of products for tropical diseases, rare diseases, and other "neglected" diseases;
6. The Reagan–Udall Foundation, made up of senior advisers from outside the federal government, to advise FDA on innovation and enhanced food and drug safety. (the foundation was not initially funded by Congress, but sustainability models are evolving):
   - More transparency regarding possible conflicts of interest is required for potential Advisory Committee participation; and
   - The clinical trials database was expanded.

21st Century Cures Act

The 21st Century Cures Act was passed by Congress and then signed into law on December 13, 2016. The stated intent of this legislation was to accelerate innovative medical product development and get advances to patients who need these products more efficiently.

The law encourages FDA to consider the perspectives of patients in FDA's decision-making process in medical product development. This encompasses innovation in drugs, therapeutic biologics, vaccines, and medical devices. The legislation encourages new approaches to scientifically-sound clinical trial designs and clinical outcome assessments.

The law also provides new authority to facilitate recruitment and retention of a broad base of highly qualified personnel to execute these innovative programs. The legislation contemplates new approaches to expedite innovation, including the following:

- **Regenerative Medicine Advanced Therapy (RMAT):** This describes an expedited option for certain eligible biologics products;
- **The Breakthrough Devices Program:** This is intended to speed the review of certain innovative medical devices.

In addition, this legislation directs FDA to create cross-center initiatives to coordinate activities in strategic areas, e.g., diseases with a major public health impact. These activities cascade to the regulation of combination products. It also establishes an FDA Oncology Center of Excellence (OCE), which supports patient-centered decision-making and an integrated approach to the evaluation of drugs, biologics, and devices medical products for the treatment of cancer. The OCE works with centers and offices across the FDA.

This Act authorized an additional US$ 500 million for FDA over 9 years to implement the legal requirements.

FDA Reauthorization Act of 2017

FDA Reauthorization Act (FDARA) was signed into law on August 18, 2017 and it extended the user fee programs for drugs, medical devices, generic drugs, and biosimilar biological products through FY 2022 (and added other obligations). It reauthorized PDUFA for the fifth time. In addition, the Medical Device User Fee Amendments (MDUFA) was reauthorized for the third time, and included both the Generic Drug User Fee Amendments (GDUFA) and the Biosimilar User Fee Act (BsUFA) for the first time.

Selected provisions of FDARA include the following:

- An enhanced ability to capture patient preferences in drug development;
- Flexibility to inspect medical device facilities based on risk, while encouraging predictability and transparency in the inspection process;
- A focus on treatment of rare diseases (especially in pediatrics);
- Additional resources for review of breakthrough therapies;
- "Real world evidence" to inform decision-making (including use of the Sentinel System);
- Enhanced partnerships with patients;
- More flexibility in the regulatory pathway for certain medical device accessories;
- New opportunities for scientific advice on surrogate endpoints;
- Cross-center coordination of combination product review;
- Enhanced hiring and retention of well-qualified staff.

Bottom line: The reauthorization of PDUFA, MDUFA, GDUFA, and BsUFA support FDA's organizational ability to focus on improved health outcomes while promoting biomedical innovation.

The Sentinel System and ARIA

Launched by FDA in 2008 as a result of 2007 legislation, the Sentinel System is a US National medical product safety monitoring system that taps into electronic medical records across the country. It is an active electronic safety surveillance system that strengthens FDA's ability to monitor the safety of marketed medical products. The program began as a pilot, which reached a milestone of 100 million covered lives by 2011. As of June 2018, the Agency had 17 distributed data partners with 178 million covered members, each of whom had pharmacy and medical coverage. It is a large system with longitudinal medical records and an analytic center in Boston which handles coordination among the data partners. Data partners retain control of the medical records to protect privacy and maintain security; FDA prepares analytic queries to explore questions, but they do not have a centralized data repository for this system. Queries can be developed by FDA and anonymized results from more than 178 million covered lives can be obtained from these distributed datasets in a matter of days.

All of FDA's centers have access to the Sentinel System through OSE.

To strengthen FDA's ability to better utilize the Sentinel System, the 2007 legislation required FDA to establish an analysis tool, ARIA (Active Risk Identification and Analysis). ARIA contains validated modular programs that have re-usable analytical tools for rapid safety analyses of healthcare data. There are three levels of output: (a) Simple counts; (b) Complex descriptive analyses; and (c) Inferential analyses. ARIA was launched at the beginning of 2016 and several hundred analyses were run in the first 2 years.

The 2007 legislation also gave FDA the authority to issue Post-marketing Requirements (PMRs). However, FDA is required to consider the sufficiency of ARIA to address the question before requiring an applicant to conduct a PMR: "The Secretary may not require the responsible person to conduct a study under this paragraph, unless the Secretary makes a determination that the reports under subsection (k)(1) and the active post-market risk identification and analysis system as available under subsection (k)(3) will not be sufficient to meet the purposes set forth in subparagraph (B)." So, for concerns that might result in a post-marketing obligation for an applicant, FDA must use available tools before imposing a requirement.

The Sentinel System is made available to others through a public-private partnership. From an organizational perspective, the Reagan–Udall Foundation offers access for FDA through the Innovation in Medical Evidence Development and Surveillance (IMEDS) program. The goal is to make the system a broader resource for public health and medical evidence generation. IMEDS and Sentinel share the same analytic coordinating center in Boston. Private users of IMEDS have access to the same data as FDA and also the same analytic tools. This approach also provides funding for sustainability of the Sentinel System.

FDA continues to expand Sentinel and integrate capabilities into the post-market safety monitoring system.

In addition, there are other related projects, such as the following:

- European Network of Centers for Pharmacoepidemiology and Pharmacovigilance (ENCePP), a network consisting of research and medical care centers, healthcare databases, electronic registries, and existing networks to strengthen post-marketing monitoring and to facilitate the conduct of safety-related post-authorization studies (particularly observational studies);
- Innovative Medicines Initiative (IMI), a public–private partnership, has multiple projects that focus on improving drug safety and other aspects of drug development, for example, one project focused on developing validated tools and methods that will enhance adverse event data collection, active signal detection, standards for pharmacoepidemiology studies, and integration of data for evaluation of benefit-risk;
- EU-ADR, a project to design, develop, and validate a computerized system that exploits data from electronic healthcare records and biomedical databases for the early detection of ADRs, which will be complementary to existing systems with early detection of safety signals; and
- Drug Safety and Effectiveness Network (DSEN), a virtual network to assess the risks and benefits of marketed drug products.

Thus, the FDA will be able to initiate queries of multiple databases to obtain safety information and to do active and proactive surveillance using current and emerging methods.

In March 2003, the FDA published proposed new and comprehensive safety rules, sometimes referred to as "The Tome" because of their breadth and length. See "Safety Reporting Requirements for Human Drug and Biological Products", 68FR12405–12497, March 14, 2003. The proposal is now mostly of historical interest. However, it did outline FDA's thinking in that timeframe and consisted of extensive and complex changes to the current IND and NDA safety regulations. Major new obligations on the part of the pharmaceutical industry were proposed.

The FDA invited comments and received many thousands. Many parts of the proposal are now clearly out of date, especially with regard to electronic transmission, risk management, and FDAAA requirements. However, some changes and new requirements have been put in place via separate Federal Register Notices.

In late 2012, the FDA issued a new final rule that covers clinical trial safety reporting (21CFR312). Subsequent guidance was issued to clarify requirements of the rule. The rule is not fully consistent with ICH E2A and requirements of other key regulators. This presents special challenges for sponsors who entertain possibilities for global development programs.

FDA has indicated that it will periodically issue updated post-marketing regulations, as appropriate.

One concept in particular from the Tome is worth noting and may eventually be enacted: the "Always Expedited Report". This new category requires submission of an ICSR within 15 calendar days of first awareness, whether expected (labeled) or not, for these events:

Congenital anomalies;
Acute respiratory failure;
Ventricular fibrillation;
Torsades de pointe
Malignant hypertension;
Seizures;
Agranulocytosis;
Aplastic anemia;
Toxic epidermal necrolysis;
Liver necrosis;
Acute liver failure;
Anaphylaxis
Acute renal failure;
Sclerosing syndromes;
Pulmonary hypertension;
Pulmonary fibrosis;
Transmission of an infectious agent by a marketed drug/biologic;
Endotoxin shock; and
Any other medically significant "serious" adverse events requested by FDA for specific investigational products or protocols.

■ What is Expected from Drug Companies by the FDA?

The federal regulations noted above describe what the FDA expects to receive from biopharmaceutical companies regarding the reporting of drug safety information. In all cases, sponsors are expected to be 100% compliant with regulations, i.e., submit complete reports on time and do follow-up with due diligence to get complete medically-relevant information:

- Clinical trials — AEs reported to the IND
  - *In 7 calendar days*: deaths/life-threatening (at presentation), serious, unexpected, associated with the drug;
  - *In 15 calendar days*: serious, unexpected, associated with the drug;
  - *For both 7- and 15-day reports*: FDA requests that sponsors submit one ICSR to the "parent" IND rather than to all open INDs. (The "parent" IND is the open IND for the subject active substance that has the earliest filing date.) This is to avoid duplicate reports that could confound safety signal detection; and
  - *In annual periodic reports*: summary of all studies, tabular summary of the most serious and most frequent serious AEs, deaths, discontinuations due to AEs, and the 15-day reports submitted since the last aggregate report. The general acceptable format for the annual reports in the US is now the DSUR format, originally adopted in the EU. The content and format of the DSUR is more comprehensive than the requirements of the US IND Annual Safety Report and is now generally accepted by the FDA.
- Marketed biopharmaceuticals — AEs reported to the NDA
  - *In 15 calendar days*: serious, unexpected. Note that all spontaneous reports are considered to be "associated with the drug". The reasoning is that if the reporter did not believe there was at least some level of association (causality) with the drug, he or she would not have reported it. This comes from an earlier CIOMS recommendation.
  - *In 15 calendar days*: Reports from the medical literature that are serious and unexpected.
  - *In the quarterly or annual periodic reports (PADERs) or PSURs*: A narrative summary and analysis of the 15-day alert reports submitted since the last periodic report plus all other reports that are not serious and not unexpected. Foreign non-serious AEs do not have to be reported. In general, clinical trial AEs do not have to be reported to the NDA. Note that, currently, ICH E2C PSURs are

not required by FDA and PADERs are required by regulations. FDA does accept PSURs with the PADER-specific appendices; the ICH PSUR (PBRER format) may be made obligatory at some point in the future.

Solicited reports: AEs that are received from customer engagement programs with the possibility of two-way communication, e.g., disease management programs, patient support programs, etc., should be reported as 15-day reports to the NDA if they are serious, unexpected, and associated with the drug. It is the latter causality assessment that differentiates solicited reports from spontaneous reports (FDA Guidance for Industry, August 1997).

What is Expected from Consumers and Healthcare Professionals by the FDA?

Safety reporting by consumers and the healthcare community is purely voluntary, but strongly encouraged. (Exception: The US National Childhood Vaccine Injury Act (NCVIA) requires healthcare providers to report: (a) Any event listed by the vaccine manufacturer as a contraindication to subsequent doses of the vaccine; and (b) Any event listed in FDA's Reportable Events Table that occurs within the specified time period after vaccination (see www.fda.gov for the latest Reportable Events Table).) Reports may be made to the FDA directly via MedWatch (mail, online, fax, etc.) or to the pharmaceutical company that manufactures, sells, or packages the product. Once a manufacturer (NDA holder or "Applicant") or distributor, etc., learns of an adverse event for one of its products, reporting to FDA is mandatory.

FDA Publications and Updates

FDA has various publications and feeds freely available without cost online, such as e-mail alerts and as RSS feeds. "What's New (Drugs)" comes out several times a week with new drug-specific information. The relevant publications are well worth receiving, particularly the MedWatch and CDER notifications.

Others include the following:

1. **CDER New:** New items posted to the CDER website;
2. **Drug Information:** Occasional drug information updates on hot topics, frequently asked questions, and more;
3. **Marketing and advertising communications:** Drug marketing, advertising, and communication regulation information; updates to the Office of Prescription Drug Promotion web pages, which occasionally involve fair balance with safety matters;
4. **Drug Safety News (Podcast alert):** Emerging safety information about drugs, broadcast in conjunction with the release of Public Health Advisories and other drug safety issues;
5. **Drug Safety Newsletter:** Post-market information for healthcare professionals on new drug safety information and reported adverse events;
6. **FDA Patient Safety News (video):** TV broadcasts for healthcare professionals about recalls, alerts, and ways to improve the safety of drugs, medical devices, vaccines, and diagnostic products;
7. **MedWatch Safety Alerts:** Product safety alerts, Class I recalls, market withdrawals, and public health advisories;
8. **FDA Guidance Documents** for the industry;
9. **FDA Warning Letters:** FDA Warning Letters and untitled letters issued to companies, investigators, IRBs, etc.; and
10. **Good Clinical Practice:** Information about the development of final rules related to FDA's regulations on good clinical practice and clinical trials. These reference the ICH E6 guideline, as revised.

The reports may change from time to time, with new ones introduced and old ones phased out. Check the FDA web site for updates. There are other alerts on biologics, CBER, and specific diseases and conditions, including HIV and infectious hepatitis, women's health, medical devices, research, food contamination, and cosmetics.

This site offers sign-up for multiple subscriptions at the same time from various health and human services agencies and divisions, including the CDC, NIH, Med-Line Plus, and others.

The FDA, the industry, and nearly everyone else is now struggling with the newly and rapidly arising social media (Twitter, Facebook, LinkedIn, Buzz, blogs, blog-inars, eCards, podcasts, widgets, virtual worlds, etc.). As of this writing, FDA had several Twitter feeds and a Facebook page, and is expanding its use of social media.

The FDA's influence on life in the United States is extensive. The Agency oversees and regulates drugs, biologics, vaccines, dietary supplements, radiation-emitting devices, certain foods, cosmetics, and tobacco. They cover both human and veterinary products. FDA's influence outside the United States is obviously less strong than within the United States but, nonetheless, is felt through direct and indirect actions in international entities (e.g., ICH, CIOMS, where FDA is a major player either directly or indirectly), formal and informal interactions and memoranda of understanding with other health agencies (Europe, Canada, Japan, China, etc.), and as a thought and action leader (e.g., a drug safety restriction or withdrawal in the United States must be addressed, in practice, rather quickly elsewhere around the globe). FDA also has an extensive network of offices outside the US (Mexico City, San Jose, Santiago, London, Brussels, New Delhi, Beijing, among others).

For those in industries regulated by the Agency, the FDA has an impact on actions every moment of the day in just about all areas of business:

- Approval of INDs and NDAs, 510Ks, and so on;
- Regulations covering all aspects of manufacturing (current Good Manufacturing Practices), clinical research (Good Clinical Practices), animal research (Good Laboratory Practices), quality systems, drug safety (Good Pharmacovigilance Practices), the supply chain(s), and so on;
- Inspections (often unannounced) of factories, clinical trial sites, safety divisions, clinical trial divisions, licensing partners, contract research organizations, and so on;
- Drug safety;
- Product labeling and packaging;
- Product advertising, sales promotion, and other professional communications;
- Advice to the public; and
- Communication to all stakeholders.

The FDA has multiple "clients" to which it must answer: the Secretary of Health and Human Services (in the President's cabinet), the Congress (which provides funding and oversight), the American public, activist groups (consumer groups, lobbies, etc.), the media (press, TV, Internet, blogs, etc.), the pharmaceutical industry, other healthcare players, and, indirectly, foreign health agencies.

Pharmaceutical companies also have multiple clients but some are different: the stockholders (owners) of the company, the Securities and Exchange Commission, the American public, activist groups, the media, licensing partners, academic collaborators, trade groups, the FDA, and, for multinational companies, other health agencies, insurance companies and other payers, and foreign media.

The FDA's fundamental viewpoint and *raison d'être* differ from those of pharmaceutical corporations. The FDA's prime concern is protecting the American public (and animals). They are, in theory, not concerned with the viability or profitability of corporations or market share, whereas companies, again in theory, have a primary fiduciary goal of increasing shareholder value. Obviously, a company would not want to increase its stock price at the expense of the public health. But, in practice, decisions on what is good or bad for public health are almost never black and white. Rather, they are the subject of debate on the risks and benefits that usually fall somewhere in the gray area between the extremes. Nevertheless, it is in the interest of the public health for the public and healthcare community to have access to medical products when needed; all stakeholders should strive to ensure that the benefits of these products outweigh their risks.

Other factors come into play. In general, salaries and bonuses, particularly for professionals, are often better in private sector companies than in the FDA or academia. However, benefits, pensions, and retirement packages are often better in government service. Private sector companies tend to have more resources (people, computers, parking spaces, etc.) than government agencies.

As with other federal agencies, there is often a steady flow of personnel leaving the Agency to go to the private sector and, with the FDA, occasionally vice versa. This is generally viewed as a good phenomenon because it allows government workers to understand the functions and pressures in private industry and for private industry personnel to understand how government agencies function. Others feel this is a bad concept as it binds the regulators and the regulated too closely together and influences the actions of regulators who may want to get a job in industry after leaving the Agency. Many people enter the industry or the FDA from academia, often just after finishing training (in medicine, pharmacy, nursing, pharmacology, toxicology, statistics, IT, etc.) and, thus, the "first job" provides basic training that is essential for success in either industry or the government.

There is a continuing debate, which varies in intensity and persistence over time, on whether the FDA works too slowly ("drug approval lag") or too quickly ("releasing dangerous drugs onto the market without adequate evaluation") and whether there are too many regulations ("the biopharmaceutical industry is one of the most regulated or over-regulated industries in the United States"). This was very evident in the Covid era with drugs and vaccines permitted for use often with less than usual testing via waivers.

Most pharmaceutical companies live with a low-level dread of the FDA and other health agencies coming into their safety departments (or other departments) to do an inspection (unannounced as a rule when done by the FDA). The inspection may be routine, done periodically (often every 1 to 2 years) or "for cause" (wherein the FDA has a suspicion that all is not right). The inspection may last from a few days to months if major issues are found. The FDA may go to sites outside the United States, if appropriate. Conversely, the EMA and other agencies abroad inspect in the United States. However, most companies now understand that building quality management systems is now obligatory, not just in safety, but throughout the organization. They also realize that periodic audits (including self-audits) and governmental inspections are now part of the norm and "a cost of doing business". Such inspections not only provide markers for compliance, but also serve to promote trust in medical products and the regulatory system.

There has been much controversy after the withdrawal of Vioxx and other products from the US market as well as contaminated products (e.g., heparin) for safety reasons. Some (both from within the FDA and from the outside) have accused the FDA of not sufficiently protecting the American public from "dangerous" drugs, food, and other products. There have been accusations of too rapid approval of drugs, insufficient analysis of data submitted to the FDA, companies' not submitting complete or sufficient data to the FDA, and other charges. Similar controversies have been seen with other regulatory agencies in regard to financial regulation, air transport safety, and so forth. The PDUFA, FDAAA, and other changes are a result of these controversies. More will come.

■ Drug Safety Inspections

The FDA has an extensive role in doing drug safety and PV inspections. This is covered in a subsequent chapter in this manual.

■ Frequently Asked Questions

Q: Is there too close a relationship between the FDA and the pharmaceutical industry?

A: The answer depends on whom you ask. The FDA would (most probably) say that they are not compromised by maintaining correct and formal communications with the industry. Indeed, close communication promotes an understanding of regulatory expectations as well as practical challenges. The industry supplies FDA with much of the post-marketing safety data and nearly all of the pre-marketing safety data. There must be communication between the industry and the Agency to clarify ambiguous points, get further information on critical cases, and so forth. The FDA also encourages (and legislation even requires in some cases) meetings with the industry during the development of regulation and guidance. The FDA also regularly tracks drug development and meets with sponsors to discuss progress and next steps with investigational drugs (in the IND phases) and in post-marketing situations where safety issues arise. It is a professional-to-professional exchange of information to ensure the safety of the American public.

The industry would say that its influence on the FDA is slight. Companies go out of their way to be sure the FDA gets what it needs (and wants) and companies often submit more than regulations require to be sure that the FDA gets what it wants and that the companies are not accused of hiding or under submitting data. The industry often (privately) believes that the FDA is rather tough and tends to not give the industry a fair shake or a level playing field. Some feel the FDA treats big pharma differently from small pharma or start-up companies, cutting the latter a little more slack and giving them more "hand-holding".

There has been speculation that the substantial PDUFA fees provided by industry for scientific assessment of new data by FDA "guarantee" new product approval, i.e., payment for a positive opinion. For example, in 2017 the fee for review of an application with clinical data was $2,038,100. Of course, integrity and objectivity of FDA reviewers is not adversely influenced by payments to the Agency (not to individuals) for operational expenses that improve efficiency of the drug review process.

Others claim that there is too much interchange of personnel between the FDA and industry, wherein some people start their careers or spend some time at the FDA and then move on to work for pharma companies, or vice versa, carrying with them their contacts and inner knowledge (which often becomes outmoded quickly) of the other. Some feel that this may influence a person's actions in the company or FDA since his or her next job may be for the "other side".

The consumer groups and activists believe that the FDA is indeed in bed with the industry and point to the various "fiascos" in safety that have occurred, such as Vioxx, Fen-Phen, suicide in pediatric patients on antidepressants, and contaminated heparin, Oxycontin and other opioids, and vaping among others. The FDA and the industry would (probably) counter by saying, quite the contrary that these episodes have shown that the drug safety system in place is indeed functioning and functioning well; the real challenge is to identify these problems earlier and manage the emerging risks.

These criticisms have been made for many other federal agencies, including regulators of banks, insurance companies, Wall Street, the airline industry, and car manufacturers. This is a fascinating and controversial area that is and will remain a work in progress for the foreseeable future.

Q: Should the FDA be broken up into an approving body and a safety body, similar to some other federal regulatory agencies?

A: This proposal has been advanced in the last several years. The argument is that the people who approve a drug have a vested (and emotional) interest in seeing their drug stay on the market and may not act vigorously on safety matters as this might be a tacit admission that their original approval decision was incorrect or too hasty. Organizationally, these functions are already split, but within CDER. It is claimed that separate reviewers should oversee safety, as they have no interest in defending an approval decision and they would be able to better interpret real world evidence, i.e., understand impact of bias and confounders, in data from the post-marketing phase. Thus, the medical skill set involved in post-marketing safety review is arguably different from that required in pre-approval safety review, which focuses on controlled clinical trial data. In all instances, however, safety assessment must always be considered in the context of benefit. Separating the functions would discount the knowledge the reviewing group has obtained over months and years of review of a product, moving post-marketing follow-up to people unfamiliar with the drug. This also would increase the bureaucracy and be more costly. In addition, complete separation would introduce additional challenges in the pre-approval phase when non-routine safety interventions, e.g., REMS, are under discussion. Clearly, each side has valid points. What will evolve will most likely be a political decision. There has also been talk of separating the food part of FDA into a separate agency. This too is under evaluation. It is possible, given the many issues on vaccines, waivers, communication with the public, new untested or minimally tested products that appeared during the Covid period in the early 2020s, that a whole new look at FDA and CDC will occur.

CHAPTER

5

The European Medicines Agency

In 1995, the European Medicines Evaluation Agency (EMEA), now called European Medicines Agency (EMA) but also "the Agency," was created and based in London, England but was moved to Amsterdam, The Netherlands after Brexit. Now, over two decades later, the face of drug regulation in Europe has totally changed. In 2010, a new PV Regulation was issued generating hundreds of associated Directives, Guidances, Q&A, etc. This "tsunami" continues to evolve with ongoing new or updated regulatory documents which continue to be published. See the very extensive website of the EMA. In addition to English, the EMA website is available in official languages of the EU. Regulators in the Member States have their own websites. We will examine the EMA in detail and take a brief look at one Member State's Health Agency: France.

■ Introduction

Like the US FDA, the EMA's main responsibility is the protection and promotion of public and animal health through the evaluation, supervision, and safety monitoring of medicines throughout the European Union. The EU comprises 27 countries (Member States), as well as the three European Free Trade Area (EFTA) nations of Iceland, Liechtenstein, and Norway. These 30 countries are also referred to as the European Economic Area (EEA).

Switzerland also works closely with the EMA, particularly in areas regarding inspections, but is not within the EU.

■ Due to Brexit, the EMA moved from London to Amsterdam, The Netherlands and the number of EU countries is back to 27. Note that there is a pathway for additional jurisdictions to enter the EU. Registration Procedures in the EU

All medicines must be authorized ("approved") before they can be marketed. There are two main ways for authorizing medicines: a centralized process and a national one (that is, non-centralized).

Centralized Authorization Procedure (CAP): Pharmaceutical companies submit one single Marketing-Authorization Application (MAA) to EMA. EMA's Committee for Medicinal Products for Human Use (CHMP) then, using scientific resources provided by the Member States), carries out a scientific assessment of the application and makes a recommendation (an "opinion") to the European Commission on whether the medicine should be marketed or not, i.e., the EMA functions as a coordinating agency and does not have direct authority to authorize medicinal products.

Once granted by the European Commission, the centralized MA is valid in all EU Member States as well as in the European Economic Area (EEA). The new or innovative medicines pass through the centralized authorization procedure in order to be marketed in the EU. This allows the marketing authorization holder (MAH) to market the medicine throughout the EEA on the basis of one single marketing authorization. The centralized process is required for certain medicines, e.g., biosimilars, gene therapies, etc.

National Authorization Procedures: Many medicines available in the EU have been authorized at national level, either because they were authorized before EMA's creation (1995) or they were not within the scope of the centralized procedure. Each EU Member State had, and still has, its own national authorization procedures. If a company wishes to request a MA in several EU Member States for a medicine that is outside the scope of the centralized procedure, it may use one of the following routes:

- Mutual Recognition Procedure (MRP), whereby a marketing authorization granted in one Member State can be recognized in other EU countries; or
- Decentralized procedure, whereby a medicine that has not yet been authorized in the EU can be simultaneously authorized in several EU Member States.

Note: For issues that occur after authorization (e.g., safety concerns), the CHMP handles centrally-licensed products. The Coordination Group for Mutual Recognition and Decentralized Procedures — human (CMD(h)) handles nationally-registered medicines and reports to the Heads of Medicines Agencies (HMA). The Pharmacovigilance Risk Assessment Committee (PRAC) (see below) is the senior committee that then handles all authorized products and makes recommendations to both CHMP and CMD(h).

■ European Medicines Agency

The EMA serves a market about 510 million people living in the EEA. The terminology in Europe can be a bit confusing as the EU/EEA is not the European equivalent of the United States. The EEA is composed of sovereign nations, which still retain many powers and functions. They are linked by a variety of treaties. Some governmental functions are devolved in full or in part to the "central" authority (in Brussels and Strasbourg) and others are retained by the national governments. Not all countries devolve the same functions to the central authority. Thus, the EU/EEA's handling of drugs and drug safety is like but, in many ways, quite different from that of the FDA or other single, national health agency.

Organization and Structure

The EMA handles human and veterinary medicinal products (but not food, unlike the FDA). Whatever the registration status, the EMA goal is to ensure harmonized safety surveillance for all EU countries.

The EMA principle is based on a central organization (~900 EMA permanent employees), supported by ~4,500 experts, who conduct the detailed, work of the Agency by sitting on scientific and medical committees, working groups, and assessment teams. These experts are made available by the Member States, and usually reside in the Member States but may attend periodic meetings in the Member States, at the EMA, or elsewhere.

The EMA is headed by an executive director with seven reporting divisions: The Advisory Functions, the Human Medicines, the Veterinary Medicines, the Stakeholders and Communication, the Task Forces, the Information Management and the Administration and Corporate Management. "Inspections, Human Medicines Pharmacovigilance & Committees Division" handles drug safety. The other Divisions are "Human Medicines Research & Development Support", "Human Medicines Evaluation", "Veterinary Medicines", "Administration and Corporate Management", "Information Management" and "Stakeholders & Communication". See the organization chart below or on the EMA website for an organogram snapshot as of late 2023. As with any organization, changes occur over time (http://www.ema.europa.eu/ema/). As of 2023, seven scientific committees, with members from all 31 EU/EEA states, handle the main scientific work of the Agency:

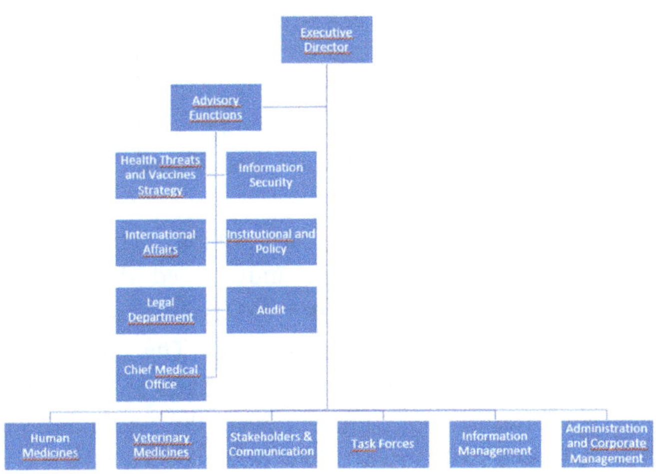

- Committee for Medicinal Products for Human Use (CHMP);
- Pharmacovigilance Risk Assessment Committee (PRAC);
- Committee for Medicinal Products for Veterinary Use (CVMP);
- Committee for Orphan Medicinal Products (COMP);
- Committee on Herbal Medicinal Products (HMPC);
- Paediatric Committee (PDCO);
- Committee for Advanced Therapies (CAT).

Note 1: Within these committees, the role of each EU country representative is not to defend a local recommendation but to ensure that the EU decision is actually applicable to and valid for all EU countries.

Note 2: The EMA has a number of working parties and related groups in place. They advise EMA's scientific committees on issues relating to their fields of expertise (e.g. Biologics or Biosimilar Working Parties, etc.).

Note 3: The CMD(h) covers a variety of issues related to new applications, variations, renewals and pharmacovigilance activities for nationally-authorized medicines. It is not strictly-speaking an EMA Committee even if CMD(h) meetings are held at the EMA.

The highest-level committee handling human medicines is the Committee for Medicinal Products for Human Use (CHMP). It is responsible for the following:

- Conducting the initial assessment of EU-wide (i.e., centralized process) marketing authorization applications,
- Assessing modifications or extensions ("variations") to an existing marketing authorization.
- Considering the recommendations of the Agency's PRAC regarding the safety of medicines on the market and, when necessary, recommending to the European Commission (EC) changes to a medicine's marketing authorization, or, in extreme instances, its suspension or withdrawal from the market. The EC is the senior level of management, is above the CHMP and PRAC, and can act on the opinions of the CHMP, i.e., has the authority to authorize a product.

Risk Management

The EU has developed a comprehensive risk management strategy for all products in the EEA. This is a strategy that covers the entire life cycle of a product, and a risk analysis is required for every product upon approval (or during its marketing). A specific committee (PRAC), replacing the former PV Working Party, was set up in 2012 (see below). The goal is to have a set of pharmacovigilance activities and potential non-routine interventions designed to identify, characterize, prevent, and minimize risks relating to medicinal products, including the assessment of the effectiveness of these interventions.

EudraVigilance — The EU Safety Database

In 2001, an EU-wide central database, called the EudraVigilance System, was created. This database serves as a repository and "clearinghouse" to ensure that all appropriate cases are available to the appropriate Member States. It is used to capture SAEs electronically as Individual Case Safety Reports (ICSRs) both pre- and post-authorization as well as spontaneous non-serious AEs. It has been designed to manage and analyze information on suspected adverse reactions to medicines which have been authorized or are being studied in clinical trials in the European Economic Area (EEA).

The EMA operates the system. This allows for a single European Pharmacovigilance database accessible to the Member States' HAs. Individual cases (ICSRs) must now be reported electronically from both public and private PV organizations (using the gateway or a web reporting application).

The pharmaceutical industry can only access detailed, proprietary data for medicines for which they hold a marketing authorization. This restriction is in place to remain in compliance with EU personal data protection and privacy legislation. They can, of course, access the high level summary information available to the general public on all medications in EudraVigilance (http://www.adrreports.eu/en/index.html). Simple queries can deliver online summary tables or figures depending on the selected criteria.

The European pharmacovigilance issues tracking tool (EPITT) is a database developed by EMA for the communication of pharmacovigilance and risk-management issues between the Agency and Member States. It provides access to documents related to the safety of products/substances authorized in the EEA. The EPITT provides the functionalities for national regulatory authorities in the EEA and EMA to track signals at EU level. It is not available to the public or the pharmaceutical industry.

Other computerized systems have been developed by the EMA:

- EudraVigilance Medicinal Products Dictionary (XEVMPD), also known as the Article 57 database. This is the EU drug dictionary.
- SIAMED II is the Agency's product information and application tracking system which will be soon migrated into the PMS (Product Management Service) hub.
- The European Clinical Trials Database (EudraCT) is the EU's electronic database of clinical trials. It contains information submitted by sponsors and informs users about ongoing clinical trials in all EEA countries, enabling an overview of multi-state trials.
- The European Network of Centres for Pharmacoepidemiology and Pharmacovigilance (ENCePP — https://www.encepp.eu/structure/index.shtml) databases contain independent (from pharma companies) post-authorization studies focusing on safety and on benefit–risk, using available expertise and research experience across Europe.
- Studies database is the E-Register of Studies (EU Post-authorization Studies (PAS) register) aims to provide a publicly accessible resource for the registration of pharmacoepidemiological and pharmacovigilance studies; they are hosted in the ENCePP system.
- PSUR/PBRER repository is a single, central platform for PSURs/PBRERs and related documents to be used by all regulatory authorities and pharmaceutical companies in the EU. The use of the PSUR Repository is mandatory for all PSUR/PBRER submissions as of June 2016 (via the e-submission Gateway).

In addition to the EMA, each European country has its own national Health Authority (HA) or authorities that handle drug safety. They are often called "competent authorities (CA)" in EU regulatory jargon. The EU is still evolving and the Lisbon Treaty (2005) and other subsequent treaties have altered some of the basic structures and functions of the EU governing bodies. The EU remains still a work in progress. The interplay between the central authority (primarily in Brussels but with various agencies scattered throughout the EU, such as the EMA in Amsterdam and the European Central Bank in Frankfurt, Germany) and the individual countries is dynamic and often changing. Note also that the EMA does not have jurisdiction over food. The European Food Safety Authority in Parma, Italy handles those matters.

As noted, for drug safety, some functions are primarily centralized in the EMA and some remain in each member state. Some national authorities are very large and powerful and exert strong influence over smaller member states. This division and, in many cases, duplication of labor, as well as the multitude of languages involved in the EU, produce a challenge for safety reporting both for the pharmaceutical industry and for the member states themselves. Most of the work in drug safety is done at the international level in English, but, obviously, at the local level the national languages are still used. The comparison with other countries, particularly the US, where the drug safety function is clearly centralized, is striking. The closest analogy would be if each of the 50 states in the US had its own mini-FDA and used languages other than English. With the UK leaving the EU, there remain only two countries that have English as a native, national language: Malta and Eire (Ireland). There has been some talk of now using more French and German. "A voir". "Bleibt abzuwarten". We shall see.

In terms of pharmacovigilance, the EMA has largely harmonized along the lines of ICH. They have codified the pre-marketing requirements in a document known as Regulation (EU) No. 536/2014 of the European Parliament and of the Council of 16 April 2014 and the post-marketing requirements in Regulation (EU) Nos. 1235/2010 and 1027/2012. Each is discussed in detail below. Nonetheless, there are still differences, particularly for clinical trial pharmacovigilance, from country to country.

With the regulation updated in 2010, a major effort has been made for an accurate communication and transparency. Numerous tools and publications have been set up to comply with this commitment including the EMA web portal, the publishing of committee meetings' agendas and minutes, *ad hoc* newsletters such as "What's new in Pharmacovigilance QPPV Updates", public hearings, etc.).

For more information on the EMA, see the following websites (Current as of late 2024):

- EMA website (http://www.ema.europa.eu/ema/);
- EMA PV System Manual (http://www.ema.europa.eu/docs/en_GB/document_library/Other/2014/07/WC500170226.pdf);
- Eudravigilance (https://www.ema.europa.eu/en/human-regulatory/research-development/pharmacovigilance/eudravigilance/eudravigilance-system-overview);
- PV Q&A web page (http://www.ema.europa.eu/ema/index.jsp?curl=pages/regulation/q_and_a/q_and_a_detail_000135.jsp&mid=WC0b01ac058066e97a%20-).

What Is Not in the Scope of EMA?

EMA does not perform the following:

- Evaluate the initial marketing authorization application of all medicines in the EU (as many drugs have been approved in each EU country before the creation of the EMA in 1995, the vast majority of medicines registered in the EU are authorized at a national level). However, the centralized process must be used for new products, e.g., biosimilars, gene products, etc.
- Evaluate applications for the authorization of clinical trials. The authorization of clinical trials occurs at Member State level, although the Agency plays a key role in ensuring that the standards of good

clinical practice are applied. The EMA also manages the database of clinical trials carried out in the EU.
- Evaluate food supplements and cosmetics. These are evaluated at national level, except for products having a pharmacological activity.
- Carry out research or develop medicines.
- Make decisions on the price or availability of medicines. This is done at the national level.
- Control medicines advertising. Also done at the national level.
- Control or have information on pharmaceutical patents.
- Develop treatment guidelines.
- Provide medical advice to any stakeholder group.
- Develop laws concerning medicines. The European Commission develops EU legislation concerning medicines and the European Parliament together with the Council of the European Union adopt the legislation. The European Commission also develops EU policies in the field of human or veterinary medicines and public health.
- Issue marketing authorizations. The legal decision to grant, suspend or revoke a marketing authorization for any medicine falls under the remit of the European Commission for centrally authorized products, and the national competent authorities of the EU Member States for nationally authorized products.

Note 1: The EMA is, since 2021, now responsible for some Medical Devices (see https://www.ema.europa.eu/en/human-regulatory/overview/medical-devices)

The Pharmacovigilance Risk Assessment Committee

The Pharmacovigilance Risk Assessment Committee (PRAC) has experts from each member state; it provides its advice and recommendations to the EU network, and for many procedures these recommendations are considered by the CHMP before they become legally binding. They meet for 3–4 days each month.

The PRAC was formally established in July 2012, replacing the former PV Working Party (PhVWP); it is responsible for assessing all aspects of risk management of human medicines, including the following:

- The detection, assessment, minimization and communication of the risk of adverse reactions, while taking the therapeutic effect of the medicine into account to evaluate the benefit/risk balance;
- The design and evaluation of post-authorization safety studies (PASS);
- Pharmacovigilance audits/inspections.

The PRAC also advises the EMA on the development of guidelines, standards, and provides advice on operational aspects of the EU pharmacovigilance system.

The PRAC provides recommendations on questions involving pharmacovigilance and risk management systems, including the monitoring of their effectiveness, to the following:

- CHMP for centrally authorized medicines and referral procedures;
- CMDh for mutual recognition and decentralized procedures;
- The EMA secretariat, Management Board, and European Commission, as applicable.

The PRAC's primary duties include evaluation of potential signals arising from spontaneous reports and or PSURs/PBRERs, advising on risk and risk management (including regulatory options) and monitoring regulatory actions. Their domain is largely in the post-approval area, but they do have authority for drugs under study.

The PRAC's member contact information and declarations of interest are published on the EMA website. The PRAC includes independent experts from all EU member states in pharmacoepidemiology, clinical pharmacology, biologics, signal detection, risk communication, and vaccine vigilance. The Detailed Rules for PRAC procedures have been published (see the EMA Website).

A yearly PRAC work plan is published during the first quarter of the year. They issue work programs in advance of their monthly meetings and publish meeting highlights and meeting minutes which usually involve safety issues on specific drugs. The meeting highlights are posted on the EMA website the day after the meeting and the minutes are published after PRAC's about a month later. You can find the meeting minutes by accessing the EMAs website, by going to "Committees" and then to "PRAC".

An analysis of the first 18 months of PRAC activities has been published and concluded positively: "Early signs, ... based on process indicators such as those reported here for RMPs, ADRs, signals, PSURs and EU Pharmacovigilance Referrals, point to more systematic and proportionate risk management planning, the promotion of reporting (including from patients), greater coordination of real-time signal management, faster assessment and decision-making, and thus strengthening of the link between pharmacovigilance assessments and regulatory actions such as labelling changes to optimize safe and effective drug use."[1]

■ Post-marketing PV EU Regulation

Four different kinds of documents exist at the EU level as follows:

- **Regulations:** These are mandatory requirements and are applicable in all EU countries as written. They are translated exactly into national languages but cannot be altered. They are usually high-level documents.
- **Directives:** These, too, are mandatory requirements as well, but can vary in each EU country depending on the local translation/adaptation. Often the member states have up to three years to put these directives into effect as national legislation.
- **Guidances/Practices/Decisions:** These are also mandatory requirements. They are more focused on a specific topic or theme. Note that in the US, the term *guidance* or *guideline* represents FDA's current thinking on a topic but, unlike the EU, they are not mandatory.
- **Recommendation/Opinion:** These are not mandatory and are usually more general documents (e.g., healthcare policy, providing priorities).

[1] Peter Arlett *et al.*, Proactively managing the risk of marketed drugs: experience with the EMA Pharmacovigilance Risk Assessment Committee, *Nat Rev Drug Discov* 2014; 13: 395–397.

The previous legally-binding document covering post-authorization PV was called EudraLex Volume 9A. It covered all EU PV Regulations. It was amended in 2010 and since then thousands of pages of documents have been issued to update the EU PV Regulation. This new legislation aims to rationalize, simplify and improve workflow, to stop useless tasks, to be more consistent, to focus on risks, to improve transparency to all stakeholders, to help ensure that commitments made are actually done and to involve patients and the public.

It is impossible to provide here an exhaustive list of these numerous documents, below are listed the key ones to consider:

- Regulations (EU) Nos. 1235/2010 and 1027/2012
- Directives 2010/84/EU and 2012/26/EU
- Good Vigilance Practices (GVP)
  - *Note* 1: Modules XI, XII, XIII and XIV have been cancelled. Their content has been incorporated into other documents.
  - 2: These are living documents. They are periodically updated, submitted to PV stakeholders (including the pharmaceutical industry) for comments/proposals, validated, and then published.

These documents require the EMA, the member states, and others to set up systems to handle the collection, verification, exchange, and presentation of adverse reaction reports within the European Union but also to identify safety signals and manage risks.

The roles and responsibilities of the MAH are spelled out and require that an appropriate system of PV is put in place by the MAH. All information regarding the benefit–risk profile must be promptly and fully sent to the competent authorities. And most critically, it describes the role of the EU Qualified Person for Pharmacovigilance (EU QPPV), to be appointed by the MAH and to be continuously (24/7) available for safety matters.

Table 1. EU Good Pharmacovigilance Practice (GVP) Modules and Annexes.

GVP Module	GVP Title	Details
GVP Introductory Cover Note	—	This module introduces all GVPs and annexes and details the following: ■ Background to GVP; ■ History of the GVP development process and latest updates; ■ Objectives of pharmacovigilance; ■ Pharmacovigilance in the EU: roles of different actors; ■ Legal basis, scope and process for GVP; ■ Maintenance and further development of GVP; ■ Structure of GVP; ■ Referencing of legal requirements in GVP; ■ Practical advice for the public consultation.
GVP Module I	Pharmacovigilance Systems and Their Quality Systems	This module contains guidance for the establishment and maintenance of quality assured PV systems for MAH, competent authorities of Member States and the Agency (EMA). How the systems of these organizations interact while undertaking specific PV processes is described in each respective Module of GVP. The PV system is a system used by the MAH and by Member States to monitor the safety of authorized medicinal products and detect any change to their risk-benefit balance. The Agency likewise maintains a PV system to fulfil its pharmacovigilance activities.
GVP Module II	Pharmacovigilance System Master File	A pharmacovigilance system master file (PSMF) is a detailed description of the PV system used by the MAH with respect to one or more authorized medicinal products. This module provides detailed guidance regarding the requirements for the PSMF, including its maintenance, content and associated submissions to competent authorities.
GVP Module III	Pharmacovigilance Inspections	This module contains guidance on the planning, conduct, reporting and follow-up of PV inspections in the EU and outlines the role of the different involved parties.
GVP Module IV	Pharmacovigilance Audits	This module provides guidance on planning and conducting the legally required audits, and in respect of the operation of the EU regulatory network, the role, context and management of PV audit activity. This module is intended to facilitate the performance of PV audits, especially to promote harmonization, and encourage consistency and simplification of the audit process. The principles in this Module are aligned with internationally accepted auditing standards, issued by relevant international auditing standardization organizations and support a risk-based approach to PV audits.
GVP Module V	Risk Management Systems	The aim of a risk management plan (RMP) is to document the risk management system considered necessary to identify, characterize and minimize a medicinal product's important risks. To this end, the RMP contains: 1. The identification or characterization of the safety profile of the medicinal product, with emphasis on important identified and important potential risks and missing information, and also on which safety concerns need to be managed proactively or further studied (the "safety specification"). 2. The planning of PV activities to characterize and quantify clinically relevant risks, and to identify new adverse reactions (the "pharmacovigilance plan"). 3. The planning and implementation of risk minimization measures, including the evaluation of the effectiveness of these activities (the "risk minimization plan").

Table 1. *(Continued)*

GVP Module	GVP Title	Details
		This Module includes the principles of risk minimization and should be read in conjunction with GVP Module XVI and GVP Module XVI Addendum I on educational materials. A RMP template has been developed by the EMA (see EMA Website): it is not considered as part of the GVPs.
GVP Module VI	Collection, Management and Submission of Reports of Suspected Adverse Reactions to Medicinal Products	This module of GVP addresses the legal requirements which are applicable to competent authorities in Member States, MAHs and the Agency (EMA) as regards the collection, data management and submission of individual reports of suspected adverse reactions (serious and non-serious) associated with medicinal products for human use authorized in the European Union (EU).
GVP Module VI — Addendum I	Duplicate Management of Suspected Adverse Reaction Reports	The guidance in this document proposes methods for detecting, confirming and managing duplicate cases suitable for organizations receiving PV data in various different formats and describes methods for stakeholders to collaborate with the Agency (EMA) in the detection and management of duplicate cases; it is also provided for situations where individual cases might be reported by different senders.
GVP Module VII	Periodic Safety Update Report (PSUR/PBRER)	This guidance specifies scope, objectives, format and content of the PSUR/ PBRER. Further details and guidance for the submission of PSURs/PBRERs in the EU, including the list of Union references dates and frequency of submission, are provided. The process to follow for a single assessment of PSURs/PBRERs in the EU for different medicinal products containing the same active substance or the same combination of active substances authorized in more than one Member State for which a Union reference date and frequency of submission of PSURs has been established, is also detailed.
GVP Module VIII	Post-authorization Safety Studies (PASS)	This module concerns both interventional and non-interventional PASS, with a main focus on non-interventional ones. It does not concern pre-clinical safety studies. Non-interventional PASS concerned by this guidance are those initiated, managed or financed by a MAH voluntarily or pursuant to an obligation imposed by an EU competent authority. The purposes of this module are to: ■ provide general guidance for the transparency, scientific standards and quality standards of non-interventional PASS conducted voluntarily or pursuant to an obligation imposed by an EU competent authority; ■ describe procedures whereby an EU competent authority may impose on a MAH an obligation to conduct a PASS; ■ describe procedures that apply to non-interventional PASS pursuant to an obligation imposed by an EU competent authority for the protocol oversight and reporting of results and for subsequent changes to the marketing authorization.
GVP Module VIII — Addendum I	Requirements and Recommendations for the Submission of Information on Non-interventional Post-authorization Safety Studies	This addendum provides additional information on legal requirements and recommendations for the submission of study protocols, progress reports and final study reports of non-interventional PASS to national competent authorities and the Agency (EMA). It also provides additional information as regards the registration of non-interventional PASS in the EU PAS Register. It does not provide recommendations for the transmission of information to ethics committees, national review boards or other bodies in place according to national legislation.

(Continued)

Table 1. (*Continued*)

GVP Module	GVP Title	Details
GVP Module IX	Signal Management	The objectives of this module are to: ■ provide general guidance and requirements on scientific and quality aspects of signal management; ■ describe roles, responsibilities and procedural aspects in the setting of the EU signal management process overseen by the PV Risk Assessment Committee (PRAC). This module applies to all organizations involved in signal management, i.e., MAHs, national competent authorities and the European Medicines Agency.
GVP Module IX — Addendum I	Methodological Aspects of Signal Detection from Spontaneous Reports of Suspected Adverse Reactions	This addendum lists some of the methodological aspects that should be considered in detecting potential signals. The proposed approach complements the classical disproportion-ality analysis with additional data summaries, based on both statistical and clinical considerations.
GVP Module X	Additional Monitoring	This module is divided in two sections: ■ X.B. provides general principles for assigning additional monitoring status to medicinal products and on communication and transparency aspects; ■ X.C. describes the operation of the EU network regarding the supervision of additional monitoring status, the communication strategy and the impact on PV activities.
GVP Module XI	Cancelled — Included in other GVPs	Not applicable
GVP Module XII	Cancelled — Included in Other GVPs	Not applicable
GVP Module XIII	Cancelled — Included in Other GVPs	Not applicable
GVP Module XIV	Cancelled — Included in Other GVPs	Not applicable
GVP Module XV	Safety Communication	This module provides guidance to MAHs, competent authorities in Member States and the EMA on how to communicate and coordinate safety information concerning medicinal products authorized in the EU. Section XV.B of this module describes principles and means of safety communication. Section XV.C provides guidance on the coordination and dissemination of safety communication within the EU network. Both sections give particular consideration to direct healthcare professional communications and provide specific guidance for preparing them.
GVP Module XVI	Risk Minimization Measures: Selection of Tools and Effectiveness Indicators	The guidance provided in this Module should be considered in the context of the wider GVP guidance, in particular in conjunction with GVP Module V.
		This Module provides guidance on the principles for: ■ The development and implementation of additional risk minimization measures, including examples of risk minimization tools; ■ The evaluation of the effectiveness of risk minimization measures.

Table 1. *(Continued)*

GVP Module	GVP Title	Details
		Section XVI.B describes the development, implementation and coordination of risk minimization measures and the general principles of the evaluation of their effectiveness. Section XVI.C considers the application of those measures and principles in the setting of the EU regulatory network.
GVP Module XVI — Addendum I	Educational Materials	This addendum to GVP Module XVI provides further guidance for MAHs on the submission of draft educational material(s) to the competent authorities of Member States, as well as, guidance for these authorities to support the assessment of such materials, in particular with regard to format and content. Because of the specificities of the national healthcare systems and of how particular risk(s) are managed within these systems, individual Member States may have additional requirements. In this case, the guidance in this addendum to GVP Module XVI should be followed together with national guidelines.
Draft GVP Module XVI Addendum III	Pregnancy prevention programme and other pregnancy-specific risk minimisation measures	Pregnancy prevention program; when such program is needed; risk-minimisation measures to be considered Anticipated date for coming into effect after finalization: 2023
Product- or Population-Specific Considerations I	Vaccines for Prophylaxis Against Infectious Diseases	The objective of this GVP Considerations Chapter is to strengthen the conduct of PV for vaccines. It should be noted that the overall objectives and processes of PV are similar for vaccines and other types of medicinal products and this guidance does not replace the information provided in the process-focused modules of the Good Pharmacovigilance Practices (GVP). This document focusses on vaccine-specific aspects and unique challenges that should be borne in mind when designing and implementing PV activities for vaccines.
Product- or Population-Specific Considerations II	Biological Medicinal Products	This document applies to all biological medicinal products regardless of the regulatory pathway of approval or market exclusivity status, i.e., it applies to reference biological medicinal products, to biosimilars and to products which contain the same or closely related active substance but not authorized as biosimilars (e.g., different versions of interferon beta-1a, factor VIII or normal human immunoglobulin). The legal requirements for PV and the good PV practices (GVP) apply to biologicals just as they do for other medicines. The guidance of this Module does not replace any of these. However, biologicals are associated with several specific challenges in PV. This module is intended to be read and followed alongside the process-related GVP Modules when developing and implementing PV for biologicals to ensure that these challenges are addressed. Section P.II.A describes some of the specific issues and challenges; section P.II.B provides guidance on addressing these in the context of the main PV processes described in the GVP and Section P.II.C provides guidance related to operation of the EU network.
Product- or Population-Specific Considerations III	Pregnant and breastfeeding women	This document aims to provide guidance to MAA/MAH, competent authorities of Member States and the Agency for facilitating appropriate pharmacovigilance for medicinal products that may be used in pregnant or breastfeeding women Anticipated date for coming into effect after finalization: 2023

(Continued)

Table 1. *(Continued)*

GVP Module	GVP Title	Details
Product- or Population-Specific Considerations IV	Paediatric Population	This guidance provides details on paediatric PV activities, including ICSRs management, signal detection and risk management. The guidance contained in this Chapter is addressed to MAHs, the competent authorities in Member States and the Agency (EMA). It covers all paediatric age groups. The paediatric use of vaccines and safety surveillance of paediatric outcomes after exposure to medicines in utero are outside the scope.
GVP Annex I	Definitions	This document details all commonly used PV terms, from "Abuse of a medicinal product" to "Validated signal"
GVP Annex II — Templates	Templates: Cover Page of Periodic Safety Update Report (PSUR)	Template providing the detailed information which is to be displayed on the cover page of each PSUR/ PBRER.
GVP Annex II — Templates	Direct Healthcare Professional Communication (DHPC)	This template should be used for the preparation of a core EU Direct Healthcare Professional Communication (DHPC).
GVP Annex II — Templates	Communication Plan for Direct Healthcare Professional Communication (CP DHPC)	This template lists the stakeholders to be involved/informed in case of DHPC.
GVP Annex III — Other Pharmacovigilance Guidances	Guideline on the Exposure to Medicinal Products During Pregnancy: Need for Post-authorization Data	This guideline provides criteria to select medicinal products for which active surveillance for collecting post-authorization data in pregnancy is necessary. It provides guidance on how to monitor accidental or intended exposure to medicinal products during pregnancy and specific requirements for reporting data and adverse outcomes of pregnancy exposure.
GVP Annex III — Other Pharmacovigilance Guidances	EudraVigilance Access Policy	The guideline also includes detailed recommendations regarding presentation of data collected on exposure in pregnant women. The guideline relates in particular to new products, for which a summary of the potential risks of exposure in pregnancy and of the potential need for the product during pregnancy should be included in the RMP (Safety Specifications). The aim of these specifications is that the MAH proposes a PV Plan in order to evaluate the potential risk of a product and/or to provide missing information on the safety of the product in pregnancy. The Agency (EMA) is granting medicines regulatory authorities in the EEA unrestricted access to all ICSRs held in EudraVigilance. Since May 2012, healthcare professionals, the public, MAHs and academia have certain levels of access to spontaneous reports focusing on centrally authorized medicinal products. This access is provided through the adrreports.eu portal of the Agency and was extended in September 2014 to all active substances contained in medicinal products authorized in the EEA. This Access Policy defines the overall principles for providing access to ICSR data held in EudraVigilance in line with the EU legal framework and taking into account that the interest in and the use of the data may vary between stakeholders.
GVP Annex V	Abbreviations	This document lists all acronyms used in the EU regulation from "A-CASI: Audio computer-assisted self-interviewing" to "XEVPRM: eXtended EudraVigilance Product Report Message"

In brief, the QPPV establishes and maintains the PV system, has an overview of all the products and safety issues pending, and makes sure all safety functions are handled properly. The QPPV's roles are discussed in detail elsewhere in this manual. The QPPV must ensure that all suspected ADRs are collected, collated, reported, and accessible within the EU. The MAH must prepare, update, and have available a "Pharmacovigilance System Master File" (PSMF). Requirements for risk management systems, expedited reporting, PSURs/PBRERs, special situations, databases, documentation, company post-marketing safety studies, quality assurance/control and regulatory matters are also addressed (Regulations and Directives). These topics are covered in detail in this manual in the individual chapters.

Specific obligations for member states' national health agencies are similar to what is required for pharmaceutical industry; how PV is to be done, handling of ICSRs, PSURs/PBRERs, signal detection, medication errors, benefit–risk analyses, communication, data exchange, crisis management plans relating to safety matters, inspections, rapid-alert and non-urgent information communication system, how referrals to the EMA are to be done.

The Practices Annexes to the Modules include a glossary, abbreviations, terminology, references to guidelines and templates for the EU Risk Management Plan, the PSUR/PBRER sections, and distribution requirements for reporting to competent authorities.

In summary, this is a complete and well-prepared set of documents that shapes a consistent PV System at the EU level. The documents are rich in explanations and background and anyone in the field of PV, whether in the EU or elsewhere, should read and be familiar with these documents. Many of the principles and procedures are used throughout the rest of the world as they are based on the common seminal antecedent documents of PV, namely, the Council for International Organizations of Medical Sciences (CIOMS) and ICH documents.

Volume 10 Clinical Trial PV

As with the post-marketing requirements, the regulation of drug safety surveillance during clinical development has been updated over the last several years. The changes are not as dramatic as those put in place for post-marketing surveillance but are significant. EudraLex Volume 10 has been amended and new Regulations have been put in place (2019) (see w: Regulation (EU) No. 536/2014. Contrary to Post-marketing Regulation for which specific PV documents (Directives, Practices, Q&A, etc.) are issued, the drug safety surveillance rules during clinical studies are part of the clinical study regulation.

Regarding clinical trial PV, the main changes represent a simplification of the rules on safety reporting as follows:

- The protocol may provide that not all adverse events (AE) and suspected serious adverse events are recorded and reported as part of the safety assessment if they are used as efficacy endpoints, for example.
- For a clinical trial involving more than one investigational medicinal product (IMP) it is now possible to submit a single safety report on all the IMPs used in the trial to the EudraVigilance database.
- Suspected unexpected serious adverse reactions (SUSARs) are reported to the Clinical Trial Eudravigilance database:
  - *Note* 1: For multinational trials, all SUSARs, whether occurring within the EU or in a third country, are reported to the Agency.
  - *Note* 2: Fatal or life-threatening SUSARs are within 7 calendar days. Non-fatal or non-life-threatening SUSARs within 15 calendar Days.
- The regulation requires Member States to collaborate in assessing the annual Development Safety Update Reports (DSURs) and SUSARs:
  - *Note*: Unexpected events which affect the benefit–risk balance of the clinical trial must be reported within15 calendar days.

The sponsor's responsibilities are described in terms of collecting, recording, handling, and communicating. Additional requirements are explained regarding ethics committees, interactions with investigators, issues unique to trials (e.g., unblinding), expedited reporting, annual reporting, inspections' outcomes disclosure, and other details.

The Clinical Trials Information System (CTIS), launched in January 2022, supports the flow of information between clinical trial sponsors, European Union (EU) Member States, European Economic Area (EEA) countries and the European Commission.

The EMA Website

The EMA website (https://www.ema.europa.eu/en) contains much useful information: Regulations, Directives, Practices, Q&A Documents, PRAC meetings, presentations, position statements, videos and Standard Operating Procedures (SOPs). These are useful to read as there are many of them, and they cover many areas of PV. They give a flavor of how the EMA handles PV on an operational level.

There is a section on European Public Assessment Reports (EPARs), which contain summaries of product-specific information (by brand and generic/INN name) on the CHMP opinions in granting Marketing Authorizations. There is often interesting safety information in each document, including the SmPC and labeling as well as the scientific reviews.

There is a very useful section on inspections for GCP, GLP, GMP, and pharmacovigilance. The PV section contains information on relevant documents, scope and mission, Inspectors Working Group, and specific procedures and guidances governing inspections. The EU Risk Management Strategies site can be found within the EMA website.

There is an up-to-date page of links to the HAs of the EU and elsewhere, as well as other regulatory agencies and scientific organizations (https://www.ema.europa.eu/en/partners-networks/eu-partners) As the EMA was originally aimed primarily at industry and regulators, there is less consumer information compared to the FDA website or other national websites within the EU. Nevertheless, more information has been added to the website aimed at patients and the general public.

The websites of member states vary in completeness and utility even if they are now required to maintain clear communication and full transparency. They are in the native language of each country, though many have some sections in English (not always the PV section). The website of the French HA, the *Agence Nationale de Sécurité du Médicament* (ANSM), is useful but is in French (http://ansm.sante.fr/). The Dutch Agency's website (https://www.igj.nl/) has a section on PV in English, as does the German Agency (https://www.bfarm.de/DE/Home/home_node.html). However, many of the key documents are in the national languages and are not translated into English.

European Network of Centers for Pharmacoepidemiology and Pharmacovigilance

European Network of Centers for Pharmacoepidemiology and Pharmacovigilance (ENCePP) is a network of centers throughout Europe (not just the EU) with nearly 100 centers in 21 plus countries, including medical centers, healthcare databases, electronic registries, and other existing networks. Their goal is to further strengthen PV and pharmacoepidemiology in the EU by facilitating the conduct of high quality, multi-center, independent post-authorization studies (PAS), both safety and efficacy (PASS or PAES), with a focus on observational research. They have worked on several projects, including a checklist of operational research standards, a code of conduct, the means to promote research in PV and pharmacoepidemiology, an EU resources database with information on data sources and research centers, a study database, and the development of methodology to promote PV research.

They are collaborating with the FDA's Sentinel Project and Health Canada's Drug Safety and Effectiveness Network.

It is also well worth subscribing to the e-mails from the agencies as well as various blogs and news services to stay up to date on these matters.

For more information https://www.encepp.eu/.

■ Newsletters and RSS Feeds

The EMA has multiple free subscriptions available from its website as RSS feeds https://www.ema.europa.eu/en/news-event/rss-feeds). There are many feeds available, and it is well worth subscribing to several of them. The ones that may contain safety-related news are: Ongoing public consultations, Events, Pending EC decisions and European Public Assessment Reports (EPARs) on human medicinal products, What's new, Regulatory and procedural guidelines, Inspections, and Scientific guidelines.

■ Comments

The operational issues involved in drug safety in the EU are far more complex and numerous than those in the US because of the multiplicity of member states and requirements. The regulation launched in 2010–2012 dramatically improved the consistency of requirements for post-marketing surveillance. The clinical trial PV requirements are markedly less harmonized than the post-marketing requirements at this writing, as specific national requirements are still in force despite the EU regulation.

Remaining in compliance with all of the ever-changing reporting requirements, new drug approvals, safety issues, and such in the 27 member states plus the EMA plus the affiliated countries presents enormous practical and logistical problems. The EU, like the US and Japan, is now undergoing and will continue to undergo changes in many aspects of AE reporting (electronic reporting, new risk management initiatives, drug dictionary, social media, smartphone app reporting, and "wearable" eHealth technology, etc.). The EMA and the member states are also becoming much more active in inspecting companies' and vendors' drug safety practices, both on a routine basis and on a "for cause" basis. The EU authorities conduct PV inspections within Europe and also abroad, which is a particularly important consideration, since inspections are used as a source of income and funding for health agencies.

In practice, what this means now is that any company that does studies or sells (or distributes) products within the EU must either have subsidiary or affiliated offices within the EU (and sometimes even within each country in which they sell or study). Failing this, the company needs to engage, with a written contract, a company (i.e., business partner or a contract research organization, CRO) to handle these functions for it. There must be an EU QPPV physically living and operating in the EU, and he or she must have direct and immediate access to the database (ICSRs, PSMF, PSURs/PBRERs, etc.) to deal with the EMA's and individual member states' queries and requests for information on marketed products. Language issues also oblige a company to be sure it has personnel who can deal with local HAs and others in the language of the country. The cost of doing business within the EU to handle all the regulatory requirements is high. Conversely, European companies wishing to do business in the US and in Canada must also open offices in these countries, though the US and Canada still have, to a large degree, "one-stop shopping" at the health agencies.

We now give an example of one of the major EU member states' drug agencies: France. This will give you an idea of what a large national agency may look like and handle in the EU.

■ Agence Nationale de Sécurité des Médicaments et Produits de santé

The French Agency (today called National Agency for Medicines Safety, ANSM) dramatically updated its organization (and name) over the past years, mainly in 2012 and 2016. As with the EMA, the principles are based on a centralized organization with permanent ANSM employees, supported by regional structures or experts. The ANSM works under the care of, and is funded by the French Ministry of Health. The website is: https://ansm.sante.fr/. It is in French.

Missions

The main missions are assigned to the ANSM as follows:

- Provide a fair access to innovation for all patients;

- Guarantee the safety of medicines throughout their life cycle, from the first-in-human use until the post-marketing surveillance.
- Inform and exchange with other Healthcare stakeholders

Scope

The products in the scope are drugs, blood-derived medicines, narcotic & psychotropic agents, vaccines, homoeopathic compounds, herbal medicines, customized preparations, biologicals (organs or tissues used as medicines, cell- gene-therapies, blood products) medical devices (therapy, *in vivo* or *in vitro* diagnosis, medical software), cosmetics, tattoo agents, and biocides.

Even if many decisions are now taken at the EMA level, each EU local agency can make its own decision as long as it does not dispute the EU measures. These measures can lead to decisions in the French public health interest such as: Drug registration approval, withdrawal or suspension; Clinical Trials green light; Named patient basis use (individuals or cohort); Batch release for vaccines or blood-derived medicines; Batch/Product recall; Medical device ban; Import agreement; Advertising approval or refusal.

In line with the EU regulation updated in 2010/2012, the ANSM improved information for patients, healthcare professionals, media and increased transparency and close collaboration with other healthcare organizations (regional healthcare agencies, health insurance, other food and healthcare agencies, scientific societies) and patients/consumers.

Organization

A matrix organization has been set up over the past several years as follows:

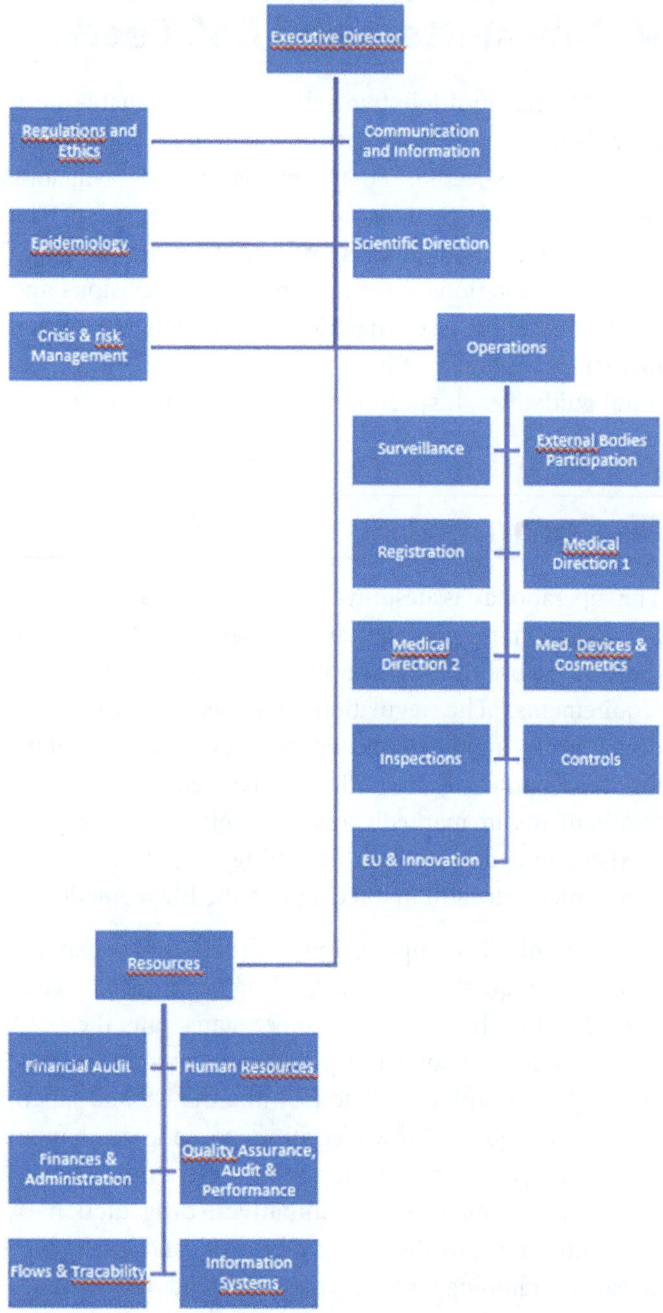

- **Four support departments Departments:** These are accountable for the activities and missions for:

  Regulations and Ethics (including General Data Protection Regulation)
  Epidemiology and PharmacoEpidemiology
  Communication & Information
  Scientific Direction (transversal department enriching the scientific strategy)
  Crisis & risk Management

- **Nine Operation Departments:**

  Surveillance: transversal activities in line with pharmacovigilance, addictovigilance, biovigilance, medical devices, surveillance during clinical development

External Bodies Participation: national and international committees and boards
Registration
Medical Direction 1 and Medical Direction 2 through therapeutic areas
Med. Devices & Cosmetics
Inspections
Controls
EU & Innovation

- **Six Resources Departments:**
  Financial Audit
  Human Resources
  Finance and Administration
  Quality Assurance, Audit and Performance
  Flows and Traceability: flows mastering & Electronic Document Management Information Systems,

The surveillance department handles pre-registration and post-marketing surveillance with the following missions:

- Monitor signals/alerts with the support of regional and local surveillance systems/organizations;
- Ensure organization and coordination of regional and local vigilance structures;
- Monitor signals/alerts assessment and risk management;
- Enlist internal and external experts to support the other departments in their decision-making process in the PV field;
- Maintain approval and control of advertising;
- Handle a secured process for medicines supply;
- Assesses the drug's market with a medico-economic viewpoint in a public healthcare perspective;

To support the ANSM Surveillance department, 31 regional PV centres are collecting ICSRs from hospital records or case reports provided by GPs and other specialized healthcare professionals or patients. Based within a hospital and university desk, they are collecting case reports, informing healthcare professionals on the drug safety profile and prescription rules. In addition, at the request of the ANSM Surveillance department, they are involved in the safety signal detection and assessment process, in benefit–risk assessment dossier, in labeling update assessment, in PSURs/PBRERs review and assessment; depending on their specialty/center of interest, they also are part of various working groups (drug–drug interaction, pregnancy, safety database, etc.).

Other bodies:

The Scientific Committee:

- Ensures the scientific strategy is in line with the latest scientific knowledge
- Is made up of ten experts nominated by the ANSM and six by the Ministry of Health

Permanent Scientific Committees:

- Focused on specific domains of interest (cardiology, dermatology, oncology, pharmacovigilance & surveillance etc)
- Set up each for about four years, they provide advices on specific questions

Ad hoc Scientific Committees

- Set up upon request for a specific and unanticipated topic / concern

Medicines Information Committee

- Consultative Committee about information and communication for medicines
- Made up of external expert (communication, healthcare professional, patients etc)

Liaison Committees

- Various Committees willing to maintain a good transparency and communication with healthcare stakeholders
- Applicable for GPs, Pharmacists, patients, pharmaceutical companies etc

Frequently Asked Questions

Q: Is it likely that the EU, the US, and the rest of the world will "settle down" and stabilize their rules and regulations anytime soon?

A: Probably not. There are several factors at work. First, the entire world of drug safety and risk management is in a state of flux. New technology (e.g., social media, smartphone medical apps) and regulations are being put in place as a result of many influences, including the following:

- Consumer awareness;
- Political pressures and globalization;
- Economic pressures and outsourcing;
- Changes in the structure of HAs (e.g., the may expand beyond its current 27 members);
- Critical safety issue(s) that have caused product restrictions or withdrawals; and
- Use of artificial intelligence sites;
- Capacity limitations of governments.

The changes would be aimed at making each member state requirements 100% consistent with the clinical trials regulation and ICH E2A. Another change would remove some of the ambiguity in the causality determination requirements for SUSARs. Currently, the investigator or sponsor makes causality determinations, though this is often difficult to do for any particular individual case. The EU may move toward requiring the sponsor to consult with the investigator to determine a possible causality. If there is disagreement between the sponsor and investigator, then the submitted SUSAR must contain both causalities.

It is not clear that collective, global organizations will be any more effective in drug safety as they are in limiting arms proliferation, wars, or climate change.

Another point to note is that a decade or two ago, the major PV players were the US, the EU, and Japan. Since then, we have major new players gaining more and more influence (e.g., China and India) as well as the "discovery" of PV by most of the remaining 100 plus countries of the world on all five continents. Many countries are putting forth PV requirements, usually in their own languages, based largely on ICH and CIOMS though sometimes following EU procedures more or less. The emphasis here is on "more or less" and regional requirements are often introduced. Many of the new players have individual differences and quirks in their requirements which make PV compliance in all markets very challenging.

Q: Does one need to know any other languages besides English if one is doing PV?

A: A delicate question. Obviously, in countries where English is not the official language, one must know the language of that country. Often, some documents, cover letters, local cases, e-mails, and other requirements must be prepared in the local language. In addition, governmental officials, patients, healthcare workers, and company employees are more comfortable in their native language. Some medical terms do not translate well language to language. Having said that, the "official" language of drug safety is English (as much as there can be an official language) and nearly all international documents (e.g., PSURs/PBRERs) are done in English. However, local submission of English language documents often requires summaries in the local language. At a high level and on the international scene (ICH, WHO, CIOMS), the main, or often only, business language is English. Thus, one can often survive rather well knowing only English, but more opportunities are available for those with linguistic skills. As noted earlier, there may be a push to use French and German as well as other languages in the EU now that the UK left the EU.

Q: Considering the EU regulations which will likely continue to change in the coming years, how can we ensure that we are up to date on the new/latest documents?

A: Obviously, one must pay attention to changes in requirements in all countries and markets where one does studies or markets drugs (or has business partners). There are various ways to do this depending on the size of the organization you are working in. Within large pharma companies, dedicated employees identify and analyze new EMA and national documents. This is often called "regulatory intelligence". These people sometimes also perform impact analyses of the new requirements.

At the very least, one should periodically review the EMA website as well as other important websites (e.g., EudraVigilance) and the national agencies' websites.

Small and mid-size companies may not have specific personnel devoted to such a task or to regulatory intelligence. For these companies it may be wise to hire a vendor that specializes in regulatory tracking. One may also attend the periodic meetings that EMA and some national health agencies hold to update the pharma companies. Some private and academic organizations (e.g., the Drug Safety Research Unit (DSRU) in the UK, The DIA, also holds periodic meetings).

CHAPTER

6

Council for International Organizations of Medical Sciences (CIOMS)

This chapter summarizes the functions of the Council for International Organizations of Medical Sciences (CIOMS) and the reports (relevant to pharmacovigilance) issued by working groups created by CIOMS. These reports have been crucial for the International Council on Harmonization (ICH) and the development of safety regulations in North America, Europe, Japan, and elsewhere. This chapter provides an in-depth historical context on how CIOMS has been shaped over the years, helping those with a desire to understand foundational aspects of key drug safety and pharmacovigilance regulations. Remember that not all proposals from the CIOMS reports were adopted, and those were not necessarily adopted directly and without change by ICH and national regulatory authorities. CIOMS currently has an observer liaison relationship with ICH.

Keep in mind that unless these documents are directly put into law in a country or region, they do not constitute legal requirements.

■ Introduction

From the CIOMS website (www.cioms.ch): "CIOMS is an international, non-governmental, non-profit organization established jointly by World Health Organization (WHO) and United Nations Educational, Scientific and Cultural Organization (UNESCO) in 1949." The membership of CIOMS includes 60 international member organizations, representing many of the biomedical disciplines, national academies of sciences, and medical research councils. No individual persons are members of CIOMS, although individual experts serve on working groups to develop consensus reports. The remit of CIOMS is broad, although two areas of concentration are pharmacovigilance and biomedical ethics. The main objectives of CIOMS are:

- To facilitate and promote international activities in biomedical sciences, especially when the participation of several international associations and national institutions is deemed necessary;
- To maintain collaborative relations with the United Nations and its specialized agencies, notably WHO and UNESCO;
- To serve the scientific interests of the international biomedical community in general.

CIOMS has several long-term programs, including one on drug development and use. Starting in the early 1980s, working groups composed of experts from industry and governments have been examining gnarly issues in drug safety. They have issued many reports, several of which have served as seminal documents for procedures that ICH, the US Food and Drug Administration (FDA), regulators in the European Union and Japan, and other drug safety authorities have issued. Key pharmacovigilance documents issued by CIOMS working groups are summarized in the following sections. Individuals may also access the current and former working group documents by accessing the website and subscribing to email updates.

From an operational standpoint, when a company is developing and or reviewing their SOPs relevant to some of the topics described within, it would be in their best interest to download and obtain copies (often free) of these working groups as they are working hand-in-hand with the regulators and often have shaped the current thinking and general practice of these topic areas.

■ CIOMS I (1990): International Reporting of Adverse Drug Reactions

The goal of this working group was "to develop an internationally acceptable reporting method whereby manufacturers could report post-marketing adverse drug reactions rapidly, efficiently, and effectively to regulators". It noted the fact that post-marketing surveillance is necessary because pre-marketing studies in animals and humans have "inherent limitations". It noted the need for standardization internationally.

The report established several conventions that have largely been adopted, including the following:

1. The concept and format of a paper-based case safety report ("a CIOMS I report") from the manufacturer receiving the event to the regulators.
2. "Reactions" are different from "events". "Reactions" are reports of clinical occurrences that have been judged by a physician or healthcare worker as having a "reasonable possibility" that the event was caused by a drug. "Events" have not had a causality evaluation made, and thus may or may not be related to or associated with the drug.
3. Causality is discussed with an emphasis on clinical judgment. No method of assessing causality is recommended. The working group recommends that manufacturers not separate out those spontaneous reports that they receive (for marketed products) into those that seem to be drug-related and those not seemingly drug-related. The physician, by voluntarily making the report to the manufacturer, indicates that there is some level of causality possible in the report. This is a "suspected reaction". This has become a fundamental concept in most spontaneous reporting systems around the world, wherein all spontaneous reports from physicians (now extended to all healthcare providers, and in most countries, such

as the United States, and Canada, to consumers) are to be considered possibly related to the drug; that is, they are "reactions", not "events".

4. Because labels for marketed drugs differ from country to country, it is recommended that all reactions be collected at one point and then submitted to local authorities on a country-by-country basis based on whether the reactions are labeled locally. If labeled, the reaction is considered "expected" in that jurisdiction (But see Core Data Sheet, below, for the distinction between "listed" and "labeled." Note that a distinction between these two terms is not consistently applied.)
5. The report discusses the four minimum requirements for a valid report: (1) an identifiable source (reporter), (2) a patient (even if not precisely identified by name), (3) a suspect drug, and (4) a suspect reaction.
6. The report recommends that all case reports be sent in as soon as received and no later than 15 working days after receipt, to create a common worldwide deadline. This concept has been adopted, but the 15 working days has been changed to 15 calendar days because of differences in the designation of "working days" and non-working days (holidays) around the world. The reporting clock starts the date the report is first received by anyone anywhere in the company.
7. The CIOMS I form was created. It is essentially the same form still used now for paper-based exchange of case reports. This form is to be used for reporting to regulatory authorities, unless superseded by electronic transmission of reports.
8. Reactions are to be reported in English.

CIOMS II (1992): International Reporting of Periodic Drug-Safety Update Summaries

This working group proposed a standard for Periodic Safety Update Reports (PSURs) of reactions received by manufacturers on marketed drugs. This standard, with modifications from the ICH and other organizations, has been widely adopted. The document defined several key terms:

1. CIOMS Reportable Cases or Reports: "serious, medically substantiated, unlabeled ADRs with the four validity elements (reporter, patient, reaction, suspect drug)".
2. Core Data Sheet (CDS): A document prepared by the manufacturer containing all relevant safety information, including adverse drug reactions (ADRs). This is the reference for "labeled" and "unlabeled". This concept, which has been widely accepted, has since gotten more complex, and one should distinguish labeling from listing (e.g., unlabeled and unlisted).
3. International Birth Date (IBD): The date that the first regulatory authority anywhere in the world has approved a drug for marketing.
4. Data Lock-Point (Cut-Off Date): The closing date for information to be included in a particular safety update.
5. Serious: Fatal, life-threatening, involves or prolongs inpatient hospitalization.

Other fundamental concepts were established:

1. Reports should be semiannual and not cumulative (unless cumulative information is needed to put a safety issue into context).
2. The same report goes to all regulatory authorities on the same date irrespective of the local (national) approval date of the drug.
3. Reactions reported should be from studies (published and unpublished), spontaneous reports, published case reports, cases received from regulatory authorities, and other manufacturers. Duplicate reports should be eliminated.
4. The manufacturer should do a "concise critical analysis and opinion in English by a person responsible for monitoring and assessing drug safety".
5. A sample simulated PSUR is included based on a fake drug, "Qweasytrol".

CIOMS III (1995 and 1998/1999): Guidelines for Preparing Core Clinical Safety Information on Drugs (1995), Including New Proposals for Investigator's Brochures (1998/1999)

The CIOMS III guideline is now out of print but established and extended several fundamental concepts now in use in much of the world. The idea of the CDS introduced in CIOMS II was extended to the Core Safety Information (CSI). The CDS contains all key core data (not just safety data) on a drug. The CSI contains (only) core safety information and is a subset of the CDS. Several fundamental concepts were introduced:

- The CSI is the core safety information that should appear in all countries' regulator-approved labeling for that drug. Additional information could be added at the national level, but the core information should be included in all countries' labels. The CSI (and national labels) are guides for healthcare professionals and contain the most relevant information needed for the drug's use.
- Marketing considerations should not play a role in preparing the CSI.
- The CSI was proposed primarily as a medical document and not as a legal or regulatory document.
- Every drug should have a CSI prepared and updated by the manufacturer.
- Adverse events (AEs) due to excipients should be included.
- AEs that have no well-established relationship to therapy should not be included.
- The CSI should include important information that physicians are not generally expected to know.
- As soon as relevant safety information becomes sufficiently well established; it should be included. The specific time when it is included occurs when the safety information crosses the "threshold for inclusion", which is defined as the time when "it is judged that it will influence physicians' decisions on therapy".
- Thirty-nine factors were proposed that can be ranked and weighed for an AE for a particular drug to assess whether the information has crossed the threshold. An extensive discussion on the threshold is given as follows:
  1. The threshold should be lower if the condition being treated is relatively trivial, if the drug is used to prevent rather than to treat disease, if the drug is widely used, or if the ADR is irreversible.
  2. Hypersensitivity reactions should be noted early.
  3. Substantial evidence is required to remove or downgrade safety information.

Ten general principles were proposed as follows:

1. In general, statements that an adverse reaction does not occur or has not yet been reported should not be made.
2. Generally, clinical descriptions of specific cases should not be part of the CSI.
3. If the mechanism is known, it should be stated whether a potentially major, new safety signal signifies a shift, calling for significant action in the established relationship between benefits and risks; it also provides guidance for deciding what options for action should be considered and on the process of decision-making should such action be required.
4. As a general rule, secondary effects or sequelae should not be listed.
5. In general, a description of events expected as a result of progression of the underlying treated disease should not be included in the CSI.
6. Unlicensed or "off-label" use should be mentioned only in the context of a medically important safety problem.
7. The wording used in the CSI to describe adverse reactions should be chosen carefully and responsibly to maximize the prescriber's understanding. For example, if the ADR is part of a syndrome, this should be made clear.
8. The terms used should be specific and medically informative.
9. The use of modifiers or adjectives should be avoided unless they add useful important information.
10. A special attribute (e.g., sex, race) known to be associated with an increased risk should be specified.

Where possible, frequencies should be provided, although it is admitted that this is very difficult with spontaneous safety data. A proposed classification is as follows:

- Very common: >1/10 (10%);
- Common (frequent): 1/100 and <1/10 (1% and <10%);
- Uncommon (infrequent): 1/1000 and <1/100 (0.1% and <1%;
- Rare: 1/10,000 and <1/1000 (0.01% and <0.1%);
- Very rare: <1/10,000 (<0.01%).

Many of these recommendations have been adopted in one form or another around the world, though not in their totality. The revised edition (1998/1999) of this document appeared as CIOMS V (see below).

CIOMS IV (1998): Benefit–Risk Balance for Marketed Drugs: Evaluating Safety Signals

From the preface of the report: "CIOMS IV is to some extent an extension of CIOMS II and III. It examines the theoretical and practical aspects of how to determine whether a potentially major, new safety signal signifies a shift, calling for significant action in the established relationship between benefits and risks; it also provides guidance for deciding what options for action should be considered and on the process of decision-making should such action be required."

The report looks at the general concepts of benefit–risk analysis and discusses the factors influencing assessment, including stakeholders and constituencies, the nature of the problem (risk), the indication for drug use and the population under treatment, constraints of time, data and resources, and economic issues. Several examples of benefit–risk analyses are given (quinine and allergic hematologic events, felbamate and blood dyscrasias, dipyrone and agranulocytosis, temafloxacin and renal impairment and hypoglycemia, remoxipride and blood dyscrasias, clozapine and agranulocytosis, sparfloxacin and phototoxicity).

No example of a real benefit–risk report is given using this format. This type of report seems eminently possible in situations where the risk is small and there is no urgent or immediate action needed to protect the public health. However, in situations in which immediate action is needed, usually in multiple markets around the world, the preparation of such a report is probably not feasible.

Since this CIOMS IV report, several other guidelines and documents on benefit–risk analysis have been published by the FDA, European Medicines Evaluation Agency, ICH, and others. Most of these documents use similar conceptual frameworks for benefit–risk analyses but do not follow or propose the rigid CIOMS IV format. Clearly, however, this document served as a stimulus to a much closer and intense examination of benefit–risk analyses around the world. The document is worth reading, particularly for the case studies noted above.

CIOMS V (2001): Current Challenges in Pharmacovigilance: Pragmatic Approaches

The CIOMS V report is a 380-page document that covers a wide variety of issues in drug safety. A summary of some of the proposals follows. Not all these recommendations are universally accepted or required.

The sources of individual case reports are recommended as follows:

Traditionally, the primary source of safety information on marketed drugs has been spontaneous reports, with occasional literature reports also appearing. New types of reports are now appearing, including Internet reports, solicited reports from patient support programs, surveys, epidemiologic studies, disease registries, regulatory and other databases, and licensor and licensee interactions. In the past, consumer reports were often not analyzed unless medical validation was obtained.

The CIOMS V report makes various recommendations, some of which are as follows:

1. **Consumer reports**
    a. Consumer reports should be scrutinized and should receive appropriate attention.
    b. The quality of a report is more important than its source.
    c. Spontaneous reports are always considered to have an implied causal relationship to the drug.
    d. Respect privacy and the laws and regulations governing it.
    e. If a report is received from a third party, that party should be asked to encourage the consumer to report the information to his or her physician or to authorize the sponsor/authority to contact the physician directly.
    f. All efforts should be made to obtain medical confirmation of serious unexpected consumer reports. The regulators may be in a better position to get this information if companies have been unsuccessful.
    g. If an event is considered not to be drug related, it should be retained in the company database but not reported.
    h. Even in the absence of medical confirmation, any ADR with significant implications for the medicine's benefit–risk relationship should be submitted on an expedited or periodic basis.
    i. Consumer reports should be included in PSURs in an appendix or as a statement indicating they have been reviewed and do or do not suggest new findings.

2. **Literature**
    a. Cases may appear in letters to the editor.
    b. There may be a long lag time between the first detection of a signal by a researcher and his or her publication of it.
    c. Publications may be a source of false information and signals.
    d. Companies should search at least two internationally recognized literature databases using the International Normalized Nomenclature name at least monthly.
    e. Broadcast and lay media should not ordinarily be monitored. If such information is made available to the company, it should be followed up.
    f. Judgment should be used in regard to follow-up, with the strongest efforts made for serious unexpected ADRs.
    g. If the product source or brand is not specified, a company should assume it was its product. The company should indicate in any report that the specific brand was not identified if this is the case.
    h. If there is a contractual agreement between two or more companies (e.g., for co-marketing), the contract should specify the responsibility for literature searches and reporting.
    i. English should be the standard language for literature report translations.
    j. Regulators should accept translation of an abstract or pertinent sections of a publication.
    k. References cited in a publication on apparently unexpected/unlisted and serious reactions should be checked against the company's existing database of literature reports. Articles not previously reported should be retrieved, translated to English (as needed), and reviewed as usual. Routine tracking down of all such sources is unrealistic unless faced with a major safety issue.
    l. The clock starts when a case is recognized to be a valid case (reporter, patient, drug, event).

3. **The Internet**
    a. Protection of privacy is particularly important regarding Internet cases.
    b. A blank ADR form should be provided on a website to facilitate reporting.
    c. A procedure should be in place to ensure daily screening of a company's or regulator's website(s) to identify potential case reports.
    d. Companies and regulators do not need to routinely surf the net beyond their own sites

other than to actively monitor relevant special home pages (e.g., disease groups) if there is a significant safety issue.

e. The message should be consistent around the world because the Internet does not respect geographic (or linguistic) boundaries.

4. **Solicited reports**

a. Solicited ADR reports arising in the course of interaction with patients should be regarded as distinct from spontaneous unsolicited reports.

b. They should be processed separately and so identified in expedited and periodic reporting.

c. To satisfy post-marketing regulations, solicited reports should be handled in the same way as study reports: causality assessments are needed. Serious unexpected ADRs should be reported on an expedited basis.

d. Serious, expected and non-serious solicited reports should be kept in the safety database and reported to regulators on request.

e. Signals may arise from solicited reports, so they should be reviewed on an ongoing basis.

5. **Aspects of clinical trial reports**

a. In general, safety information reported expeditiously to regulatory authorities should be reported to all phase I, II, and III investigators who are conducting research with any form of the product and for any indication.

b. It is less important to notify phase IV investigators; they should ordinarily use the available up-to-date local official data sheet as part of the investigator's brochure.

c. Quality of life studies should be handled like clinical trial data.

6. **Epidemiology: Observational studies and use of secondary databases**

a. Structured epidemiologic studies should have the same reporting rules for suspected ADR cases as clinical trials.

b. For epidemiologic studies, unless there is specific attribution in an individual case, its expedited reporting is generally not appropriate.

c. If relevant, studies should be summarized in PSURs.

d. Promptly notify regulators (within 15 days) if a study result shows an important safety issue (e.g., a greater risk of a known serious ADR for one drug versus another).

e. For manufacturers, expedited reports from comparator drug data should be forwarded to the relevant manufacturer(s) for their regulatory reporting as appropriate.

7. **Disease-specific registries and regulatory ADR databases**

a. A registry is not a study. Cases should be treated as solicited reports (causality assessment required).

b. Although there are numerous ADR databases created by regulatory authorities, it is unnecessary to attempt to routinely collect them for regular review. If a company possesses data from a regulatory database, it should review those data promptly for any required expedited reporting. Careful screening should be done to avoid duplicates.

c. It is advisable to mention in the PSUR that the databases have been examined even if no relevant cases have been found.

8. **Licenser–licensee interactions**

a. When companies co-develop, co-market, or co-promote products, it is critical that explicit contractual agreements specify processes for exchange of safety information, including timelines and regulatory reporting responsibilities.

b. The time frame for expedited regulatory reporting should normally be no longer than 15 calendar days from the first receipt of a valid case by any of the partners.

c. The original recipient of a suspected ADR should ideally conduct any necessary follow-up; any subsequent follow-up information sent to the regulators should be submitted by the same company that reported the case originally.

9. **Clinical case evaluation**
   a. The company or regulatory authority staff can propose alternate clinical terms and interpretations of the case from those of the reporter, but unless the original reporter alters his or her original description in writing, the original terms must also be reported.
   b. When a case is reported by a consumer, his or her clinical description should be retained even if confirmatory or additional information from a healthcare professional is obtained.
   c. There is an important distinction between a suspected ADR and an "incidental" event. An incidental event occurs in reasonable clinical temporal association with the use of the drug product but is not the intended subject of the spontaneous report (it did not prompt the contact with the company or regulator). There is also no implicit or explicit expression of possible drug causality by the reporter or the company's safety review staff. They should be included as part of the medical history and not be the subject of expedited reporting. Incidental events should be captured in the company database.

10. **Assessing patient and reporter identities**
   a. When cases do not meet the minimum criteria (patient, reporter, event, drug) even after follow-up, the case should be kept in the database as an "incomplete case".
   b. The regulatory reporting clock starts when a valid case is initially reported to the company, even by a consumer.
   c. One or more of the following pieces of information automatically qualify a patient as identifiable: age, age category (e.g., teenager), sex, initials, date of birth, name, or patient number.
   d. Even in the absence of such qualifying descriptors, a report referring to a definite number of patients should be regarded as a case as long as the other criteria for validity are met. For example, "Two patients experienced…" but not "A few patients experienced…."
   e. For serious, unexpected, suspected reactions, the threshold for reporting in the absence of confirmatory identity should be lowered.

11. **Criteria for seriousness**
   a. Hospitalization refers to admission as an inpatient and not to an examination or treatment as an outpatient.
   b. All congenital anomalies and birth defects, without regard to their nature or severity, should be considered serious.
   c. There is a lack of objective standards for "life threatening" and "medical judgment" as seriousness criteria; both require individual professional evaluation that invariably introduces a lack of reproducibility.
   d. Within a company, the tools, lists, and decision-making processes should be harmonized globally.

12. **Criteria for expectedness**
   a. The terminology associated with expectedness depends on which reference safety document is being used and for what purpose:
      - "Listed" or "unlisted" refers to the ADRs contained in the CSI for a marketed product or within the development CSI (DCSI) in the investigator's brochure.
      - "Labeled" or "unlabeled" refers to the ADRs contained in official regulator-approved product safety information for marketed products (e.g., summary of product characteristics in the European Union or the package insert in the United States).
   b. Determining whether a reported reaction is expected is a two-step process: first, is the reaction term already included in the CSI? Second, is the ADR different regarding its nature, severity, specificity, or outcome?
   c. Expectedness should be strictly based on inclusion of a drug-associated experience in the ADR section of the CSI. Special types

of reactions, such as those occurring under conditions of overdose, drug interaction, or pregnancy, should also be included in this section.

d. Disorders mentioned in "contraindications" or "precautions" as reasons for not treating with the drug are not expected ADRs unless they also appear in the ADR section.
e. If an ADR has been reported only in association with an overdose, it should be considered unexpected if it occurs at a normal dose.
f. For a marketed drug CSI, events cited in data from clinical trials are not considered expected unless they are included in the ADR section.
g. For expedited reporting on marketed drugs, local approved product information is the reference document for expectedness (labeledness).

   For periodic reporting (PSUR), the CSI is the reference document for expectedness (listedness).

   Disclaimer statements for causality (e.g., "X has been reported but the relationship with the drug has not been established") are discouraged; however, even if used, the reaction X is still unexpected.

   Class labeling does not count as "expected" unless the event in question is included in the ADR section.

   Lack of expected efficacy is not relevant to whether an AE is expected.

   If the treatment exacerbates the target indication, it would be unexpected unless already detailed in the CSI.

   Unless the CSI specifies a fatal outcome for an ADR, the case is unexpected as long as there was an association between the reaction and the fatality.

13. Case follow-up approaches

a. Highest priority for follow-up are cases that are serious and unexpected; followed by serious, expected; and non-serious, unexpected.
b. Cases "of special interest" (e.g., ADRs under active surveillance at the request of the regulators) also deserve high priority, as do any cases that might lead to a labeling change.
c. For any cases with legal implications, the company's legal department should be involved.
d. When the case is serious and if the ADR has not resolved at the time of the initial report, it is important to continue follow-up until the outcome has been established or the condition stabilized. How long to follow up such cases requires judgment.
e. It is recommended that collaboration with other companies be done if more than one company's drug is suspected as a causal agent in a case.
f. Follow-up for unexpected deaths and life-threatening cases should be done within 24 hours.
g. If a reporter fails to respond to the first follow-up attempt, reminder letters should be sent as follows:
h. A single follow-up letter for any non-serious expected case.
i. For all other cases, a second follow-up letter should be sent no later than four weeks after the first letter.
j. In general, when the reporter fails to respond or is incompletely cooperative, the two follow-up letters should reflect sufficient due diligence.

14. Role of narratives

a. A company case narrative is different from the reporter's clinical description of a case, though the reporter's comments should be an integral part of the company narrative. The reporter's verbatim words should be included for the adverse reactions.
b. Alternate causes to that given by the reporter should be described and identified as a company opinion.
c. The same evaluation should be supplied to all regulators.
d. Narratives should be prepared for all serious (expected and unexpected) and non-serious unexpected cases but not for non-serious expected cases.

e. Narratives should be written in the third person past tense. All relevant information should be in a logical time sequence.
f. In general, abbreviations (except laboratory parameters and units) and acronyms should not be used.
g. Time to onset of an event from the start of treatment should be given in the most appropriate time units (e.g., hours), but actual dates can be used if helpful to the reader.
h. If detailed supplementary records are important to a case (e.g., autopsy report), their availability should be mentioned in the narrative.
i. Information may be supplied by more than one person (e.g., initial reporter and supplementary information from a specialist); all sources should be specified.
j. When there is conflicting information provided from different sources, this should be mentioned and the sources identified.
k. If it is suspected that an ADR resulted from misprescribing (e.g., wrong drug or wrong dose) or other medication error, judgmental comments should not be included in the narrative because of legal implications. Only the facts should be stated (e.g., "four times the normal dose was administered", "the prescription was misread and a contraindicated drug for this patient was given").
l. The narrative should have eight sections that serve as a comprehensive stand-alone "medical story":
   - Source of the report and patient demography.
   - Medical and drug history.
   - Suspect drug(s), timing and conditions surrounding the onset of the reaction(s).
   - The progression of the event(s) and their outcome in the patient.
   - If the outcome is fatal, provide relevant details.
   - Rechallenge information, if applicable.
   - The narrative preparer's medical evaluation and comment.

15. **PSURs: Content modification**
   a. For reports covering long time periods (e.g., 5 years), it is more practical to use the CSI current at the time of PSUR preparation.
   b. Clinical trial data should be supplied only if they suggest a signal or are relevant to a possible change in the benefit–risk relationship.
   c. If there are more than 200 individual case reports, submit only summary tabulations and not line listings (which may be supplied on request by the regulator).
   d. For 5-year reports, follow-up information on cases described in the previous report should be provided only for cases associated with new or ongoing safety issues.
   e. Inclusion of literature reports should be selective and cover publications relevant to safety findings, independent of listedness.
   f. For PSURs with large numbers of cases, discussion and analysis for the overall safety evaluation should be by system organ class rather than by listedness or seriousness.
   g. An PSUR saves time and resources if little or no new safety information is generated during the time period covered. Criteria for an abbreviated report:
      - No serious unlisted cases
      - Few (e.g., 10) serious listed cases
      - No significant regulatory actions for safety
      - No major changes to the CSI
      - No findings that lead to a new action
      - The term "abbreviated PSUR" as used here should not be confused with "abbreviated PSURs" prepared at short intervals, e.g., monthly line listings during pandemic influenza outbreaks.

16. **PSURs: A bridging report**
   a. A summary bridging report is a concise document that provides no new information and integrates two or more previously prepared PSURs to cover a specified period.
   b. Its format follows that of a regular PSUR, but the content should consist of summary

high-lights of the reports being summarized. Note that bridging PSURs no longer have a role per the ICH E2C(R2) guideline.

17. **PSURs: An addendum report**
    a. This report is prepared on special request of the regulators to satisfy regulators who require reports covering a period outside the routine PSUR reporting cycle (e.g., if the reports are based on the local approval date in that country rather than on the IBD).
    b. It updates the most recently completed PSUR.
    c. It follows the usual PSUR format.

18. **PSURs: Miscellaneous proposals**
    a. A brief (e.g., one-page) stand-alone overview (executive summary) should be provided.
    b. Manufacturers should be allowed to select the IBDs for their older products to facilitate synchronization of PSURs.
    c. If there is no CSI for an old product, the most suitable local labeling should be considered for use.
    d. The evaluation of cases in a PSUR should focus on unlisted ADRs, with analyses organized primarily by system organ class (body system).
    e. Discussion of serious unlisted cases should include cumulative data.
    f. Complicated PSURs and those with extensive new data may require more than 60 days to prepare adequately and the regulators should be flexible.
    g. The possibility of "resetting" the PSUR clock (from annual to semiannual reports as the result of a new indication or dosage form) should be allowed by the regulators.

19. **PSURs: Population data**
    a. Detailed calculations on exposure (the denominator) are ordinarily unnecessary, especially given the unreliability of the numerator; rough estimates usually suffice, but the method and units used should be explained clearly.
    b. Drug exposure data are approximate and usually represent an overestimate.
    c. For special situations, such as dealing with an important safety signal, attempts should be made to obtain exposure information covering the relevant covariates (e.g., age, gender, race, indication, dosing details).

CIOMS VI (2005): Management of Safety Information from Clinical Trials

The CIOMS VI working group focused on clinical trial safety, which represents a departure from the focus of the earlier working groups that concentrated primarily on post-marketing safety issues. The report, available from the CIOMS office in Geneva, like the CIOMS V report, runs some 300 pages. The most important points are summarized here. The reader is referred to the report for further detail. Keep in mind that these recommendations have not been put into regulations in all jurisdictions.

20. **General Principles and Ethical Considerations**
    a. The concepts of pharmacovigilance presented here apply to trials in phase I–IV.
    b. Any study that is not scientifically sound should be considered unethical.
    c. Informed consent is the cornerstone of human subject research, but there are situations in which it is either not possible or appropriate (such as in anonymous tissue sample studies, epidemiologic research, or emergency treatment protocols).

21. **Systematic Approach to Managing Safety Data**
    a. The concepts of pharmacovigilance, risk management, assessment, and minimization should be applied to the study phases and

the post-marketing period. Sponsors must have in place a well-defined process to readily identify, evaluate, and minimize potential safety risks. The process should start before the first phase I study. A formal development risk management plan should be developed.

b. A dedicated safety management team should be formed for each development program to review safety information on a regular basis so that decisions can be made in a timely manner. The review should be at least quarterly, and the team should consider changes to the investigator's brochure, informed consent, and protocol as needed.
c. When licensing partners are involved, a joint safety committee should be created, with clear roles and responsibilities. This should ideally be defined in the initial contract. A project management function should be set up to ensure scheduling, tracking, and timelines.
d. All pertinent data must be readily available from the clinical trial and safety databases as well as non-clinical toxicology, mutagenicity, pharmacokinetic, pharmacodynamic, and drug interaction data.
e. Epidemiology should be incorporated into the planning process.
f. Certain toxicities should be considered for all new drugs, including abnormalities of cardiac conduction, hepatotoxicity, drug interactions, immunogenicity, bone marrow toxicity, and reactive metabolite formation.

22. **Data Collection and Management**

a. The investigator should report to the sponsor (immediately if judged critical) any information considered to be important regarding safety even if the protocol does not call for it. The sponsor must carefully train the investigative site in this matter.
b. The collection of "excessive" data can have a negative impact on data quality. Case report form fields should collect only those data that can be analyzed and presented in tabular form. All other data should be collected as text comments.
c. Safety monitoring in phase IV studies may not require the same intensity as for phase I–III trials, but the same principles and practices should apply.
d. If a company provides any support for an independent trial it does not sponsor (investigator-initiated studies/trials), the company should still obtain at a minimum all serious suspected adverse reactions. The company should do its own causality assessment and, if appropriate, report it to the health authorities, even if the investigator has already done so.
e. In the early phases of drug development, it is often necessary to collect more comprehensive safety data than in post-marketing studies. Some studies may require longer follow-up.
f. Phase I data are especially important because these data are collected in healthy volunteers and are critical to the future development of the drug.
g. There is no definitive way to determine causality of a particular AE. That is, its attribution to the drug or to a background finding with only a temporal association cannot be definitively done. Thus, the following is recommended.
h. All AEs, both serious and non-serious, are collected whether believed to be related or not. This applies to the experimental product, placebo, no treatment, and active comparators.
i. Similarly, studies initiated during the immediate post-approval period should continue this practice. Once the safety profile is judged to be well understood, it may be possible to collect less data (e.g., omitting non-serious AEs believed not to be due to the drug).

23. **Other Points**

a. The use of herbal and other non-traditional treatments should be sought when data are being collected in all studies.

b. Although causality assessments based on aggregate data or case series are usually more meaningful than those based on individual cases, the investigator causality assessment should be done and may play a role in the early detection of significant safety events, especially rare ones.
c. The investigator should be asked to use a "simple binary decision" for drug causality of serious AEs: related or not related, reasonable possibility or no reasonable possibility, and so on. The use of the words "unknown" or "cannot be ruled out" should be avoided.
d. Causality for non-serious AEs should not be requested from investigators routinely.
e. Where appropriate, the investigator should supply a diagnosis rather than signs and symptoms. However, when a diagnosis is supplied for a serious AE, the accompanying signs and symptoms should be recorded.
f. Before starting a study, AEs of special interest and anticipated AEs (if known) should be communicated to the investigator. This is less critical for non-serious AEs unless they are prodromes of more serious conditions (e.g., muscle pain and creatine phosphokinase elevation as a possible prodrome of rhabdomyolysis).
g. Medically serious clinical events recorded in a trial as clinical efficacy outcomes or endpoints should be reviewed by the sponsor and data monitoring committee even though they are not considered AEs.
h. It is preferable to frame questions to patients in general terms rather than suggest that the study treatment was responsible for reported AEs. Although a "laundry list" of AEs should not be read to the patient, patients should be alerted to known issues of medically important suspected or established AEs so they can alert the investigator as soon as possible.
i. Data collection should start from the time the informed consent is signed.
j. Safety data event collection should continue after the last dose of the drug for at least an additional five half-lives of the experimental product.

24. General Rules for Data Quality

a. Cases should be as fully documented as possible.
b. There should be diligent follow-up of each case.
c. The reporter's verbatim terms should be captured and retained.
d. If the reporter's terms are considered inaccurate or inconsistent with standard medical terminology, attempts should be made to clarify them. If disagreement continues, the sponsor should code the AE terms according to its judgment but identify them as distinct from the reporter's terms and note reasons for differences.
e. Primary analyses of the data should be done using the reporter's terms. Additional analyses may be done using the sponsor's terms. Any differences must be noted and explained.
f. Individual case safety reports should be categorized and assessed by the sponsor, using trained individuals with broad experience. Investigators should obtain specialist consultation for clinically important events that fall outside their expertise.
g. AE tables may display both the reported investigator's verbatim term and the sponsor's terms.
h. The sponsor (as well as health authorities) may wish to consider the use of a listing of event terms always regarded as serious and important. Such events then routinely trigger special attention and evaluation.
i. Cases should not be "overcoded" using more terms than minimally necessary to ensure retrieval of the cases. Similarly, cases should not be "undercoded", where the terms chosen downgrade the severity or medical importance of events.

25. **Risk Identification and Evaluation**
   a. *Ongoing Safety Evaluation*
      - Sponsors should develop a system to assess, evaluate, and act on safety information on a continuous basis during drug development to ensure the earliest possible identification of safety concerns to allow risk minimization.
      - The integrity of the studies should not be compromised by the safety monitoring and analysis.

   b. *Safety Data Management*
      - Safety data should be handled using consistent standards and criteria, with care and precision.
      - Safety evaluations must be individualized for each product because there are no standard approaches to evaluating or measuring "an acceptable level of risk".

26. **Review of Safety Information**
   a. Safety data analysis should involve both individual case reports as well as aggregate data. Individual cases should be reviewed within specified time frames and aggregate data periodically.
   b. The evaluation should be done in the context of the patient population, the indication studied, the natural history of the disease, and currently available alternative therapies.
   c. Causality determinations should be done for all reported cases. The investigator causality assessment should be taken into account when the sponsor is reviewing the safety information.
   d. AEs of special interest (AESI) should be identified in the protocol and handled as if they are serious even if they do not meet the regulatory definition of serious.
   e. Non-serious AEs should be reviewed to see whether there are events of special interest, with particular attention paid to those associated with subject discontinuation from the study.

27. **Frequency of Review of Safety Information**
   a. Safety review of all data should be done frequently:
      - *Ad hoc* for serious and special interest AEs;
      - Routine periodic review of all data whose frequency varies from trial to trial or program to program;
      - Reviews triggered by specific trial or program milestones;
      - At the time of study completion and unblinding.

28. **Analysis and Evaluation**
   a. Subgroup analysis, though possibly limited by small sample size, should be done for dose, duration, gender, age, concomitant medications, and concurrent diseases.
   b. Data pooling should include studies that are of similar design. This can include all controlled studies, placebo-controlled studies, studies with any positive control, studies with a particular positive control, and particular indications.
   c. If the duration of treatment varies widely among participants, data on the effect of treatment duration should be analyzed.

29. **Statistical Approaches**
   a. The techniques for use of statistics for analyzing safety data are less well developed than for efficacy.
   b. Statistical association (probability values) alone may or may not be of clinical value. Examination of both statistical and clinical significance must involve a partnership between the statistical and clinical experts.
   c. It may be necessary to acknowledge when the data are insufficient to draw conclusions on safety: "Absence of evidence is not evidence of absence".
   d. There are several large sections of this report devoted to specific statistical situations and techniques, and the reader is referred to the report for further detail.

Regulatory Reporting and Communications of Safety Information from Clinical Trials

The working group notes, in bold type, that these recommendations are only proposals and do not supersede current regulations. They represent proposals for discussion.

- The group endorses ICH Guideline E2A and recommends the harmonization of criteria for expedited reporting, whereby such reporting to authorities should include only suspected ADRs that are both serious and unexpected. Only under exceptional circumstances should other cases (i.e., expected cases) be submitted as expedited reports. If reporting without regard to causality is required, it should be done on a periodic basis with clearly defined timelines and format.
- The regulators should adopt the phrase "a reasonable possibility of a causal relationship" and not use the ICH E2A phrase of "a causal relationship cannot be ruled out" in regard to suspected ADRs.
- Once a drug is marketed, the company CSI (CCSI) document should be used as the reference safety document for determining expectedness for regulatory reporting of phase IV trials. For new indication trials, the DCSI document should be used. The two documents should be aligned as much as possible.
- As with spontaneous reports, reportability for case reports from trials should be determined at the event level. That is, a case would be expedited if there is a suspected adverse reaction that is serious and unexpected.

  Suspected ADRs that are serious and unexpected and, thus, meet criteria for expedited reporting should, in general, be unblinded (unblind the single case, not the entire study). There may be certain circumstances where this should not occur, however (e.g., serious AEs that are also efficacy endpoints). Such exceptions should be agreed on by the regulatory authorities and be clearly described in the investigator brochure and the protocol.
- Unblinded placebo cases should not be reported to regulatory authorities as expedited cases. Unblinded (and open-label) comparator drug cases should be reported to the regulatory authorities or the company owning the comparator on an expedited basis, whether or not expected.
- Seven-day reports should be limited to cases from clinical trials and not spontaneous reports. This should apply both in countries where the drug is approved and where it is only under clinical study.
- The sponsor should develop clear standard operating procedures for the expedited or prompt reporting of other safety issues, with special attention to when the clock starts for:
  - Non-clinical safety issues that might have implications for human subjects.
  - A higher incidence of a serious AE for the drug compared with the comparator or the background rate in the general population.
  - An increased frequency of a previously recognized serious adverse reaction.
  - A significant drug interaction in a pharmacokinetic study.
  - AEs that are deemed not to be drug-related but are considered study-related.
- Contrary to established regulations, the working group recommends that routine expedited cases reported to investigators and Institutional Review Boards (IRBs)/ethics committees (as opposed to reports to regulatory authorities) be eliminated and replaced with regular updates of the evolving benefit–risk profile highlighting new safety information.
- For unapproved products, the reports to investigators and IRBs should include a line listing of unblinded clinical trial cases that were expedited to regulatory agencies during this time period, a copy of the current DCSI with an explanation of changes, and a brief summary of the emerging safety profile. Quarterly updates are the "default" with other frequencies as appropriate.
- For approved products, the reports to investigators and IRBs should be quarterly if the product is in

phase III trials. For well-established products, a less frequent interval would be acceptable. At some point, only investigators and IRBs would need to be updated for significant new information. For phase IV investigators and IRBs, only changes to the CCSI would be needed.

- The reports, whether for approved or unapproved products, should include in the line listings only unblinded expedited reports from trials and include only interval data (i.e., changes since the last update). A summary of the emerging safety profile should be included with cumulative data as needed. MedDRA® should be used. The listings should not include spontaneous reports, which should be described in narrative form in the update.
- Should a significant safety issue be identified (i.e., an issue that has a significant impact on the course of the clinical trial or program or warrants immediate update of the informed consent), the sponsor should promptly notify the regulatory authorities, investigators, IRBs, and, if relevant, data safety monitoring committees.
- A safety management team should review all safety data on a regular basis: quarterly before approval and coordinated with the PSUR schedule post-approval. *Ad hoc* meetings would occur as needed to address urgent safety issues and signals. They would review the overall evolving safety profile to make changes to the DCSI, informed consent, and protocol as needed.
- A single Development Safety Update Report (DSUR) should be submitted to regulators annually. The format and content would be defined and would cover the drug product, not just a single study.
- For marketed products with well-established safety profiles and for which most trials are in phase IV in the approved indications, the PSUR would replace the DSUR.
- Sponsors should incorporate the DCSI into every investigator brochure, either as a special section of the investigator brochure or as an attachment. The sponsor should clearly identify the events for which the company believes there is sufficient evidence to suspect a causal drug relationship. These events would be considered expected ("listed") for regulatory reporting criteria.
- The investigator brochure and DCSI should be reviewed and updated at least annually.
- If the developer or manufacturer of a product is not the sponsor of a particular trial but rather supports an external clinical or non-clinical investigator-sponsored study, a provision of any agreement should be the prompt reporting to the company of all serious suspected ADRs in humans or significant findings in animals.
- As with the CCSI for marketed drugs (see CIOMS III/VI), the same threshold criteria should be applied to the DCSI and informed consent in preapproval drugs.
- Informed consent should be renewed with the subjects whenever there is new information that could affect the subjects' willingness to participate in the trial. In certain circumstances, more immediate communication may be appropriate.

CIOMS VII (2006): Development Safety Update Report (DSUR)

This working group created the concept of the DSUR, which is the pre-marketing equivalent of the Periodic Safety Update Report for marketed products. Most agencies have implemented their own guidance documents on how to adhere and develop the DSUR locally, therefore it is in one's best interest to be familiar with local regulatory guidance surrounding this report.

There should be one DSUR for one chemical entity. The goal is to include all new, pertinent, clinical, and non-clinical safety information, that is, the drug's safety profile. It will include cumulative and interval summaries of key safety data and try to evaluate safety data in the context of subject exposure. It will describe new safety issues, summarize known and potential risks, and give an update on the status of the clinical development program. It will note any urgent or emerging issues and will note changes to clinical trial protocols, consent forms, and the IB. It is not meant to be a signal detection tool or a means to document or discuss individual cases. The DSUR should be prepared in parallel to the PSUR if the drug is already on the market. The first authorization anywhere in the world to conduct a clinical trial will be the developmental international birth date, in the same way that the first approval anywhere in the world creates an international (marketing) birth date. It will be prepared annually by the sponsor and submitted to the regulatory agencies within 60 days of the data lock point. An executive summary plus line listings of serious ADRs are sent to IRBs and ethics committees. The reference labeling document will be the investigators' brochure in place at the beginning of the reporting period. It may contain some proprietary information, which may need to be redacted if the document is sent to places other than regulatory agencies.

■ CIOMS VIII (2010):

Signal Detection (Points to Consider in Application of Signal Detection in Pharmacovigilance) This working group has developed and published a consensus document on signaling for consideration by sponsors, health agencies, and others who deal with drug safety. It takes a life cycle view of signaling. This is a well-written summary of the principles of signaling. It is not prescriptive in the sense of mandating a "one-size-fits-all" policy but rather comes forward with conclusions and recommendations to be tailored to the particular product and situation. Chapter 6 provides a more in-depth discussion regarding the application of Signal Detection in Pharmacovigilance.

■ CIOMS/WHO Working Group on Vaccine Pharmacovigilance (2012): Definitions and Applications of Terms for Vaccine Pharmacovigilance

The working group, composed of senior scientists from developed and emerging countries, prepared a consensus report general terms and definitions for vaccine pharmacovigilance. The report also considers practical aspects of how to apply these in vaccine safety surveillance. The report proposes several case definitions for common vaccine-associated AEs. See the chapter in this Manual for further information on "Vaccinovigilance" which takes many of the principles created by the CIOMS/WHO Working group & Brighton Group into consideration and how to operationalize them in daily practice.

■ CIOMS IX (2014): Practical Approaches to Risk Minimization for Medicinal Products

This consensus working group report focuses on how to minimize the wide variety of risks, serious and non-serious, that are encountered with today's medicines. All medicines have risks as well as potential benefits and routine risk minimization measures are adequate to manage the risks of most drugs. However, some products require non-routine tools to ensure that their benefits outweigh risks. Such risk minimization tools are used to prevent harms from occurring or mitigating them when they occur.

The application of these tools are the topics covered in this thoughtful and practical report. The recommendations are intended for consideration by sponsors/applicants, drug regulators, the healthcare community, and other drug safety stakeholders. The report emphasizes that, when necessary, these non-routine risk minimization tools should be customized to the product and situation. Further, the report recommends selecting risk minimization tools that will be the least burdensome on the healthcare system, while achieving the intended goals. Metrics should also be applied periodically to measure effectiveness of the tool(s) and possible triggers for program modification.

■ CIOMS X (2016): Evidence Synthesis and Meta-analysis

Systematic data reviews and meta-analysis have an increasingly important role for healthcare decision-makers and many other stakeholders. A well-done systematic review can inform many aspects of drug development. This report provides important principles, considerations, rationale, and recommendations for appropriate systematic reviews and meta-analysis to understand the overall best evidence in regulatory decision-making.

Both pre-marketing and post-marketing phases are considered and conditions for combining evidence and the limits of summarizing results. This working group has carefully described application to both efficacy data and, separately, to combining evidence on adverse events. The emphasis of this report is on safety aspects and adverse events. Much of the report describes highly technical statistical approaches, important tools for systematic analysis of safety data for drugs, although there may be broader conceptual application to other medical products.

■ CIOMS SMQs (2016): Development and Rational Use of Standardized MedDRA Queries: Retrieving Adverse Drug Reactions with MedDRA — Second Edition Japanese Translation Available

Biopharmaceutical companies, drug regulatory authorities, vendors, and other stakeholders use MedDRA® to code, exchange, and analyze regulatory information for medical products. MedDRA is used, particularly with large amounts of drug safety data stored in databases. Because of the granularity of MedDRA, detailed search strategies are needed to identify and retrieve individual case safety reports of interest from these databases. Standardized MedDRA Queries (SMQs) have been developed over more than a decade by senior scientists from many countries in a cooperative effort of CIOMS and ICH. SMQs focus on clearly defined conditions of interest to support a consistent approach to developing a series of individual safety reports to help answer a safety question. This second edition of the "Red Book" provides historical perspectives and "how to" develop, execute, and interpret output from a query using an SMQ. It is important to have a good understanding of SMQs and other safety queries, as there is the possibility to monitor safety risks and use results in benefit–risk assessments.

MedDRA® is a product of the International Conference for Harmonization (ICH) owned by the International Federation of Pharmaceutical Manufacturers Associations as trustee for ICH.

■ CIOMS (2017): Guide to Active Vaccine Safety Surveillance

This working group developed a guide for vaccine surveillance in resource-constrained areas. This project is particularly important for national public health programs when safety of a newly introduced vaccine must be addressed in low and middle-income countries. This guide contains consensus principles relevant for Objective #8 of WHO's Global Vaccine Safety Initiative regarding public–private information exchange. More vaccine products are focused on unmet needs and these products are reaching previously under-served populations sooner. The guide has practical advice on steps to consider if gaps in safety data prompt additional safety surveillance.

■ CIOMS ICH Terms and Definitions

This glossary, most recently updated and published in February 7, 2024, combines the terms and definitions included in the guidelines of the International Council for Harmonization of Technical Requirements for Pharmaceuticals for Human Use (ICH). It was compiled by CIOMS from the publicly available guidelines found on the ICH website. The guidelines themselves are owned by the International Council for Harmonisation of Technical Requirements for Pharmaceuticals for Human Use (ICH).

While every effort has been made by CIOMS to ensure the accuracy of this glossary, there may be unintentional errors or omissions. Please refer to the original ICH guidelines to verify the information provided. As ICH adopts new guidelines and introduces new terms on an irregular basis, CIOMS intends to review and update this document, e.g., quarterly, or as warranted.

CIOMS (2020) Drug Induced Liver Injury (DILI)

The consensus report of the CIOMS DILI Working Group aims to provide a critical framework and essential set of tools to detect, diagnose, and manage DILI during drug development and in the post-marketing setting. The report is intended for clinical and basic pharmaceutical industry investigators who capture, analyze, and communicate liver safety data in drug development. It is also intended for regulatory scientists and expert consultants who comprehensively evaluate new products and emerging biomarkers for their association with DILI risk, and for health care professionals who monitor and manage patients treated with potentially hepatotoxic drugs in clinical practice.

CIOMS XI Patient Involvement in the Development, Regulation and Safe Use of Medicines (2022)

This report describes the importance of systematically involving patients throughout a medicine's life — from its early development through the regulatory process to ongoing monitoring and safe use in everyday healthcare. It provides a comprehensive overview of the current knowledge about the benefits of patient involvement and existing initiatives, gives many examples and recommendations, and addresses the remaining challenges and practice gaps. The report prompts readers to implement its best practice recommendations according to how well they fit in with their organizational and national needs.

The report combines the experience and expertise of the CIOMS Working Group XI on Patient involvement in the development, regulation and safe use of medicines. It also incorporates views gathered from an open meeting in Switzerland and a workshop in Uganda, which both brought together members of the public, patient organization representatives, regulators, drug development experts, industry, academia, health professionals and other related stakeholders. The report was finalized following public consultation.

CIOMS XII (2023, Draft) — Benefit-Risk Balance for Medicinal Products

This working group was launched in September 2019 and includes participants from industry, regulators, academia and the World Health Organization. The goal is to update CIOMS IV on *Benefit-Risk Balance for Marketed Drugs: Evaluation of Safety Signals*, originally published in 1998, and potentially to extend the scope to include pre-approval as well as post-marketing considerations for medicinal products.

Additional Working Groups

Several additional projects ongoing as of late 2023 include:

- Working Group XIII on Real-World Data & Evidence in Regulatory Decision-Making;
- Working Group XIV on Artificial Intelligence in Pharmacovigilance;

- Working Group XV on Pharmacoepidemiology for Public Health;
- Working Group on MedDRA Labelling Groupings;
- Working Group on Severe Cutaneous Adverse Reactions (SCARs);
- Working Group on Good Govenance Practice for Research Institutions;
- Working group on Recommended Standards of Education and Training for Health Professionals Participating in Medicines Development.

CHAPTER

7

International Council for Harmonization of Technical Requirements for Pharmaceuticals for Human Use (ICH)

ICH is a global consensus organization composed of industry, regulators, and others currently operating as an association under Swiss law to develop technical guidelines for drug development. ICH guidelines are non-binding until adopted by regulators at the local level as guidance or regulation. This chapter summarizes key ICH activities at a high level and some of the guidelines issued by the various working groups related to drug safety. These guidelines have been used as the basis for creating certain safety guidance and regulations in North America, Europe, Japan, and elsewhere. They are worth taking the time to review online. Keep in mind that not all consensus guidelines issued by ICH have been adopted as requirements at the national level. Further, some ICH proposals have been modified by national regulatory authorities prior to adoption. Check current local regulations for specifics of what is required in each regulatory jurisdiction.

ICH was started by drug regulators and industry from Europe, Japan, and the US in 1990 as a voluntary consensus organization to improve and harmonize the drug development process. ICH was conceived as a forum for bringing together regulatory authorities, academic experts and pharmaceutical industry to discuss scientific and technical aspects of drug registration. The overall mission is to ensure that safe, effective, and high quality medicines are developed and then made available in the most resource-efficient manner. The original name of the organization was the International Conference on Harmonization of Technical Requirements for Registration of Pharmaceuticals for Human Use. The name was changed as part of a reorganization and expansion in late 2015 to the International Council for Harmonisation of Technical Requirements for Pharmaceuticals for Human Use.

Along with the name change, ICH expanded participation beyond the founding regions to include additional organizations and extend the benefits of harmonization. This required a series of organizational changes. These changes included greater international outreach, a new governance structure, and broader communication of ICH processes and work products. The governance structure evolved from a "six pack" Steering Committee, which was limited to the six founding parties and a few observers, to an Assembly and a Management Committee. Further, ICH is now a legal non-profit entity under Swiss law. Additional details regarding the current structure and processes are published on the ICH website (www.ich.org).

ICH has organized drug development topics into four categories: Efficacy (E), Quality (Q), Safety (S), and Multidisciplinary (M). ICH topic codes are assigned according to these categories. Note that "S" topics deal with non-clinical safety; clinical safety is covered under "E" topics. Experts from the various parties are appointed to comprise a working group, which produces technical documents. These documents usually take the form of guidelines or Q&A. An established multi-step process, including public consultation, is used to achieve final consensus.

Since technology and regulatory science are not static, ICH guidelines are periodically updated to reflect this. Revisions are indicated by an "R" in the ICH topic code. In certain instances, Q&A documents are developed to provide clarification.

The subset of ICH topics directly relevant to pharmacovigilance are:

- E1: The Extent of Population Exposure to Assess Clinical Safety for Drugs Intended for Long-Term Treatment of Non-Life Threatening Conditions;
- E2A: Clinical Safety Data Management: Definitions and Standards for Expedited Reporting;
- E2B(R3) and E2B(R2): Maintenance of the Clinical Safety Data Management, including the Maintenance of the Electronic Transmission of Individual Case Safety Reports Message Specification (Note: ICH has published several documents in an implementation package for E2B(R3));
- E2C(R2): Periodic Benefit-Risk Evaluation Report (Note: Relevant parts of a separate document, E2CA, Addendum to E2C, has been incorporated into the E2C(R2) guideline);
- E2C(R2) Q&As: Questions and Answers: Periodic Benefit-Risk Evaluation Report;
- E2D & E2D(R1) EWG: Post-Approval Safety Data Management: Definitions and Standards for Expedited Reporting;
- E2E: Pharmacovigilance Planning;
- E2F: Development Safety Update Report;
- E19: Optimisation of Safety Data Collection; and
- M1: MedDRA® Terminology (Medical Dictionary for Regulatory Activities).

While the subset above is primarily focused on safety and pharmacovigilance topics, other ICH Efficacy guidelines are relevant and would be important for any well-rounded safety & pharmacovigilance professional. These include:

E3: Clinical Study Reports
E6: Good Clinical Practice
E8: General Considerations in Clinical Trials
E9: Statistical considerations in Clinical Trials
E15: Definitions for Pharmacogenetics/ Pharmacogenomics
E19: Safety Data Collection

In addition to the efficacy guidelines, it would be prudent for those in study to also familiarize themselves with the other subset of guidelines in quality (such as Q7 Good Manufacturing Practice, Q8 Pharmaceutical Development, Q9 Quality Risk Management and Q10 Pharmaceutical Quality Development.

The ICH consensus documents, as well as information on ongoing work, can be found on the ICH web site (www.ich.org) and, if adopted into local regulatory requirements (with or without modification), on web sites of concerned regulators.

E1: The Extent of Population Exposure to Assess Clinical Safety for Drugs Intended for Long-Term Treatment of Non-Life Threatening Conditions

This guideline was finalized in 1994. It summarizes principles for safety evaluation of products intended for chronic use (or repeated intermittent use) of six months or longer for treatment of non-life-threatening conditions. The duration of drug exposure and its relationship to both time and magnitude of occurrence of adverse events are important considerations in determining the size of the data base necessary to characterize and quantify the safety profile of such a product. It is recommended that safety data derived from studies of shorter duration be analyzed separately from studies of longer duration. Also, the guideline suggests that events where the rate of occurrence changes over a longer period of time may need to be characterized depending on their severity and importance to the risk-benefit assessment of the drug. Safety data obtained during clinical development would not be expected to characterize rare adverse events, for example, those occurring in less than 1 in 1,000 patients.

E2A: Clinical Safety Data Management: Definitions and Standards for Expedited Reporting

E2A combines many concepts from the Council for International Organizations of Medical Sciences (CIOMS) I and CIOMS II reports covering the development of standard definitions and terminology for safety reporting and the appropriate mechanism for handling expedited (alert) reporting. This document was originally developed to cover primarily the investigational phase of drug development, but its concepts have been extended to cover post-marketing (approved) drugs also (see the E2E guideline, referenced below).

The definitions and recommendations for expedited reporting developed in this document have largely been accepted throughout the world. However, some of the recommendations have been tried and withdrawn (e.g., increased frequency reporting in the United States), inconsistently applied (e.g., breaking the blind), or never applied (reporting an expedited case to all open Investigational New Drug Applications [INDs]).

Definitions

Note on Definitions: Most regions have adopted the same, or similar definitions for these events terms and it is important for companies to note the differences between what is defined in ICH versus FDA, EMA, and agencies world wide. It is within a companies best interest to decide and define in writing and procedural documents which definitions they will abide by for consistency amongst personnel and health care professionals. Ideally, and in a perfect world, we wouldn't have even "slight" differences in these definitions, however it is in the nature of agencies to interpret terms on their own.

Adverse event or adverse experience (AE): "Any untoward medical occurrence in a patient or clinical investigation subject administered a pharmaceutical product and which does not necessarily have to have a causal relationship with this treatment."

Adverse drug reaction (ADR): "In the pre-approval clinical experience with a new medicinal product or its new usages, particularly as the therapeutic dose(s) may not be established: all noxious and unintended responses to a medicinal product related to any dose should be considered adverse drug reactions. For marketed products: A response to a drug which is noxious and unintended and which occurs at doses normally used in man for prophylaxis, diagnosis, or therapy of disease or for modification of physiological function."

Unexpected ADR: "An adverse reaction, the nature or severity of which is not consistent with the applicable product information (e.g., Investigator Brochure for an unapproved investigational medicinal product)." Note that this applies to non-marketed drugs. This definition was extended to marketed drugs in the E2D guideline (see below).

"Serious" and "severe": The terms serious and severe are differentiated. The term "severe" is often used to describe the intensity (severity) of a specific event (as in mild, moderate, or severe myocardial infarction); the event itself, however, may be of relatively minor medical significance (such as severe headache). This is not the same as "serious," which is based on patient/event outcome or action criteria usually associated with events that pose a threat to a patient's life or functioning. Seriousness (not severity) serves as a guide for defining regulatory reporting obligations.

Serious: "A serious adverse event (experience) or reaction is any untoward medical occurrence that at any dose results in death, is life-threatening, requires in-patient hospitalization or prolongation of existing hospitalization, results in persistent or significant disability/incapacity or is a congenital anomaly/birth defect."

"Medical and scientific judgment should be exercised in deciding whether expedited reporting is appropriate in other situations, such as important medical events that may not be immediately life-threatening or result in death or hospitalization but may jeopardize the patient or may require intervention to prevent one of the other outcomes listed in the definition above. These should also usually be considered serious." Note that "cancer" and "overdose" have been removed. These terms appeared in various pre-1995 definitions of "serious."

What Should Be Reported to Regulatory Authorities as Expedited Reports?

All suspected ADRs that are both serious and unexpected are subject to expedited reporting. This applies to reports from spontaneous sources and from any type of clinical or epidemiologic investigation, independent of design or purpose.

Note that this means all suspected adverse reactions (i.e., possibly causally related to the drug) that are serious and unexpected. Thus, it requires all three categories (causality, seriousness, and unexpectedness) for clinical trial cases. Although not explicitly stated in this document, for post-marketing cases the causality is implied (i.e., all spontaneous reports are presumed to be causally related), and, thus, only two criteria need to be met: seriousness and expectedness. Note:

- No international consensus standard exists for causality determination;
- An increased frequency of a known serious suspected ADR should be reported in an expedited fashion;
- A significant hazard to the patient population, such as lack of efficacy with a medicinal product used in a life-threatening disease; and
- A major safety finding from a newly completed non-clinical (e.g. animal) study.

Reporting Time Frames — Sponsor to Concerned Regulator(s)

- Fatal or life-threatening suspected ADRs: Alert within 7 calendar days, followed no more than 8 calendar days later with an expedited 15-day report;
- Other serious unexpected suspected ADRs: 15 calendar days after the first knowledge by the sponsor that the case meets the minimum criteria for reporting.

Minimum Criteria for Reporting

- An identifiable patient;
- A suspect medicinal product;
- An identifiable reporting source; and
- An event or outcome that is serious and unexpected and, for clinical trial cases, a reasonable suspected causal relationship.

Follow-up information should be sought and reported as soon as it becomes available. The CIOMS I form should be used to report the cases. (Notes: (a) Now with electronic transmissions, E2B-format submissions are required in many jurisdictions; (b) "Once a 15-day report, always a 15-day report" — including for medically important follow-up information obtained after the initial report.)

Managing Blinded Cases

E2A recommends that, although it is advantageous to retain the blind for all patients before study analysis, when a serious adverse reaction is reportable on an expedited basis, the blind should be broken only for that specific patient by the sponsor, even if the investigator has not broken the blind. The blind should be maintained where possible for the personnel in the company responsible for the analysis and interpretation of the overall study results. There may be circumstances where not breaking the blind is desirable, and in these circumstances, an agreement with the regulatory authorities should be pursued.

Note: This is generally not the current case for individual case reports, although for periodic active moiety reporting, i.e., aggregate reporting, all information is in scope. Reporting is usually to only one IND or premarketing dossier in most countries should multiple INDs or dossiers exist;

- Post-study AEs are usually collected for a defined interval described in the protocol, perhaps 28 days after last dose, but are otherwise not collected or sought by sponsors. Nevertheless, investigators may send reports to the sponsor after the protocol-specified follow-up period. These events should be treated as if they were study events and reported as expedited reports should they qualify to be such.

E2B: Clinical Safety Data Management: Data Elements for Transmission of Individual Case Safety Reports

Two working groups were set up in the ICH to develop the means for the electronic transmission of individual case safety reports (ICSRs) between or among companies and regulators, regulators and regulators, and companies and companies. There are two series of related documents.

The first set has the E2B documents, which were prepared by safety experts. These documents specify the medical and administrative data elements, as well as coding, required for the transmission. The second set has technical specification documents (ICH M2 or HL7), prepared by either ICH or HL7 informatics experts (see below). These documents provide technical specifications for structured messaging; electronic data interchange; data definitions to incorporate structured data formats (e.g., XML); security to ensure confidentiality, data integrity, authentication, and nonrepudiation; documents to handle heterogeneous data formats; and physical media for storage and transferability of data.

The E2B(R3) and M2 Documents

The terminology here has been confusing, as there have been multiple other designations for earlier versions of these documents, including E2B, E2B(M), E2B(R), and others. The documents were first developed in 1997 and finalized (more or less) in 2001. The ICH E2B(R3) implementation package is based on standards developed by ISO and HL7 to support ICH business requirements and includes provisions for experience gained over the last several years (see below).

There are several initiatives under way that aim to standardize data transmission of health data, including ICSRs, of which E2B is the current standard. Ultimately, it is expected that the Health Level 7 (HL7) standards will support the International Organization for Standards (ISO) standards, local regional requirements, and ICH requirements for interoperability with electronic medical records (see below).

The relevant ICH documents are:

- E2B(R3): Revision of the E2B(R2) ICH Guideline on Clinical Safety Data Management: Data Elements for Transmission of Individual Case Safety Reports;
- E2B(R2): Maintenance of the Clinical Safety Data Management, including Data Elements for Transmission of Individual Case Safety Reports (previously designated as E2B(M));
- M2: Electronic Standards for the Transfer of Regulatory Information (ESTRI); and
- M1: MedDRA and MedDRA Points to Consider documents.

Personnel involved in drug safety should be familiar at a high level with the E2B and M1 (MedDRA) documents; in addition, the informatics personnel supporting them should be familiar with M2. The contents of the E2B transmissions determine to a certain degree how data are handled and stored in a company's or business partner's database. For example, decisions must be made on whether to enter laboratory data as free text or as coded, structured data.

The E2B(R3) and ISO/HL7 Documents

In 2003 ICH re-assembled the E2B EWG to update and revise the E2B(R2) guideline; the revised guideline, E2B(R3), was released for public comment in 2005. In a similar timeframe, ICH decided that collaboration with standards development organizations (SDOs) would be incorporated as part of the process of developing technical specifications for ICH use. The intention was to enable wider inter-operability amongst stakeholders in the broad regulatory and healthcare domains. The first ICH topic to be developed under this process was E2B(R3). The ICH E2B(R3) business requirements were used to underpin an SDO Joint Initiative to develop consensus standards for the safety and acknowledgment messages. A double-badged standard for ICSR message exchange, ISO/HL7 27953-2, was developed via the SDO process and then the ICH E2B EWG created an implementation guide (IG) "package" for the E2B(R3) data elements and the ICH message specification.

■ E2C(R2) Periodic Benefit-Risk Evaluation Report and E2C(R2) Q&As

The E2C guideline was first adopted by ICH in November 1996. An addendum was published in 2003 and relevant points have been incorporated into the most recent revision, E2C(R2). ICH experts have also produced a Q&A document to facilitate understanding and consistent implementation of E2C(R2). These documents give guidance on the format and content of safety updates, which need to be provided at intervals to regulatory authorities after products have been marketed. The guideline is intended to ensure that the worldwide safety experience is provided to authorities at defined times after marketing with maximum efficiency and avoiding duplication of effort.

PSURs (either in E2C(R1) or E2C(R2) format) have been adopted by many countries, including those in the European Union, Japan, Canada, and others. In the United States, they are not yet obligatory, but most NDA holders submit PSURs rather than the older NDA Periodic Reports (PADER format), as long as the PADER content, particularly appendices, are included as required in the regulations. Companies wishing to submit PSURs in place of New Drug Application periodic reports must contact the FDA to obtain a waiver and FDA consent for their submissions in this format.

The general principles are as follows:

1. One report for one active substance. The PSUR should cover all dosage forms, formulations, and indications for a given active moiety. There may be separate presentations of data for different dosage forms or populations, as appropriate. The PSUR should be a "stand-alone" document;
2. For E2C(R1) format reports, only interval data will be included, but for E2C(R2) format reports, both interval and cumulative data will be included;
3. For combination products also marketed individually, safety information may be done as a separate PSUR or included in the PSURs prepared for one of the components, with cross-referencing;
4. The report should present data for the interval of the PSUR only, except for regulatory status information, renewals, and serious unlisted ADRs, which should be cumulative;
5. The report should focus on suspected ADRs. All spontaneous reports should be assumed to be suspected reactions (i.e., possibly related). Reporters are not restricted to healthcare professionals. For clinical trial and literature reports, only those cases believed by the reporter and sponsor to be unrelated to the drug should be excluded (ex-US). For reports submitted to the US FDA, causality assessment is solely the responsibility of the sponsor;
6. Lack of efficacy reports (which are considered to be AEs) should not be included in the tables but should be discussed in the "other information" section;
7. Increased frequency reports for known reactions should be reported, if appropriate;
8. If more than one company markets a drug in the same market, each Marketing Authorization

holder (MAH) is responsible for submitting PSURs. If contractual arrangements are made to share safety information and responsibilities, details should be specified in a written pharmacovigilance agreement;

9. Each product should have an international birth date (IBD), usually the date of the first Marketing Authorization anywhere in the world. This date should be synchronized around the world for PSUR reporting such that all authorities receive reports at the appropriate interval based on the IBD;
10. See the ICH E2C(R1), E2C(R2), and local requirements for the required submission timeline, e.g., submission within 60- or 90-days of the data lock-point;
11. The reference safety information document for expectedness ("listedness" in PSURs as opposed to "labeledness" in ICSRs) should be the company core data sheet (CCDS), the safety section of which is known as the company core safety information (CCSI);
12. The verbatim reporter term as well as the ICSR coding term (i.e., term selected for coding to MedDRA, which was approved after E2C was finished) should be used; and
13. Suspected ADR cases should be presented as line listings and summary tabulations. That is, individual CIOMS I or MedWatch forms are not included. Required individual cases are transmitted via E2B to accompany an E2C(R2) format report, not as included paper cases. Some jurisdictions may require supplementary line listings for E2C(R2) reports.

The sections of a PSUR in E2C(R1) format are as follows:

1. Introduction
2. Worldwide market authorization status
   a. Update of regulatory authority or MAH actions taken for safety reasons
3. Changes to the Reference Product Information
   a. The version of the CCDS in place at the beginning of the PSUR interval as the reference document. If there is a time lag between changes to the CCDS and local labeling, this should be commented on when submitting to that local health authority.
4. Patient exposure
   a. The most appropriate method should be used and an explanation for its choice provided. This includes patients exposed, patient-days, number of prescriptions, and tonnage sold.
5. Presentation of individual case histories from all sources (except non-medically confirmed consumer reports)
   a. Follow-up data on previously reported cases should be presented if medically significant.
   b. Literature should be monitored and cases included. Duplicates should be avoided. If a case is mentioned in the literature, even if obtained also as a spontaneous or trial case, the citation should be noted.
   c. If medically unconfirmed cases received from consumers are required to be submitted in the PSUR, they should be submitted as addenda line listings and summary reports.
   d. Line listings should include each patient only once. If a patient has more than one suspected ADR, the case should be listed under the most serious adverse drug experience/ADR, with the others also mentioned there. If appropriate, it may be useful to have more than one line listing for different dosage forms and indications.
      - Line listings should include the following cases:
   e. Spontaneous reports: all serious reactions, non- serious unlisted reactions.
   f. Studies or compassionate use: all serious reactions (believed to be serious by either the sponsor or the investigator).
   g. Literature: all serious reactions and non-serious, unlisted reactions.
   h. Regulatory authority cases: all serious reactions.
   i. If non-serious, listed ADRs are required by some authorities, they should be reported as an addendum.
6. Summary tabulations
   a. Each line listing should have an aggregate summary that will normally contain more terms than patients. It may be broken down by serious and non-serious and listed and unlisted, as well as other breakdowns, as appropriate. There should also be a summary for non-serious listed spontaneous suspected reactions.

   b. For E2C(R1) format, data in summary tabulations should be non-cumulative, except for ADRs that are both serious and unlisted, for which a cumulated figure should be provided in the table. Cumulative data are required in E2C(R2) submissions.
7. MAH analysis of individual case histories
   a. This section may contain brief comments on individual cases. The focus here is on individual cases (e.g., unanticipated findings, mechanism, reporting frequency) and should not be confused with the global assessment as described below.
8. Studies
   a. All completed studies (non-clinical, clinical, epidemiologic), planned or in-progress studies, and published studies yielding or with potential to yield safety information should be discussed.
9. Other information
   a. Lack of efficacy information should be presented here.
   b. Late-breaking information after database lock should be presented here.
10. Overall safety evaluation
   a. The data should be presented by system organ class and should discuss
      - A change in characteristics of listed reactions
      - Serious unlisted reactions, placing into perspective the cumulative reports
      - Non-serious unlisted reactions
      - Increased frequency of listed reactions
      - New safety issues Drug interactions
      - Overdose and its treatment
      - Drug misuse or abuse
      - Pregnancy and lactation information
      - Experience in special patient groups
      - Effects of long-term treatment
11. Conclusion
12. This section should indicate which safety data do not remain in accord with the previous cumulative experience and with the company CSI:
   a. Any action recommended or initiated
   b. Appendix: Company Core Data Sheet (CCDS)
   c. The Addendum provides clarification and guidance on E2C(R1) format PSURs and addresses some concepts not in E2C, such as Proprietary Information (Confidentiality), Executive Summary, Summary Bridging Report, Addendum Reports, Risk Management Program, and Benefit–Risk Analysis.
13. International Birth Date (IBD)
   a. PSURs should be based on the IBD (one per active moiety). To transition to a harmonized IBD, the MAH may submit its already prepared IBD-based PSUR plus (1) line listings and/or tabular summaries for the additional period (3 months if submitting a 6-month PSUR or 6 months if submitting a longer PSUR) with comments, or (2) an Addendum Report (see below) with the same duration limits as in (1).
   b. In attempting to harmonize IBDs, it is possible that a drug will be on a 5-year cycle in one country and a 6-month cycle in another. If harmonization is not possible, the MAH and regulators should try to find a common birth month and day so that reports can be submitted on the same month and day whether every 6 months, yearly, or every 5 years. (Note that many regions have changed the frequency from 5 years to 3 years.) In the EU, periodicity of PSURs is determined by the Pharmacovigilance Risk Assessment Committee (PRAC) and varies product-to-product in a risk-proportionate manner.
14. Addendum Reports
   a. An addendum report is used when it is not possible to synchronize PSURs for all authorities requiring submissions. The addendum report is an update to the most recently completed PSUR. It should be used when more than 3 months for a 6-month PSUR and more than 6 months for a longer PSUR. It is not intended as an in-depth report (which will be done in the next regularly scheduled PSUR). It should contain an introduction, any changes to the CCSI, significant regulatory actions on safety, line listings, and summary tabulations and a conclusion.

Addendum Reports are not contemplated for the E2C(R2) format.

15. Restarting the Clock
    a. For products in a long-term PSUR cycle (e.g., 5 years or more), the return to a 6-month reporting schedule may occur if a new clinically dissimilar indication is approved, a previously unapproved use in a special population is approved, or a new formulation or route of administration is approved. Restarting the reporting clock should be discussed with the regulatory authorities.
16. Time Interval Between Data Lock-Point and the Submission
    a. For E2C(R1) format reports, the MAH has 60 days to prepare a submission after the data lock-point. An issue that arose was review and comment by the regulatory authority(ies), which took a long time to do and was sent back to the sponsor at a date very close to the submission of the following PSUR. If this review contains new requirements or other obligations for the MAH, the MAH may not be able to adequately complete the additional analyses requested in time for the next PSUR. Hence, the Addendum notes that the regulatory authority will attempt to send comments to the MAH.
    b. As rapidly as possible if any issues of non-compliance with format and content are noted.
    c. As rapidly as possible and before the next data lock-point if additional safety issues are identified that may require further analysis in the next PSUR. Such analyses could also be sub-mitted as a separate stand-alone report instead of in the next PSUR.
17. Additional Time for Submissions
    a. In rare circumstances, the MAH may request an additional 30 days to submit a PSUR. This might occur if there is a large number of case reports and there is no new safety issue, if issues are raised by the authorities in the previous PSUR for which additional time is needed for further analysis for the next PSUR, or if issues needing further analysis are identified by the MAH.
18. Reference Safety Information (RSI)
    a. The MAH should highlight differences between the CCSI and the local product labeling in the cover letter that accompanies the PSUR.
    b. For 6-month and 1-year PSURs, the CCSI in effect at the beginning of the period should be used as the reference document.
    c. For PSURs longer than 1 year, the CCSI in effect at the end of the period should be used as the reference document for PSURs and Summary Bridging Reports.
19. Other Issues
    a. The title page of the PSUR should have a confidentiality statement because proprietary information is contained in the report.
    b. An executive summary should be included right after the title page in each PSUR.
    c. Patient exposure data
        - It is acknowledged that these data are often difficult to obtain and not always reliable. If the exposure data do not cover the full period of the PSUR, extrapolations may be made. A consistent method of exposure calculations should be used over time for a product.
    d. Individual case histories
        - Because it is impractical to summarize all cases as narratives, the MAH should describe the criteria used to describe the cases summarized.
        - The section should contain selected cases, including fatalities, presenting new and relevant safety information and grouped by medically relevant headings or MedDRA system organ class.
    e. Consumer listings
        - If required by regulators, consumer listings should be done in the same way that other listings and summary tabulations are prepared.
    f. The "comments" field
        - This field should be used only for information that helps to clarify individual cases.
    g. Studies
        - This section should contain only those company-sponsored studies and

published safety studies (including epidemiology studies) that produce findings with potential impact on safety. The MAH should not routinely catalogue or describe all studies.

h. The "other information" section
   - Risk management programs may be discussed in this section.
   - When a more comprehensive safety or risk — benefit analysis has been done separately, a summary of the analysis should be included here.
   - Discussion and analysis for the "Overall Safety Evaluation" section should be organized by system organ class and not by listedness or seriousness.

E2C(R2) Periodic Benefit-Risk Evaluation Report (PBRER)

The ICH E2C(R2) guideline is titled "Periodic Benefit-Risk Evaluation Report," but, like earlier versions of E2C, provides guidance on the format and content for the Periodic Safety Update Report (PSUR). The original E2C guideline for the PSUR was finalized in 1996 and an addendum, subsequently designated E2C(R1), was released in 2003. The addendum was based, in part, on recommendations in the report of the CIOMS V Working Group. E2C(R2), a major revision, was finalized in 2012. The E2C(R2) guideline broadens the scope of the PSUR; it contains updated concepts and principles for aggregate post-market safety analysis and reporting integrated information. It represents a conceptual evolution from the original PSUR (an interval safety report with a focus on ICSRs and risks) to a cumulative, analytical benefit-risk report. One of the reasons ICH decided to revise the guideline was the desire to decrease overall duplication of effort in document preparation. This revision permits a "modular" approach to corresponding sections of the PSUR, the Development Safety Update Report (DSUR, ICH E2F), and safety specification of a risk management plan (ICH E2E). Sections of these documents can be essentially identical in format and content. The PSUR is required for registered products by many regulatory authorities at various intervals after authorization. The primary goal of such reports is to provide a periodic, comprehensive, benefit-risk assessment that is based on: A safety evaluation, an evaluation of all relevant available information accessible to the marketing authorization holder (MAH), and a conclusion on the product's benefit-risk balance. A PSUR (E2C(R2) format) is intended to be a concise analytical document that covers the designated interval plus the cumulative experience.

A Q&A document for E2C(R2) was published in 2014 to facilitate practical implementation of the guideline.

E2D: Post-Approval Safety Data Management: Definitions and Standards for Expedited Reporting

This guideline was finalized in 2003 and provides a standardized procedure for post-approval safety data management, including expedited reporting to the relevant authorities. It parallels and adds to the E2A document, which covered pre-approval (clinical trial) safety data management, by covering post-marketing safety data management. This document standardizes data management of cases from consumers, literature, Internet, and other types of post-marketing cases.

Sources of Individual Case Safety Reports

1. Unsolicited sources: Spontaneous reports
   a. These are unsolicited communications by healthcare professionals or consumers to a company, regulatory authority, or other organization (e.g., World Health Organization, Regional Centers, Poison Control Center, etc.) that describe one or more ADRs in a patient who was given one or more medicinal products, and that does not derive from a study or any organized data collection scheme.
   b. "Stimulated reporting may occur in certain situations, such as a notification by a 'Dear Healthcare Professional' letter, a publication

in the press, or questioning of healthcare professionals by company representatives. These reports should be considered spontaneous." (Note this contradicts to a certain degree the FDA's guidance of August 1997, which requests that such cases be considered as if they were obtained from a post-marketing study and thus requires the triple criteria of seriousness, causality, and expectedness.)

c. Consumer reports should be handled as spontaneous reports irrespective of any subsequent "medical confirmation," a process required by a very few authorities for reportability. Emphasis should be placed on the quality of the report and not on its source. Even if reports received from consumers do not qualify for regulatory reporting, the cases should be retained in the database.

2. Unsolicited sources: Literature
   a. The MAH is expected to regularly screen the worldwide scientific literature by accessing widely used systematic literature reviews or reference databases according to local requirements or at least every 2 weeks. Cases of ADRs from the scientific and medical literature, including relevant published abstracts from meetings and draft manuscripts, might qualify for expedited reporting.
   b. The regulatory reporting time clock starts once it is determined that the case meets minimum criteria for reportability.
   c. If the product source, brand, or trade name is not specified, the MAH should assume that it was its product, although reports should indicate that the specific brand was not identified.
3. Unsolicited sources: The Internet
   a. MAHs are not expected to screen external websites for ADR information. However, if an MAH becomes aware of an adverse reaction on a website that it does not manage, the MAH should review the case and determine whether it should be reported.
   b. Unsolicited cases from the internet should be handled as spontaneous reports.
   c. Regarding e-mail, identity of the reporter needs to be evaluated to see whether it refers to the existence of a real person. That is, determine if it is possible to verify that the patient and reporter exist.
4. Unsolicited sources: Other sources
   a. Cases from nonmedical sources, such as the lay press, should be handled as spontaneous reports.
5. Solicited sources
   a. This refers to cases from organized data collection systems, which include clinical trials, post-approval named patient use programs, other patient support and disease management programs, surveys of patients or healthcare providers, or information-gathering on efficacy or patient compliance. AE reports obtained from any of these should not be considered spontaneous. For safety purposes, reporting solicited reports should be handled as if they were study reports and therefore should have an appropriate causality assessment.
6. Contractual agreements
   a. If companies make contractual arrangements to market a product in the same or different countries or regions, explicit agreements must be made to specify the processes for exchange of safety information, including timelines and regulatory reporting responsibilities, though the MAH is ultimately responsible. Duplicate reporting should be avoided.
7. Regulatory authority sources
   a. Individual serious unexpected ADR reports originating from foreign regulatory authorities are always subject to expedited reporting. Resubmission of serious ADR cases without new information to the originating regulatory authority is not usually required, unless otherwise specified by local regulation.

Good Case Management Practices

1. Assessing patient and reporter identifiability
   a. One or more of the following automatically qualifies a patient as identifiable: age (or age category, e.g., adolescent, adult, elderly), gender, initials, date of birth, name, or patient identification number. In the event of secondhand reports, every reasonable effort should

be made to verify the existence of an identifiable patient and reporter;

b. All parties supplying case information or approached for case information should be identifiable (minimum of one per ICSR);

c. In the absence of qualifying descriptors, a report referring to a definite number of patients should not be regarded as a case until the minimum four criteria for case reporting are met.

2. The role of narratives

a. The objective of the narrative is to summarize all relevant clinical and related information, including patient characteristics, therapy details, medical history, clinical course of the event(s), diagnosis, and ADR(s), including the outcome, laboratory evidence, and any other information that supports or refutes an ADR. The narrative should serve as a comprehensive stand-alone "medical story." The information should be presented in a logical time sequence; ideally, this should be presented in the chronology of the patient's experience rather than in the chronology in which the information was received. In follow-up reports, new information should be clearly identified.

b. Abbreviations and acronyms should be avoided, with the possible exception of laboratory parameters and units.

3. Clinical case evaluation

a. An ADR report should be reviewed by the recipient for the quality and completeness of the medical information. This should include, but is not limited to, the following: Is a diagnosis possible? Have the relevant diagnostic procedures been performed? Were alternative causes of the reaction(s) considered? What additional information is needed?

b. The report should include the reporter's adverse event verbatim terms (and, in the case of consumer reports, the consumer's description of the event). Staff receiving reports should provide an unbiased and unfiltered report of the information from the reporter. Clearly identified evaluations by the MAH are considered acceptable and, for some authorities, required.

4. Follow-up information

a. The information from ADR cases when first received is generally incomplete. Efforts should be made to seek additional information on selected reports;

b. The first consideration should be prioritization of case reports by importance: cases that are (1) both serious and unexpected, (2) serious and expected, and (3) non-serious and unexpected. In addition to seriousness and expectedness as criteria, cases "of special interest" also deserve extra attention as a high priority (e.g., ADRs under active surveillance at the request of regulators), as well as any cases that might impact the benefit-risk assessment, i.e., lead to a labeling change decision;

c. Follow-up should be obtained by a telephone call, a site visit, or a written request. The MAH should provide specific questions it would like answered. The MAH should tailor the effort to optimize the chances of obtaining the new information;

d. Written confirmation of details given verbally should be obtained whenever possible. Ideally, healthcare professionals with thorough pharmacovigilance training and therapeutic expertise should be involved in the collection and the direct follow-up of reported cases.

5. Pregnancy exposure

a. MAHs are expected to follow up all reports, from healthcare professionals or consumers, of pregnancies where the embryo/fetus could have been exposed to one of its medicinal products.

6. How to report

a. MedDRA should be used for coding relevant E2B fields. E2B(R3) format is preferred rather than E2B(R2), and E2B(R3) should be implemented for electronic transmission of individual cases when partners are ready.

7. Recommended key data elements

a. The reader is referred to the Appendix of the E2D report for a list of recommended key data elements that should appear in all expedited reports.

■ E2E: Pharmacovigilance Planning

This guideline was finalized in 2004 and is intended to aid in planning pharmacovigilance activities, especially in preparation for the early post-marketing period of a new drug. The main focus of this guideline is on a Safety Specification and Pharmacovigilance Plan that would be submitted at the time of the application for marketing.

Background and Scope

All three founding regions of the ICH (the European Union, Japan, and the United States,) have been turning their attention to risk management and pharmacovigilance planning throughout the life cycle of a drug. This document reflects ICH's views.

The guideline is proposed for new chemical entities, biotechnology-derived products, and vaccines, as well as for significant changes in established products (e.g., new dosage form, new route of administration, or new manufacturing process for a biotechnology-derived product) and for established products to be introduced to new populations or for new indications, or where a new major safety concern has arisen.

It is recommended that company pharmacovigilance experts get involved early in product development. Planning and dialogue with regulators should also start long before license application. A safety specification and pharmacovigilance plan can also be developed for products already on the market (e.g., new indication or major new safety concern). The plan could be used as the basis for discussing pharmacovigilance activities with regulators in the different ICH regions and beyond.

For products with important identified risks, important potential risks, or important missing information, the pharmacovigilance plan should include additional actions designed to address these concerns. For products for which no special concerns have arisen, routine pharmacovigilance should be sufficient for post-approval safety monitoring, without the need for additional actions (e.g., safety studies). During the course of implementing the various components of the plan, any important emerging benefit or risk information should be discussed and used to revise the plan.

The Sections of a Pharmacovigilance Plan

A pharmacovigilance plan for a product has three sections: (1) Safety Specification, (2) Pharmacovigilance Plan, and (3) Annex — Pharmacovigilance Methods.

The safety specification is a summary of the important identified risks of a drug, important potential risks, and important missing information. It should also address the populations potentially at risk (where the product is likely to be used) and outstanding safety questions that warrant further investigation to refine understanding of the benefit–risk profile during the post-approval period.

The format and contents should focus on the identified risks, important potential risks, and important missing information. It should refer to the three safety sections in the Common Technical Document. The following elements should be considered for inclusion.

1. Non-clinical
   a. This section should present non-clinical safety findings that have not been adequately addressed by clinical data, for example, toxicity (including repeat-dose toxicity, reproductive/developmental toxicity, nephrotoxicity, hepatotoxicity, genotoxicity, carcinogenicity, etc.), general pharmacology (cardiovascular, including QT/QTc interval prolongation, nervous system, etc.), drug interactions, and other toxicity-related information. If the product is intended for use in special populations, consideration should be given to whether specific non-clinical data need to exist.
2. Clinical
   a. Limitations of the human safety database (e.g., related to the size of the study population, study inclusion/exclusion criteria) should be considered and discussed. Particular reference

should be made to populations likely to be exposed during the intended or expected use of the product in medical practice;

b. The worldwide experience should be briefly discussed, including the extent of the worldwide exposure, any new or different safety issues identified, any regulatory actions related to safety, and populations not studied in the pre-approval phase (for example, children, elderly, pregnant or lactating women, patients with relevant co-morbidity, such as hepatic or renal disorders, patients with disease severity different from that studied in clinical trials, subpopulations carrying known and relevant genetic polymorphism, patients of different racial or ethnic origins);
c. AEs/ADRs: This section should list the important identified and potential risks that require further characterization or evaluation. Discussion of risk factors and potential mechanisms should draw on information from the Common Technical Document and other relevant information, such as other drug labels, scientific literature, and post-marketing experience;
d. Important identified risks that require further evaluation:
   - More detailed information should be included on the most important identified AEs/ADRs, which would include those that are serious or frequent and that also might have an impact on the balance of benefits and risks of the product. This information should include evidence bearing on a causal relationship, severity, seriousness, frequency, reversibility, and at-risk groups, if available. Risk factors and potential mechanisms should be discussed. These AEs/ADRs should usually call for further evaluation as part of the pharmacovigilance plan (e.g., frequency in normal conditions of use, severity, outcome, at-risk groups).
e. Important potential risks that require further evaluation:
   - Important potential risks should be described and the evidence that led to the conclusion that there was a potential risk should be presented. It is anticipated that for any important potential risk, there should be further evaluation to characterize the association;
   - Identified and potential interactions, including food–drug and drug–drug interactions, should be discussed with consideration of the evidence, and potential health risks posed for the different indications and in the different populations should be discussed.
f. Epidemiology
   - The epidemiology of the indication should be discussed, including incidence, prevalence, mortality, and relevant comorbidity, and should take into account whenever possible stratification by age, sex, and racial or ethnic origin. Differences in the epidemiology in different regions should be discussed (because the epidemiology of the indication(s) may vary across regions), if this information is available;
   - For important AEs that may require further investigation, it is useful to review the incidence rates of these events among patients in whom the drug is indicated (i.e., the background incidence rates).
g. Pharmacologic class effects
   - The safety specification should identify risks believed to be common to the pharmacologic class;
   - Summary: This should include the important identified risks, important potential risks, and important missing information on an issue-by-issue basis.

Pharmacovigilance Plan

The pharmacovigilance plan should be based on the safety specification and developed by the sponsor. It can be discussed with regulators during product development, before approval of a new product (i.e., when the marketing application is submitted or in advance of submission), or when a safety concern arises post-marketing. It can be a stand-alone document (in the U.S., this document is the Package Insert).

For products for which no special concerns have arisen, routine pharmacovigilance should be sufficient for post-approval safety monitoring, without the need for additional actions (e.g., safety studies). However, for products with important identified risks, important potential risks, or important missing information, additional actions designed to address these concerns should be considered. It should be updated as important information on safety becomes available and milestones are reached.

The format and content should include the following:

1. Summary of ongoing safety issues, including the important identified risks, important potential risks, and important missing information;
2. Routine pharmacovigilance practice should be conducted for all medicinal products, regardless of whether additional actions are appropriate as part of a pharmacovigilance plan. This routine pharmacovigilance should include the following:
3. Systems and processes that ensure that information about all suspected adverse reactions that are reported to the personnel of the company are collected and collated in an accessible manner;
4. The preparation of reports for regulatory authorities, including expedited ADR reports and periodic aggregate reports;
5. Continuous monitoring of the safety profile, including signal detection and management, issue evaluation, updating of labeling, and liaison with regulatory authorities;
6. Other requirements, as defined by local regulations.
7. Action plan for safety issues:
   a. The plan for each important safety issue should be presented and justified according to the safety issue, objective of the proposed action, non-routine action proposed, rationale for proposed action, monitoring by the sponsor for the identified safety issue and proposed action, and milestones for evaluation and reporting. Any protocols for specific studies may also be provided.
8. Summary of actions to be completed, including milestones:
   a. An overall pharmacovigilance plan for the product, bringing together the actions for all individual safety issues, should be presented and organized in terms of the actions to be undertaken and their milestones;
   b. It is recommended that milestones for completing studies and for submitting safety results be included in the pharmacovigilance plan. The milestones should reflect when exposure to the product will have reached a level sufficient to allow potential identification/characterization of the AEs/ADRs of concern or resolution of a particular concern and when the results of ongoing or proposed safety studies are expected to be available;
   c. These milestones might be aligned with regulatory milestones (e.g., PSURs, annual reassessment, and license renewals) and used to revise the pharmacovigilance plan.
   d. Pharmacovigilance methods
      - The best method to address a specific situation can vary, depending on the product, the indication, the population treated, and the issue to be addressed. When choosing a method to address a safety concern, sponsors should use the most appropriate design.
   e. Design and conduct of observational studies
      - Carefully designed and conducted pharmacoepidemiologic studies, specifically observational (non-interventional, non-experimental) studies, are important tools in pharmacovigilance;
      - A protocol should be finalized and experts from relevant disciplines (e.g., pharmacovigilance experts, pharmacoepidemiologists, and biostatisticians, etc.) should be consulted. It is recommended that the protocol be discussed with the regulatory authorities before the study starts (in many cases this is required). A study report after completion, and interim reports, if appropriate, should be submitted to the authorities according to the milestones within the pharmacovigilance plan;
      - The sponsor should follow good epidemiologic practice for observational studies and internationally accepted guidelines, such

as the guidelines endorsed by the International Society for Pharmacoepidemiology.

f. Annex
g. A detailed discussion of pharmacovigilance methods is appended to the document to which the reader is referred for further details.

E2F: Development Safety Update Report

This document has been formally adopted in many regulatory jurisdictions and is accepted in most jurisdictions. The contents of the DSUR in E2F are very similar to those in the CIOMS DSUR report.

The DSUR is intended to be the common standard for annual clinical trial safety reporting and would replace other required pre-market periodic safety reports. It presents an annual review and evaluation of pertinent interval safety information: (1) to summarize the current understanding and management of identified and potential risks, (2) to describe new safety issues that could have an impact on the protection of clinical trial subjects, (3) to examine whether the information obtained during the reporting period is in accord with previous safety knowledge, and (4) to provide an update on the status of the clinical investigation/development program. This is similar to the CIOMS proposal. Full details on the contents can be found in the E2G guideline on the ICH website.

E19: Optimization of Safety Data Collection

Work on this topic began in late 2016 and the guideline was in development as of mid-2018. According to ICH, when this guideline reaches ICH step 5, it will "provide harmonised guidance on when it would be appropriate to use a targeted approach to safety data collection in some late-stage pre-marketing or post-marketing studies, and how such an approach would be implemented. Recognising that protection of patient welfare during drug development is critically important, unnecessary data collection may be burdensome to patients and serve as a disincentive to participation in clinical research. By tailoring safety data collection in some circumstances, the burden to patients would be reduced, a larger number of informative clinical studies could be carried out with greater efficiency, studies could be conducted with greater global participation, and the public health would be better served." This reflects applications of risk-based principles by ICH and a systematic approach to product development.

M1: MedDRA® Terminology (Medical Dictionary for Regulatory Activities)

The development of a regulatory terminology, Medical Dictionary for Regulatory Activities, was approved by ICH in 1997 and it was launched in 1999 with English as the base language. In addition to the terminology, which is available by subscription, ICH created "Points to Consider" documents that are available from the sole-source MedDRA provider of the terminology (see www.meddra.org). As of mid-2018, MedDRA was available in eleven languages (Chinese, Czech, Dutch, English, French, German, Hungarian, Italian, Japanese, Portuguese, and Spanish). Note, however, that not all terms are translated in each language. For example, English word order ("neck red" vs "red neck") does not translate to two unique terms in Japanese.

The Points to Consider documents are updated on a regular basis, as relevant for each new version of MedDRA. Both documents are maintained in English and Japanese; summaries are provided in the other languages that are otherwise available in MedDRA.

CHAPTER

8

The Uppsala Monitoring Centre

The Uppsala Monitoring Centre (UMC) is a non-profit foundation that operates the WHO Programme for International Drug Monitoring and maintains both a drug dictionary, WHODrug Global, and a post-marketing safety database, VigiBase. An obsolete third UMC tool was WHO-ART, an adverse reaction terminology database that is currently only available to regulators who specifically request access from the UMC. The UMC also provides many research publications and services related to pharmacovigilance. These activities have been essential in expanding the concepts and principles of pharmacovigilance beyond the traditional ICH regions and have paved the way for ICH expansion. The UMC has a variety of services related to research including signal detection, general education and training, tools for managing pharmacovigilance communications, a pharmacovigilance reference library and glossary of terms for reference. They also play a crucial role in global efforts to standardize the way products and substances are identified by helping implement the Identification of Medicinal Products (IDMP) standards which "aim to increase clarity and efficiency in communications about medicines and provide greater certainty to patients no matter where they are".

UMC and the WHO Program for International Drug Monitoring

Ten founding government safety organizations (Australia, Canada, Czechoslovakia, Federal Republic of Germany, Ireland, Netherlands, New Zealand, Sweden, United Kingdon, USA) created the WHO Programme for International Drug Monitoring in 1968 following the thalidomide birth defect tragedy. To prevent recurrence of another such tragedy, the concept was to systematically collect spontaneously reported drug safety information from around the world regarding the harm caused by medicines.

Since 1978, the programme has been managed from Uppsala, Sweden, by the UMC and today over 170 government drug safety organizations participate in the network (as full or associate members), along with the WHO in Geneva, and the UMC.

The reach of the WHO Programme for International Drug Monitoring is extensive and Individual Case Safety Reports in VigiBase originate from across the globe. Countries have started to contribute cases in a staggered manner. It is worth noting that the pharmacovigilance capacity of some countries is more robust than in others. Nevertheless, these data are a key part of the global pharmacovigilance system.

UMC is one of the five WHO collaborating centers in the network. Member countries submit domestic suspected serious and non-serious adverse reactions electronically to VigiBase at UMC. Suspected reactions are pre=coded with either MedDRA® or legacy WHO-ART (A UMC coding terminology that is now largely out of date and is no longer maintained). However, enhanced capabilities for VigiFlow, the interface for electronic reporting to VigiBase, were introduced in 2017 and require MedDRA-coded adverse reactions. Fortunately, a one-way "cross-walk" is available for conversion of WHO-ART terms to MedDRA. Consistent with legislation, the interface also accommodates direct reporting from healthcare professionals, public health programs, patients, and the pharmaceutical industry.

As of 2023, VigiBase contained more than 30 million reports of suspected adverse reactions for marketed medicines, including vaccines. VigiBase is continuously updated with new reports on a periodic basis. Importantly, UMC has developed vigiMatch, an automatic algorithm in VigiLyze that has been available since early 2017 for detection of suspected duplicates in VigiBase. vigiMatch uses a statistical model that scores pairs of reports, taking into account the amount of matching and mismatching information. This is a complex system and much more information is available from the UMC.

Key Functions of UMC

- Maintenance and operation of an international safety database, VigiBase, which contains spontaneous reports submitted by Member State regulators (or local equivalent) and interaction with contributing Member States.
- Identification and analysis of aggregate data by scientific staff to detect new safety signals from VigiBase, primarily via a data mining tool, VigiLyze.
- Information exchange between WHO and national pharmacovigilance centers, mainly through "VigiMed," a restricted Internet forum set up in 1997 for rapid e-mail information exchange among government safety agencies on pharmacovigilance matters. This is not generally available to the public or industry.
- Publication of periodic newsletters (e.g., "Uppsala Reports"), guidelines, and books on the topics of pharmacovigilance and risk management. Some are available on the Internet and in languages other than English. Some are available at no charge, others not so.
- Supply of tools for management of clinical information, including adverse drug reaction case reports. The main product is the WHO Drug Dictionary (- UMC formerly provided and maintained the WHO Adverse Reaction Terminology (WHO-ART). This terminology and system is no longer being maintained, and is obsolete. Most users should now user MedDRA as their preferred dictionary.

- Training and consulting support to national centers and countries for establishing and helping pharmacovigilance systems mature.
- Computer software for case report management, designed to suit the needs of national centers and consistent with the enhanced VigiFlow electronic interface.
- Annual meetings for representatives of national centers, at which scientific and organizational matters are discussed.
- Methodological research for the development of pharmacovigilance as a science, particularly in resource-constrained settings, but also customized research to complement mature pharmacovigilance systems (at a fee).
- Publication of scientific articles in pharmacovigilance. Note that all scientific papers by UMC authors have been freely available online at no charge since 2015 (www.who-umc.org).

The UMC has played a major role in the development and propagation of the concepts and techniques of pharmacovigilance, particularly pragmatic approaches in less developed countries. For many years, it was a lone international voice. It has now been joined by others to advance the field of pharmacovigilance. The key publications on its website are well worth reviewing.

Benefits of the UMC

There are many benefits to familiarizing oneself with the UMC, its offerings, and its relevance within the industry. Safety and Pharmacovigilance professionals, along with those in Clinical Development, Drug Manufacturing, Labeling, Regulatory, Data Management, Marketing and Communications, and many other areas, should be familiar with what UMC has to offer. Training from the UMC is offered via self-paced e-learning on YouTube channels and can be found by simply visiting their website and doing a search for relevant offered training, which currently includes videos and material on general Pharmacovigilance, Signal Detection, adverse drug report (ADR) reporting, and pharmacovigilance communications. Why create your own training when this is readily available (one might ask)?

Pharmacovigilance Communications

The UMC "strives to meet a global need for better communication practices in our field". Their activities focus on raising awareness of the importance of pharmacovigilance, and the basics of how adverse drug reactions occur and should be handled. They have also taken on the mission to strengthen communications capacities within the global pharmacovigilance community, by conducting training and lectures, social science-based research, and by producing and sharing innovative campaign materials and information packages.

Pharmacovigilance professionals as well as those in marketing and communications, should take advantage of the efforts of the UMC and consider implementing the recommendations outlined from the organization when it comes to communicating risks and how to effectively communicate those risks to the public.

The UMC also publishes "Uppsala Reports" which are pharmacovigilance focused and available for free, as well as a podcast called Drug Safety Matters which hosts new speakers and focuses on relevant and hot topics within drug safety and pharmacovigilance.

Why a chapter on the UMC?

We have dedicated a chapter solely to the UMC because we feel it is important for professionals to understand its functions, its impact on product development and research, and its utilization in the ongoing pursuit of pharmacovigilance.

CHAPTER 9

Biopharmaceutical Companies

There are many types of companies and institutions in the pharmaceutical world with responsibilities regarding drug safety. A general summary of various types of institutions follows, although there is a wide variety of business approaches that result in a myriad of hybrid combinations. The creative organizational structures can (and do) morph over time. The common feature is a requirement to comply with regulations or go out of business.

Introduction

There are many large drug companies in the world that sell billions of dollars of products each year. Although the number of companies has decreased through mergers and acquisitions, there still remain more than 50 publicly traded companies with annual sales of more than US$1.5 billion per year and roughly another 400 with sales less than $1 billion per year. The largest public company has sales of more than $100 billion per year in 2022 (including approximately $30 billion attributed to the COVID 19 pandemic). In addition, there are several very large and many other small and mid-sized companies that are privately held (not traded on the stock exchange). As noted throughout this book, companies are obligated to report animal and human safety data (among other information) to health authorities, ethics committees, investigational review boards, and so on. Companies also have a fiduciary duty to timely report material facts to the investment community.

Big and Somewhat Big Pharma

Big pharma generally refers to the dozen or so large, "full-service" companies with global reach and revenues in the billions to tens of billions of dollars. These companies are multinational, with headquarters primarily in the United States or Europe, but with some located in Japan and elsewhere (India, China, or Israel). They usually have scientists doing drug discovery to come up with new patentable drugs that will, it is hoped, become "blockbusters" (drugs with sales of more than a billion dollars a year by some definitions). Some of these highly capitalized companies have adopted a strategy of developing a larger number of products that are not blockbusters to avoid a "patent cliff", i.e., when revenues decline as a major product goes off patent.

The big innovative companies have the capacity to do their own pre-clinical studies (pharmacology and toxicity) and clinical trials (phase I–IV) though many of them now out-source parts of these complex processes. Many now also have generic divisions that develop and market generics, both of their own branded products and of other companies' products that are off patent. Another active area is switching prescription products to non-prescription status.

These companies have large marketing and sales divisions with hundreds to thousands of "representatives", "sales reps", or "detailers". The big pharma company does some of its own manufacturing in factories throughout the world, sometimes with active pharmaceutical ingredients (APIs) from contractors, as well as outsourcing full or partial production from other countries (often India or China). There are large departments to handle regulatory issues, legal issues, patents, and other key activities. Since pharmacovigilance touches many different functions, it is essential to have a well-established communication network to support coordination of activities amongst the various functions. Many companies have subsidiaries in the major markets (50 or more) throughout the world. Some subsidiaries are only sales organizations, whereas others are staffed to do clinical research and medical affairs as well. Some functions may be located outside the mother country (e.g., home office in the United States but a phase I clinical research unit in the EU or Asia, or vice versa). These often-far-flung contributors to safety are frequently in different time zones and have different holiday periods when facilities are essentially closed, and routine pharmacovigilance is handled by a slimmed down "skeleton" team.

Of course, there is a large drug safety department. The safety department is often, but not always, located in the corporate headquarters in the mother country. This is the major center for drug safety, with receipt of some or all of the individual case safety reports for data entry as well as preparation of MedWatch and CIOMS I forms, electronic submissions (E2B), Common Technical Documents (eCTDs), Marketing Authorizations, PSURs/PBRERs, NDA periodic reports, IND annual reports, DSURs, Risk Management Plans/REMS, signal management, reference safety information, clinical trial reports, and other aggregate reports. There is usually a large IT department and dedicated IT staff to support drug safety as much of the work is now electronic rather than paper based. There is often a large IT department based in the US if the company is not headquartered there. Since pharmacovigilance touches many different functions, it is essential to have a well-established communications function to coordinate. This also facilitates workload-sharing across time zones and geographies. Servers for the safety database and back-up servers are located at a central location as a rule as well as data storage in the Cloud, often through third parties. There are usually drug safety departments (or at least a person) in most or all subsidiaries to receive local safety reports (in the local language) and make submissions (sometimes in English, sometimes in the local language) if electronic E2B reporting is not done centrally. If not otherwise required, a local person may be needed to perform expectedness determinations based on the local reference safety information.

These subsidiaries, depending on size and function, may have a separate physician, pharmacist or other health care professional serving as safety officer or have the medical director (often the only medical doctor in the local company) also serve as the safety physician. Many jurisdictions have a legal requirement for an individual who is "responsible" for pharmacovigilance functions. The subsidiaries often serve as "pass through" points for AEs to be sent to central or regional data centers for data entry into the safety database. Sometimes a subsidiary (or regional center) will have expanded functions covering multiple countries. For example, some companies (e.g., whose headquarters are in the US or Japan) will set up a major center in the EU to do data entry and to prepare PSURs/PBRERs and other documents for submission to the EMA and EEA national health authorities or elsewhere. In some instances, work is segmented and done on several continents and then synthesized into an aggregate report, e.g., PSUR/PBRER. In addition to routine (e.g., periodic) reports, these activities are often required on short notice when an Urgent Safety Measure is contemplated.

In other situations, where the corporate headquarters are in a smaller country (e.g., Switzerland), one of the "subsidiaries" may become the dominant center for drug safety (e.g., in the EU or US). There is a tendency for safety departments to now be located in major English-speaking countries, such as the US or the UK, which, coincidentally or not, are the regulatory sites for the two major world pharmaceutical markets, the United States and the European Union (*Note*: The move of EMA from London to Amsterdam (Brexit) impacted drug safety centers covering the EU if they were/are based in the UK).

Things are changing, however, in biggish pharma. The large companies are getting larger, following mergers and acquisitions (e.g., Merck, Pfizer, Novartis, Sanofi, Roche, Eli Lilly, etc.). There is now a trend in the very big companies to have some functions remain centralized for the entire corporation, such as IT and the safety database, but for the drug safety functions to be separate. That is, there may be several relatively independent drug safety groups (one for prescription products, another for OTC, another for vaccines, etc.) doing individual case processing and aggregate reporting but sharing common supportive functions, i.e., IT, epidemiology, risk management, etc. Thus, big companies may function as "holding companies" for multiple smaller safety subunits. Others remain rigidly monolithic. There is no single model applicable to all. The use of outsourcing vendors, for the holistic safety function overall or a specific activity, such as data entry or writing case narratives, is also increasing.

There are several trends evident. One is that drug discovery has been somewhat slow of late in big pharma, with fewer novel blockbusters and many old blockbusters going off patent ("the patent cliff"). Many firms, both large and mid-sized, have been "rightsizing" or "downsizing" (i.e., firing workers and replacing them, if at all, with temporary workers and consultants or outsourcing some activities). Thus, they tend to do less research and more development as "R&D" components are now becoming distinct. Research is, to a significant degree, being left to the small biotech companies that do the early development and then sell the product to the bigger pharmas for the late phase II and III development for submission of the New Drug Application (NDA) or Marketing Authorization (MA) dossier. Advanced high-tech therapies have tended to be discovered by smaller biotech firms with larger pharma companies purchasing or co-developing the drug (or even the whole biotech company) in phase II or III and beyond.

Another trend is the use of generics in the developed world as well as in developing countries. 85% of the drugs sold in the United States are now generics and this trend will continue as many older drugs go off patent (https://www.statista.com/) and payers balk at ever-increasing reimbursement schedules. Europe is following this trend, too; but with lower percentages (around 20% in France and Germany and 55% for Poland). Some national and multinational companies are devoted only to generic products and, thus, have little or no drug discovery or clinical research capacity. They may do small, required studies to show bioequivalence. Occasionally, if needed, they do formal phase II, III, or IV clinical trials but these activities are usually outsourced. The generic companies create safety departments according to the functions required, but they tend to be less involved with critical issues than the companies that deal with new chemical entities. By the time a drug is generic, most of the safety issues have already been addressed. AE reporting and pharmacovigilance tends to be a "maintenance function", with few unique data or new and clinically important signals appearing. Many of the safety reports are, in fact, literature cases with few spontaneous AEs received. In addition, because it is often hard to identify the manufacturer of a generic product, the AEs tend to get reported to the originating company that first created and sold the product whether the actual AE occurred with that product or not. An interesting situation occurs when the originating company no longer exists or no longer makes or markets the product and has closed its NDAs and INDs. In that situation, in the US, generic drug labeling must be the "same as" the last approved reference listed drug. Thus, the "reference product" may not be the originator and the innovator may not maintain the reference labeling. In the US, when the innovator withdraws the product, FDA may assign one of the generic manufacturers to this role. Generic labeling has been controversial in regard to making changes in labeling. There are also now branded generics which make up some 5% of the US market.

Some big pharma companies have generic divisions in addition to the innovator divisions. This is done, of course, to make money but also to create generic versions of their branded products to sell after the branded products go off patent. That is, a company may sell a branded and a generic version of the same product.

Some companies are also investing in "nutraceuticals." Many such companies have one single drug safety group or they have separate teams to handle these products as well as a process for innovator products. The regulation of nutraceuticals in most jurisdictions is much more limited than for drugs. Companies are organized to address the level and breadth of their obligations (including those with business partners).

Biosimilar products are an expanding part of product availability. These are in a sense "generic biologics" but clearly are not since they are not relatively simple molecules but rather "advanced therapeutics". Many biologics are complex proteins that cannot be created, assembled, and "folded" except in living organisms. Regulatory agencies and companies realize these biosimilars cannot be handled like generic drugs of small molecules. The rules are evolving, and it is likely that pharmacovigilance ("biovigilance") will need to be done at the level of innovator products. In the US generally some sort of clinical trial is usually required for a biologic to be approved by FDA.

Another trend is the outsourcing and offshoring of many functions that formerly remained entirely within the company as core competencies. Drug safety falls into this category. The operational aspects of drug safety, particularly case processing, are sometimes strong candidates for this. Processing individual case safety reports has now become something of a commodity (Definition: "a good or service whose wide availability typically leads to smaller profit margins and diminishes the importance of factors [like brand name] other than price" — *Merriam-Webster's Collegiate Dictionary*), whereby the place and personnel who do the case processing, data entry, and follow-up are chosen almost entirely on the basis of lowest cost; aggregate reports for older drugs in particular are also more and more often outsourced to these low cost countries. Thus, much of this drug safety work is now being done in India, China, Brazil, the Philippines, Costa Rica, Hungary, and elsewhere. Manufacturing, toxicology, computer programming, and other services are also following this route. The major business, signal management, risk–benefit assessment, and epidemiologic and management decisions tend to remain in the home office. Although there is a trend to automate and outsource some components of these core activities (among others signal detection steps), artificial intelligence will at some point be playing a major role in safety with expected changes in the routine processes described above.

■ Mid-sized and Small Pharma

Some pharmaceutical companies are mid-sized (sales in the hundreds of millions of dollars) and are sometimes located in a single country. They thus do not have to establish worldwide expertise in the safety department and can concentrate on the safety analysis and reporting in their one or two markets only. These companies range from those that have significant sales figures (e.g., hundreds of millions of dollars) down to small biotech start-up companies with only one product in clinical research, no marketed products, and no sales. These companies usually establish a safety function either as a stand-alone unit with a handful of people if the volume warrants it, or they combine the function with the medical/clinical research group or the regulatory affairs group. Sometimes the drug safety department is one single person, often with other functions! (Usually Regulatory, Quality and/or Medical). The trend is to outsource some or all of these functions (e.g., data entry, aggregate report writing, etc.) to clinical or contract research organizations (CROs) or other outsourcing firms, though the pharma company will retain the final say and accountability for the cases. In certain instances, e.g., when a bolus of reports appears, the established safety group will require supplementation with temporary resources to remain in compliance. Examples of such situations include toxicology or registry reports or emergence of a pandemic. Likewise, seasonal appearance of influenza, etc., may cause pharmacovigilance staff (company, vendors, regulators, etc.) to fall ill and be unable to work

Sometimes, these companies have contractual agreements for research or sales with other companies both inside and outside their home country. These contracts oblige the company to conform to safety and regulatory requirements if the partner is outside the home country. A separate, detailed pharmacovigilance agreement and relevant training are required. That is, the second (or third, etc.) partner must send AEs and other safety information to the contracting business partner in a timely manner and in the proper format so that the business partner can remain in compliance with its local laws and regulations. These safety functions may be kept inside the company or outsourced in whole or in part.

Note: If a pharma company (large, middle-size or small) has at least one medicinal product authorized/registered in the EU, it must have an EU Qualified Person for Pharmacovigilance and set up this function (EU QPPV). For EU centrally authorized products, many EU countries require a Local Person for PV (even if the product is not marketed in these territories).

Contract/Clinical Research Organizations (CROs)

CROs are companies that handle some or all clinical and regulatory functions that pharmaceutical companies do, including phase I–IV studies, regulatory submissions, safety data, pharmacovigilance, IT matters, eCTD, IND, NDA preparation, and so forth. There are large "full-service" CROs that are almost mini-pharmaceutical companies, and there are "niche", or "boutique", CROs that specialize in one or two functions in the pharma world, such as drug safety or pharmacovigilance CROs or IT vendors supporting safety.

These CROs usually set up whatever safety system(s) are needed for their functions. If they are doing primarily clinical research, they often set up a database for entering or uploading the individual case safety reports (ICSRs) that are either sent to the sponsoring company or to the Health Authorities (U.S. FDA, EMA, etc.) For the "major" authorities, ICSRs can be sent directly in structured electronic format (E2B). For some clinical trials (per contract), the CRO sends case report forms (CRFs) as electronic data capture files (EDC). They may prepare IND or European Union DSURs/PBRERs or handle investigator notification, IRBs/Ethics Committees, and so on. Others that handle safety as their primary function may set up multiple safety databases so that they are able to use the same ones that the sponsoring company(ies) use, both for clinical trials and post-marketing data. Many of the CROs will have to support multiple databases, as their clients may use different safety databases and do not want their data transferred to a new system. Other CROs will use one single database for drug safety and arrange for data imports or data reentry between their database and the clients' databases. The trend is to one database with storage in The Cloud. There are many, many levels of complexity in the business arrangements with CROs (or other partners).

There are multiple other types of service organizations that serve the pharmaceutical industry. A listing in the DIA's (Drug Information Association) publication "Contract Service Organization Directory" includes companies providing the following services: abstract preparation; advertising; specific types of trials (e.g., AIDS); analytic laboratories; bibliography preparation; contract management; validation of assays and laboratories; specimen storage; preparation of NDAs, Biologic License Applications, PSURs/PBRERs, clinical study reports, investigator brochures, expert reports, publications, drug master files; creation and maintenance of

Pharmacovigilance System Master Files, cardiovascular monitoring; case report form preparation; central laboratories; chemistry–manufacturing–control issues; studies: phases I–IV, investigator-initiated trials, compassionate use trials, epidemiology trials, pharmacoepidemiology studies, claims support studies, safety studies; information technology services (server management, programming and software development, data migration, data management, validation); clinical pharmacology; clinical packaging; clinical supply management; study management; focus groups and consumer testing; auditing; ethics committees and investigational review boards; data safety monitoring boards; adjudication committees; digitized QTc analysis; dissolution testing; DNA diagnostics; document imaging; paper and electronic data management; translations; environmental assessments; formulation development; compliance with Good Clinical Practices, Good Manufacturing Practice, Good Laboratory Practice, Good Pharmacovigilance Practices; home infusions; intranet, internet, and website development; investigational site finding; setting up investigator meetings; licensing and acquisitions; market research; patient support programs; medical communications; medical information/call centers; medical science liaisons; microbiology testing; nursing; patient compliance, education, recruitment; preparation of labeling and patient information leaflets; process validation; project management; quality assurance and quality control; quality of life assessment; randomization; regulatory affairs; registries; remote data entry; prescription to over-the-counter switch; stability testing; standard operating procedure development; statistical services; toxicology; training; transportation; and reengineering and process redesign. New to the game are social media niche companies that deal in X (formerly Twitter), Facebook, blogs, and other evolving communication methods. Not all these organizations deal with safety or pharmacovigilance issues, although occasionally issues do come up, and the drug safety department may need to work with these companies on safety-related projects. Even if the primary purpose of a social media program is not safety-related, the company still has an obligation to assess any safety information from two-way social media communication. Artificial intelligence services are now being created to handle many of these roles and the landscape is expected to change significantly in the next few years.

The business models in the pharmaceutical world are changing. Some of the bigger CROs are actually becoming pharma companies as they in-license or purchase early or even late-stage drugs and then continue the development on their own.

Innovation is tending to come now from small start-ups and biotechs as well as from large pharmaceutical companies. The large pharma companies are now downsizing in some areas in order to specialize more deeply in fewer areas (e.g. cardiology) and outsourcing many functions to CROs and other vendors that they formerly kept in-house. They are, thus, transforming into development and marketing companies, leaving much of the innovative discovery to the smaller companies. Similarly, when large pharmas purchase small biotechs, they often inadvertently (or expressly) transform the smaller innovator into a more classic company, hobbling the innovation atmosphere. Any acquisition will force changes in the handling of safety data as one or both companies must adapt to the new products, procedures, and relationships.

Mergers, Acquisitions, and Bankruptcies

For better or worse, the pharma world is one where companies join, split, merge, and occasionally go bankrupt. No matter what the outcome of such situations, the responsibility for drug safety and pharmacovigilance remains in place, even when production and marketing cease.

When a corporate change occurs, it is the responsibility of the company (in the European Union of the QPPV) to ensure that a clear transition of responsibilities occurs and that all drug safety activities are maintained. Specifically, there must be clarity on who will be the new EU QPPV and when, what database(s) are in place, and, if more than one is in use at one time, how is compliance assured? Are all safety data exchange agreements still in place and valid with other entities? If the MA or NDA changes ownership, how is this handled to ensure that all clinical trial and post-marketing SAEs, PSURs/PBRERs, IND safety, or periodic reports are submitted correctly and on time? In other words, there must be a smooth transition to ensure that no safety issues or responsibilities are missed.

The transition teams (both internal and external, including consultants) must ensure a robust transition and make it a very high priority. There must be total continuity. Safety activities cannot stop or diminish during the handover or transition period. The concerned health authorities should be kept informed and assured that all issues have been successfully dealt with and other obligations, e.g., corrective actions, have been fulfilled.

As the merger or acquisition is usually done for financial and business reasons, safety and PV are often an afterthought and may not be addressed until very late in the negotiations, or sometimes not until after the deal is concluded. A pharmacovigilance agreement is usually a document separate from the commercial contract. This can produce operational challenges for all parties. It is desirable to have a separate document so that it can be modified when pharmacovigilance requirements change without renegotiating commercial aspects of the arrangement.

Expect a governmental inspection from one or more of the health authorities after a merger to ensure that all the requirements and systems for drug safety have been and are still in place and functioning well — during and after the transition phase; health authorities actually know that such a situation is challenging for drug safety departments.

Bankruptcies (also called liquidations) can be especially tricky if the company ceases to exist. Legal counsel should be obtained where necessary and the health agencies contacted, as needed. As always, the safety functions must continue uninterrupted.

Note: Whatever the policy defined by the pharma company regarding the organization and/or outsourcing arrangements, one main principle remains valid for any drug safety group: have real and robust oversight on all activities which are directly or indirectly part of the PV roles and responsibilities. This is a required quality function.

CHAPTER

10

The Safety Department's Role in Cross-Functional areas

The safety & PV department works closely with many other teams within and outside the Pharmaceutical Company.

■ Introduction

Historically, those who worked in clinical safety and or pharmacovigilance were locked away in their own department and office space and rarely interacted with other functional areas. Our job was mainly to receive and process safety cases, maintain the safety database, and report information to the regulatory authorities and sites, the end. Thankfully, this mindset has changed, and it will continue to develop as the cross-functional areas are educated as to what safety and pharmacovigilance truly is.

We will outline in this chapter the cross-functional areas with which the safety and pharmacovigilance function should interact and describe in what capacity they should be working together. The relationship between the safety department and others is improving in the larger scale organization space; however, this symbiotic relationship is not always realized or appreciated in small to mid-size biotech and pharmaceutical companies.

When companies and institutions truly understand the purpose of what pharmacovigilance is, and how to monitor for it throughout the life-cycle of the product, we can then understand how this function relates to CMC and pre-clinical departments, Clinical Operations, Clinical Development, Data Management, Medical Affairs, Quality & Supply, Regulatory, Labeling, Epidemiology, Biostatistics, Business Development, Marketing, Health Economics and Outcomes Research (HEOR), Legal, and so on.

If there is one chapter you could give to your Chief Medical Officer or CEO, this would be the one.

General Remarks

During the development stage of a product, safety data such as AE, SAE, pregnancy, overdose/underdose, AE of Special Interest (AESI), and other special situation reports are collected in a clinical trial database and further collected and reported in a safety database. Some other events, such as product quality events associated with AEs, events from animal and in-vitro studies, and reports of pregnancy are collected and reported outside a clinical trial database but must have the means of getting into the safety database for further evaluation and reporting. Once a product is on the market, the sources of safety data are less controlled and come from a variety of areas, most of which are not in a formalized database or system. When we start to look at the flow of safety data wholistically, we can start to appreciate how important it is for cross-functional areas to interact with pharmacovigilance groups to ensure the data is flowing to the appropriate channels.

Clinical Operations & Development

The clinical research (or medical research) department, sometimes referred to as Clinical Operations, is the section of a company (or CRO) that oversees the clinical trials and studies. There are many ways to structure such departments. Some companies have their research department do only phase 2 and 3 (developmental) trials, with a separate group handling phase 1 (clinical pharmacology and early safety studies mainly) and another group handling phase I4 (post-marketing) studies and commitments. Alternatively, there may be separate groups handling different types of products: biologics, drugs, devices, or over-the-counter (OTC) products. Other structures are by country or geographic region: US studies, EU studies, and "rest of the world" (ROW) studies. Multiple hybrids of these models exist with and without outsourcing of some of the functions.

Whatever the structure of the research division(s) may be, the drug safety department must play an active and continuous role in these groups' day-to-day activities because clinical studies almost always produce adverse events (AEs). The main areas of interaction between the two groups would be the following:

1. Project Planning and Development
   a. Drug Safety should be a primary reviewer of the protocol and Investigator Brochure, DSMB Charters and TFL documents, and protocol and site training materials
   b. Secondary reviewer of the Clinical Trial Management Plan, Medical Monitoring Plans, trial master file plans, clinical trial monitoring plans, etc.
2. Interactions regarding Signal Detection and Benefit Risk Assessment
3. Annual and Aggregate Reporting

The drug safety group must ensure that it receives all appropriate AEs from all trials. "Appropriate" usually means all serious AEs (SAEs), some or all non-SAEs, and all pregnancy cases (pregnancy is not an AE, of course, but in practice handled like AEs from a logistic point of view). In most regions there is a requirement to report certain events to the health authorities in either 7- or 15-calendar day (expedited reports) or periodically (e.g., yearly). Unless the clinical research divisions are able to receive and process such AEs themselves, these cases must be sent to the drug safety department.

The clinical research and drug safety groups must establish a process to ensure that all SAEs are reported to the company by the investigator within 24hours after occurrence at a clinical site. Note that the obligation of the investigator to report SAEs to the sponsor is clearly stated in almost all countries' regulations; e.g., FDA regulations: "An investigator must immediately report to the sponsor any SAE, whether or not considered drug-related, including those listed in the protocol or investigator brochure and must include an assessment of whether there is a reasonable possibility that the drug caused the event" (21CFR312.64(b)). This allows the company to process them and report the cases to the appropriate health authorities, particularly for the 7- or 15-calendar day SAEs.

Investigator Training and Meetings

The investigators must be trained to report SAEs, or other events of special interest according to the protocol. This is typically done during an Investigator Meeting prior to the conduct of the trial and through Site Initiation Visits (SIVs) where general protocol, product, and trial conduct information is shared. What does this mean? The safety group should be involved in the review and dissemination of safety reporting for the protocol at the Investigator Meeting and should also be involved in the development of the SIV slide decks.

Interim Analysis, Annual and final study reporting

The drug safety group should generally be involved in the creation and review of reports generated for interim analysis and for annual and final study reporting (such as DSURs and final Clinical Study Reports (CSRs)), including the final integrated safety summary for the submission dossier (e.g., CTD, MAA or NDA). This includes data reconciliation as well as supplying the "narrative" (or "capsule summary") or other data sets prepared for each case to clinical research to aid them in preparing their final study reports. Some companies now use an "automated case narrative" for SAEs. They are usually included in the CSR and the CTD/MA dossier. They are derived from the recorded information in the ICSRs in the company drug safety database. If there are post-marketing data held by drug safety, these will usually need to be supplied to the dossier as well. Any analysis or summary of data which includes AE event summaries should include a review by the appropriate drug safety and pharmacovigilance team members for accuracy and completeness. The annual and periodic reports are generally overseen by the PV groups along with regulatory, with input from the clinical operations and development groups; whereas the final clinical study reports (CSRs) are generally owned by the clinical operations and development groups. Regardless of how this is structured at a company, it is imperative that drug safety and pharmacovigilance place a significant role in the generation and review of data included in each type of report.

Signal Detection & Benefit Risk Assessment

The clinical operations, clinical development, and drug safety groups usually collaborate when a signal is being worked up or an *ad hoc* health authority question is received. For example, if a health agency asks about a particular AE or groups of AEs (e.g., acute pancreatitis or all pancreatic AEs), it is usually necessary to pull the non-SAEs from the clinical research database and the SAEs from the drug safety database to capture all similar AEs in question. Because of the way data are entered into the clinical research database (either at the end of the study or when batches of data arrive at the data entry site), the drug safety database is usually more up to date for SAEs at any one time because drug safety usually enters data immediately upon receipt, and clinical research may enter data periodically, when a group of CRFs arrives, or even at the end of the study. If EDC is used and the data are efficiently collected and distributed to both databases, this problem may be largely alleviated.

In addition, the clinical research group deals with both safety and efficacy and may feel they have a better appreciation of the balance between risk and benefit compared with the drug safety folks, who tend to see the risk side and rarely are involved in the benefit side. However, the drug safety personnel usually have better understanding of seriousness, labeledness, and (perhaps) causality, because they have more experience across many drug classes. From a practical point of view, a system of adjudication, escalation, and resolution of disagreements (e.g., serious versus non-serious) must exist and must function rapidly. In most, but not all situations, drug safety tends to have the final say on reportability of cases to the health authorities. The company does not want to be in a position where clinical research does not want a case reported as a 7- or 15-day report and drug safety does. A paper trail showing that the company did not take the most conservative position (i.e., reporting the case when there is some doubt) may be embarrassing at best and harmful at worst.

Project Planning & Development

The clinical research department and the safety department also interact at development, project planning, and risk management meetings as well as on signaling, training sessions, preparation of annual reports, investigator brochure updates, and so on. The drug safety group is also frequently charged with sending blinded or unblinded safety information to Drug Safety Monitoring Boards (DSMBs) or other data monitoring committees. These are outside independent groups that evaluate the safety profile and status of a study on an ongoing basis during the study to ensure patient safety and data integrity. This may become tricky if the drug safety group breaks individual patients' blinding codes to report the case unblinded to the health agencies and data committees but, at the same time, endeavors to maintain the blind for the clinical research and biostatistics departments. Drug safety may also assist the clinical research department in preparing data for meetings with health authorities, health agency advisory committee meetings, responses to *ad hoc* queries, and so forth.

Abstracts and Poster Presentations

Throughout product development, companies may choose to publish abstracts, white papers, and present at scientific conferences on the status of their clinical trials. This may be done to support additional funding from outside sources and to show advancement and benefits of their product compared to other competitors. Typically these presentations are developed by the clinical development team, but should be reviewed by the safety department for accuracy and care of reporting any statistics or reported outcomes relevant to perceived/potential benefits and risks. Often

Sometimes the dealings between the two departments may become strained. The clinical research physicians and staff dealing with the drug in question often feel it is "their baby" and become protective and defensive about it. This may be because they "believe" in the drug and want to give it the benefit of the doubt clinically but also for potential financial reasons: bonuses and rewards are better for drugs that succeed in clinical trials and get approved for marketing. They also may feel (sometimes correctly) that they are much more familiar with the drug, its activity, safety, and behavior, than the drug safety group, which may handle a whole array of drugs and must, of necessity, devote less time to the drug in question.

Data Management

Another area for cross-functional collaboration involves the Data Management group, along with Clinical Operations and safety. The question we generally ask is "how we will collect the AE data on the Case Report Form (CRF) in the electronic data capture (EDC) system"? How does this information get to the safety team and when? What are the desired outputs for various working groups such as DSMBs and IRBs? How will queries be addressed to the sites, via email or EDC? These groups must all work together in order to build the clinical trial database in such a way that supports the protocol design and also allows for appropriate measurement of the primary and secondary endpoints, of which often include safety data. Data Management and the clinical operations team should include safety and PV in the design, review, and edit check process when building CRFs in any database. Safety should be allowed to also review any other associated forms such as the product page where the site will capture dosing and dispending information, death pages where the site will report on fatal outcomes, as well other pages relevant to the reporting of safety information such as laboratory results, medical history, concomitant medication, and drug dosing pages. Setting up such systems requires much thought and work up-front before the study starts. Drug safety should insist on being involved in creating the system, processes, and data rules from the beginning.

Examples of such documents which collaboration is imperative include:

1. EDC development such as eCRF development and completion guidelines, User Acceptance Testing for electronic reporting of safety data Tables, Figures and Listings (TFL) review and development for summary data
2. Safety Reconciliation Plans
3. Secondary reviewer on Data Management Plans, data migration documents, data coding techniques, and any other operational document supporting the clinical trial database.

The process for collection and reporting of AEs involves the capture of the AE on the Case Report Form (CRF) or in the Electronic Data Capture (EDC) system, with transmission of the information to the company or CRO. Transmission to the company or CRO is done either electronically in the EDC system or by the older means of written case report forms or dedicated SAE collection forms that are faxed or e-mailed. This information must contain all the data necessary for the SAE case to be entered into the safety database and for preparation of an E2B transmission or a MedWatch or CIOMS I form for submission to the concerned health authorities, the clinical investigators, IRBs/Ethics Committees when required, and IDMC/DSMB if applicable. This process often involves queries to the investigator (done either by drug safety directly or via the clinical research department, or CRO). Care must be taken to avoid having multiple company departments sending repetitive questions to the investigator; usually a single point of contact is best from the company and instructions should be stated in the protocol as well as discussed at investigator meetings. This process can become exceedingly complex if SAE volume is very high, if multiple worldwide sites are involved, if a clinical research organization or other intermediaries are involved, if a cooperative group is involved (e.g., in oncology studies), or if a governmental agency (e.g., National Institutes of Health) or (non-governmental organization (NGO) is involved.

Some studies generate very large numbers of SAEs, such as oncology studies in very ill patients receiving toxic study drugs. If studies run long enough, just about every patient (whether on study drug, comparator, or placebo) will have an AE (though not necessarily an ADR) at some point during the trial. Normally, all SAEs are transmitted to the company within 1 or 2 days. However, for some studies, various protocol customizations may be done to ensure that the critical and important SAEs (those that are unexpected or related to the study drug) reach the company within 1–2 days and the health agencies within 7–15 days, though all SAEs should be sent to the sponsor immediately. Non-serious AEs may be reported to the company in a less urgent fashion (e.g., FDA requires monthly reviews, although observational data may be collected at the end of the study) and to the agencies in the annual or special periodic reports.

In some cases, arrangements may be made with the health agencies overseeing a study to report certain expected and occasionally unexpected SAEs periodically rather than as expedited reports. Most health agencies (including the FDA and EU agencies) are willing to negotiate such arrangements. For large multi-national trials, this may require negotiations with multiple national health authorities to reach a workable consensus that meets all needs. For example, a protocol might state that, because drug X in previous trials has been shown to produce mild gastrointestinal, urinary, and pulmonary hemorrhage in this patient group, these cases will not be reported until the end of the trial unless the patient dies or the patient requires a transfusion (for example). Hemorrhage from other body sites would be SAEs and reported to the company in 1–2 days. Nevertheless, before setting up such an option, careful analysis should be done regarding the implications of this. It means the company must run a continuous signal detection process on SAEs and maybe non-serious AEs. The goal is to ensure that no signal will be missed from these non-reported cases.

Many companies, especially the larger ones, maintain two "safety databases". One very common model has a safety database maintained by the drug safety department and a clinical trial database maintained by the clinical research/statistics groups. The drug safety database holds two sets of data: (1) the SAEs from clinical trials and (2) all spontaneous serious and non-serious reports; that is, most non-serious clinical trial

AEs are not kept in this safety database. This database is used for the regulatory reporting of spontaneous and clinical trial SAE expedited reports, Periodic Safety Update Reports (PSURs/PBRERs), and annual clinical trial safety reports (e.g., IND annual reports, DSURs). The clinical research department maintains the other database that holds all safety and efficacy data from clinical trials (but no spontaneous reports) and is used in preparing the final clinical study report for each study as well as safety sections for Marketing Authorization dossiers and integrated safety summaries for New Drug Application (NDA) submissions.

The data in the two databases for any given clinical trial patient may (unfortunately) be different. One reason is due to different mechanisms of data collection and collection at different times. In paper-based (non-EDC) trials, the drug safety database usually receives data from the investigator using a dedicated SAE reporting form rather than multiple pages from the case report form. The clinical trial database receives the data on the pages in the CRF that are used for SAE/AE data collection.

The data may differ if the SAE collection form is not filled in at the same time or by the same person as the CRF. Thus, the same SAE information is collected in two different places for each patient and may not be fully reconciled at the investigator site. Also, follow-up information may be entered into the CRF and not sent on the separate SAE collection form or vice versa. In addition, the drug safety group receives a clinical trial SAE within 24–48 hours after the investigator first notes it. The clinical trial database may not receive the CRF data for several weeks if the CRFs are "harvested" only every four weeks or so by the medical monitor. The use of EDC usually alleviates this problem if all the safety data are collected in the EDC and transmitted to the drug safety group. If the EDC system only collects safety data and notifies the company by an e-mail alert that a new SAE has been collected, the investigator may still end up sending a separate SAE sheet to the company, which could differ from the EDC data. So unless the safety data are collected and transmitted in only one place and manner, there is the risk of differing and incorrect or out-of-date information being present in the two company safety databases.

Other differences between the databases may occur if different people (one person in the drug safety department and one in the clinical research department) code each case differently. Follow-up information or corrected data may reach one database and not the other. More subtle differences may arise in the data that are collected. For example, for the clinical research department, the drug compliance (what percentage of the study drug was actually taken by the patient and which doses were missed) is critical. To the safety department, it is less important that the patient took 75% of the study drug versus 85% or 95%. To drug safety, it is a much more binary (yes/no) question of whether or not the drug was ingested at all (though, of course, dose-related effects may occur). Drug safety usually spends less time clarifying the dosing schedule followed by the patients than the clinical research department does.

It is thus necessary to reconcile the cases within the two databases to ensure that the data, or at least the key data, are identical. The process of reconciling the two databases, clinical and safety, is typically called Safety Database Reconciliation and should be conducted at regular intervals throughout the conduct of the trial based on either volume or timelines associated with interim reviews by DSMBs/IDMCs or internal groups. This can be a very time-consuming procedure requiring detailed case review by the drug safety and clinical research groups. Differences must be ironed out, and sometimes new queries to the investigative sites are generated from the reconciliation. The reconciliation process is simplified thanks to the EDC (one single source); but if a handwritten CRF has been used during the clinical trial, a detailed comparison is to be led: for each difference, a decision has to be taken to know which database is to be updated. Follow-up expedited SAEs can then be sent to health authorities depending on the updated information. Successful reconciliation needs to result in a high degree of medical consistency and interpretation between the two datasets, but not necessarily a 100% letter-for-letter match.

■ CROs

If the sponsor is using one or more CROs for various clinical research (or safety or regulatory or drug supply functions), the safety department should be in close and continued touch with the external CRO(s). If the

CRO is handling some or all of the safety functions for the company, there must be a clear written agreement between the parties. One or more internal groups should track, both in real time and with periodic audits and quality reviews, how the safety work is being handled. Although outsourced, the pharmaceutical company still has the legal (and moral) responsibility for the safety of its drug. It is, therefore, critical to ensure that a very detailed contract specifying which tasks are to be covered by whom with timelines is put in place prior to the start of work.

Marketing and Sales

Drug safety and marketing/sales interact in various ways. At some level in each company, a medical group (sometimes drug safety, sometimes medical affairs, sometimes regulatory, sometimes another group) must review advertising and promotional copy for drugs to be sure that the medical and safety claims are correct. That is, the claims made by the company must correctly reflect the information contained in the official labeling (approved Package Insert in the US, SmPC in the EU, etc.).

Marketing will often ask drug safety for information on AEs for their own uses (to help sell more product). Although it is hard to refuse to supply such data, drug safety should remind the marketers that spontaneous drug safety data cannot, as a rule, be used for promotional activities or safety claims.

Drug safety may also be asked to supply data that the customer relations department (often within marketing, where technical and scientific questions are directed) uses to prepare responses to patients' or healthcare professionals' medical queries ("Have you ever seen pulmonary emboli with this drug in young women? If yes, how did the patients do and how were they treated?"). Some companies might make the safety data available to more groups in the company than drug safety. This may be a dangerous course to take if the data are used for inappropriate (if not flat-out illegal) purposes. It is a wise policy to let the drug safety group be the gatekeeper for the drug safety data.

In the evaluation of signals and in the production of certain reports (PSURs/PBRERs, PADERs, etc.) and other required reports for regulatory agencies, it is necessary for drug safety to obtain drug use data, such as sales data, patients using the drug, tonnage shipped, or prescriptions written, to estimate a reporting frequency of AEs. These data are usually obtained and kept by the marketing and sales departments. Sometimes they are generated internally and sometimes they are purchased from outside vendors who track prescriptions and sales. This is another area of interaction between drug safety and marketing/sales.

Drug safety often does training of sales representatives, advertising copywriters, and others in the marketing and sales departments in regard to the reporting of AEs. Although the sales force generally believes that its job is to sell drugs and not collect AEs, it is now generally understood by all parties that sales representatives (as well as all company employees, agents, etc.), when they hear of AEs on their products, have an obligation to report them to the safety department for follow-up and regulatory reporting. For example, when the commercial groups conduct customer engagement programs, e.g., disease management, patient support programs over the Internet or by phone or by personal visits, etc., they must have a way to assess the risk of these programs for non-compliance. If there is the possibility for two-way communication between the company and its customers, there is the possibility for the company to receive safety information. Such information will usually be considered "solicited", which requires a validity check, labeledness and seriousness determinations, and also a causality assessment. Even though the main purpose of the program is commercial and unrelated to safety data collection, if the company becomes aware of safety information on its products, there is a safety obligation to address. This usually requires extensive training.

In a more subtle way, drug safety must also influence and reinforce its ethical and legal role with marketing and sales. Many salespeople, particularly those handling over-the-counter products, do not fully comprehend that the pharmaceutical industry, along with the financial and nuclear power industries, is among the most regulated industries in the world. The limitations, reporting obligations, and safety issues are often not in the mindset of marketers and salespeople, whose job and pay depend on product sales. It is drug safety that often must set the limits on what marketing and sales can and may do. For this reason, the marketers often call the drug safety department the "sales prevention department" and the head safety physician "Dr. No". If the company management does not appreciate this and does not ensure that safety is handled properly, the company may suffer severe regulatory, legal, and sales consequences, particularly if a safety issue arises.

The drug safety department is a cost center that never produces revenue and profit for a company. This tends to produce, in some drug safety people, a siege mentality because they carry little weight in the corporate hierarchy and are continually "fighting" to get their message out. The primary goal of the safety department, of course, is to prevent patient harm, ensure compliance, and protect the public health. This viewpoint is sometimes not shared by others in the company who believe that the safety department's primary job is to protect the company's products at all costs. In fact, by doing correct and complete safety work, the safety department proactively protects the company's products so that, at some point down the road, when the safety issues arise, they will not produce drug withdrawals, lawsuits, and patient harm. However, this is often a hard concept to "sell to the sales department". Potential dollars not lost in the future do not appear on balance sheets or get people raises and bonuses.

■ The Labeling Department

The drug safety department will have some role in label creation and maintenance. Labeling is defined broadly and includes the marketed labeling (Package Insert, SmPC, PIL, CCDS/CCSI, wording on the box or package, etc.) as well as the Investigator Brochure for drugs in clinical trials (many companies still prefer the IB to be created and updated by Clinical Development). At the simplest level, drug safety supplies AE information to the department (e.g., regulatory affairs, medical writing, dedicated label departments) that creates and maintains the label. The safety department may also be charged with periodic or continuous label review to ensure that the label contains the latest scientific and medical information. This may mean that the safety department must notify the appropriate departments of new AEs worthy of being put into the label (usually with due process and prior approval by a labeling or safety committee), changes in the pregnancy status of a drug, new warnings, contraindications, and precautions both for the product and for the whole class of drugs ("class labeling"). It is also worthwhile for the drug safety or labeling department to scan the drugs labels of other companies' products for the appearance in these other drugs' labeling of a new drug interaction with other marketed drugs. The actual division of these duties is not clearly standardized and varies from company to company.

■ The Legal Department

The drug safety department may be involved with the legal department when AEs are reported in cases under litigation or when there is threat of litigation. In such instances, the lawyers usually forbid the drug safety department to have direct contact with the patient or healthcare providers. All contact to obtain further safety information is usually done through the company's legal department. In addition, one or more people from the drug safety department (usually physicians) may be subpoenaed to testify in cases involving the company and safety issues related to its products. This involves "witness training" for those at risk to be called on to testify in court or to give depositions.

It is also common, when a company is being sued, for the plaintiff's attorneys to request copies of safety information. This process is called "discovery". The safety department may be forced to stop work to prepare or assist in preparing paper or electronic copies of hundreds to thousands of pages of material needed in a very tight time frame. In the worst case, the drug safety department may have its paper or electronic files sealed to prevent any changes or the adding of new information. Drug safety is also heavily involved in preparing the company's defense in such cases and in evaluating claims that have not yet reached litigation.

In some companies, the legal department may have some say in review of the expedited reports, PSURs/PBRERs, RMPs/REMS, submissions (MAAs, NDAs), PVSMF and other documents and reports produced by the safety department. This may be a two-sided coin, as the legal department will not want drug safety to indicate that the drug may have caused an AE. This can be very problematic as companies are expected to make judgments in signaling reports, expedited reports, PSURs/PBRERs, and other documents in regard to causality. The legal department may not want such "admissions" made that could come back to bite the company should a court case arise.

The legal department may be helpful in setting up safety data exchange agreements with other companies to ensure that the company receives all appropriate safety information. In the same spirit, any outsourced PV activity must be contracted with the support of the legal department. Likewise, co-development and co-marketing agreements must have clear responsibilities written in a Pharmacovigilance Agreement (PVA).

In practice, when wisdom prevails, the drug safety group and the legal department are allies in the desire for the facts and the science to be handled correctly, transparently, and honestly. This is always the best policy for the company, the patients, the healthcare professionals, and the stockholders, though in the heat of battle and fog of war this may not be evident.

■ Regulatory Affairs Department

The drug safety department's function is primarily regulatory. In some companies, particularly small ones, the regulatory group may also handle some drug safety functions, such as the submission of safety and aggregate reports to the authorities.

Drug safety is typically responsible for the preparation and submission of expedited reporting (7- and 15-day reports, MedWatch for IND/CIOMS I reports, E2B reports), IND Annual Reports/DSURs, PSURs/PBRERs, and NDA periodic reports and such to the health agencies and similar reports to business partners and others. However, sometimes the regulatory department will own the actual submission and maintain the communication between the company and the agencies. The regulatory department may sometimes have a role in reporting cases to the health agencies depending on the size and structure of the company (e.g., sometimes assigning a special number to each submission, such as a serial number for FDA reporting) or tracking such cases. This requires careful and detailed procedures to ensure that reports are not lost or sent in late. Regulatory affairs is usually the intermediary in any direct contact between health agencies and the safety department and other departments in the company, because most companies prefer to carefully control and monitor all communications with health authorities. Most company employees are not permitted to contact the health agencies directly but must go through regulatory affairs, whether in the home office or in subsidiaries or affiliates. Nevertheless, some functions/positions can free themselves of such company constraints. For example, the EU QPPV role, as designed by the EU regulations, must be available 24/7 by the EMA and is required to provide answers directly to the health agency contacting him/her.

Some issues may arise if a company has been operating in only one country (studies and sales) and expands to one or more other countries. The regulatory department may be totally versed in US requirements but not in the requirements elsewhere. Drug Safety and Regulatory will have to rapidly come up to speed on external requirements.

The health authorities may approach the company and request that a labeling change be made. Such communications will usually go to the regulatory department (whether in the home office or in the local affiliate, partner, or subsidiary) as the point of entry into the company. This usually results in the company's invoking an SOP-defined process or setting up a rapid response team or task force, including drug safety, clinical research, regulatory, medical affairs, legal and animal toxicology, to respond to the request.

■ The Quality and Compliance Department

The drug safety group interacts with the quality group and the compliance group (which may be the same group or different groups) both in regard to the safety department's duties and in regard to assisting in technical matters when these groups are dealing with safety issues in other departments.

For drug safety functions, the quality/compliance group may assist and oversee preparation of SOPs, processes, and interactions within the company to be sure the group is handling its functions correctly. They may also audit the drug safety group periodically and assist in or oversee any Corrective Action/Preventive Action Plans (CAPAs) that might be the outcome of the audit. They will also assist in and sometimes take the operational lead in handling and responding to external audits and governmental inspections of the drug safety group. They may be involved in audits of investigator sites, vendors and contract research organizations, business partner standard operating procedures and safety data, and manufacturing safety issues. This is highly variable from company to company and with the terms of the business agreement. As with legal, the quality and compliance group should, ideally, work as partners with the drug safety group rather than purely as overseers and "police".

■ New Business Due Diligence

When a company wishes to purchase or in-license or out-license or co-develop a product, good business practice requires examination of the data set for the product to be acquired or divested. This includes the review of manufacturing data, standard operating procedures, animal toxicology and pharmacology data, clinical data, regulatory correspondence with the health agencies, and so forth. The drug safety department may be called in during this "due diligence" review to examine the clinical safety data, including expedited reports (E2B, MedWatch and CIOMS forms), risk management plans, PSURs/PBRERs and NDA periodic reports, clinical trial annual reports and IND annual reports, health agency queries and other interactions, documentation, archives, and all sorts of other safety information. Sometimes the needed data are available electronically, sometimes on paper, or both. Sometimes it is aggregate data primarily, and other times it is less well-organized individual patient safety information. For a drug that has not been tested in humans or only minimally so, the data may be sparse; for a marketed drug, it may be extensive.

In general, the safety evaluation of a drug should include all clinical trial and post-marketing safety data, regulatory correspondence, and animal toxicology data. Attention should be paid, in clinical trial data, to drop-outs, deaths, lack of efficacy, and lost-to-follow-up cases and any other areas where safety data might be lurking. The safety department should take the view that the information supplied to them is data intended to "make the sale" and as such it will highlight favorable information and put less favorable data in the background. Although the outright hiding of safety data is rare, it is not unheard of, and the safety reviewer should approach the due diligence duty with healthy skepticism. The safety reviewer cannot say yes or no to the company's in-licensing a product but must spell out the safety and risk part of the "benefit–risk" analysis that the company performs.

■ Pre-Clinical Toxicology and Pharmacology

According to US FDA 21 CFR 312.32.c.iii, IND safety reports are also required when there are findings from animal and invitro studies. The regulation states: "*The sponsor must report any findings from animal or in vitro testing, whether or not conducted by the sponsor, that suggest a significant risk in humans exposed to the drug, such as reports of mutagenicity, teratogenicity, or carcinogenicity, or reports of significant organ toxicity at or near the expected human exposure. Ordinarily, any such findings would result in a safety-related change in the protocol, informed consent, investigator brochure (excluding routine updates of these documents), or other aspects of the overall conduct of the clinical investigation*". This means that companies should have procedures in place to review findings from such studies and make a determination of any of them pose a risk to humans. Individuals within the safety and pre-clinical teams should ideally be asking the following questions:

1. Is there an ongoing communication between these two groups so that each are aware of the number and type of animal and invitro studies ongoing?
   a. Is there a list of these types of studies?
   b. How is safety informed of the outcome of these studies?
2. Do we define what will constitutes a "significant risk" when we are evaluating animal and invitro data?
   a. If defined in a SOP, who will review the cumulative data to identify these risks and at what frequency?
   b. If a safety concern is identified, has the company defined day 0 for reporting purposes? It generally is the date the decision was made that the event may suggest a possible risk in humans. This means that there should be a documented decision tree, form, or minutes that can clearly identify the time course for identifying, evaluating, and then determining a specific finding poses human risk.

Drug safety and PV must interact with these groups when animal and laboratory testing results are needed for safety evaluations and in ongoing drug life cycle risk management evaluations. Sometimes the drug safety group will need to go back to the animal data to analyze a signal or safety issue to see whether there were any early clues in the pre-clinical data. Other times, the toxicology group may call on drug safety should they find a striking safety concern in an animal study that may produce a 15-day expedited report. Sometimes, the drug safety group is called on to assist, as these reports are generally quite rare and the toxicology groups ask for assistance from drug safety and regulatory in preparation of the submissions. But too often, the drug safety group is forced to remind non-clinical team to contact them if important toxicology or pharmacology finds are noted which could impact the clinical safety.

In the EU regulations, the EU QPPV is expected to be informed of such findings. The company may be chastised if he/she is not informed in due time of such safety issues.

■ Signaling and Epidemiology Groups

Drug safety will often interact on a very tight basis with these groups to supply data as well as to sit in on sessions that analyze, evaluate, and prepare further actions (e.g., clinical trials, epidemiology studies, registries). Coordination regarding signals noted in PSURs/PBRERs or other reports prepared by drug safety should be done with the signaling and epidemiology groups. Joint meetings are usually held periodically. This varies from company to company. In large pharma companies, a Pharmacoepidemiology/Epidemiology group, at the corporate level, is now a standard; this helps to manage newly identified signals in the best and rapid manner.

■ The Medical Information/ Medical Affairs Department

Drug safety may interact with the internal or external groups handling communications into and out of the company. For incoming questions, this will include complaints, AEs, product quality issues, and queries from patients, consumers, and healthcare professionals. The safety group should ensure that SOPs are in place that will get AEs, particularly SAEs, to the drug safety group in a timely manner with all the appropriate information allowing follow-up by the safety group. The medical information department may also handle after-hours communications. That is, they may set up either internal or outsourced systems (e.g., phone centers, poison control centers) to receive after-hours AEs and complaints. Drug safety should be sure that all processes are in place to ensure that such AEs and complaints get to drug safety promptly.

Drug safety may also supply safety information for queries to the medical information department that go beyond the official labeling. That is, most companies do not allow their staff to make medical judgments or give clinical advice on their drugs. The usual responses follow the officially approved labeling and go no further. However, sometimes, physician-to-physician requests come into the company, asking certain questions that go beyond the labeling (e.g., "Have pulmonary emboli been seen with this drug and if so, what was the course and treatment?"). The drug safety group may be requested to supply data from its database to answer such questions.

Manufacturing (Product Quality Complaints)

In the signal analysis of a product, it is not sufficient to simply examine AE data. The signal reviewer must also review product quality complaints. It is entirely possible that the AE is due to a problem in the manufacturing process that produced an impurity, an unstable product, an excipient issue, a manufacturing process, a counterfeit product, or a vendor change that produced unforeseen bad effects. This is surprisingly common, as companies change vendors frequently for raw materials and product containers and make process changes when efficiencies or new machines are available. These are all done under appropriate change control (or should be), but unintended consequences can occur. For this reason, the signal review must include product quality complaints and drug safety must communicate frequently with colleagues in the manufacturing area when issues arise.

Falsified products (counterfeits) may lead to product complaints or safety issues. There must be an established process for the safety group to rapidly communicate information on suspected or possible counterfeits to the product complaint group. Whether the initial report turns out to be a product complaint or a safety concern the loop must be closed and supply chain security will often engage, depending on initial findings.

General Remarks

Integrating pharmacovigilance and safety professionals across a company is difficult and often challenging, no matter the size of the company. One may find themselves often vying for "a seat at the proverbial table", if only to ensure the company is protected and adhering to specific regulations. One of the ways to improve cross-functional engagement is to first train and educate those in other areas. It may simply be a result of others not knowing what our purpose is and how the data and interactions between other GxP areas impact pharmacovigilance. Giving the power of knowledge to others will improve cross-functional outcomes and we have found that by approaching other groups with an attitude of "why we are asking these questions" instead of "we must" and "we have to" attitudes, will lend to a more productive and collaborative conversation. It is also important that senior management is aware of the need for cross-functional collaboration. Educating them will also likely smooth the way for success.

CHAPTER

11

Organization of a Typical Drug Safety Department

This description covers a "standard" safety department found in a large or mid-sized (multinational) pharmaceutical company. Some functions and divisions do not exist in smaller companies or in companies that do not have international or research functions. Some functions are combined with others. Some functions may work with other divisions in the corporation in addition to the safety department. In a smaller company, one individual may need to wear the proverbial "many hats." Finally, we summarize the skills needed to work in pharmacovigilance (PV).

Introduction

There is not one single valid organization structure for a pharmacovigilance (PV) department; each pharma company has its own history, product types, territories, licensing partners, etc. which can explain or justify differences in each organization. The main principle remains to ensure that the DS department head (or the EU qualified person for pharmacovigilance (QPPV) or the Chief Medical Officer) has real and robust oversight of the DS organization and its performance. The goals here are to (1) Ensure the best possible protection for patients and the public health (2) Maintain all PV roles and responsibilities in accordance with current regulations and practices, and (3) Meet all PV obligations with licensing partners. Below is an overview of the main functions that are needed. Depending on the company's size and reach, some can be grouped or split, but generally, all of these areas should be covered in some fashion.

Organization

The department which collects, studies, and reports on safety information gathered from clinical trials and postmarketing data can be called a variety of names: Drug Safety Department, Clinical Drug Safety & Pharmacovigilance, Global Safety & Pharmacovigilance, Safety and Risk Management, Product Safety and Development, etc. There isn't one right or wrong way, but the department title should reflect its goals and purpose within an organization and should also have a clear position and structure just like any other functional area.

Generally, companies have a physician who is designated "chief safety officer", "chief medical officer", or "QPPV" who is (usually) a senior-level physician (e.g., executive or senior vice president) and is responsible for the final decision on medical issues for the corporation. This job includes decisions on product restrictions and withdrawals, stopping clinical trials, amending protocols, changing product labeling, and so forth, for safety reasons. This person is either in the senior management of the company or in regulatory affairs or clinical research. In many companies, the QPPV is different from the senior medical officer and is sometimes not a physician.

There is also a functional head of drug safety, who ensures that the department runs in a timely, orderly, and professional manner. In smaller companies, the chief safety officer and the functional head may be the same person. That person is usually a healthcare professional. In larger companies, they tend to be separated, especially if the company has several major safety units around the world.

A typical chain of command within a safety organization would be that the unit reports directly into the Chief Medical Officer and is overseen by a Head of Safety, or President/Vice President of Global Safety Operations. The remaining composition of the department will depend on its size, the current stage of development, and the number of products and types of products it has. It will also depend on if the company has developed an in-house (most safety activities are performed by company employees) or primarily outsourced (most safety activities have been outsourced to vendors and CROs) model.

Small to Mid-Size Companies

Small to mid-size companies can often function with around 5–15 employees, but will also highly depend on the structure. At a minimum, a safety department should be overseen by a Head of Safety, reporting into the CMO, and supported by at least 2 individuals for business continuity purposes. Most companies in the Phase 1 and 2 spaces will outsource these roles to consultants or contractors until they are confident in their products ability to meet primary and secondary endpoints.

Large Companies

Larger sized companies, typically more than 800–1000 full time employees, will have a wider range of positions within the safety department, and may also have different "arms" that focus on a particular product, compound, or device. Larger companies will also tend to bring more of the safety operations in-house and primarily outsource safety case processing, database management, literature searching and social media monitoring to vendors, keeping safety case medical assessment, reporting, signaling, and benefit risk in-house.

Triage Unit

The triage unit is responsible for receiving and reviewing, often at a single central point, all incoming adverse events (AEs), plus, in many situations, product complaints, requests for information from consumers and healthcare professionals, requests for reimbursement, and other medical information functions. Each incoming contact is routed to the appropriate department (person) for handling. Decisions have to be made if a single incoming contact has several components: "I took your pill, which was red instead of its normal blue color; I had chest pain after I took it — is that normal? And I want my money back." This is a product quality complaint, an AE, a question, and a request for reimbursement. In general, the priority should go to the AE and quality issue. Routes of entry of AEs are changing. Formerly, phone calls and letters were predominant. Now, phone calls, e-mail, websites, social media, and other electronic avenues bring in many post-marketing AEs. "Snail mail", case reports of clinical trial AEs, reports from a health authority, medical literature screening, lawsuits, and other assorted sources also supply AEs.

Some drugs have more AEs reported by healthcare practitioners and others by consumers and patients. Triage must be rapid and in real time because expedited (7- and 15-day) reports need to be acted on immediately. Serious AE cases should be reviewed with more urgency than non-serious cases.

The triage is usually made up of both professional and clerical personnel whose job is to do the first-level screening of all incoming contacts. Telephone calls are usually screened initially by call centers with or without medically trained personnel (pharmacists, nurses) as the initial responders. E-mail, website information and social media as well as any other electronically arriving AEs may first be seen by clerical or IT staff but must be routed rapidly to medical professionals to perform the medical triage. Snail (postal) mail with possible AE information must be handled rapidly by personnel in the mailroom. The clock for expedited reports begins ticking when the information hits the mailroom or when it is available to a member of company staff on a computer, etc.

In multinational companies, there is usually a triage group locally to handle phone calls and written communications arriving in the local language. US phone centers often are able to handle calls in English and often Spanish and sometimes other languages. In Canada, English and French are required. Many companies are now moving call centers "offshore", especially to India, the Philippines, Eastern Europe, and other English-speaking countries, as well as to Latin America for Spanish-language calls. Cost savings can be substantial, though time zone and cultural differences may also present significant challenges. Obviously, these centers must function at the same level and under the same regulatory requirements as if they were in the US. The FDA will hold them to US standards if they receive calls from US patients and physicians. Similarly, other health agencies will require domestic standards to be applied to external centers as well.

At this stage, many companies require the Triage Unit team to record the basic information (mainly administrative) for each case report in an IT system (tracking tool or safety database). The purpose is not to record exhaustive information but to check for duplicate reports and to ensure that all case reports received are actually recorded and not lost. If, when first received, a report is not considered "valid", i.e., does not include the four validity criteria (identifiable patient, suspect medication, AE and identifiable reporter) the report should still be entered into the database in anticipation of follow-up information. This will also facilitate the next steps (assessment, prioritization, data entry, processing, medical review, transmission) in the case handling process.

■ Case Assessment and Prioritization

A medical professional should rapidly review the cases for seriousness, expectedness (labeledness), and causality (for clinical trial cases). Priority then goes to AEs that are potentially 7- or 15-day expedited reports. The personnel must have all the needed tools (computer access and training, latest labeling and investigator brochures, etc.).

■ Data Entry Unit

After triage, cases must be medically evaluated (if not already done) and entered into the safety database (if not already done either manually or electronically). Cases that come in electronically, such as from clinical trial electronic data capture programs or post-marketing cases from online data entry forms, partner databases, and so forth, usually do not need to be reentered unless the sending database and the receiving safety database cannot "talk" to each other. Rather, these cases may sit in an electronic "holding area" and must be screened by the triage or medical personnel for minimum validity criteria, correct drug identification, duplicates, quality and so forth, before being uploaded into the safety database. Uploading is normally instantaneous when done electronically and has implications for the "clock start date". Some companies may allow direct upload into their safety database from trusted, validated, and virus-free sources, such as partner companies or CROs.

Paper cases (including faxed, PDF, or other "paper cases" that arrive "electronically" but not in files that are directly uploadable as structured data) must be manually entered into the database. Cases that are identified at triage to be expedited reports are usually prioritized for immediate data entry. Cases that are not expedited reports are put into a queue for handling and data entry. Serious cases that are to be manually entered are usually "databased" within 7–15 days and non-serious cases within 30 days. Companies' procedures vary widely. The EU requires non-serious cases to be submitted electronically within 90 days.

The initially received information is entered into the drug safety database after screening for the four minimum criteria, the correct drug, and duplicates. Data entry is usually performed by clerical personnel who have been trained on how to enter cases into the company's safety database and sometimes after training in medical terminology. Some companies do manual data entry at a single site or at multiple sites (e.g., one on each continent). Most data, though not all, are entered in English. Some documents may need to be translated. Source documents may also be entered (either summarized or scanned in or both), catalogued, and stored in the database. Some data may need to be anonymized or redacted to remove personal information. See the chapter on Data Privacy.

■ Case Processing Unit

This unit is made up of health professionals, usually nurses and pharmacists, but occasionally also podiatrists, dentists, and other healthcare professionals. This group does the initial evaluation for expedited cases (as noted above, usually before data entry) and then reviews and/or prepares the case medical information. In particular, this involves the creation of the "narrative" (which is a stand-alone chronological text summary of the case that appears in the electronic case [E2B] or on the MedWatch and CIOMS I forms if still used), and the verification of drug names, dosages, past medical history, and so on. The case-processing group also prepares medical queries (with the assistance of the physicians) to be sent to the reporter or investigator to obtain further information if the initial data are incomplete, including the final outcome for ongoing cases.

■ Medical Case Review

This group is usually composed of physicians with expertise in drug safety and case review. They generally review the assessment, the AE coding, and the medical content of the narrative to ensure that the medical story is cogent and that it is a true reflection of the source data supplied. These physicians may also handle other work, including the preparation and review of signals, aggregate reports, and *ad hoc* queries.

■ Transmission Unit

This group ensures that the appropriate cases are sent to the appropriate recipients. Expedited reports either go directly to the health agencies (usually by electronic E2B transmission or paper) or to the regulatory department for transmission to the health authorities. Cases may also be sent within the company to other interested parties (e.g., clinical research, legal) and to associated business partners who market or study the drug. This function may be assumed by a unit that handles all safety "traffic" matters, including triage, routing, and transmission. If the transmission is via E2B there may not be a separate transmission unit, though someone must still track what goes where and handle electronic acknowledgement of receipt.

PV Regulatory Intelligence

Usually part of Regulatory Affairs, but sometimes within PV departments, a regulatory intelligence unit is needed to identify new and future regulations or guidances. (This is the responsibility of the EU QPPV in the EU). A PV department must always be up to date on new or updated regulations to remain compliant. In addition, the responsibility of this team is to assess the consequences for the PV team (organization, processes, tools, goals, etc.) of a new or future regulation.

Regulatory Unit

Usually, this unit is not a part of drug safety but is a separate division, at least in larger companies. In some companies, expedited cases are reviewed by the regulatory group before transmission to the health authority as a final quality check. Many companies prefer to have all communications to and from the health authorities handled by the regulatory division rather than by drug safety and other groups to ensure tight tracking of all governmental contacts.

Legal Unit

This unit is never a part of drug safety. The legal unit interacts with drug safety in three primary areas.

First, in some companies, the legal department reviews all cases that are sent to health agencies to ensure that "troublesome" statements will not be included and, thus, avoid statements that could inadvertently produce difficulties for the company. (This is controversial, as it may mean that the company cannot make a causality assessment on cases, as that might mean admitting the drug and the company are "guilty" of causing that ADR.)

The second area involves litigation or potential litigation based on AEs. In these cases, the drug safety and legal areas work tightly together in defending the litigation and in obtaining any follow-up from the suing party. Such follow-up is often done via the attorneys rather than directly from drug safety. The legal unit may also be a source of AEs that arise in lawsuits against the company that first arrive in the legal department.

The third area is in negotiating agreements with external parties for in- or out-licensing, outsourcing, co-marketing, and so forth. The two groups work together to ensure that all safety obligations to all health authorities and business partners are met.

Signaling, Pharmacovigilance, Pharmacoepidemiology, Medical Information or Medical Affairs Unit

Although this function may be called many things, as noted in the heading, its primary job is to look for new safety signals. This unit is made up of physicians and other healthcare workers. Their main function is to review the safety data (AEs, medical errors, and product quality complaints) collected by the company and to evaluate whether new signals are popping up or old ones are resolving or worsening. They may use tools available commercially or developed in-house for data mining When an issue is found, they begin an initial safety investigation that includes a review of the published literature, the company's clinical research database (if different from the safety database), external databases, medical literature (which must be searched weekly under EU regulatory requirements), toxicology, pharmacology, and any other relevant information, to prepare a summary report for presentation to the decision-makers (e.g., the senior corporate safety committee) for resolution.

They may handle other functions, including review of individual cases, preparation of Investigational New Drug Application (IND) annual report, New Drug Application (NDA) periodic reports (PADERs), Development Safety Update Reports (DSURs), Periodic Safety Update Reports (PSURs/PBRERs), integrated safety summaries, responses to queries from health authorities, pharmacoepidemiology studies and analyses, advertising review for medical content, review of communications to the public ("Dear Doctor" or "Dear Healthcare Professional" letters), review of labeling (e.g., Package Inserts or SmPCs, etc.), medical testimony in litigation, and consultation on drug restrictions or withdrawals. Some of these functions may be split into separate groups, such as a PSUR/PBRER preparation group, a pharmacoepidemiology group, and so forth, particularly in large companies.

This group may also handle the preparation of risk management documents such as REMS or RMPs.

■ Aggregate Report Preparation

This unit, comprising physicians and other healthcare professionals, sometimes separate from the PV unit, prepares aggregate or summary reports of data derived from ICSRs and sometimes other sources. These reports include IND annual, NDA periodic reports, DSURs, PSURs/PBRERs, benefit–risk assessment reports, *ad hoc* and PSUR/PBRER-derived queries from health authorities, and other corporate departments or business partners. They will sometimes prepare white papers or literature reviews for internal and external scientific requests for information.

Large and mid-sized pharma companies are out-sourcing more and more of these tasks.

■ Labeling Review and Update for Safety

This function is sometimes done within drug safety and sometimes separately by the labeling group or regulatory affairs. It usually involves the clinical department and requires the continuous monitoring of the labeling of the company's products to ensure that all the safety (and other required labeling information) is fully up to date and the transition to new labeling format and content requirements in various countries is being performed accurately and in a timely manner. This includes examination of the reference safety information (CCSI or regulator-approved professional labeling), as well as local labeling documents (e.g., US PI, the EU SmPC, etc.) and patient information leaflets. Areas of interest include AE, warnings, precautions, contraindications, pregnancy and lactation, overdose, drug interactions, and off-label use. This may be a very substantial task if the company sells multiple drugs with multiple formulations in many countries around the world.

For labeling updates, the PV department is responsible for identifying and managing the safety signals, being a part of the team making proposals for any possible labeling updates, as well as helping to deliver a rationale supporting the proposed labeling update.

It may also require the monitoring of the safety labeling of products of other companies' drugs in the same class as well as drugs that may have interactions with the company's drugs. For example, if company B adds a statement to its drug's labeling stating that there is a drug interaction between the company B drug and a company A drug, company A should determine whether it should add a similar statement to its labeling. In most jurisdictions a generic product must follow the labeling of the innovator product.

Qualified (Responsible) Person for Pharmacovigilance

This is a critical role for companies with marketing authorizations in the EU and a large number of other countries. This important role is discussed in greater detail elsewhere in this manual. (See Specific Chapter on EU QPPV)

■ Archive/File Room

Archiving involves several issues. First, there is now an enormous amount of electronic information, including e-mails, electronic case reports, lab data, and computer files and programs. This is critical data that must be backed up and archived. This is usually an IT function, which is transparent to the drug safety group. This has become, with the advent of electronic storage and data security and privacy rules, a very complicated matter. Hacking may now become a problem.

In terms of paper, although there is a trend toward the so-called paperless office, the amount of paper and the number of photocopy machines used for drug safety appear to be decreasing only marginally. The safety department must make sure they have an adequate archive/file room system (including shredders to securely dispose of draft documents), such that all relevant safety information is saved in the appropriate place and is readily available for immediate review, whether by the company or during a health authority inspection. In terms of electronic data, secure server parks (or "The Cloud") with backup and all appropriate privacy and data protection must be in place. If multinational data are stored in a server or the Cloud then all applicable laws and requirements from the data's source country must be in place.

Several logistical decisions need to be made for both paper and electronic archiving concerning the following things:

1. The storage of documents in a multinational company where serious AE reports may come in multiple languages: Should they be kept in the country where they are received (and are able to be read) or centrally or both? What should be translated? And if translated, what must be "officially" translated and what can be translated using a fast but inaccurate computer translation program?
2. Are the storerooms adequately protected from fire, flood, insects, vermin, and other hazards? Should sprinkler systems specifically not be installed but rather an alternative system used for fire protection?
3. Storing paper charts for tens of thousands of cases per year (in a large company) can require large physical storage areas. Should these cases be kept on site or archived in a document storage facility off-site?
4. What tracking system will be used? Should bar codes or chips be used for paper files, and, if so, for the folder jacket or for every document inside? If a case has some parts stored as paper and some as electronic files, should they be merged and all stored electronically? How should they be indexed and tracked? How will follow-up data be stored and indexed?
5. How long should documents and electronic files be retained? Note that retention rules differ for various jurisdictions. In general, documents should be retained for the longest time required by any country whose documents are stored in that archive. Some companies keep all safety data forever.
6. Who has access to and control of the file room and electronic files? Access should be for appropriately qualified persons and only on a need-to-know basis.
7. What backup methods are used (e.g., in case of fire or water damage, etc.) for paper and electronic records?
8. Are all privacy and anonymization regulations being followed? Are the new EU requirements in place?
9. If contract facilities (outside vendors) are used, who supervises them and ensures the safe keeping of the files and the ability to retrieve needed files (e.g., for a health authority inspection) within 24 hours?
10. Are paper and electronic files reconciled?

Note 1: One of the best options is to scan, or upload and attach relevant documents to each ICSR within the safety database. A decision must be made on whether to retain the paper copy. Ideally, no, but there may be legal and regulatory implications.

Note 2: Employee emails are often backed up on a daily (or more frequent) basis and retained in an archive according to company retention policy. The usual retention policy is ordinarily placed on indefinite hold when litigation is involved for any given product.

Information Technology/ Informatics Liaison

Almost all drug safety departments use a commercial database to store safety data and produce required output in prescribed timeframes. There is usually a dedicated informatics/information technology (IT) support and development group that works with drug safety ("the business owners") to support the database and handle changes, bugs, new hires and access levels, upgrades, MedDRA® and other dictionaries, testing, and validation. Sometimes the IT support person(s) report directly to the drug safety group and sometimes not.

Usually, the IT group is fully versed in the IT aspects of the database but needs business input from a "superuser" or drug safety expert who understands the safety business and issues and who can speak the "IT language" to facilitate communication. This IT liaison function has various titles from company to company but is found in nearly all companies because the need to bridge the gap between the computer experts and the safety experts is real and ongoing.

In large companies, the 24/7 maintenance of the multiple databases involved in safety in one way or another (clinical trial database, ePRO-electronic patient recorded outcomes, safety database, telephone call tracking database, product complaint database, labeling database, etc.) requires IT departments of scores or even hundreds of persons all around the world (wherever someone has a computer or smart-phone, etc.). Linking databases and ensuring database-to-database communications (E2B), internally as well as with business partners, and keeping up to date on other data standardization matters, is now a major operation in most companies.

■ Quality Documents Creation and Maintenance

Written formal SOPs, working documents, and guidances are obligatory in drug safety departments under Good Clinical Practices (GCP) requirements from the International Conference on Harmonization (ICH), the FDA, the European Medicines Agency (EMA), and other agencies and bodies. In addition, there may be manuals, guidances, and job aids that accompany the SOPs (e.g., a data entry manual).

The first thing an FDA, EMA, inspector or internal company auditor will ask for at the start of an inspection or audit is often a copy of the organizational chart of the safety department and list of the Quality Documents in place. The SOPs govern the handling of everything in PV: safety data, report preparation, training, database and computer issues, crisis management, and so forth.

It is not uncommon for a company to have 50 or more such SOPs and guidances. The creation, review (yearly at least), maintenance, and updating of SOPs is a function that must be ensured in a safety department and must reflect any changes in regulatory requirements. The issue of version control of quality documents must also be addressed so that everyone has access to and is working from the latest versions of the SOPs and work instructions. This means controlled distribution of electronic (or paper copies) of the latest and applicable quality document (QD) for each particular job function.

■ Training

Another requirement of GCP and quality systems is that training be done and documented *before* the SOP or process is put in place or the person starts work. The training, based on the SOPs, guidances, and working documents, covers the following:

- The concepts of drug safety, PV, and risk management;
- The laws, guidances, and regulations currently in place;
- The specific procedures in that organization or division and others, if appropriate (e.g., clinical research);
- Communication and escalation pathways for concerns; and
- The computers and software.

In addition, there is the more general training the organization offers, on corporate values and workplace behavior, equality issues, physical safety in the workplace, and so on.

There is usually a formal training function or department within drug safety with a dedicated trainer (sometimes "certified" by some training body or organization either internal to the company or outside), who develops formal curricula and courses for the various people (based on job function), who need to be trained. This applies to both new hires and update training for current employees. The training involves the drug safety department workers as well as others in the organization who might receive AEs in the course of their own jobs (e.g., in clinical research, regulatory, legal, telephone operators, customer relations). Each person in the safety department should have an up-to-date and accurate training folder documenting all training that person has had. This will often need to be produced during a health authority inspection or a third party or internal audit.

Much training is now done online with elegant self-pacing and self-testing modules, allowing the individual to do the training at his or her own pace and timing (though by a certain due date). There are multiple organizations that offer courses, both in-house and externally.

■ Quality Assurance/Control

The concept of "quality assurance/control (QA/QC) and quality systems" is relatively new to drug safety and GCP compared with their use in the manufacturing and laboratory areas. However, regulatory agencies in the US, EU and elsewhere insist upon a formal quality function and will inspect and audit to ensure this is in place and functioning well. Quality is broadly broken up into two phases.

The first is QA, which, as we refer to it in drug safety, refers to actions taken during the process of handling safety data to ensure that the work is correct and complete. During the preparation of an ICSR for submission to a health authority by a pharmacist, the QA might be done by his or her supervisor. This is quality that must be built in up-front and executed during the process. The view is that, if something bad has to be picked up at the end of the workflow, when everything is completed, it is too late. Corrections should be made during the process and in real time.

The second phase is QC, which usually refers to a review of the (final) deliverable. This is done to ensure that the deliverables (e.g., the completed E2B file or PSUR/PBRER) were correctly and completely prepared and that no data are lost or changed along the way. QC may include formal audits by third parties from outside or inside the company or organization. Such audits/inspections are routinely done at the end of the process. The difference from QA is that the review is usually done after the work product is completed. Note that confusion exists since some use QA and QC interchangeably or use QA to mean "after-process quality" and QC to mean "in-process quality". Others consider QA to be a component of the overall QC system. In any case, quality must be done both during and after no matter what we label it!

Organizations should have both quality functions in place. During the processing and analysis of safety data, quality checks should be performed at the appropriate stages in the process. After the work is done, a review or an audit may be done on selective cases routinely or periodically (e.g., monthly) to see that the entire process is done correctly. Key performance indicators (KPIs) and other metrics should also be built in. With these periodic KPIs and associated metrics, oversight can be maintained using real-time data. These metrics will also ensure that corrective and preventive measures (CAPAs) are set up, sustained and are effective. Many safety departments in companies have a yearly audit done by their corporate quality group (separate from the drug safety group) or by an external PV auditor/consultant. Of course, the health agencies (the FDA, EMA, and Medicines and Healthcare Products Regulatory Agency [MHRA] in particular) do periodic PV inspections to check the quality of the safety department's work.

■ Safety (AE) Exchange Agreement Function: Creation and Maintenance

Many pharmaceutical companies, both large and small, now enter into agreements with other companies to out-source or share certain responsibilities, such as co-marketing in the same country, marketing in other countries, clinical trials (including development, monitoring, and data analysis), manufacturing, and safety data handling.

As with other business arrangements, it is obligatory that all parties involved have written contracts specifying the safety functions and requirements of all partners. The contract should set specific terms for the exchange of all needed safety data, both individual case safety reports and aggregate reports such as PSURs/PBRERs and NDA periodic reports as well as labeling, investigator brochures, advertising, and regulatory communications. This must be done so that all partners are able to stay in full compliance with all regulations and laws. In the European Union, the QPPV must ensure that this function is done completely and correctly.

■ Literature Review

United States and European Union regulations, as well as those elsewhere, require periodic review of the worldwide literature to ensure that published reports of safety information on a company's products are found and reported to health authorities. This involves a computerized literature search (weekly as required in the European Union) of large databases that scan hundreds to thousands of medical journals and then report on "hits" (i.e., citations containing the drug in question or any other keywords designated in the search).

Once a safety case is found that meets reporting criteria (drug, AE, patient, reporter), the usual reporting requirements (e.g., 15-calendar days for an expedited report) apply. The safety department must ensure that this function, usually done in conjunction with the corporate library or an outside vendor, is performed in a correct and timely manner. This can be a complex task as it is required that both branded and generic cases be included in the literature search and reported in PSURs/PBRERs. Issues of timing, clock start, and translation must be worked through.

In the EU, the EMA has set up a literature review for many products that they perform and make public. However (and unfortunately) even with this medical literature monitoring by the EMA, pharma companies still must check literature on a weekly basis. When a literature case report is identified, it must follow the "classical" rules for recording and reporting (same criteria and timeframes as for spontaneous reports).

■ Data Dictionary Maintenance

In this sense of the word, a "dictionary" is a listing of standardized and fixed terms that companies and regulators agree to use. This is particularly important when data are exchanged electronically. If an unknown term is used in sending a case from one company or health authority to another, the receiving computer system often rejects (or at least notes, or "flags") the case for attention.

MedDRA is the standard dictionary used for the coding of AE terms. Other (now largely outmoded) AE dictionaries include COSTART, WHO-ART, and HARTS. Dictionaries exist for the standardization of drug names (e.g., WHO's Drug Dictionary), abbreviations, laboratory measurements and units, and so forth.

A more global dictionary now being used primarily in the United States, the United Kingdom, Canada, Australia, Denmark, Netherland, Sweden is SNOMED CT. SNOMED CT stands for Systematized Nomenclature of Medicine–Clinical Terms and is claimed to be the most comprehensive multilingual clinical healthcare terminology in the world. The US Department of Health and Human Services is using SNOMED to build "a national electronic healthcare system that will allow patients and their doctors to access their complete medical records anytime and anywhere they are needed, leading to reduced medical errors, improved patient care, and reduced healthcare costs". It is likely that at some point SNOMED will be used with or instead of MedDRA. It is also likely that a mapping of MedDRA into and out of SNOMED will be done at some point.

■ Coding Unit

Again related to dictionaries, in particular to MedDRA, the use of a standardized coding dictionary also implies the use of this dictionary in a standardized manner. That is, every member of the drug safety staff (and any other unit that does coding, such as clinical research) should be taught to code in the same manner using the same methodology and conventions to achieve internal consistency. This is done through a central coding unit (within or outside of drug safety) that either does the actual coding or verifies the coding done by the drug safety personnel. Not all companies have this function and those that do not will often suffer through coding reconciliation at the end of a study or at the time aggregate reports are prepared.

Planning and Project Management/Operations

Many pharmaceutical companies are now integrating project planning directly into the drug safety unit to oversee and facilitate the multiple and ongoing changes that now seem to be a part of daily life in drug safety. This includes ensuring a smooth integration of ongoing safety work by introducing new procedures, software and hardware, and dictionaries. For example, regulations change frequently around the world and all of them must be adhered to even though they may sometimes be contradictory. Other usual occurrences include MedDRA upgrades twice a year, safety database upgrades or transfer to a new platform, and new contracts signed with business partners.

To coordinate the successful implementation of these ever-changing requirements, a solid operations and project planning/management function must be in place to manage contingencies, timing, personnel, and communications. Many of these functions are being combined with or handled by the life cycle risk management groups so that they address global planning for all aspects of a drug's "needs", including drug safety and PV.

Risk Management

Risk management throughout the entire life cycle of a drug is now obligatory and looked at during HA inspections. Companies now form an internal (or use an external) function to handle risk management analysis and planning. At the early stages of a drug's life cycle the risk management functions may be small. However, as the drug enters clinical testing, real-time serious risk management must be done at all stages to ensure that patients are protected, that the drug is developed rationally, and that no major risks that could have been found earlier are discovered at the last minute. Risk management and minimization is now obligatory in the United States, the European Union, and elsewhere. This is discussed elsewhere in this manual.

Liaison to External Organizations/Drug Safety Intelligence

Many companies and health authorities regularly attend meetings held by international organizations that examine and develop new guidances and procedures. These include the ICH, CIOMS, Pharmaceutical Research Manufacturers of America (PhRMA), EFPIA, CDISC, HL-7, the International Society of Pharmacoepidemiology, the Drug Information Association, and many others as well as FDA, EMA and national health authorities. Pharmaceutical companies send personnel from their drug safety units to these meetings. Attendees are either employees whose sole or primary function is to represent the company at external organizations or *ad hoc* representatives chosen because of the duties they perform in their companies. The use of Zoom, webcasts and other electronic meeting options are making attendance at some meetings easier and less expensive by eliminating travel time and costs.

Participation in these meetings is critical for the future of PV because these organizations continue to spearhead the changes and advances in drug safety. ICH has produced many guidances that now form the basis for pharmaceutics in the United States, the European Union, and Japan. CIOMS developed the "CIOMS I form" and "CIOMS II line listings", among others.

This group may also serve as a "safety intelligence unit", gathering information on new laws, regulations, and guidance that touch drug safety. They then disseminate this information to relevant departments in the company. If this function is not done here, it must be done elsewhere in the company to be sure that the company is up to date and in full compliance with all rules and requirements.

PV Worker Education, Skills, and Profile

The needed PV education, skills and profile can vary depending on the company's products, the size of the department, the organization, affiliate versus corporate role, etc. The purpose of this section is to give an overview on the "nice to have" education, skills and profiles, to achieve the PV mission, but also to ensure full control of all PV activities at both affiliate and corporate levels. Most of the information below is applicable to a person leading a PV team (alone or with a team of co-workers). This topic represents one facet of a quality system that keeps patient safety as the main priority of the organization.

Education

More and more often, regulations ask for a medically qualified person (i.e. physician) to head the PV department. This means that if not medically qualified (basic medical training at academic level which usually but not always means a physician), this person must have permanent access to a physician (access shall be duly documented). Training in a specialty (internship & residency) is very desirable but not obligatory.

Whether based at the local or corporate level, the person leading the PV team must actually have expert knowledge on the most frequent drug-induced diseases and safety issues. In addition, he/she must ideally have robust knowledge of Leadership, Regulatory Affairs, QA, IT/IS project management and be able to work in English.

Note: Within large PV organizations, specific safety-related units are set up: case assessment, data entry, QA and PV compliance, pharmacoepidemiology, aggregate/periodic report preparation and delivery, IT/IS support, etc. For jobs within these units, PV members should have an education which is focused on their activities. They do not necessarily need to have an MD or PharmD education. We are seeing many excellent employees now with health-related training such as nurses, nurse practitioners, physician assistants, as well as occasional dentists, podiatrists, "biologists", etc. The job description for each position should carefully state the needed and "nice to have" education, training, and experience. These should be customized and tailored to the specific roles and responsibilities within the PV group.

Skills

Junior PV persons need to handle basic roles within PV departments: answer phone calls from healthcare professionals (HCPs) or patients, document case reports, analyze ICSRs, record ICSRs within the PV database, provide HCPs and patients with additional written information on the case reports, work on safety issue analysis, prepare safety aggregate reports, work on risk management plans and implementation, participate in the defense of submissions of safety dossiers and reports in front of Health Authorities (HAs), etc. These are very interesting tasks that personnel who are making a career in PV should learn. With such experience, personnel will better understand the daily tasks, missions and objectives of the PV team and provide more accurate proposals, recommendations or requirements. This is the way to advance in PV.

A broader training than just PV is usually a clear positive. Employees coming from Regulatory Affairs, Clinical Development, Medical Affairs or other functions can move into PV and advance equally well. In addition, getting people with affiliate experience when working in a corporate environment (or vice versa) is always useful. Achieving a high level of PV is intrinsically linked to the availability of an adequate number of competent and appropriately trained personnel. In addition, to trained personnel, the organization has an obligation to provide appropriate facilities and equipment so the work can get done.

English: Good knowledge fluency in English is, in practice, needed in most situations even though there are few, if any, actual regulations or laws requiring this. English is the *de facto* language used by all or almost all PV employees, both in private and public environments.

Therefore, a good English level, even if working in an affiliate, is needed. Any exchange between affiliates and Headquarters must usually be written in English. If English knowledge or usage are insufficient, PV employees should continue English language training. Obviously, care must be taken to avoid incorrect or unclear English. This could lead to problems or misunderstanding in ICSR narratives or, which could negatively impact or delay the conclusion, the decisions to take and/or the measures to implement.

Crisis experience: PV employees must be able to work under pressure and react quickly when needed, in case of safety crisis for instance. PV crises often have common elements but each one is different. Each crisis can have nuanced aspects relating to the product in question but also to the company, whether the issue is in one or multiple countries, were there deaths, is there a recall required, etc. Considering the current bad image of pharmaceutical companies, having PV employees experienced in crisis management (by education or by experience or by both) is very important. Many companies have employees trained in crisis management, media communications, etc. There should be an SOP for crisis management (though it's not always called this) and PV employees should be familiar with it.

Clinical development strategy and methodology: Thanks to their knowledge of overall safety and PV, more and more pharmaceutical companies are involving PV employees in the management of safety during clinical development. They not only handle the processing and analysis of serious AEs but safety personnel also provide support in safety data analysis, including the safety analysis plans, signal detection, benefit–risk assessment, and project management. They may also set up and manage Data Monitoring Committees, Safety Committees, etc. Personnel moving from clinical development to PV can then be of added value for the PV team.

Epidemiology and pharmacoepidemiology: PV, epidemiology and pharmacoepidemiology are now closely interlinked partners in the pharma world. Considering the permanent evolution in this area, it is illusory for a PV expert to reach a top level and think he or she can keep it for the long term! Continuous changes occur and one must never stop learning. Nevertheless, mastering the basics of epidemiology and pharmacoepidemiology is needed to evaluate and perhaps challenge the proposals made by these partners.

Regulations: Most PV employees, being MDs and PharmDs and other medical professionals, are usually not fans of regulations and lawyers! Nevertheless, as highlighted in many chapters in this manual, regulations become more and more constraining. Often, they are contradictory or have many loopholes or possibilities for "waivers". Sometimes they are written with enormous detail, e.g., the EU GVP modules, and sometimes they are very high level, e.g., FDA regulations compared to the EU modules. Oftentimes they are written in arcane language. Yet they must be known, understood, and complied with in any PV department. Having PV employees with a previous professional background in a regulatory environment can help.

Profile

Availability and reactivity: In most countries, the PV department's head is supposed to be available 24/7 in case of major/critical safety issue occurrence. Even if rare, an urgent safety issue can actually occur at any time. This generates an unscheduled workload for which people must be fully dedicated on an urgent basis. We therefore must be available but also very reactive to manage such tasks in the best possible way. If not feasible within the company, an external group, e.g., CRO or poison control center, etc., must be available. Ultimately the responsibility still falls on the company, e.g., MAH, NDA or IND holder, etc.

Rigorousness: No matter what one's background and training, PV requires rigor and compulsiveness to be sure all the appropriate data, follow-ups, analyses, etc., are obtained to ensure a fair and complete review of any safety issue and a balanced benefit–risk assessment. Note that many safety matters must be decided quickly and a full and complete dataset is rarely available.

But, as highlighted in many chapters of this manual, the PV business (1) is strongly regulated, (2) involves many stakeholders, and (3) can have serious penalties for misbehavior. This justifies why, for most of PV tasks or processes, PV employees must be rigorous and follow a clear methodology.

Communication and negotiation ability: PV issues are always sensitive for all stakeholders. Transparency and good communication abilities are needed to ensure that correct, accurate messages and information are provided and understood. Keep in mind that PV workers are "birds of ill omen" and often considered as responsible for the safety issue even if they only are the recipient of data from the outside! Yes, sometimes they do "kill the messenger". One of us was known in the company as "Dr. NO" as he often brought bad news. This applies to senior management, health authorities, marketing/commercial, healthcare professionals, patients, media, etc. Scapegoats are sometimes sought and sometimes they will be the safety folks.

Note: In the authors' experience, PV employees are often not good communicators though there are, of course, exceptions. This is particularly challenging, even for good communicators because the safety message is often a negative one. It is, therefore, usually recommended for PV employees not to take the lead on communication tasks but to remain experts with abilities to provide advice. Most companies have communication departments and designated spokespersons to handle external media.

Perseverance and resistance to stress: PV is still often perceived as a regulatory and cost constraint by top managers, which moreover is costly. Getting the needed resources to take on PV missions can be challenging. Resistance to the safety department's actions and opinions can often come in subtle or subliminal ways from others in the company, particularly those with career or money invested in the drug in question.

When convinced that a specific measure or plan or report is needed, PV needs to know it could face a battle. If not successful immediately, long term obstinacy will sometimes succeed. However, some can face situations where frankly illegal and/or unethical requests are made; then, the best course is to leave the position or company in situations where this truly cannot be resolved.

In addition, PV activities can generate a very stressful environment both in safety crises, but also in activities that have regulatory deadlines, management "interest" and controversial medical judgments. Sometimes this is seen in soft and subtle ways ("You don't mean the causality is "probably related" what you mean is "possibly related"). To work in such an environment, perseverance, a thick skin, and resistance to stress are needed. It is not uncommon for external pressures, e.g., politicians, the media, etc., to interject influence that is not evidence-based.

Quick analysis and prioritization: Safety data comes continuously into a PV department. Big companies with many studies and/or products can have cases and safety issues flowing in 24/7. Some data will have an urgent and critical impact which must be assessed immediately. In such circumstances, PV employees must be able to make an immediate analysis of the available data, including important missing information, and make a choice of actions to be taken, people to be notified, etc. using a prioritization model (from very urgent to non-urgent, considering also what can, or cannot, be delegated to other PV colleagues). This usually requires skill and experience, but the escalation scheme should have a clear chain and SOP.

Authority and weight: Being experienced in PV is not sufficient to lead a team. Some decisions or measures can sometime be difficult to for partners or personnel within the PV team to accept. Handling a major safety issue that arises during a clinical development program can be a challenge. The clinical team is very protective of its "baby"! If the PV team is well recognized as competent and professional by all within the company, such tasks will be less difficult. Having a strong authority and weight within the organization is needed to succeed in this area. It also requires strict fairness and impartiality. A calm and non-combative style is a major asset.

Politics: One must realize that all jobs, companies, life situations, etc., involve politics and dealing with other people. Some people are not nice or even downright nasty or evil. Some do not have your best interests or even the company's best interests in mind. Some people are not as rational or clear thinking as you might be. This is obviously not unique to PV but is a part of normal daily life. It is wise to try to identify who one's friends are, who one's "enemies" are, who is obstructive and who can be sought to help resolve problematic situations.

Vision and strategy: Regulations and data sources are constantly evolving and technical solutions are to be envisaged for many PV tasks in the future (artificial intelligence is an obvious domain which will bring solutions for some PV tasks). This explains why PV is and will be for a long time in a permanent evolutionary mode, though it is not clear that a Darwinian survival of the fittest will triumph. Organization, tools, processes, needed skills or education are actually permanently to be challenged and updated. To succeed in this area, PV workers must be creative and able to guide all stakeholders, while maintaining a positive mindset mode. This is possible only if they easily share their vision and strategy.

■ Frequently Asked Question

Q: Should PV employees be "Superman" or "Superwoman"?

A: Yes! And try to find out as soon as possible who has the kryptonite! All kidding aside, ideal candidates would have a wide variety of cross-functional knowledge in order to succeed in these roles.

CHAPTER

12

Clinical Trial Phases and Investigator-Initiated Trials

To obtain government approval to market an innovative drug, i.e., a new molecular entity (NME) in the United States, Canada, the European Union, and most countries, a series of clinical trials on patients is required. The extent of the trials depends on the drug (already approved for other uses or formulations, a new breakthrough product for use in a therapeutic void, expected to be very toxic, etc.), the disease or indication treated (severe diseases, such as advanced cancer versus mild allergies, diseases with no known treatments, rare diseases with few patients afflicted, etc.), the nature of the patients studied (healthy, very ill, young, old, organ impairment, etc.), experience in other countries where it is already available and other factors. The data collected through these clinical trials and other such studies are a critical source of safety data and should be carefully monitored and tracked within a company to ensure all available information regarding the product is properly collected and reported as required.

■ Introduction

A universally accepted tenet is that safety and pharmacovigilance representatives should be engaged contributors across the entire continuum of product development (i.e., during due diligence, program planning, development, implementation, and analysis). This is essential, as all types of studies have the potential to uncover safety information and is important when developing the safety profile of the product, as well as obligations to investigators, ethics committees, and regulatory authorities. All clinical studies are subject to scrutiny for adherence to Good Clinical Practices (GCP) and compliance with legal obligations. Safety must advocate and prosecute strong positions for comprehensive pharmacovigilance, even though other groups, e.g., business development, commercial, co-development partners, etc., may bring opposing views to discussions and wish to incorporate minimalist approaches to pharmacovigilance aspects of the program. In addition to meeting government and ethical requirements, robust pharmacovigilance represents good product stewardship and will support successful use of the product. Pharmacovigilance is essential across the entire continuum of product development and use.

Initiating the Research

After the appropriate pharmacology and toxicology testing *in vitro* and in animals, development of small-scale and sometimes (even at this early stage) larger-scale manufacturing procedures, and other preparatory testing, the drug is ready to be used in humans in the so-called "first in human" study. Permission must be requested from the regulators and ethics committees to proceed. In the United States, a company (sometimes an individual investigator or an academic center) submits an Investigational New Drug Application (IND) to the Food and Drug Administration (FDA). The IND contains preparatory data that support administration of the investigational medicine to humans. The EU Regulation requests a Clinical Trial Application (CTA) dossier, made available to all concerned Member States through a single submission portal (as of 2019); one single authorization is given for all concerned countries before starting the clinical trial. Elsewhere, an equivalent data package is submitted to the local health authority, as may be required. This package ordinarily contains data that are proprietary and not available to the public, however recent changes in EU regulations will change what is and is not publicly available.

In addition, the submitter includes in the package a protocol for a clinical trial in humans. The protocol must address a specific scientific question. If the trial is successful, the trial data will be part of the basis for regulatory approval of the product and will specify conditions for use if the product is eventually approved for marketing. It is extremely important for a safety representative to get engaged as early in the process as practical to address relevant safety parameters in the protocol. Outside the US, this administrative package is categorized as a "CTA". In some countries, the regulator must issue a positive opinion to the applicant before the first human trial can begin and in others, there is a waiting period and if no refusal to proceed is received from the authority, the trial may begin. In such situations, "CTA" may also refer to clinical trial authorization.

Although clinical drug development is often described as four phases, both referred to as Phase I, II, III, and IV or 1–4, it is important to appreciate that the phase concept is a description and that phases of development may overlap or be combined. There are many different study designs, such as single-arm (noncomparative) trials, placebo-controlled trials, crossover trials, noninferiority trials, factorial trials, observational studies, and adaptive design trials, etc.

Some development programs may refer to **phase 0 trials**, which were introduced by FDA in 2006. These are exploratory in nature and these studies are usually designed to deliver subtherapeutic doses. The main goal of phase 0 trials is to evaluate basic effects of a potentially toxic effects of an experimental drug. One common example of the use of phase 0 trials is in neuro-oncology, wherein participants receive a full therapeutic dose for a short duration of time prior to a scheduled tumor resection.

In rare instances, a physician may request an Emergency Use IND for a specific patient. In the US, this is handled by the FDA. Similar programs elsewhere are known by different classifications, e.g., Compassionate Use, etc. Drug trials are heavily regulated, and multiple layers of protections and precautions have been developed to protect the participants. These include oversight by investigational review boards, data safety monitoring boards, sponsor and health authority scrutiny, and usually some level of public notification and publicizing of the study on the Internet (e.g., clinical trial registries). Trials are ordinarily divided into four phases, each accommodating greater participant enrollment and increasing complexity, although there is usually some overlap.

Academic centers are doing more and more of this work as well as other earlier discovery research. The goal has been to create a multi-disciplinary approach from lab to bedside for new and better therapies. This is now called Translational Research and many medical centers and some of the more influential regulators now have departments of Translational Research.

For awareness, once an innovative product loses patent protection, the generic "copies" usually have a relatively less complex dossier for registration (or licensure) consisting primarily of manufacturing details, dissolution, and bioavailability studies, etc., rather than the extensive clinical trials required for the first-to-market product. Clinical trial data and numbers of participants of the innovator are included by reference. Prescribing information for generic products is the same as the innovator product. In the US the dossier for a marketing approval of generic drug product is known as an Abbreviated New Drug Application or "ANDA."

■ Phase I

Phase I trials ("First in Human" or FIH, sometimes also called "First in Man") actually belong to human pharmacology, in contrast to animal pharmacology. These are the first steps in determining the profile of both the beneficial and the untoward effects in humans. They are designed mainly to find the maximum tolerated dose and the pathways for metabolizing and eliminating the drug. Safety is more important in this phase than efficacy. The first study is often a single-dose trial in a small number (e.g., a dozen) of healthy, often male (to avoid any possible pregnancy issues) volunteers. If tolerated, a multiple-dose study and a dose escalation study follow. The aim of phase I trials is to study Absorption, Distribution in the body, Metabolism, and Excretion (the so-called "ADME" studies), as well as safety and toxicity.

Other things that may be examined include the proposed formulation to be used in subsequent trials and marketing (as they may be different, and usually are) and the dosing frequency or schedule. Drug interaction studies may be done in phase I or later in phase II. If the drugs are known to be toxic or have severe and predictable ADRs, these studies are often done for ethical reasons in patients with the disease to be treated rather than in healthy volunteers, e.g., cancer chemotherapy or AIDS. Each study is short, often running no more than a few days to a few weeks at most. The trial design is usually simple and open label. They may or may not be controlled, i.e., designed with a comparative agent(s). Several phase I studies often take a year or so and may include around 100 patients in total.

There is usually no benefit to the participants in the trial, and they participate either because of generosity of spirit or because they are paid. Because there is no gain to the individual participants, all efforts are made to minimize the risk of toxicity. Serious adverse events (SAEs) are usually rare in phase I trials and, if SAEs do occur, they often result in suspension or modification of the study protocol (sometimes a single SAE will stop further development of a compound.) participants are often "housed" for these studies in special clinical research centers run by academic medical centers or clinical research organizations (CROs). These research centers provide constant supervision and participants are carefully monitored. Note that the term *participants* in this context usually refers to "normal people", not patients. However, the term *subjects* is ordinarily also used to refer to people, with the disease in question, who are enrolled in clinical trials.

Hence, phase I trials usually involve healthy participants, and phase II, III, and IV trials involve participants with the disease to be studied. This distinction is not always followed, and some use the terms *patient* and *subject* interchangeably. For example, it is common to refer to any person enrolled in any study phase to be referred to as a study subject or participant. These terms will be used interchangeably in this book to refer to an individual in a trial. The preferred use is "participant" for anyone in a study and "patient" for anyone otherwise seeking or receiving care in the healthcare system.

Adverse events (AEs) seen in phase I trials are always noteworthy because the participants are usually normal and a low starting dose of the drug in question is usually used. Because few participants are studied in phase I, any AE should be investigated thoroughly. SAEs and the rare death seen in phase I trials should be looked at immediately and consideration should be given to stopping further dosing or enrollment, or protocol modification.

Some countries now require that the next participant is dosed only when the previous participant ends the surveillance period scheduled in the protocol; this minimizes the risk of tragic adverse experiences in several subjects at the same time. Note that the FDA now requires all SAEs (whether labeled or not, whether felt to be due to the drug or not) to be submitted as expedited reports. In addition to the toxicity of the drug preparation, subjects have been known to hide serious medical problems or medical history to participate in the study, especially if the subjects are compensated. Participants who are motivated by money payments may confound the safety profile if they mask safety data, enroll in several studies simultaneously or in close succession.

■ Phase II

Phase II trials are done after the drug has successfully passed through all or parts of phase I trials. Phase II trials are sometimes performed in patients afflicted with the disease for which that drug was developed. Many phase II trials are done in normal volunteers (subjects). Whereas phase I trials are usually done for tolerance and safety, phase II trials are done for both efficacy and safety. The goal is to find the minimal effective dose that retains efficacy with the minimum number of AEs and safety issues. These studies may also continue the ADME investigations of phase I. In addition, they may also be used to develop safety and efficacy markers and tests for subsequent larger phase III trials. The studies may include up to hundreds of participants and are usually double blinded (and controlled). They may run several weeks or months.

Sponsors and investigators engaged in phase II trials must pay particular attention because unexpected SAEs, including deaths, may occur. Neither investigator nor participant knows the randomization. Severe and unexpected toxicity may force the immediate stopping of the study or a midstream alteration of the protocol and informed consent. Participants in phase II trials usually are not compensated for their participation, although they routinely receive study medication and study-related medical care.

Special studies may be done in phase I, II, III, or IV, such as drug-interaction studies (sometimes in healthy volunteers, sometimes in patients with the disease), food or alcohol interaction studies, and evaluation studies in renal failure or liver failure patients. These special studies, however, are usually required for the MAA or NDA submission and so must be done at some point.

Some drugs or products, e.g., oncology drugs or herbals, may not fully undergo phase I and II testing as is classically done and as described above. Oncology drugs, which are often very toxic, are rarely studied in normal subjects, but are used directly in patients with malignancy. Similarly, "orphan drugs", which are drugs developed for rare diseases, may undergo abbreviated testing. The FDA Orphan Drug Designation program provides orphan status to drugs and biologics which are defined as those intended for the safe and effective treatment, diagnosis or prevention of rare diseases or disorders that affect fewer than 200,000 people in the US, or that affect more than 200,000 persons but are not expected to recover the costs of developing and marketing a treatment drug. A similar situation exists in the EU where an orphan drug designation is given to products aimed at treating diseases that afflict no more than 5 in 10,000 people or where the potential profit is insufficient to justify research and development costs.

■ Phase III

Phase III is often divided into phases IIIA and IIIB. Phase III trials include hundreds to thousands of patients, and the whole phase may take several years to complete, depending on the treatment duration and outcomes of the disease studied. Each individual trial may include multiple sites on one or more continents and run months to a year or more. (Survival studies may take even longer because the study usually does not end until the last patient dies.)

For oncology products, protocols are often designed to follow patients for disease progression-free survival after completion of treatment for a set timeframe, such as five years. Certain advanced therapies, e.g., gene-based therapies, may also require long-term follow-up for delayed appearance of AEs. Based on a variety of scientific criteria, FDA guidance suggests consideration of a minimum of 15 years for follow-up in gene therapy protocols.

The goal in phase III is to obtain sufficient clinical trial data to support regulatory approval to market the drug. However, it may be possible to obtain product approval prior to completion of all follow-up activities. Indeed, many regulatory jurisdictions have legislative authority to make important products available on an "emergency use" basis. This authority was used during the COVID-19 pandemic.

Phase IIIA trials are usually the key (the old term is "pivotal") studies to be submitted for regulatory approval, and they are incorporated in the NDA submission or "MAA dossier". The design used in these trials is usually double blind, but many other varieties are used. Depending on the drug and disease under study, each study arm will get the currently accepted therapy ("standard of care") plus the study drug and the comparator is the "standard of care". This is usually obligatory in almost all cancer, infection, severe pain trials. There are many variants of this model that are used. In some cases, the FDA and other agencies may require a placebo-controlled trial. This is becoming more and more controversial in terms of the ethics of using placebo if there is an established standard of care. Many health agencies and payers often require trials against the standard of care rather than placebo. Although both have a place in drug development, placebo trials are felt to be less and less acceptable. In infectious diseases, for example, it is considered ethically unacceptable to exclude an active comparator from the protocol.

Phase IIIB trials are additional (usually) large-scale studies that may be started during the examination and review of the initial dossier by the health agency and may end before or after the approval for marketing (NDA or MA). Because the total elapsed review time by the health agency may take a year or more, sponsors may continue studies during this review period. These studies may focus on pharmacoeconomic or risk evaluation issues as well as cost-effectiveness and studies against competitor drugs. Sometimes, surprising or unexpected results of phase IIIA studies force late changes in phase IIIB studies. As most products now have full life cycle risk evaluation and management programs in place, additional testing may be added to phase III trials to evaluate risks that are unclear or that need further evaluation. By doing such testing in phase III, it may be possible to achieve more rapid marketing approval though post-marketing studies and other commitments (or requirements) for risk evaluation, management, and mitigation may continue in phase IV. Alternatively, FDA permits selective safety data collection of non-serious events in late phase studies for products that have an otherwise well-characterized safety profile. Examples where this has been permitted are primarily in line extensions for oncology products.

Other approaches to making clinical trials more efficient include adaptive clinical trial designs, which permit modification of protocol parameters (or statistical procedures) after study initiation according to a prescribed schedule. There are several types of adaptive designs that can be applied in various settings while maintaining the integrity and validity of the study.

In some jurisdictions, Health Technology Assessment (HTA) data are required to demonstrate product value before payers, e.g., governments, insurance companies, etc., will reimburse for use of the product, even after approval for marketing by the appropriate drug regulator. A Health Technology Assessment is the systematic evaluation of properties, effects, and/or impacts of health technology. It is a multidisciplinary process to evaluate the social, economic, organizational and ethical issues of a health intervention or health technology (WHO definition). The goal is to be sure a new technology is cost effective and that dubious products are not approved for use (Pan American Health Organization. This can be a complicated exercise that impacts the commercial viability of the product. For example, in England the National Institute for Health and Care Excellence (NICE) and in France the French National Authority for Health, review UK/French approved products to see if they improve outcomes and add to patient care. If they determine that a product does not do this, their recommendation may determine whether the product is reimbursed by the UK or French National Health Service. That is, the drug is approved in England/France but may not be reimbursed by insurance.

A full safety dataset is not always required. For example, ICH has developed guidance, "E19 A Selective Approach to Safety Data Collection in Specific Late-Stage Pre-Approval or Post-Approval Clinical Trials". This is internationally harmonized guidance for the use of selective (reduced) safety data collection that may be applied in specific situations, e.g., late-stage clinical development to improve efficiency of the trial.

■ Phase IV

Phase IV studies include different types of studies. They are done after the approval and marketing of the drug. Note that a drug may not always be marketed immediately after approval. Sometimes, the company receiving the approval may choose to sell or out-license the drug, or timing may make it wiser to wait, e.g., new seasonal allergy drugs should be marketed near the time for the allergy season to hit.

Sometimes additional studies beyond those required for approval may be desired. The company (applicant) may choose to propose and agree to additional work, i.e., a "Post-Marketing Commitment" (PMC) in the US. Many regulators also have authority to impose additional work, i.e., a "Post-Marketing Requirement" (PMR) in the US or Post-Authorization Studies in the EU. Imposed studies in the EU are the equivalent of PMRs in the US. These studies may be done to clarify some safety and efficacy issues that remained after phase III, but which the health agency believed were not sufficient to prevent or delay marketing of the drug. In the US, these studies may be included in a Risk Evaluation and Mitigation Strategy (REMS) or may be independent of REMS. In the EU, EMA and member states may require further studies in their Risk Management Plans (RMPs), i.e., Post-authorization Safety Studies (PASS) and/or Post-authorization Efficacy Studies (PAES). Failure to perform such tasks in any jurisdiction where agreed or imposed may result in penalties to the company, fines, or even withdrawal or limitation of the marketing approval. Such misbehavior is usually publicized, which can impact public trust of the company and its products. These study types are conducted to ensure benefits of the product outweigh its risks.

PMCs and PMRs are published, along with timetables for expected completion and, eventually, results, on public websites.

Phase 4 studies may also be marketing or pharmacoeconomic studies to aid in selling the product by studying head-on comparisons with competitor drugs (see HTA note, above). They may be studies looking at sub-groups of the approved group and indication, e.g., testing a drug approved for diabetes on diabetics who are elderly or are also in heart failure. They may be done in children, not only to evaluate the usefulness and safety but also to obtain, in various markets, additional patent exclusivity. In the US, a sponsor who receives an approval for a drug or biologic to treat a "rare pediatric disease" may qualify for a "voucher". This "voucher" can be redeemed later to receive a priority review of a subsequent marketing application for a different product. These vouchers are transferable and may be sold to other companies.

Phase IV studies may be done for specific safety reasons to investigate an AE or a signal that has unexpectedly been detected after marketing. Such studies may be classical clinical trials or they may be observational or epidemiologic studies done in large databases. The design and size are very variable, ranging from small open-label trials to massive, multi-center, double-blind comparator trials or "large simple safety studies" with simple protocols and minimal record-keeping. Sometimes patients are compensated for participation.

The so-called market-driven phase IV "seeding studies" are now forbidden in most parts of the world. These were pure marketing projects designed to encourage physicians to prescribe a particular product in place of a competitor's product. A protocol was usually written (to justify calling the endeavor a study), but was often of poor quality. Results were not always collected by the sponsor and, if collected, were often not analyzed. Prescribers were sometimes compensated. In a more subtle way, post-marketing trials for entirely legitimate purposes may include elements aimed at getting physicians to use the new drug in place of another product ("stealth seeding trials"). By doing this, the prescriber becomes familiar with the product, and the company hopes he or she will prescribe it for other patients after the trial is completed.

Late Phase Studies

A term that has appeared in the last few years is *late phase studies*, referring to the grab bag of requirements that agencies and companies are doing both for registration, evaluating risk, and marketing reasons. They include registries (product, disease, safety), post-marketing observational studies, classic phase 4 trials as discussed earlier, clinical effectiveness trials (i.e., real world evidence), OTC trials, community-based trials, health economic and outcomes studies (retrospective, prospective, observational), cost-effectiveness, burden of disease, patient reported outcome (PRO, Quality of Life [QoL], chart review, survey (physicians, patients), health economic piggyback trials, risk management, expanded access, drug safety, and others.

In the US, the FDA will also sometimes impose post-marketing requirements (PMRs) and post-marketing commitments (PMCs) that can be in the form or other late phase studies and additional research requirements. PMRs and PMCs are often listed in the agency approval letter received by the manufacturer after submission for approval and must be carried out according to the requirements set forth in the communication from the agency. In the EU, similar studies are called Post-Authorization Safety Studies, or PASS studies and carry similar requirements. From a pharmacovigilance perspective, it is therefore imperative that those within safety and PV are aware of the approval letter and communication with the agencies after submission as these types of late phase and post-market studies are a source of safety data and therefore are crucial to the pharmacovigilance system.

Commercially-driven "Customer Engagement Programs", e.g., patient support programs, drug delivery and treatment continuity programs, "sentiment analysis," social media "listening", etc., where there is the possibility of two-way communication, are an additional source of AEs after a product is marketed. And these programs are evolving, e.g., Patient safety is usually not the focus of such programs, but any safety data that are generated must be evaluated.

Other study designs that merit mention include pragmatic clinical trials and low interventional studies. Pragmatic trials are randomized trials designed to assess how effective a treatment actually is in routine, everyday practice. These studies have limited protocol-driven requirements so that there is minimal impact on the patient's standard treatment for the condition of interest. Following randomization, follow-up patient care is managed by the healthcare provider(s) according to their normal standard of care. Pragmatic studies address practical questions about risks, benefits, and costs of an intervention as it is used in daily practice under usual circumstances. This type of study can also be used to assess compliance, i.e., whether patients actually follow the instructions as to daily dose, timing of drug intake, avoiding known interactions with foods or other medicines, etc.

In some pragmatic studies, non-standard of care diagnostic or monitoring procedures are included, but these must not pose more than minimal additional risk or burden to the safety of patients compared to normal clinical practice. Secondary data sources (e.g., electronic health records, claims data, safety monitoring databases, etc.) may be used to obtain follow-up information.

Low interventional studies *do not* involve any protocol-required assignment to an intervention that is expected to impact a clinical outcome. However, they *do* require non-standard of care diagnostic or monitoring procedures which do not pose more than minimal additional risk or burden to the safety of patients compared to normal clinical practice. Low interventional studies are designed and conducted in real-world healthcare settings to evaluate, for example, epidemiology or natural history of a disease or the safety or effectiveness of an intervention under routine care conditions.

Various groups around the world are looking at the use of generative AI (artificial intelligence) to continue to find and/or develop new safety data on marketed products. This work may lead to additional useful safety information.

Investigator-Initiated Research

Investigator-Initiated Research (IIR) includes Investigator-Initiated Trials (IITs) and Investigator-Initiated Studies (IISs), also called Investigator-Sponsored Trials (ISTs). These usually arise from new ideas thought up by researchers in the academic world or occasionally suggested by the pharmaceutical company. New uses or ways of administering drugs are frequently proposed by academic researchers to pharmaceutical companies. Many companies actually have physicians, PhDs, or pharmacologists on staff (often called "medical liaisons"), who travel to academic medical centers and seek out such clever new uses. Such trials are usually done at single centers. Sometimes, the investigator will come up with the idea and approach the company (sponsor or patent holder) for assistance with either a grant or product supply (especially if the product is costly).

These types of studies are instrumental in the scientific development of a drug, and are also a source of safety data, therefore, making these types of studies an important component of the pharmacovigilance and safety system for any given product.

The advantages of IIR are that new ideas are found and explored, costs are usually relatively low, and the studies can often be done fairly quickly. The disadvantage is that many details that should be determined before the trials are not addressed (e.g., effective dose and safety in this population). IIR that fails usually ends that idea. Thus, if too low a dose is chosen, one might never know that a higher dose would produce positive results. Funding is usually from the pharmaceutical company in the form of a grant-in-aid, drug supply, protocol, or case report form support. It is important to understand the roles and responsibilities of the company versus investigator.

The legal bases which support the inclusion of IITs/ISTs in a pharmacovigilance system stem from US FDA 21 CFR 312.32 (c) (1) "Findings from Other Studies", which states that the sponsor must report any findings from epidemiological studies, pooled analysis of multiple studies, or clinical studies... whether or not conducted under an IND, and whether or not conducted by the sponsor, that suggest a significant risk in humans exposed to the drug. This regulation necessitates a robust communication channel between Investigators conducting their own research and the sponsor/manufacturer of the products.

Once an Investigator determines he/she will conduct research on a given product, there is typically a contract or agreement signed by both parties which outlines each party's role in the IIR, including the responsibility of reporting safety information to the agencies and within the two parties. This contract or agreement is typically called a Safety Data Exchange Agreement, or SDEA, and can be a part of the primary Master Service Agreement, or a separate document that is legally binding and subject to review during audits and inspections. In these cases, the legal sponsor of the study is not the pharmaceutical company but rather the investigator. It is he or she who opens the IND with the FDA or the equivalent in other countries (often with the help of the pharmaceutical company by giving the investigator permission to reference a company IND). The usual safety provisions are followed: Good Clinical Practices, investigational review boards, and SAE reporting to the health agency by the investigator. Note that FDA IND regulatory rules requires the investigator/sponsor to handle safety reporting to the FDA, IRB, etc., as if he/she were a typical sponsor, such as a pharmaceutical company. Most pharmaceutical companies also require the investigator to report SAEs to the company (in addition to the health authority) so that the company maintains a full safety database for all uses of a product.

The contract/agreement between the investigator and the company must be perfectly clear regarding safety responsibilities among the parties concerned. This includes a mechanism for adaptation to new regulatory or partner requirements. The company should not engage in monitoring the data, i.e., checking source documents, because this could be construed as assuming the responsibilities of a sponsor. It is less clear from FDA regulations whether the pharmaceutical company should also submit the cases if the company receives them from the IIR investigator, who is required to submit them directly to FDA. These trials would technically be phase I if a new indication, formulation, or delivery is being studied. If not, they would most probably be considered phase IV trials. Not all studies require an IND (if the use of the drug is fully covered within the approved labeling). Such studies usually have to be registered with the appropriate health authority and clinical trial database (e.g., clinicaltrials.gov in the US and EudraCT in the EU).

In earlier years, disputes occurred over ownership of data and the publication (or rather lack of publication) of negative results. These are resolved, in general, with both parties retaining "ownership" of data and with the right to publish retained by the investigator regardless of the results.

Ultimately, how a company decides to handle the oversight of such studies is up to the company, but these studies are subject to regulatory scrutiny and should be tightly controlled and understood by both the Investigator/owner of the IND as well as the product manufacturer.

Other Study-Related Issues

Study phases are often hazier than the "official" schema described above. Phase I studies that go beyond the initial dose finding and escalation studies are often done throughout the phases over several years. If a drug does not go beyond phase II because of lack of efficacy (i.e., the company "kills" it), there is little point in doing drug, food, or alcohol interaction studies. Thus, these are usually not performed early in the course of development. Likewise, it is not common for the initial studies to use a formulation that is eventually approved for marketing.

Some companies have been known to try to speed up development (and lower costs) by doing somewhat larger phase II trials that, should they succeed, are submitted to the health agencies as combined phase II and III trials for approval. For critical drugs, this may be advantageous as long as it does not compromise the safety and efficacy evaluations. In general, the more patients who are studied, the more comfortable one is with the safety profile of the drug. Smaller safety databases obtained in phases I–III may require larger post-marketing safety study commitments to obtain additional information to adequately evaluate the benefit/risk profile as larger numbers of disparate patients use the drug. Obviously, the sponsor should discuss any proposed alterations of the classic drug development with the health authorities.

Phase I studies are created and supervised in most pharmaceutical companies by a dedicated phase I group (e.g., the pharmacokinetics/pharmacodynamics group) usually run by pharmacologists (PhDs, PharmDs), nurses, and physicians. The actual study is often outsourced to CROs or academic centers (clinical research units), where the patient enrollment and dosing occur. This permits close observation and continuous monitoring of participants.

Phases II and III are usually run by "high power" clinical or medical research groups within the company led by physicians (often sub-specialists such as cardiologists, oncologists, etc.). These studies are complex and have large infrastructures supporting them in biostatistics, study-site monitoring, in-house data monitoring, clinical research, regulatory affairs, safety monitors, quality control, quality assurance, coordination of central laboratory services, independent data monitoring committees for individual protocol oversight, a Safety Assessment Committee for development program oversight across all protocols, and so on. Many companies, particularly smaller ones, also outsource the trials (or parts of the trials) to one or more CROs and other vendors. These studies are rigorously done and are likely to be audited by the health authority before marketing approval. A co-development or co-marketing arrangement will increase complexity and increase requirements for well-organized logistical arrangements. The team must agree on SOPs and training, coding conventions, record-keeping responsibilities, and a governance structure. These agreements must be reviewed periodically if changes occur in either party or new parties enter. These studies may run into tens of millions of dollars and require complex organization, project management, and information technology support.

Phase IV studies may be done by the phase II and III group or by a separate post-marketing group. If phase IV studies are done in the clinical research department, the rigor of the earlier phases usually carries over to these phase IV studies. If the phase IV studies are done by the marketing department in isolation from the clinical research group, these studies may be somewhat more variable in quality and rigor. Some companies now have separate Safety/Epidemiology/Risk Management departments that handle PMCs and PMRs, e.g., post-marketing clinical and epidemiologic trials (but not the marketing studies). Many of these are now outsourced to CROs or firms specializing in "late phase" trials.

Some company executives have argued that small phase IV marketing studies or IIR programs are dangerous because they might discover some safety "problem" and might fail to show efficacy, thus doubly hurting the drug. Safety officers often argue just the reverse: these studies may uncover a previously unknown safety issue that represents good product stewardship, i.e., the new finding can be added to the product labeling to better inform prescribers and patients. It is arguably better for a company to discover a potential issue first, so that the company has strong and useful input into the situation.

Clinical trial registries have been set up by health authorities and governments (clinicaltrials.gov in the US and EudraCT in the EU), as well as by pharmaceutical companies and others in which all or almost all research trials are now posted, in detail, on a website. It has been felt by some that this will raise the standards for all trials and allow for easier data comparisons. That is not yet clear. Several things have happened, though. Patients, disease support groups, and patient advocates are now more easily able to find and track studies involving their disease by simply searching through the databases. There is also an industry that mines various databases for information on patient and investigator availability, enrollment, completion dates, and so forth.

IIR programs have traditionally posed problems. IIR is usually encouraged by companies that have roving medical liaisons. They visit academic medical centers to provide medical information and seek out new trials. These visiting medical liaisons may or may not be trained in classic clinical research methodology. They may also do "in-service" teaching or training on the company's new products. Thus, this role combines a medical and a marketing function. In well-structured pharmaceutical companies, protocols submitted by academics are reviewed by the clinical research department, the statisticians, and the pharmacovigilance group to ensure good quality. A formal contract requiring completion, a final report within a finite period (e.g., 1 year), and SAE reporting must be done under good clinical practices. Pharmacovigilance departments in companies usually submit the SAEs to their own MAs, NDAs, and INDs, as the case may be, even if the investigator has said he or she has also done so. In less well-structured companies, the medical marketing group may be less well-connected to the other research groups and details may slip. Specifics of the contract (agreement) should be audited for compliance.

Other types of outreach programs (sometimes in combination with registries) are also used by companies for various reasons:

- To help patients finish the course of therapy when they are already taking the drug;
- As part of a REMS/RMP as an ETASU (an "element to assure safe use of the drug");
- To help sell the drug: In particular, for chronic therapy diseases such as cancer, hepatitis, and hypertension, companies have found that it is good medicine and good marketing to encourage patients to stay on their therapy to the end (until the cancer is in remission or cured, the viral titers drop, etc.). This means continued sales of the drug as well as successful patient treatment. The usual reasons for stopping therapy are AEs, dosing problems, or convenience reasons. Sometimes it is cost. Outreach programs that use nurses or pharmacists to contact patients every week or month on how to handle AEs and other issues are now common. These are a type of a Customer Engagement Program and must be linked to (or at least known to) the safety department because they are often a source of safety information. When the program is well-executed, the patient's physician is kept informed of issues and progress. The outreach team is able to work with the patient to get the patient over rough patches in the treatment regimen. AE data must be collected by the company, kept in the safety database, and reported to the health authority as required.

■ Frequently Asked Questions

Q: Does the company have to collect all AEs from all trials?

A: Basically yes. The sponsor has a responsibility to fully understand the safety profile of the product, and in order to do so, you need all of the data available. Second, it is legally required in most instances (US FDA 21 CFR 312.32(c)(1) and 312.32(c)(1)(ii) support this requirement). In practice, only SAEs must be collected from clinical trials in real time by the sponsor, i.e., the sponsor's drug safety group. The data must be evaluated and reported to the authorities either in 7 or 15 calendar days or periodically in annual reports. Tighter timelines may be required by SOPs or in certain contracts. Non-serious AEs and some SAEs (e.g., expected SAEs that the sponsor and health authority agree will be reported only at the end of the study) do not get reported until the final study report.

Q: What if the clinical trial data is in multiple databases? How can I collect all the data from various sources?

A: In many pharmaceutical companies, two or more databases contain safety information. There is the drug safety database maintained by the drug safety group for expedited and periodic regulatory reporting and the clinical research database for marketing authorization and NDA submissions. Furthermore, if you have multiple studies ongoing with different CROs, your data could end up in a variety of places that needs to be consolidated into a single system. The safety database contains all SAEs (as well as all serious and non-serious post-marketing AEs) but not non-serious clinical trial AEs. This database is dynamic and always up to date. The clinical research database contains the (paper or electronic) case report form information, including all serious and non-serious AEs.

Sometimes data are not entered into the clinical research database rapidly but rather only when paper case report forms arrive in the research department, perhaps monthly. In other cases, where electronic data capture is used instead of paper CRFs, the data entry at the site may be delayed or incomplete. Some companies using electronic data capture (EDC) also require an e-mail, fax, or direct download of EDC data into the safety department's database. Nonetheless, the use of electronic case records should make data available more rapidly than in paper-based studies.

Q: What are the challenges with having multiple systems with the same data?

A: Having two databases produces various problems. To get a full picture of the safety in the trial, one must obtain the SAEs from the safety group (their database is usually up to date) and the non-serious AEs from the clinical research group's database (which may not be up to date). The data outputs must then be reconciled (a problem if the two database outputs are not compatible or normalized) to have a full dataset. In addition, the SAEs in the two safety databases must be reconciled if the same SAE safety data are collected in two different places or in two different ways (e.g., EDC and e-mail/fax of the case to the sponsor's drug safety group).

For example, if a company has single case reports (ICSRs) in one database, and aggregate reports in another, these databases must be synchronized for coding conventions and other data points. This has been a source of regulatory findings in inspections.

Signaling investigations should be done using all serious and non-serious clinical trial data no matter where they are stored or how they are obtained. This may mean the creation of a "data warehouse" to allow access to the data contained in both databases. It is likely that, as EDC and health data standardization advance, clinical trial safety data will be collected in one place without the need for double collecting systems.

Modernizing clinical trial data collection will have many implications:

- Safety data (serious and non-serious AEs) would be received in real time.
- Electronic data entry would be done remotely at each study site rather than centrally at the company or CRO. This takes the data entry out of the direct control of the company or CRO and put into the hands of employees (of variable skill levels and

oversight) at each investigational site. Issues with training, personnel turnover, and quality maintenance at each site now become critical.

- The company drug safety database may not be linked electronically to the EDC database, and new procedures would have to be developed to get the safety data to the safety group for entry into the safety database in an accurate and timely manner.
- Source documents (e.g., laboratory tests, X-ray reports) might not be sent to the company now that studies are "paperless". In fact, source documents may now be electronic, because the classic case report form no longer exists. Where paper source documents exist, they may need to be scanned and added to the EDC, clinical trial, or safety databases.

Getting follow-up information, which continues to be a challenge, will still remain difficult. One can envisage the day when the US, the EU, and other medical systems are standardized and online. All data, including study data and safety data, will be sent electronically in real time and simultaneously to all needed databases at the company, the health agencies, the hospital, the insurance companies, and so on. Safety data will be accurate and rapidly received everywhere they are needed. Maybe. Some hope that AI will help smooth out this situation in the future.

Q: Are phase IV study SAEs reportable as clinical trial AEs (to the IND in the US) or as post-marketing AEs (to the NDA in the US), or as both?

A: If a study is done under an IND or a similar premarketing situation, then the SAEs that meet reporting criteria are reported to the IND. Note that FDA would like only "informative" reports. Further, FDA is skeptical that causality can be attributed using reports of a single subject. Thus, similar reports in the aggregate are perceived to have greater value than single cases, particularly when background rates of the event are considered. Many companies believe that the NDA/MA takes precedence over the IND and would report those SAEs to the NDA/MA, also. This may vary from country to country, so local rules and regulations must be checked. SAEs from studies not done under an IND should be reported to the NDA and in most jurisdictions treated as post-marketing AEs.

Q: If multiple companies or investigators are involved in a trial (whether it is an IIR or a formal company sponsored trial), should there be double (or even triple) reporting just to be sure the cases are not missed?

A: There is no logical reason for duplicate reporting in general and most regulators discourage this. If more than one company is involved, the protocol or other formal written document should contain an agreed-upon mechanism for a single company to handle safety reporting. In such situations, both companies may keep the AEs in their respective databases, but only one company should submit the cases to the regulatory authorities both as expedited and aggregate (annual) reports (and the companies should audit each other for compliance with the agreement).

In some situations, however, companies request that the investigator involved in IIR send a copy of each SAE ICSR to the company. The investigator, as the sponsor, must report such cases to the regulatory authority. The company, in many cases, will also report the case to the regulatory authority "just to be sure", noting in the transmission that this is an IIR and that the investigator is the sponsor and should be submitting the case. Note that in certain cases a duplicate report must be sent to an IND and an NDA at FDA.

Q: Should AEs be reported from observational or epidemiologic trials or registries?

A: This again may vary from country to country, but in general, yes, if a case meets the four validity criteria, then it should be submitted even if it is not from a classic clinical trial. The FDA clarified this issue in its IND reporting guidance by saying that such cases must be reported. For large amounts of data (e.g., "data dumps" from poison control centers), the sponsor may wish to discuss with the agency how such large numbers of cases should be handled. The study protocol should specify how these data should be identified and handled and, in some instances, by agreement, will not be reported.

Q: I thought most of the reporting requirements for clinical trial SAE cases have been harmonized, so why does it seem so complex?

A: To a degree, there has been harmonization. Clinical trial deaths and life-threatening SAEs that are unlabeled and possibly related to the study drug are reportable in 7- and 15 calendar days, respectively. However, there are substantive differences between the way these reports are handled for the US FDA and the rest of the world. Outside the US, each individual SUSAR (suspected unexpected serious adverse reaction) should be expedited; causality is per either the investigator or the sponsor. While the regulatory definition of "serious" is consistent and there is a single, worldwide Investigator Brochure for expectedness, determination of causality for reporting to the US FDA is the responsibility of the sponsor (only). Further, the term "SUSAR" is not recognized in US regulation, even though the concept is the same. Across the globe there are many exceptions or other requirements, local language requirements if the case is a domestic case, non-expedited reporting if the case is not domestic, and so forth. Some countries want or require electronic reporting and others still take or require paper reports (e.g., CIOMS I or MedWatch forms). It is likely things will harmonize eventually, but they are not yet at the level of harmonization for post-marketing case reports. Note that there are different requirements for medical devices, combination products, and, in some countries, there are different requirements for over-the-counter products, neutraceuticals, biologics, and herbals. Finally, a drug may be in clinical trials and not yet approved for marketing in one country, and approved and marketed in another country with different reporting requirements.

Note that the United States spells "harmonization" with a "z" (pronounced "zee" in the United States and "zed" elsewhere) and the UK and others as "harmonisation" with an "s". So, we have not yet even harmonized spelling and pronunciation!

Q: What if an Investigator performed the IIT and did not inform the company?

A: This happens all the time. Unfortunately, some large companies do not have a clear process for communicating with the MAH of the product. Therefor it is within the best interest of the company to develop a process to monitor Clinical Trial Listings (through ClinicalTrials.gov in the US for example) and conduct a regular (suggest monthly) search for new trials involving their products. Another suggestion would be to publicly state your company policy on how to handle IITs and how potential investigators can work collaboratively with the manufacturer on developing their product for further use. Making a company policy publicly available may help with Investigators proactively including the manufacturers in the beginning.

CHAPTER 13

Data Monitoring Committees and Investigational Review Boards/Ethics Committees

■ Data Monitoring Committees

Over the years, in addition to Investigational Review Boards (IRBs), the concept of a separate and additional independent group to monitor the safety of clinical trials has developed. This group or function is known under several names, including Data Monitoring Committee (DMC), Data Safety Monitoring Board (DSMB), Data Safety Board, Clinical Trial Safety Monitoring Committee/Board, and others. This was codified as a draft guidance by the US Food and Drug Administration (FDA) in 2001, updated in 2006 and February 2024 and by the European Medicines Agency in 2003, updated in 2005. (It must be read in conjunction with ICH Note for Guidance E3, E6, E9 but also with Directive 2001/20/EC).

These committees are typically overseen by the clinical development and regulatory teams, however the safety and pharmacovigilance department should have explicit insight into the charter and activities as it relates to the safety evaluation of data and outcomes that need reporting to agencies in either expedited reports, interim analysis, or annual reports.

As stated in the FDA document: "A clinical trial DMC is a group of individuals with pertinent expertise that reviews on a regular basis accumulating data from one or more ongoing clinical trials. The DMC advises the sponsor regarding the continuing safety of trial subjects and those yet to be recruited to the trial, as well as the continuing validity and scientific merit of the trial." Usually, a DMC/DSMB focuses on a single protocol. The FDA has more recently introduced the concept of a Safety Assessment Committee (SAC) charged with monitoring an entire development program, i.e., all protocols.

The EMA definition is similar: "A group of independent experts external to a study assessing the progress, safety data and, if needed, critical efficacy endpoints of a clinical study. In order to do so a DMC may review unblinded study information (on a patient level or treatment group level) during the conduct of the study. Based on its review the DMC provides the sponsor with recommendations regarding study modification, continuation or termination."

Even if some DMCs can be set up to assess both efficacy and safety, the primary mandate is patient safety.

The sponsor or creator of the DMC can be the holder of the IND or equivalent, a company or government agency, or any individual or group to whom the sponsor delegates authority for decision-making, including the study steering or executive committee, the contract research organization (CRO), or the principal investigator. The presence of a DMC, however, is additive to the safety precautions in the trial. All legal and regulatory obligations in all jurisdictions must still be carried out by the investigator (patient protection, AE reporting, etc.) and sponsor (expedited reporting, signaling, etc.).

The DMC must be independent, meaning that no member has any personal basis for preferring the trial outcome to be in one or the other direction, and no member has any ability to influence the trial conduct in a role other than that of a DMC member.

The committees should contain at least three members (usually those noted with an * below) and include such expertise as follows:

1. *Clinical medicine (appropriate specialty) physician
2. *Biostatistics
3. Biomedical ethics
4. Basic science/pharmacology
5. *Epidemiology/pharmacovigilance — drug safety
6. Clinical development and clinical trial methodology
7. Legal /regulatory
8. Patient advocate/community representative

These members should be on every committee. Sometimes there are more than one from these areas. The other members are not necessarily required. Sometimes ad hoc guests with expertise in these areas may attend as needed. Patient advocates are usually not included.

Ideally, there should be geographic representation, especially in international trials, demographic representation on the committee relevant to the trial (race, gender, age), personalities amenable to consensus development, reliability and time to attend meetings, and prior DMC experience. The appointment to the committee should be made by the sponsor, and, for government-sponsored trials, members should be acceptable to the health agency and the investigators. Expenses and honoraria should be paid by the sponsor, and the members should be independent and free of conflicts of interest. The DMC should not have any representation from the industry sponsor, study investigators, or individuals who stand to gain or lose financially from the study outcome, such as major consultants or investors in the sponsor or a competitor. A DMC member should not have any planned authorship of publication(s) or of study results. A DMC may cover more than one trial if the studies are very closely related (note FDA's requirement for a program-level SAC).

A DMC is needed in general for the following:

FDA criteria:

- Large, randomized multi-site studies that evaluate treatments intended to prolong life or reduce risk of a major adverse health outcome such as a cardiovascular event or recurrence of cancer;
- Any controlled trial of any size that will compare rates of mortality or major morbidity;
- When DMC review is practical; and
- When DMC review helps ensure the scientific validity of the trial.

EMA criteria:

- In case of life-threatening diseases, usually the implementation of a DMC is indicated from an ethical point of view;
- Certain patient populations (even if trial is in a non-critical indication): pediatric and mentally disabled patients;
- Prior knowledge or strong suspicion that a treatment under consideration has the potential to harm patients (even though it will be eventually more effective than other available treatments);
- Pre-planned interim analyses for early stopping (either for futility or for positive efficacy) or in case of complex study designs in which a possible

modification of the study design based on unblinded interim data is intended. In such a situation, the use of an independent DMC gives more credibility to the process.

Some trials should almost always have a DMC:

1. If more than one investigational drug is being used in a trial;
2. Trials where early stopping for efficacy is considered:
   - Treatment reduces mortality or major morbidity;
   - Treatment reduces toxicity, cost, or other important secondary factors while maintaining efficacy against mortality/major morbidity;
3. Trials raising special safety or ethical concerns:
   - Early AIDS vaccine trials;
   - Gene therapy trials;
   - Trials in especially vulnerable populations;
4. International and multi-center trials;
5. Phase III confirmatory trials;
6. Phase IIb proof-of-concept trials;
7. Trials where review by independent experts would optimize patient safety and the scientific integrity and credibility of the trial; and
8. Politically sensitive or highly "emotional" trials.

When a DMC is generally not needed:

1. Not required or recommended for most clinical studies (FDA);
2. Trials at early stages of product development, for example, phase I (FDA);
3. Trials addressing lesser outcomes, such as relief of symptoms, unless the trial population is at elevated risk of more severe outcomes (FDA);
4. A clinical study that can be performed in a short time frame that does not allow for appropriate preparation of information for a DMC or the DMC process would delay the finalization of the trial (EMA);
5. Clinical studies in non-critical indications where patients are treated for a relatively short time and the drugs under investigation are well characterized and known for not harming patients (EMA).

The DMC will have several functions during a trial, including the rapid identification of any safety problems; of logistical problems, such as inadequate subject/patient accrual, undesirable distribution of baseline characteristics, excess dropouts, or protocol non-compliance; of the continued feasibility of the trial as designed; and of whether the trial objectives have been met and the trial terminated early. The committee must maintain full confidentiality, as they will usually receive unblinded data. Health agencies typically expect that confidentiality of the interim data will be maintained even if the DMC interacts with the sponsor or trial investigators to clarify issues relating to the epidemiologic context, the conduct of the trial, potential impact on the trial of external data, or other topics, such as scientific or medical progress that eclipses the value of the trial.

To these ends, the DMC will review and approve the study protocol, assess the study conduct, evaluate accumulating data for both safety and efficacy, recommend termination or continuation of the study, recommend modifications of the study (including the informed consent), and recommend additional safety or efficacy analyses, if appropriate. Requests for additional analyses will ordinarily focus on specific parameters and results will only be distributed to DMC members on a confidential basis.

There should be an internal procedure (SOP) that discusses how each DMC is organized, the necessity for a charter, and how they will receive and report information. The SOP should be general enough to have applications to a variety of protocols and the charter should be the more precise document that governs the DMC. The DMC must have a written charter that is drafted and approved by the sponsor and DMC members, ideally before the first DMC meeting. The health agency may in some cases also be involved in the drafting and approval. The charter must include the schedule, format, and venue for meetings, including unscheduled meetings if a safety problem occurs, the format for presentation of data, the specification of who will have access to interim data and who may attend all or part (closed sessions) of the DMC meetings, procedures for assessing conflict of interest of potential DMC members, the method and timing of providing interim reports to the DMC from the sponsor or data-gathering group, the definition of a quorum for decision-making, and details on how the committee will communicate (webinars, teleconferences, face-to-face, etc.). The chosen processes and tools must allow a strong support and flexibility from DMC members; urgent ad-hoc meetings for any important safety issue must be possible to quickly bring an accurate proposal to the sponsor.

A key component (though not "officially" a voting member) of the DMC is the statistician or statistical group, who prepares, analyzes, and presents interim trial results to the DMC. The statistician may be from the company or sponsor or may be from an external CRO or independent consulting firm, but must not be engaged in the actual conduct of the study. The statistician will usually have the blinding key and will unblind study results (see below).

Each DMC meeting usually has an initial open session, followed by a closed session and then a wrap-up open session. At the initial "open" session with DMC and the sponsor, non-confidential matters are discussed, including the clinical trial program, the status of recruitment, baseline patient characteristics, ineligibility rate, accuracy and timeliness of data submissions, and other administrative data and plans. The closed session is attended by only the DMC members and the "independent" statistician who prepared and is presenting the interim analyses to the DMC. After the closed session, a wrap-up open session may be held with the sponsor to relay any recommendations from the DMC. The DMC has the option of conducting an "executive" session with no participants other than DMC members (that is, no sponsor representatives at all), though this is usually not needed.

There has been controversy over whether the DMC should see blinded or unblinded data. Most feel that DMC members should have access to unblinded data to ensure their ability to make accurate risk–benefit assessments. If this is the case, then printed reports of unblinded interim analyses should be supplied to the DMC members several days (at least) before the meeting to allow for adequate review of the information. Sometimes a partial unblinding is done, whereby treatment codes are given for each treatment group (e.g., drug X, drug Y, rather than the names of the drugs). The sponsor should supply the data in a reviewable form. For large studies, some sponsors provide the DMC with listings of individual patients' data, often in a very non-user-friendly way. When there are hundreds or thousands of patients each with multiple labs, exams, and so forth, totaling millions of data points over thousands of pages, it is hard to "eyeball" the data and find trends or issues. These reports and underlying data can also be supplied in digital format. Excellent software is available for examining trends and outliers. Many DMCs also want to see the case report forms for all serious cases or at least all expedited cases.

A terminology note: Companies that make ophthalmologic products usually do not like to use the word "blinded" and prefer to use the word "masked". So, studies are not blinded but masked.

There is a "statistical downside" to multiple reviews of interim data that the sponsor may perform in some studies, namely, that repeated statistical comparisons of event rates between the treated and control groups increases the "false-positive" rate if p values are not adjusted for multiple testing. To put it another way, the more interim data reviews that are done, the more likely that a type I error will be found. At the $p < 0.05$ level, the probability of nominally significant results occurring with three interim analyses is about 10% greater, and with 10 interim analyses about 20% greater.[1] To get around this problem, there are various options available that basically increase the p value required for significance (e.g., requiring a level of 0.018 at each interim and final analysis or 0.001 at each interim analysis and 0.05 at the final analysis). No matter what statistical techniques are used, the DMC must not rely on statistical analyses alone to reach a conclusion. Clinical judgment must also be used to evaluate the safety and efficacy information. Thus, a DMC should have one or more experienced clinicians (physicians) to make clinical judgments.

The DMC will compare AE rates in each treatment arm to see whether there are any major imbalances of concern, and which seem to be due to the intervention rather than the disease or confounding factors (e.g., all the patients in some Northern Hemisphere centers come down with a seasonal influenza). The DMC may also want to see specific patient information for critical or important cases (e.g., SUSARs, acute liver failure, all patients where the blind is broken by the sponsor

[1] See McPherson, Statistics: the problem of examining accumulating data more than once, *New Engl J Med* 1978; 290: 501–502.

or investigator for safety reasons). Again, this calls for good software and reporting tools to allow the DMC to visualize the data it needs.

All meetings should have minutes and kept as a record for the TMF at study closure. This can be tricky as there may be unblinded discussions and sections of the meeting. If the minutes are circulated to company and external individuals, unblinded information must not be included in the minutes. These unblinded discussions may need to be excluded from the minutes or a separate set of "unblinded" minutes may be kept within the DMC. Some DMCs write "minimalist" minutes in which only the topics and options (as noted in the next paragraph here) are included. Discussions are not included.

The DMC has three options after each meeting as follows:

1. Continue the trial unmodified;
2. Modify the trial (Make recommendations on clinical development):
   a. Drop a treatment arm or sub-group;
   b. Modify the treatment dose/schedule;
   c. Add additional safety tests (e.g., electrocardiograms) at screening or during the trial;
   d. Modify consent/Investigators' Brochure;
3. Terminate the trial early due to the following: Serious safety issues;
   a. The efficacy question has been answered and the results are truly compelling, with the risk of a false-positive conclusion acceptably low;
   b. The hypothesis is no longer relevant or the hypothesized benefit cannot be achieved.

There are no rigid stopping rules. Rather, the committee must exercise judgment. General rules of thumb have evolved. It is usually appropriate to demand less rigorous proof of harm to justify early termination than would be appropriate for a finding of benefit. The best is probably to develop general stopping rules in the DMC charter but also keep the door open for unanticipated signals which would justify further assessment and potential stopping.

Interestingly, there is an ongoing and probably unanswerable ethical conflict with DMCs, namely, where does their primary responsibility lie?

- **Perspective 1:** The DMC's primary responsibility is to the specific patients enrolled in the trial. This implies that the DMC should stop the trial early if further results are unlikely to change the conclusion based on interim data. That is, do not put the individual patients at further risk or subject them to placebo for longer than the minimal time necessary.
- **Perspective 2:** The DMC's primary responsibility is to the entire "patient horizon" and the practice of medicine in general. In this case, the DMC would stop the trial early only if the results are sufficiently persuasive to effect changes in medical practice based on limited data.

No single answer fits all cases.

The DMC is usually advisory to the sponsor, and the sponsor may reject the DMC's comments, though this will obviously produce controversy and multiple ethical issues. The DMC results must be communicated to the health agency and the IRBs in any case.

In practice, for large multi-year, multi-center studies, DMCs have proved very useful when well-constituted and well-run. Logistics can be costly and complex if there are thousands of patients and several studies going on at the same time. It is likely that more and more DMCs will be used. Some are even considering DMCs or their equivalent in the post-marketing setting, looking at the spontaneous data coming into the sponsor or Marketing Authorization Holder (MAH). Some have used DMCs in early phase I trials also, but this is very uncommon.[2]

Investigational Review Boards/Ethics Committees

Clinical trials require formal, external, neutral committees to review the protocol and course of the study as well as other aspects of the study. These are called either

[2]For more information on DMCs, refer to the following articles: Shein-Chung Chow, Ralph Corey, Min Lin, On the independence of data monitoring committee in adaptive design clinical trials, *J Biopharm Statist* 2012; 22(4): 853–867; Ellenberg SS, Culbertson R, Gillen DL, Goodman S, Schrandt S, Zirkle M, Data monitoring committees for pragmatic clinical trials, *Clin Trials* 2015; 12(5): 530–536.

Investigational Review Boards (IRBs) or Ethics Committees (ECs). The rules are fairly complex and vary a bit in different regions, but the concepts are all the same: patient protection and good science. These committees may be attached to medical institutions (e.g., hospitals, medical schools) or may be unattached and free-standing, which has led to some controversy. Some may be "central" (e.g., in the European Union covering all sites in one country or in the United States covering all sites) or local. Some studies use a mixture of both local and central IRBs. There are some US-based IRBs that provide service-for-a-fee.

- ICH addressed the issue in their 2016 guideline: Integrated Addendum to ICH E6(R1): Guideline for Good Clinical Practice E6(R2) (www.ich.org).

The EU addressed Ethics Committees in several places, including Directive 2001/20/EC and EudraLex Volume 10 Clinical Trials Guidelines. There are extensive FDA regulations and guidances for IRBs to follow regarding their requirements and obligations in clinical studies. See the "Detailed guidance on the application format and documentation to be submitted in an application for an Ethics Committee opinion on the clinical trial on medicinal products for human use".

The key US regulations are found at 21CFR56.109 (IRB on the review of research). Other requirements include 21 CFR 50.25, which covers protection of human subjects. An FDA summary page clinical trials and human subject protection can be found at: (https://www.fda.gov/scienceresearch/specialtopics/running clinicaltrials/default.htm).

Finally, in August 2016, the FDA issued a draft Guidance for IRBs on written procedures (https://www.fda.gov/downloads/regulatoryinformation/guidances/ucm512761.pdf). There are multiple other guidances on the FDA website which should be referred to covering various aspects of IRBs. The IRB is now expected to be sure of the following:

1. Risks to the subjects are minimized;
2. Risks to subjects are reasonable in relation to anticipated benefits, if any, to subjects, and to the importance of the knowledge that may be expected to result;
3. Selection of subjects is equitable;
4. Informed consent will be sought and appropriately documented;
5. Where appropriate, the research plan adequately provides for monitoring the data collected, to ensure the safety of subjects;
6. Where appropriate, there are adequate provisions to protect the privacy of subjects and to maintain the confidentiality of data;
7. Appropriate additional safeguards are included to protect vulnerable subjects; and
8. Where the study involves children, the research complies with 21CFR50, Subpart D.

FDA regularly audits IRBs and FDA has issued Warning Letters in instances when the IRB was not meeting its obligation to protect patients.

In the EU, the guideline specifies, "The responsibility of an Ethics Committee is to ensure the protection of the rights, safety and well-being of human subjects involved in the clinical trial."

The IRBs and Ethics Committees must review and approve clinical trial protocols to ensure the maximum possible patient protection. This includes a review of the protocol, informed consent, and other aspects of the safety procedures in these trials before the trial starts, as well as maintaining ongoing monitoring of the conduct and results of the trial at least yearly.

These requirements oblige investigators and sponsors to submit certain serious AEs to the IRBs/Ethics Committees either as they occur or in aggregate summary reports. A key controversy revolves around what data are to be sent to the IRBs and Ethics Committees. In the past, every expedited report and follow-up case was sent. This proved to be logistically problematic for the investigators and IRBs as follow-up reports often contained uninformative data (e.g., correction of height or weight). The health agencies have clarified this situation to a degree and now recommend aggregate reporting and line listings sent periodically, e.g., annually.

Individual expedited cases are still required but follow-up reports are usually not sent unless they are medically important. It is useful to discuss with the IRBs and Ethics Committees before starting the study what they wish to receive and when.

For further information, the reader is referred to these documents as well as documents in each country where a trial is being held. This is a complex and changing area as health agencies and the public are becoming increasingly concerned about patient protection.

■ Frequently Asked Questions

Q: Does it make sense to set up one single DMC for the whole clinical development program rather than one per important trial? This would be similar to the FDA concept of a Safety Assessment Committee (SAC).

A: This is a sponsor's policy/decision, although Health Agencies expect a sponsor to demonstrate due diligence across a whole program conducted under an IND. For very large international development projects, with trials in many countries, requesting DMC members to review systematically all safety data can be problematic because of a heavy amount of data to review. Nevertheless, if a DMC is covering part of the trials, in the case of an important safety issue, providing safety data from other trials to the DMC to ensure an accurate assessment should be considered. One of the authors served on a DMC that covered about 10 or 12 trials over several years. They overlapped for certain periods, and we often saw data from 6 to 8 trials. This was feasible for the group but did require a lot of time for data review. The SAC concept now seems to be a good fit for a situation like this.

Q: With the roles and responsibilities of the IRB/Ethics Committee overlapping the duties of the DMC, do we really need a DMC?

A: IRB/EC are required (by regulation) to approve the protocol and then should become an active stakeholder in case of a safety issue. Although the roles of the IRB/EC and DMC overlap, the DMC works much more in "real time" whereas the IRB/EC often sees the data in aggregate or in summary form at intervals. IRB/ECs also may work with many studies and cannot spend as much time and focus on a single safety issue from one of the many studies, perhaps only annually. The DMC can also call for additional data and analyses more easily and more quickly than the IRB/EC. In addition, the IRB/EC can usually stop a study whereas the DMC usually only makes recommendations to the sponsor and cannot actually stop a study itself. Finally, in general, in medicine, the more eyes that look at a patient or a study or data, the better.

Q: Isn't having Key Opinion Leaders (KOLs)/experts in a DMC a way to transfer the responsibility for any decision from the sponsor to the DMC?

A: From the legal and regulatory viewpoint, the sponsor remains THE responsible person/entity for the trial and is viewed that way by the regulatory agencies. From a practical viewpoint, any decision or recommendation made by the DMC, the sponsor is more or less "forced" to follow it.

In other words, setting up a DMC is an important decision and choosing the DMC members is a key part of the process. Picking members who are biased or who are expected to make only favorable decisions is a dangerous policy. Choosing "friends" of some employees can be risky. As an example, having DMC members not experienced in the clinical development field can become problematic if they force a decision which is not appropriate or if they miss a safety issue that the experts would have picked up.

It is unfortunate that many financial and stock analysts follow DMCs decisions and make buy and sell decisions based on this. They usually do not understand or have all the data. These observers can have a strong impact on a start-up company's value and financial stability. It is, therefore, critical to agree on clear roles and responsibilities between the sponsor and the DMC before the DMC kick-off meeting. Moreover, the roles, responsibilities and limits must be included in the charter and agreed on by all parties. DMC members should not talk to the press or others who might benefit from DMC knowledge about the situation; confidentially aspects must be specified in the contract.

CHAPTER 14

How an Individual Case Safety Report (ICSR) is Handled from Start to Finish

This chapter traces an adverse event (AE) through its course in a company from start to finish. The focus of this chapter is on process. A typical case handling process is outlined below. Each step varies from company to company, but all such processes must have written procedures for data receipt, case assessment for expedited reporting, data entry, coding and data review by medical professionals (initially often by a nurse or pharmacist), and a final data review by a physician. The processes illustrated here are not necessarily better than other processes used in the industry. Nor is there a mandated process from the U.S. Food and Drug Administration (FDA), European Medicines Agency (EMA), or any other health authority. Rather, whichever process is implemented, it should ensure a smooth workflow and full compliance with all laws, directives, regulations, and guidances.

Introduction

The mission of the AE processing unit is to ensure that all complaint cases (including AEs, product quality problems, tampering, packaging problems, counterfeits, etc.) are processed in a timely and accurate manner, such that all cases are of high quality and sent to the appropriate departments within the company, to business partners, and to health authorities on time. The goals are to ensure prompt handling and submission of expedited reports, periodic pre-marketing (e.g., Development Safety Update Reports (DSURs)) and post-marketing (e.g., Periodic Safety Update Reports (PSURs) reports and any other obligatory reports. Because late reports to health agencies and business partners are usually easily and immediately noted, this statistic tends to be the one that drug safety groups, management, and health authorities look at to "grade" companies. The goal is 100% compliance all the time, but the reality is that, in an imperfect world, 100% is not always attained. However, nobody will officially write or say this or give an acceptable error rate. More importantly, cases that are late should not be late by very long or for the same reason twice. A root cause analysis to find errors, failures to follow the standard operating procedures, and so on should be performed and corrective actions put in place to prevent repetition.

Many companies put maximal effort into keeping the expedited report score near 100%, often at the expense of case quality or delays in the processing of non-expedited cases — even though no one ever admits to decreases in quality. Companies often build up backlogs of unprocessed or partially processed cases when resources are insufficient to be fully compliant with both expedited and non-expedited cases. Sooner or later, this situation produces a disastrous result unless corrective actions are applied and modified processes are put in place. Adjusted processes must be workable and actually followed. Everything has to be done correctly.

There are many ways to handle cases. In some companies, there is ownership by an individual drug safety specialist (e.g., a nurse or pharmacist), who is responsible for the completion of the case from start to finish, making sure that any other personnel involved in processing the case (e.g., medical reviewers) handle the case and return it to the specialist who "owns" it. Other companies have less individual ownership of a case and instead move a case from task to task in the workflow, with a separate "pool" of workers responsible for a particular step, such as one group that just performs data entry, another that just does coding, and another that just writes narratives. There are many variations on these themes.

■ AE Sources and Arrival in the Safety Department

Serious adverse events (SAEs) and non-serious AEs may arrive in a company from multiple sources (sometimes referred to as "feeder groups"). Standard operating procedures must be in place to ensure that these AEs arrive in a timely manner (usually 1–2 days) in the drug safety department if they first arrive elsewhere in the company or at a partner company.

Spontaneous SAEs and non-serious cases arrive by telephone (the most common route of arrival in many companies); websites; electronically; e-mail; snail mail; fax; reports to sales representatives; reports to other company employees, agents, or contractors; the legal department; health authorities (e.g., FDA, EMA/ EU Agencies, MHRA, Health Canada, etc.); other companies who receive AEs on their own drugs in which one of their drugs is involved; and other miscellaneous sources such as newspaper, social media, or TV stories. They are received primarily from consumers, healthcare professionals, and lawyers. It should be kept in mind that such AEs may arrive at any location in the company, such as manufacturing facilities (especially if the product package says something to the effect of, "Manufactured by XXX Pharma in YYY City", or if an address or phone number is on the package or patient information), subsidiaries and affiliates, contractors, outsourcers, and business partners with whom safety data exchange agreements are in place.

Safety department call centers are usually staffed to receive phone calls from a particular region in a certain language. Usually, they cover a whole country but not more than one country, because labeling, indications, precautions, and warnings may differ from country to country and the appropriate information must be given to residents of the appropriate country. There may also be language issues. For example, any phone center covering Canada must be able to respond in English or French. In the US, though not required by law, many phone centers have Spanish-speaking personnel available in addition to English speakers. Phone centers may be available Monday through Friday during business hours or sometimes 24 hours a day, 7 days a week.

Multiple time zones must also be taken into account for geographically large countries (e.g. Canada, China, Russia, US). Call centers may be kept in-house or outsourced to companies that specialize in handling medical phone calls. These call centers may be within the country or far away (e.g., India, Philippines, and other English-speaking countries are now handling calls from the US and Canada in many cases). Interestingly, some call centers covering English language callers are now being placed in non-native English-speaking countries.

Call centers should be set up to receive calls from consumers, patients, physicians, and other healthcare providers. They usually cover questions about the products; requests for reimbursement; and reporting of AEs, product quality defects, and problems and emergencies regarding the drug, including tampering, counterfeiting, and overdoses. For clinical trial (non-marketed) products, the call center may need to have an emergency code break to handle an acute AE. The call center must be set up to ensure that all AEs and quality complaints are captured and sent to the appropriate departments for handling (e.g., the AEs to drug safety and the quality complaints to manufacturing). In addition, any questions or requests for reimbursement must be handled rapidly and correctly. Callers who are complaining or agitated must also be handled carefully and diplomatically. Thus, a clear protocol must be set up to ensure that customers are served quickly and well, that their requests are met, and that all AEs and complaints are captured. The call should be picked up on the first or second ring, the caller should not be kept on hold for any significant length of time, and the caller should not have to give his or her name, address, and product issue more than once. The caller should not be bounced to multiple departments. Professional call centers are able to track very precise metrics measuring all of these factors.

All this requires a well-thought-out system to handle all issues (especially when a caller has multiple issues: "I took your pill, which was supposed to be red but was blue; it smelled bad; I developed a headache; I want my money back; and I have a question."). The decision about when to have medically trained personnel take the call must be clarified: should all calls come directly to a nurse or pharmacist or should there be some level of non-medical screening before sending the call to the healthcare professional? If non-medical professionals are used, an algorithm or script is often used to ensure that no incorrect information is given to the caller. In addition, the priorities must be considered: should the AE and quality complaint be handled first (most drug safety people would say yes to this but marketers might not)? Because there are multiple company stakeholders involved (drug safety, information technology, product quality, marketing, reimbursement, medical information, etc.), the development of the call center is complex and expensive.

Other sources of AEs (and follow-up) may include the following:

- **Clinical studies:** Clinical study events may come in from the company's clinical research and clinical pharmacology departments, as well as any other group that might run studies (sometimes unbeknownst to the drug safety department). Such groups might be in marketing, subsidiaries, affiliates, market research, pharmacoepidemiology, pharmacoeconomics, or other companies that are studying the drug with your company or are studying the drug without your company's consent and knowledge. AEs may also arrive from contract research organizations.

  Often, much to the chagrin of the safety group, the first awareness that a study is being run in some far-off outpost of the company is the arrival of a serious AE. In the most egregious of such cases, an event may arrive for a drug that the safety department does not even know to be owned, studied, or sold by the company. It might, for example, be studied (or marketed) only in one subsidiary, affiliate, or a partner far away.
- **Legal:** Lawsuits are sometimes the unfortunate first notification to a company that there is a serious AE. These cases usually come in through the legal department, which should be sensitized to the fact that they must not only defend a lawsuit, but also report the AEs to the drug safety department. These AEs are usually on marketed products but may sometimes involve clinical trial subjects. Rarely, a company may be notified of an issue by the

arrival of a subpoena to provide evidence in a lawsuit to which the company is not a party, such as a malpractice case in which there is also a drug issue. Normally, the receipt of AEs via lawsuits is limited, but in certain circumstances, such cases may be voluminous, especially in class action lawsuits in the US.

- **Health agencies:** Many health authorities send to or allow companies (and sometimes the public) access to specific AE cases. The FDA has a program (MedWatch to Manufacturer) in which it sends copies of spontaneously received reports of serious AEs on newly approved products (new molecular entities or "important new biologics") to the manufacturer of the product. The drug must be a new chemical entity. This program lasts 3–4 years and is done at the request of the manufacturer. These reports do not have to be resubmitted to the FDA by the company unless additional information is obtained, but they may have to be submitted to health authorities outside the US if the drug is marketed elsewhere. Health Canada allows the public to search their database, and the FDA has a public dashboard for safety data that can be used to sort and review FAERS data.
- **Literature reports:** US and EU regulations require that companies periodically (e.g., weekly EU GVP module VI) search the medical literature for serious AEs. Such publications are usually on marketed products but may occasionally include serious AEs from clinical trials of new uses for old drugs unknown to the company. Once a drug is on the market, however, nearly anyone may do a clinical trial using the drug (following, of course, regulations, consent, ethics committee approval, etc.) without telling the company. Reports in the literature may be of serious AEs or non-serious AEs, though the former predominate. In oncology, cooperative groups may use marketed drugs in clinical trials (alone or in combination) for new indications or at different doses or schedules from the approved labeling.
- **Stimulated reports:** Many companies have "customer engagement programs", e.g., patient support programs or disease management programs, etc., in which company or outside service companies' representatives (e.g., nurses, physicians) contact patients to encourage them to continue to take their medications and give support regarding dosing, AEs, and so forth. During the course of discussions, AE reports may be obtained. If the company is involved in these support programs (internally or outsourced), a mechanism and process must be created to ensure that all AEs reach the company in a timely manner and are handled appropriately. Other programs such as speaker programs, named-patient programs, and compassionate use may also stimulate reports.
- Other sources of AEs include poison control centers and company and external internet sites (blogs, social media, etc.). In general, the company is not required to troll the internet to look for such AEs, though it must track and capture such AEs of which it becomes aware and, of course, AEs from its own websites (or websites funded by the company). If a drug is reported to another company either by mistake or expressly (e.g., a marketing competitor, another company doing a trial with your drug or in which your drug is a suspect medication in an ICSR), SAE reports may arrive unannounced from other companies on your drug. These cases may be problematic as they may arrive as completed, anonymized ICSRs from the other company. Because of the anonymization, follow-up, as a practical matter, will usually be impossible.
- Electronic receipt of ICSRs by E2B (or customized) formats is common and the company should have systems in place allowing receipt (and transmission) of such cases. This includes the most current E2B version as well as the previous version. Note that follow-up information may arrive by a different means from the original report (e.g., an initial phone report may be followed by a written e-mail/PDF or snail mail communication).

Triage

Upon arrival, by whatever route, of the case data in the drug safety department, it must be properly classified for processing. Whether the report arrives electronically with structured data or not, it must be date-stamped upon entry into the drug safety department. For paper cases, this is a manual rubber stamp with the date and time of arrival. For electronic reports, presumably whatever system is used automatically date stamps the information. Note that this then forces day 0 to be the electronic time stamp. In "the old days", if a case is delivered on Saturday but not opened in the mailroom until Monday, the date stamp and day 0 are Monday. In the "modern electronic world" if a similar case arrives by fax or other electronic means and is date-stamped electronically as Saturday, that is day 0. Follow-up information must also be handled expeditiously.

Every single report that is received should be considered an expedited report until proven otherwise. Thus, the initial triage should be to determine whether the report needs urgent processing to be transmitted to the health authorities, others in the company (e.g., manufacturing for quality issues), or business partners as an expedited report. The triage should be done by someone with a medical skill set to make an accurate determination. Many companies have nurses and pharmacists in this critical role. Triage or case assessment should be standardized. Many companies use dedicated personnel for this function and others rotate staff in to do the triage. For difficult or controversial cases, the triage personnel may request assistance from the drug safety physicians.

Triage should cover, at the least, the following:

1. Which drug(s) is(are) involved? Is it our drug?
2. Case type: spontaneous, clinical trial, stimulated, other?
3. Are the four elements of a valid case (reporter, patient, AE, drug) present and identifiable?
4. Is the AE serious or non-serious?
5. Is there evidence or plausibility for a causal relationship with the suspected drug (for serious clinical trial cases, not for spontaneous cases)?
6. Is the AE expected (labeled) for serious and non-serious cases?
7. Which reports should be expedited?
   - 7-day clinical trial report: serious and death/life-threatening (at presentation), unlabeled, and associated (possibly caused by) with the drug in question;
   - 15-day clinical trial and solicited report: serious, unlabeled, and associated with (possibly caused by) the drug in question;
   - 15-day post-marketing report: serious and unlabeled (no causality determination required);
   - Other reports requiring urgent processing, such as those cases requested by the health agency ("heightened surveillance") to be transmitted to them in an expedited fashion, but that do not meet the formal criteria above or where contracts with a business partner require rapid transmittal.
8. Pregnancy cases (some companies examine for pregnancy cases at triage and others do it later on in the case processing);
   - With an accompanying AE (serious or non-serious);
   - No accompanying AE (serious or non-serious);
9. Product quality complaints (if handled in drug safety) — urgent or non-urgent.

These criteria may be built into an electronic algorithm in the workflow component of the safety database or may be handled with a paper log and tracking form for each case. Some databases have "portals", or desktop displays, of all new and ongoing cases, which can be customized for each employee so that a person knows which cases he or she owns, as well as their workflow status. Manager-level screens may show all the cases in the staff reporting to that manager. Some companies also log all cases into a spreadsheet to track them and ensure that they are not lost in transit within the safety department or at the time of "hand-offs" at each step of the case. In particular, "incomplete cases", or those that do not yet have the four required elements for a valid case but may later on, should be tracked to ensure they are not forgotten or do not "slip through the cracks." A case number should be assigned at this point. This may be a screening case number or the definitive case number assigned by the safety database. For E2B cases, this will include the worldwide ID number. Note that if an "informal" spreadsheet is used to track cases or potential cases, it is subject to audit or inspection and should be secured so that it cannot be altered or changed inappropriately. In general, using such informal spreadsheets or non-secure databases is not a good idea.

After triage, each case should be assigned to the appropriate work channel. Each company develops various channels. They should roughly run along these lines as follows:

- Rapid processing of the death/life-threatening clinical trial cases for submission to the health authorities within 7 calendar days from first receipt by anyone in the company, business partners, CROs, and so forth. This usually means completing the case within approximately 5 calendar days. Attempts should be made immediately to get needed follow-up information, which would be included in a follow-up report to the agencies.
- Processing of 15-day expedited reports for clinical trial or marketed products. These are serious cases for which processing and submission must be completed by calendar day 15, but preferably sooner, to allow quality review, transmission to business partners, and transmission to the authorities. Many companies develop workflow such that all cases are completed by, say, calendar day 10 after initial receipt. Completion dates tend to range from 8 to 12 calendar days in companies, though most companies pick one time frame for all cases and stick to it. This makes for simpler processing and tracking within the drug safety group. CROs and companies that work with multiple partners may (unfortunately) have to tailor their processing procedures for each partner.
- Processing of other serious cases that are not expedited reports. These cases do not have to be sent to the health agencies within 15 calendar days. Rather they are sent in periodic reports at intervals that vary from 3 months to several years, depending on the status of the drug and the regulations in that country. Thus, there is usually the potential for a longer time frame for processing the case if needed. Some companies will use the same processing system for all serious cases, whether expedited or not.
- Serious cases that are to be sent to subsidiaries, business partners, and others may also require rapid processing if contractual arrangements require this. Many companies exchange all serious cases within 10 calendar days whether expedited or not.
- Sometimes a case is not an expedited report in one country but is an expedited case in other countries (e.g., the local labeling or reporting regulations are different there). This case must be transmitted to the subsidiary or business in time to meet 15-day reporting rules there. It is often the situation, especially in large multi-national companies, that the sending company (e.g., drug safety in the home office) is not able to know whether or not any particular serious case will be an expedited report in all countries where the drug is sold. Thus, many companies process these cases as if they were expedited reports and use a completion date of about 10 calendar days (as noted above).
- Non-serious cases may be processed more slowly (e.g., 30 days) because they are not reportable at all or are reportable only in aggregate reports; In the EU non-serious spontaneous ICSRs are to be reported electronically to the EMA within 90 cal. days. It is wise to screen non-serious cases rapidly upon receipt, especially if they come from "less than reliable sources," to ensure that no serious cases are misclassified (presumably not intentionally) as non-serious cases. Misclassification could lead to late expedited reports.
- Similarly, the "other" cases, such as literature, legal, and cases received from health authorities, should be processed as appropriate for the company's needs. It is a general rule of thumb that the process should be kept as simple as possible and that "exceptions to the rule" be kept limited. As few as three fundamental procedures could serve: 7-day cases, all serious cases (handled as if they are all expedited cases), and all non-serious cases.

Database Entry

At this point, the case should be entered into the computerized safety database if it has not already been entered. If the case is received electronically, it should be reviewed in a "holding area" before it is officially uploaded into the safety database unless it comes from a trusted source where such review is deemed unnecessary. Electronic edit checks can be very useful at this point. For example, clinical trial cases uploaded from a dedicated electronic data collection system for a company's studies may be uploaded directly if the case is entered in sufficient detail and there are quality checks at the investigational site.

If the case arrives manually using a standardized paper data collection form, then manual data entry should be fairly easy to do. If not, the data may arrive in any sort of form: case report forms, handwritten notes, CIOMS I or MedWatch forms, hospital records, physicians' notes, telephone reports, and so forth. Sometimes data entry is easy; sometimes it is not. Some companies have an initial review by a medical professional who highlights items for data entry; other companies have the source documents sent directly to the data entry group (nonmedical professionals) and have medical review only after that is completed.

If a case number (also called a "control number" or "medical reference number") has not been assigned to the case at the triage or logging level, it is assigned now. MedDRA® coding of AEs, medical history, and other required MedDRA fields is done either by the drug safety group or by a dedicated coding group. Drug coding using a standardized dictionary is also done. The case narrative is usually written at this point. The narrative may be difficult and complex if the case is long and complicated. There are standard ways that narratives should be written in terms of format, content, follow-up information, etc. Some companies developed "automated narratives": data are picked from other recorded fields and the database generates the narrative; it is then to be reviewed, potentially updated and validated by Medics. The narrative is the key summary of the case and should usually be a good "stand-alone" summary of the case. Much care should be taken in its preparation.

■ Quality Review

At this point, a drug safety specialist (usually a nurse or pharmacist) reviews the data entry against the source documents and prepares or reviews the case narrative. Any changes or additions to the case are made at this time. A clear methodology on the quality check should be developed so that it is done in a systematic, standardized, and repeatable way. Those fields, if any, that are not reviewed (e.g., height) should be defined in the methodology up front in addition to those fields that are. The quality review should look at content, grammar, and format. In general, one does not need to be a perfectionist regarding grammar; however, sentences that are unclear or do not convey the desired meaning should be corrected. Short simple sentences should be used because many of the readers may not be native English-language speakers.

■ Follow-Up

Follow-up information should be requested when the initial case is incomplete or unclear. Rarely does a case have complete information, especially if the AE just happened or is ongoing. Thus, it is usually required that follow-up queries be sent to the reporter to complete the case data. The need for follow-up is also mentioned in 21CFR312.32(d) for IND reports and 314.80(c)(1)(ii) for NDA reports. EU GVP module VI also notes that follow-up is necessary: "When first received, the information in suspected adverse reactions reports may be incomplete. These reports should be followed-up as necessary to obtain supplementary detailed information significant for the scientific evaluation of the cases. This is particularly relevant for monitored events of special interest, prospective reports of pregnancy (see VI.B.6.1. for guidance on the management of pregnancy reports), cases notifying the death of a patient, or cases reporting new risks or changes in the known risks. This is in addition to any effort to collect missing minimum criteria for reports validation (see VI.B.2. for ICSRs validation). Any attempt to obtain follow-up information should be documented."

Follow-up data should be entered into the database using a procedure similar to the one used for initial data. Care must be taken to ensure that the data are not mistaken for a new case but rather are clearly identified as follow-up to a case already received.

There is no "correct" number of follow-ups that should be done. Follow-ups should be done to get the needed information. Sometimes it is a single follow-up; sometimes many. Sometimes the reporter or patient refuses to give follow-up. At least two attempts should be made and documented in such situations.

Medical Review

At this point in the case, after it has been completed and reviewed by the drug safety specialist and after it has undergone a quality review, some or all cases should be reviewed by the drug safety physician. Historically, physician review was limited to serious cases, but many companies are now having all cases undergo physician review to ensure that no serious cases are misclassified as non-serious. The medical review should generally cover the medical content of the case, with particular attention paid to the narrative, the suspect and concomitant drugs (including dosages), the past medical history, and coding. It is generally not the role of the physician to do a source document quality review unless he or she needs to refer to the source documents for clarification of a medical point. This varies from company to company, however. In certain critical cases, it is often desirable that the physician review all source documents, even if this is not routine policy.

Case Closure

In one sense, a case is never really closed, as new information could arrive weeks, months, or even years later, requiring the case to be updated. But for practical purposes, once the above steps are concluded and follow-up requested, a case may be considered closed or completed for operational purposes. If and when follow-up arrives, the case can be reopened and processed. The distinction between closure (or locking) of a version and closure or completion of a case should be noted. A company may, for practical operational reasons, "lock" each case a certain number of days after the receipt of the information so that the case can be processed properly without new data arriving and being entered into the case when it is in medical review or ready to be transmitted to the health authorities.

For example, if data are received on day 0, the case is processed and locked on, say, calendar day 7 and sent to the health authorities on calendar days 12–14. Note that business partners or local country affiliates may require shorter timelines to meet obligations. Any additional follow-up data on this case that arrive after day 7 is put into a follow-up version of the case. This prevents the staff from scrambling to get last-minute data into the case with the appropriate medical review, quality control, and so forth. In such a situation, two versions of a case may be open at the same time. Most computer systems are able to handle these versioning issues. In occasional situations, additional data may indeed be added to the case at the last minute if deemed critical (e.g., death outcome has just arrived).

Case Distribution and Transmission

Cases are next distributed to those in the company who need to see them (e.g., clinical research, legal) and to other companies with whom safety exchange agreements are in place. Cases are also submitted directly to the health agencies via E2B or other direct means (e.g., certified mail, courier) or distributed to others in the company, such as the regulatory department, for submission to the health authorities. Cases may also be sent to subsidiaries or affiliates worldwide for their submission to local agencies — often with a cover letter in the local language and, in some instances, with a translation of the case itself into the local language if English is not accepted. In the EU, cases from clinical trials are submitted to the national authority. Post-marketing cases are submitted directly to EudraVigilance in E2B format. Some jurisdictions require non-coded portions of the case to be reported in the local language. When using the E2B(R3) message format, the case narrative, for example, is a repeating field, so that a translation of the narrative may be provided in the local language at the same time as the "official" English language narrative.

Tracking

It is critical to have markers in the database to track cases through the processing system. Each drug safety specialist and manager should be aware of all pending cases, their status in the trip toward completion/closure, and, in particular, the deadlines for each case.

It is critical that all 7- and 15-day reports be tracked so that none is submitted late to the health authorities, subsidiaries, or business partners. The manager can reallocate cases or other work to ensure that the time-critical cases are handled appropriately in case of absence, vacation, staff overload, or maldistribution of caseloads.

Similarly, non-expedited cases that need to be completed for aggregate reports should be tracked so that they are completed before the data lock. This can be as frequent as every 3 months for NDA periodic reports. In the EU, non-expedited cases must be submitted to EudraVigilance within 90 days from first awareness; the data lock for PSURs/PBRERs, of course, is driven by the timetable determined on a product-by-product basis by the PRAC. The dates of the periodic reports are known in advance, so there is no excuse for a case missing the report. Follow-up information may be provided in the next aggregate report.

In general, tracking should be done electronically and generated automatically from the drug safety database unless there are so few cases that manual tracking is practical. Most modern drug safety databases have a tracking function with customizable reports. Manual tracking on spreadsheets is time consuming and usually not practical once AE volume grows and the staff becomes large.

The question often arises in a small company about whether it should have a safety department and/or a database. In regard to a safety department, whether a drug is in clinical trials or marketed, the answer is yes. That department may be one person supervising the outsourced CRO or a partner handling the safety. Such a situation may be satisfactory for small companies with few AE cases. Once the volume and complexity grow (e.g., marketing in multiple countries), the need for an in-house safety function and database becomes more compelling. Although it is explicitly stated by some regulatory authorities that an electronic safety database is not necessarily obligatory, all the appropriate (templated) reporting (e.g., PSURs/PBRERs) must still be done and, without a database, this may not be feasible or practical. The question then becomes whether it is practical to rely on a CRO or partner for all safety functions with the subsequent benefits and costs (both monetary and not) to the business as well as safety. For some companies, this may be worthwhile, but not so for others.

In addition to tracking the AEs that arrive and are processed, the following key performance indicators should be tracked at a minimum:

- Total number of AEs;
- Serious AEs;
- Non-serious AEs
- Clinical trial AEs (i.e. SAEs, SUSARs);
- Spontaneous AEs (serious and non-serious);
- Overall data and data stratified by type of report;
  - Those submitted on time;
  - Those submitted late, by how much, why, and corrective actions taken;
  - Cases submitted to business partners and others;
  - Time to process cases, depending on case type (expedited, serious non-expedited, non-serious, etc.);
  - Time to submission to each major health agency (FDA, EMA, etc.);
  - Tracking by drug or class of products or drug safety teams, depending on how the drug safety group and the company are organized;
  - Timeliness of aggregate reports, e.g., DSURs, PSURs/PBRERs, IND and NDA periodic reports.

It is useful periodically to graph and publish these metrics ("key performance indicators", or "KPIs") for the entire drug safety staff. Such data can also be used for resource allocation, budgeting, projection of future work (e.g., AEs for allergy drugs peak twice a year and more staff may be needed then), and justification for more resources. The metrics may aid in identifying problems, or "rough spots," and help to institute changes to prevent recurrence of such problems. Publicly posted data should not identify individuals or point out "non-producers" to shame them into speeding up. Praise should always be done publicly, but chastisement should be done privately.

The timing, sequence, and duration of each step in processing an AE should be clearly spelled out in measurable and auditable SOPs or working documents. If the company determines that, say, all SAEs will be completed within 10 calendar days and all non-serious cases within 30 calendar days, this timing should be built into each case. This should be done automatically in the database workflow system with a tickler, e-mail, or similar reminders to the concerned individual, telling him or her of the timing and due date for each case. The due dates would be updated as needed (e.g., it is determined to be or not to be a 15-day expedited report, or a case is upgraded from non-serious to serious). Attention must be paid to weekends and holidays in calculating due dates. Note that bank holidays in the UK may be working days elsewhere and the Chinese New Year may be celebrated outside China.

Each person in the workflow must know when his or her task is due, and the manager must be able to track the case through each step to ensure its completion. Other companies have "pools" of people handling each step rather than having one drug safety specialist "own" the case. In the pool situation, the first available "pool" member handling that step processes the case.

Investigator Notification

The concept of investigator notification of expedited clinical trial reports used to be simple but has now become somewhat more complicated.

The ICH proposals in the E6(R2) guideline "Integrated Addendum to ICH E6(R1): Guideline for Good Clinical Practice E6(R2)" are somewhat ambiguous:

- "The sponsor should promptly notify all concerned investigator(s)/institution(s) and the regulatory authority(ies) of findings that could affect adversely the safety of subjects, impact the conduct of the trial, or alter the IRB/IEC's approval/favorable opinion to continue the trial." (5.16.2)
- "The sponsor should expedite the reporting to all concerned investigator(s)/institutions(s), to the IRB(s)/IEC(s), where required, and to the regulatory authority(ies) of all adverse drug reactions (ADRs) that are both serious and unexpected." (5.17.1)

The EU is more explicit:

- The sponsor shall inform all investigators concerned of findings that could adversely affect the safety of study subjects.
- The information can be aggregated in a line listing of SUSARs accompanied by a summary of the evolving safety profile of the product;
- In the case of blinded trials, the line listing should present data on all SUSARs, regardless of the medication administered (e.g., active/placebo/comparator), maintaining the blind.
- If a significant safety issue is identified, either on receipt of an ICSR or on review of aggregate data, the sponsor should immediately notify all investigators.
- A safety issue that affects the course of the clinical study or development project, including suspension of the study program or safety-related amendments to study protocols, should also be reported to the investigators (Volume 10).

Note: No time frame is specified. Many companies use the 15-day requirement used in the US.

The US regulations are also somewhat ambiguous, particularly in terms of format:

- "*IND safety reports.* The sponsor must notify FDA and all participating investigators (i.e., all investigators to whom the sponsor is providing drug under its INDs or under any investigator's IND) in an IND safety report of potential serious risks, from clinical trials or any other source, as soon as possible, but in no case later than 15 calendar days after the sponsor determines that the information qualifies for reporting..." (21CFR312.32(c)(1)).
- 21CFR312.32(c) also requires that "In each IND safety report, the sponsor must identify all IND safety reports previously submitted to FDA concerning a similar suspected adverse reaction, and must analyze the significance of the suspected adverse reaction in light of previous, similar reports or any other relevant information."

In regard to investigator notification, FDA indicated that:

- All participating investigators filed to open INDs (including investigator initiated studies) should be notified in an IND safety report of potential serious risks;

- Follow-up reports should be sent to investigators to inform and update them about an important suspected adverse reaction if it significantly affects the care of the subjects or conduct of the study;
- Minor refinements that do not significantly affect care of subjects or conduct of the study need to be sent to FDA but need not be sent to investigators; and
- Such information may be communicated to investigators in a routine update of the investigator brochure.

These requirements have been interpreted in various ways. "Participating Investigators" is ambiguous. Many companies take a conservative view and report all expedited reports to all investigators in all phase I, II, and III trials, as well as to investigators in investigator-initiated studies using this study drug whether for this indication or not. Some sponsors will also send spontaneous reports for this drug to investigators if it is also on the market. The drug safety group prepares the analysis of similar cases from the safety database and sometimes from the clinical trial database if cases are present there that are not in the drug safety database.

15 Calendar Days and Day 0 versus Day 1

The FDA in its draft guidance *Post-marketing Safety Reporting for Human Drug and Biological Products Including Vaccines* of March 2001, refers to the completion of box G4 on the MedWatch 3500A form as the date the company first awareness of the four criteria for a valid AE (reporter, patient, event, drug) and that this is day 0 of the 15-day time clock. This has been carried over to field A.1.6 (date report was first received from source) in the E2B message. It is important to pay attention to this because it triggers compliance metrics. This date then gives up to 16 calendar days for a case. Depending on the time the case is received, day 0 is usually less than 24 hours. The document also notes clearly that the case must be received by FDA no later than day 15. If the 15th calendar day is a weekend or a US federal holiday, the report may be submitted on the first working day after the weekend or holiday. However, if a company has submission obligations in countries outside the United States, the federal holiday (and possibly even the weekends) should not be allowed to permit a delay in submission.

The EU is more explicit and states in GVP module VI.B.7: "The clock for the submission of a valid ICSR starts as soon as the information containing the minimum criteria has been brought to the attention of the national or regional pharmacovigilance center of a competent authority or of any personnel of the marketing authorization holder, including medical representatives and contractors. This date should be considered as day 0." The same applies if new information on the case is received by the MAH, i.e., the reporting time clock begins again for the submission of the follow-up report from the day the MAH receives relevant follow-up information. The clock for expedited reporting starts (day 0) as soon as the minimum information has been brought to the attention of any personnel of the MAH or an organization holding a contractual agreement with the MAH including medical representatives.

CHAPTER 15

Seriousness, Expectedness, and Causality

The drug safety staff involved in individual case evaluation generally have to make several decisions regarding each case. These decisions must be made rapidly on receipt of an Individual Case Safety Report (ICSR) because this determines how the case is handled in the drug safety department and whether, how, and when it is reported to health agencies and business partners. Seriousness and expectedness are key criteria to classify, analyze and report ICSRs to the appropriate bodies. Causality has key consequences as well, but mainly for clinical trial case reports. During clinical development, these three criteria actually support the selection of ICSRs, which are SUSARs to be reported on an urgent basis to health agencies.

■ Introduction

The concept and practice of assessing and reporting if an event is serious, if it is expected, and if it has a causal relationship to a medical product, should be clearly defined in internal procedures such as SOPs, as the process of these assessment have an enormous impact on the reporting requirements to agencies as well as the interpretation of impact of the event in the patient population. Standard procedures should define and match the regulatory definition of seriousness and state that these definitions will be included in all clinical development protocols. The SOP should also define how expectedness will be determined. If the company has both developmental and approved products (perhaps the same product in different regulatory jurisdictions), then the procedure should reference the appropriate reference material such as the Investigator Brochure for developmental products, or the appropriate Labeling document (SmPC, Package Insert, Label, etc.) for the approved product. If a company does not want to put this language in a procedure (not recommended), then the protocol should at a minimum define how these criteria will be defined and determined.

■ Seriousness

Is an event Serious? This is one of the first questions asked when we receive safety information regarding an adverse event either in a clinical trial or in the post-market setting. These definitions are fairly set-in-stone, have not changed over the course of several years and are one of the major building blocks of assessing and categorizing a case.

The generally accepted definition of seriousness is as follows:

A serious adverse event (AE) (experience) or serious adverse reaction is any untoward medical occurrence that at any dose:

- Results in death;
- Is life-threatening;
- Requires inpatient hospitalization or prolongation of existing hospitalization;
- Results in persistent or significant disability/incapacity;
- Is a congenital anomaly/birth defect;
- Is medically significant; Medical and scientific judgment should be exercised in deciding whether expedited reporting is appropriate in other situations, such as important medical events that may not be immediately life-threatening or result in death or hospitalization but may jeopardize the patient or may require intervention to prevent one of the other outcomes listed in the previous definition. These should also usually be considered serious. "Examples of such events are intensive treatment in an emergency room or at home for allergic bronchospasm; blood dyscrasias or convulsions that do not result in hospitalization; or development of drug dependency or drug abuse" (ICH E2A).

Important Medical Events

The EudraVigilance Expert Working Group has coordinated the development of an Important Medical Event (IME) terms list based on the Medical Dictionary for Regulatory Activities (MedDRA®) (see GVP Annex IV in the EMA PV Modules). This IME list aims to facilitate the classification of suspected adverse reactions, the analysis of aggregated data and the assessment of ICSRs in the framework of day-to-day pharmacovigilance activities. The IME list is intended for guidance purposes only and is available on the Agency website to stakeholders who wish to use it for their pharmacovigilance activities. It is regularly updated in line with the latest version of MedDRA. *Note*: The EU and Japan also note that any suspected transmission via a medicinal product of an infectious agent is also considered serious (GVP Module VI C.2.2.5).

Over the years, these definitions have been discussed, parsed, and clarified by health agencies, companies, and other interested observers. In general, the most conservative interpretation is the one drug safety groups should use.

Some comments are as follows:

- **Death:** Although one would believe this binary concept (alive–dead) would be rather straightforward, there have been some discussions relating to the timing of the death and the circumstances around the AE and the death.

  A note on death: It is generally accepted that death is an outcome and not an actual event, which is true; something must have caused the patient's death, be it cardiac arrest or progressive disease, but something did *cause* the death. As scientists, we want to explore the cause of the death once it has been reported, To understand whether the event that caused the death was a result of the product use, some companies in the past have failed to report cases where the only event reported was "death" citing that they didn't have the minimum criteria to report, and that this situation did not fulfill case reporting. **If during clinical development, or even in the post-marketing period, an event of "death" is reported, a company**

must regard this as valid information and report what is known and attempt to assess the case as best as possible while obtaining additional information. Companies should have clear procedures in place and language within protocols that outline how events of "death" will be handled to avoid any confusion.

It is fairly clear that if a patient has a myocardial infarction (the SAE) and then over the next several hours or days goes into shock, has severe arrhythmias, and dies, this death is related to the SAE and this is a "fatal myocardial infarction". It gets trickier, however, if the patient has a myocardial infarction and during a cardiac catheterization goes into an intractable ventricular arrhythmia and dies. Is the myocardial infarction to be classified as a fatal one or is the death a sequela of the catheterization? Some will argue that the catheterization was performed because of the myocardial infarction. There is no clear answer, and it may vary from case to case. The most conservative call is often used by drug safety units; that is, the death is a part of (or consequence of) the SAE. However, if a medically defensible call is made that is less conservative, this should be noted somewhere in the case along with the reasoning behind the decision.

Another example would be that of a fall. If a patient trips while walking on a level surface, falls, and scrapes his or her knee, this is most probably a non-serious AE. If, however, he or she falls while standing on a ledge or walking down a staircase and dies as a result of the fall, the case should be reported as a serious and fatal case but how to classify it is tricky. The fall may be non-serious, but the sum of the case is clearly serious and fatal because of the fatality occurring after the fall, not the actual fall. Again, there is no clear answer; many would take the conservative approach and consider this case (if occurring during a clinical trial) as a serious, fatal, unlabeled fall (presuming "fatal fall" is not in the investigator brochure), and unrelated to the study drug (unless it is believed to be related, perhaps due to accompanying dizziness, which should also be coded). Others would argue that the AE was the fall and everything that happened after it was due to the circumstances of standing near the ledge. Had the fall occurred on the level surface none of the events leading to the death would have occurred.

In a 1996 report on a survey done at the US and EU Drug Information Association meetings in 1993, Dr. Win Castle and Dr. George Phillips reported marked transatlantic differences in the interpretation of seriousness and expectedness. For example, "total blindness for 30 minutes" was believed to be serious by 89% in the European Union survey and 44% in the US survey compared with "mild anaphylaxis", which was believed to be serious by 37% of the EU responders and 98% of the US responders. Whether this is still the case remains to be seen, but the results nonetheless are most interesting and suggest the need for harmonization and training of safety reviewers.[1]

- **Life-threatening:** *Note*: The term *life-threatening* in the definition of *serious* refers to an event in which the patient was immediately at risk of death at the time of the event; it does not refer to an event that hypothetically might have caused death if it were more severe. This concept also has interpretation issues revolving around whether the SAE would truly kill the patient if untreated. A non-severe myocardial infarction with no cardiac function compromise or arrhythmias might be considered serious (medically significant if not hospitalized) but not life-threatening, whereas a myocardial infarction that progresses over the next hour or two to pulmonary edema would be considered life-threatening. This definition thus may overlap to a degree with "medically significant". Again, most would take a conservative approach. Note that for clinical trials, FDA changed the definition effective March 2011 to include the requirement that the idea of whether an AE is life-threatening should be commented upon by both the investigator and the sponsor and that if either one feels it is, then the AE should be so considered.
- **Hospitalization:** Much debate occurred over what actually constitutes "hospitalization" or "inpatient

[1] Castle, Phillips, Standardizing "expectedness" and "seriousness" for adverse experience case reporting. *Drug Inform J* 1996; 30: 73–81.

hospitalization". Some patients may be kept overnight (even up to 24–36 hours) in the emergency department for observation and treatment but not "formally" admitted to the hospital as an inpatient. Thus, this patient would not qualify as serious based on a stay in the emergency room (see the Food and Drug Administration's 2001 draft guidance on AE reporting, Section IV.A.3). In the EU, Directive 2001/83/EC refers to the definition of SAE, including "inpatient" hospitalization. Generally, an event meets the criteria for hospitalization if the patient was admitted to the hospital for more than 24 hours. Most clinical trial protocols will even go so far to state that if the hospitalization was due to an elective procedure, or pre-planned operation not relevant to the disease under study, that these events would not meet the criteria for hospitalization. The easiest way to figure this out is to ask "Was the person hospitalized unexpectedly for an adverse event or procedure that was unanticipated or unplanned?"

- **Significant or persistent disability/incapacity:** A relatively uncommon criterion in practice andnot formally defined. The FDA gives an interesting example in its 2001 draft guidance: *Persons incarcerated because of actions allegedly caused by a drug (e.g., psychotropic drugs and rage reactions) have sustained a substantial disruption in their ability to conduct normal life functions. Thus, these adverse experiences would qualify for the significant or persistent disability/incapacity outcome.* Note the change referred to earlier in this chapter about FDA's addition of this concept directly into the definition of "serious". The FDA slightly altered the definition of "serious" effective March 2011 for clinical trials by adding the concept of "disability" directly into the definition, including the phrase: "substantial disruption of the ability to conduct normal life functions".
- **Congenital anomaly/birth defect:** Usually rather straightforward. It would include even mild birth defects, when detected. The FDA also notes that this includes those defects "occurring in a fetus", thus covering abnormalities discovered before birth.
- **Important Medical Events (IME):** This criterion has often been difficult to handle for pharmacovigilance departments because the definition relies on medical judgment. The examples given (allergic bronchospasm, blood dyscrasias, or convulsions) do not necessarily help to clarify other less dramatic situations. The FDA also gives the examples of drug dependency or drug abuse as important events. Often, cases elicit hours of debate in drug safety units on whether to consider them medically important. Is a mild focal seizure medically important? Is a platelet count 10% below the lower level of normal medically important? Other examples abound. Various rules of thumb have developed as follows:

- If it happened to you or a family member, would you consider it important or medically significant?
- If you discuss or debate whether a case is medically important, it is.
- The EudraVigilance Working Group developed an IME (Important Medical Events) list\https://eudravigilance.ema.europa.eu/human/textforIME.asp which is updated twice a year in step with new versions of MedDRA and can be downloaded at the site listed above. Use of the IME list is voluntary and not required by regulation.
- If a member of the marketing or sales department or a non-medical professional believes it is not important, it is important. This "rule", though somewhat jocular and cynical, has developed to note the real observation that sometimes there are non-medical pressures put on personnel in the safety department to interpret cases or make decisions based on sales, financial, or other non-medical criteria. This is an unfortunate fact of life — not just in the pharmaceutical world but in the world of clinical medicine, where many judgments are now made on a cost-effectiveness basis. Always keep in mind that the primary mission of the drug safety department is to protect public health.
- As a rule, we must never forget the purpose of such criteria: the goal is not just to ensure we are (or not) sticking to the regulations (obviously we must); but to select the cases which are the most clinically-relevant/important to identify a signal, if any, to protect the public health. Moreover, if one of the seriousness criteria can be

checked off, then the others are less important as the case report becomes serious. The point is to ensure that the case is correctly assessed as serious or not. Therefore, in case of doubt, it is wise to call the case/AE as serious and avoid endless discussions between co-workers; let's not waste any more time!

■ Expectedness

Is the event expected? Have we seen this event before in the nature and severity is has occured? Is this event known to occur in the patient population or in association with the product in use? These are some of the questions we aim to answer when determining Expectedness.

The regulations governing expectedness are fairly straightforward:

For a pre-marketed product: Any adverse drug experience, the specificity or severity of which is not consistent with the current investigator's brochure; or, if an investigator brochure is not required or available, the specificity or severity of which is not consistent with the risk information described in the general investigational plan or elsewhere in the current application, as amended. For example, under this definition, cerebral thromboembolism and cerebral vasculitis would be unexpected (by virtue of greater specificity) if the investigator brochure only listed cerebral vascular accidents (21CFR312.32(a)). FDA added to this definition effective March 2011 by noting in 21CFR312 that "Unexpected, as used in this definition, also refers to AEs or suspected adverse reactions that are mentioned in the investigator brochure as occurring with a class of drugs or as anticipated from the pharmacological properties of the drug, but are not specifically mentioned as occurring with the particular drug under investigation". That is, an AE in the class labeling section of the brochure without specific mention for the study drug is considered unexpected.

> **For marketed products:** Any adverse drug experience that is not listed in the current labeling (PI or SmPC or local labeling) for the drug product. This includes events that may be symptomatically and pathophysiologically related to an event listed in the labeling, but differ from the event because of greater severity or specificity, outcome, or frequency. For example, under this definition, hepatic necrosis would be unexpected (by virtue of greater severity) if the labeling only referred to elevated hepatic enzymes or hepatitis.
>
> AEs that are "class-related" (i.e., allegedly seen with all products in this class of drugs) and mentioned in the labeling (PI or SmPC) or Investigator Brochure, but which are not specifically described as occurring with this product, are considered unexpected" (21CFR314.80(a)).

In the European Union, expectedness is addressed in Regulation 536/2014 for clinical trials and Directive 2001/83 for registered products. "Unexpected serious adverse reaction means a serious adverse reaction, the nature, severity or outcome of which is not consistent with the Reference Safety Information" (RSI) (i.e., Investigator Brochure for an unauthorized investigational product and SmPC for an authorized product). In addition, the regulation specifies that "Expectedness shall be determined on the basis of events previously observed with the active substance and not on the basis of the anticipated pharmacological properties of a medicinal product or events related to the subject's disease". Severe must not be misunderstood or confused with serious: the word severe is used to assess medical intensity while serious helps to identify regulatory reporting obligations.

In theory, this concept is rather straight forward, but in practice, it becomes somewhat harder when synonyms and overlapping concepts are considered. In the report cited previously by Castle and Phillips, 72% of the EU responders believed that if the labeled event is "dizziness", then "vertigo" would also be considered expected (labeled), but only 50% of the US responders believed vertigo was labeled. Similarly, 18% of the EU responders and 3% of the US responders believed that if "hypotension, wheezing, and urticaria" are labeled, then a reported term of *anaphylaxis* would also be expected. Whether these differences persist, many years after the survey, is unclear. However, it does highlight the fact that well-trained experienced medical personnel doing pharmacovigilance can take the same set of facts and come up with differing and even opposing views. This study also highlighted the potential differences of interpretation due to language: non-native English speakers may actually misinterpret case-reports.

In general, one should decide expectedness without thought to seriousness. That is, just because a case is non-serious and the AE in question is mildly severe and of little medical import (e.g., a maculopapular rash) compared with a serious AE (e.g., severe hepatitis), the decision on expectedness should be made purely on the basis of the wording in the label and not on the seriousness. Give each AE its due.

With clinical trial drugs, especially those not yet marketed, there may be minimal or no human experience (e.g., the first study in humans or the first phase II study after phase I studies showed no AEs). In this case, there are no labeled events in the investigator brochure, and everything is thus "new" and unexpected. Anticipated events based on the pharmacologic properties of the drug should not be considered expected until actually reported in a patient and put into the brochure.

In some cases, it is necessary to consider the route of administration, dosage, or indication being studied when assessing the expectedness. This usually depends on how the investigator brochure or marketed labeling is written. Some describe a different set of AEs for different indications, dosages, or routes of administration. Care must be taken to apply the correct label to each case when doing expectedness. Note that benefit–risk assessments are performed indication-by-indication, both for marketing approval and in the post-marketing phase. The general advice would be, as with seriousness, to decide on the side of conservatism. Thus, if there are questions on whether an AE is expected, consider it unexpected.

■ Relatedness (Causality)

Was the event associated with the use of the product? Did the product cause the event to occur?

Of the three criteria revolving around the regulatory reportability of an individual case (seriousness, expectedness, and relatedness), this one is often the most difficult to do for the multiple reasons explained next. Causality may be determined initially at the individual case level, after the receipt of an individual case safety report, but probably more importantly, again after the review of aggregate data in a case series as for signaling, risk management, and various regulatory reports with aggregate data, such as PSURs/PBRERs.

First, some basic "housekeeping" points should be cleared up to ensure that cases are always handled and collected in the same manner. In doing case assessment of ICSRs, one should be sure that cases are coded using the current MedDRA® version and codes (some older dictionaries may still be used outside the ICH regions and some labeling for older drugs may not be in MedDRA). Coders should be trained on coding conventions aligned with the current version of MedDRA and there should be consistent methodology, current coding conventions, and synonym lists. MedDRA Labeling Groupings, when used, should have clear (updated) lists of included terms.

For aggregate reports, the search criteria for the case series should be complete and normalized to the current (i.e., same) MedDRA version and drug dictionary for all ICSRs in the aggregate analysis. This may require migration from earlier versions if the aggregate report spans more than one MedDRA version. If queries are required to obtain similar cases for a specific medical concept of interest, Standardized MedDRA Queries (SMQs) developed by CIOMS and published by the MSSO in step with each version of MedDRA, should be used in accord with CIOMS guidance. Cases should be followed up (rapidly upon receipt, not at a later date), as appropriate, to ensure the maximum amount of high-quality and useful data.

In practice, many companies have two sets of standards and classifications for causality assessment of individual case safety reports. The first is used in clinical trials by the medical research group and the investigator (a separate causality assessment for each case should be done by the investigator and the sponsor as noted by many health authorities FDA, EMA, etc.). The second is used in the drug safety unit. In the EU, "The causality assessment given by the investigator shall not be downgraded by the sponsor. If the sponsor disagrees with the investigator's causality assessment, the opinion of both the investigator and the sponsor shall be provided (to health authorities) with the report."

A decision on causality for regulatory reporting is binary: yes or no, a causal relationship is possible or not. The NCI CTCAE Guidance on AE reporting suggests and simplifies causality using the bimodal assessment of yes and no.

RELATIONSHIP	ATTRIBUTION	DESCRIPTION
Unrelated to investigational agent/intervention[1]	Unrelated	The AE *is clearly NOT related* to the intervention
	Unlikely	The AE is ***doubtfully related*** to the intervention
Related to investigational agent/intervention[1]	Possible	The AE ***may be related*** to the intervention
	Probable	The AE **is** ***likely related*** to the intervention
	Definite	The AE **is** ***clearly related*** to the intervention

For other reasons, however, as explained below, various categories (usually three to six) are included in clinical trial protocols and case reports, as follows:

- Related
- Probably related
- Possibly related
- Unlikely related
- Unrelated
- Unassessable

This methodology is useful in later analyzing signals and in creating tables for Investigator Brochures, product labeling, and monographs to give a feel for the certainty or lack thereof about the causality of AEs by the drug in question. However, for the drug safety group, which must determine whether a clinical trial case meets the three criteria (seriousness, expectedness, causality) for expedited reporting, the decision is yes or no. That is, the drug safety group must make the choice between unrelated and related. There is no middle ground or gray zone for causality here. Thus, the drug safety group has to make a rapid decision on whether the case is clearly unrelated (absolutely, positively) or everything else (possibly, probably, unlikely, weakly, etc.). Some drug safety groups consider "unlikely related" to be unrelated and other groups consider it in the broad "related" category. Whichever way is decided, it should be made clear what will be done in the SOP or working document (or the protocol for clinical trials) to everyone in the company. Many drug safety officers believe that unless a case is clearly and absolutely unrelated, the causality should be, for reporting purposes, "related". To put it another way, the default causality for all cases is "possibly related" until there is evidence that the case is "unrelated". It is realized that this may not ultimately agree with the case analysis in the final clinical research study report, where a more nuanced opinion may be recorded. So, to summarize, in drug safety there are two causality choices for reporting purposes: unrelated (thus making the case not reportable as an expedited case) and everything else (viz. related for reporting purposes).

In March 2011, the FDA changed the causality regulations, introducing the concept of "reasonable possibility" (21CFR32): Suspected adverse reaction means any AE for which there is a reasonable possibility that the drug caused the AE. For the purposes of IND safety reporting, "reasonable possibility" means there is evidence to suggest a causal relationship between the drug and the AE. Suspected adverse reaction implies a lesser degree of certainty about causality than adverse reaction, which means any AE caused by a drug. This wording changes the older concept of "possible association" to "reasonable possibility". It is not clear that this has made a major difference in practice.

■ Methodology

Because there are no clear standards or classifications for causality, two broad methods have been developed for causality assessment. (Bayesian analysis is a third method, but this has not proved practical yet.)

Global Introspection

The first (and most widely used) method for causality is known as "global introspection." This is a somewhat jocular description of having one or more smart experienced drug safety experts (usually physicians) read the case details, in particular the narrative, and decide on "introspective" grounds whether the case was caused by the drug. Obviously, all the anticipated difficulties exist when the decision is left to one or more human beings using subjective criteria: different training, different experience, untested inter-rater reliability, biases, and pressure from others within the company or institution. A French group in a 2005 publication on causality found that the overall agreement among five senior experienced experts using global introspection was poor and varied according to level of causality.[2] So, in practice, companies try to get solid, smart, ethical individuals with thick skin and a strong desire to protect the public health to do the job of making the causality judgments.

These criteria are used in global introspection:

1. Reasons to suspect the AE was caused by the drug.
2. The AE occurred in the expected time frame (as a function of the drug's pharmacologic or clinical half-life);
3. No problems or symptoms before exposure;
4. No other medical conditions that could cause this AE;
5. No concomitant medications that could cause this AE;
6. A positive dechallenge and (better) a positive rechallenge;
7. The AE is consistent with the established mechanism of action of the product ("biologic plausibility");
8. A known class effect;
9. Lack of alternative explanation;
10. A dose response;
11. A "typical" adverse drug reaction (e.g., low background rate), such as a fixed drug reaction that would not generally be seen except when due to a drug;
12. A "clean subject" (e.g., a child);
13. Consistency of time to onset (e.g., early for immediate hypersensitivity or long term for tumorigenesis);
14. Similar findings in toxicity studies;
15. Positive *in vitro* test (e.g., immunoglobulin E antibodies to allergen and elevated serum tryptase in anaphylaxis);
16. Positive *in vivo* test (e.g., intradermal or prick test for immediate hypersensitivity or patch test for delayed hypersensitivity);
17. Identified subset at risk or pre-disposing factor;
18. Lack of protopathic bias: a drug given to treat early symptoms may appear temporally associated with the subsequent illness, particularly if the drug's efficacy is low. Source: Adapted from the Report of CIOMS Working Group III, Guidelines for Preparing Core Clinical Safety Information on Drugs 1995.

Algorithms

Algorithms represent the second method and the usual alternative to global introspection. They have in general not succeeded as well as global introspection when used alone, though they can be useful when used in conjunction with global introspection. Algorithms represent a decision tree that is computerizable and allows yes/no answers to preset questions to determine a causality result. Obviously, the algorithm is only as good as the questions asked and the data provided. Because of the inability to make a "one size fits all" algorithm, there is usually a final human review to ensure that the algorithm results are "reasonable" for the situation. More than 30 algorithms have been developed for both manual and computerized causality assessment of individual cases in pharmacovigilance. One of the earlier used algorithms was developed by Professor J. Venulet in 1980 and updated in 1986.[3]

In a study to evaluate agreement between various algorithms and those obtained from an expert panel using the World Health Organization method, 200 reports were studied. The rates of concordance between assessments made using the algorithms and those of the expert panel were 45% for "certain", 61% for "probable",

---

[2] Arimone, Bégaud, Miremont-Salamé, *et al.*, Agreement of expert judgment in causality assessment of adverse drug reactions, *Eur J Clin Pharmacol* 2005; 61(3): 169–173.

[3] Venulet, Ciucci, Berneker, *Int J Clin Pharmacol Ther Toxicol* 1986; 24: 559.

46% for "possible", and 17% for drug-unrelated terms. Correcting for confounding variables did not significantly improve the results. The authors concluded that full agreement with global introspection was not found for any level of causality assessment.[4]

This area continues to become more robust with advances in artificial intelligence and its application to causality and signaling.

■ Comment

Finally, there is another general rule: If there is disagreement between two or more evaluators (e.g., the clinical research team, the investigator, and the drug safety department), the most conservative judgment should be used; that is, if one believes the case is not related and the other believes it is possibly related, the case is considered to be related. The European Regulation 536/2014 for clinical trials notes that "If the sponsor disagrees with the investigator's causality assessment, the opinion of both the investigator and the sponsor shall be provided with the report"; therefore, the more conservative causality is used for reporting purposes and both opinions should be provided in the narrative of the case when submitted.

FDA also wants both the investigator and the sponsor to make a judgment, **but only the sponsor is responsible for the final determination.** Although this has been clarified for situations in which the investigator disagrees with the company, it probably should also apply within the company when there is disagreement.

Some sponsors have organized an adjudication committee (with rules and SOP) for escalation of disagreements so that timely resolution can be reached, including for possible 7- and 15-day reporting. It is not recommended to engage in dialogue with an investigator to convince them to change his/her opinion when it differs from the company's position. Conservatism and over-reporting is preferable to underreporting of SAEs in our view. The FDA, however, does allow the sponsor to override the investigator's judgment of possibly/probably related and NOT report the case as an expedited report. In our view this can be problematic.

The first highly unlikely SAE (e.g., vaginal cancer in the daughter of a woman taking DES 14 years earlier) is often felt to be unrelated to the study drug but after the second and third and additional cases, the causality now becomes possible or even probable. It is again our view that overriding an investigator's related call is often not a good path to take; it should be justifiable, taken deliberately, and with an abundance of caution. In practice, this occurs rarely, if ever. After all, the investigator knows the study subject from the bedside perspective. Another problem is that if the ICSR is reported as an expedited report in the EU but not in the US, the company is saying different things to different regulators at the same time — always an unfortunate and dangerous thing to do. The regulators talk to each other!

Criteria Table

Comparison of EU and US application of causality determination to expedited single case reporting from interventional clinical trials.

Table 1. Causality Table

	Investigator causality	Sponsor causality	Causality for regulatory reporting
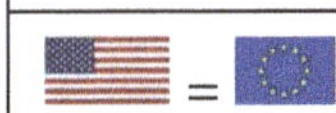	Not related	Not related	Not related
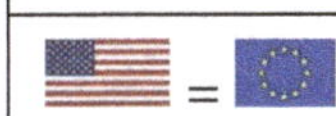	Related	Related	Related
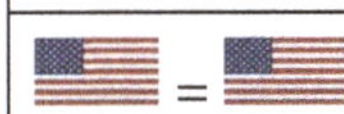	Not related	Related	Related
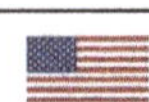	Related	Not related	Not related
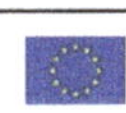	Related	Not related	Related

For a short and useful summary on how an expert on pharmacovigilance approaches causality from a clinical, pharmacologic, and epidemiologic perspective, see the article article by Diemont.[5] and the 2012 article by Edwards (Int J Risk Saf Med,

[4] Macedo, Marques, Ribeiro, *et al.*, *J Clin Pharm Ther* 2003; 28: 137.

[5] Diemont, *Netherlands J Med* 2003; 63: 7.

2012;24(1):41–54. Considerations on causality in pharmacovigilance, Ralph Edwards).

Health Authority Guidance and Requirements

There is no international standard for causality assessment or classification. The US and EU recommendations are summarized in the following sections.

United States FDA

Current United States regulations require a causality assessment for IND expedited 7- and 15-day reports. These regulations require an IND safety report (21CFR312):

> The sponsor must notify FDA and all participating investigators (i.e., all investigators to whom the sponsor is providing drug under its INDs or under any investigator's IND) in an IND safety report of potential serious risks, from clinical trials or any other source, as soon as possible, but in no case later than 15 calendar days after the sponsor determines that the information qualifies for reporting. In each IND safety report, the sponsor must identify all IND safety reports previously submitted to FDA concerning a similar suspected adverse reaction, and must analyze the significance of the suspected adverse reaction in light of previous, similar reports or any other relevant information.
>
> An unexpected AE or unexpected suspected adverse reaction is defined by FDA in the regulations as unexpected if it is not listed in the investigator brochure or is not listed at the specificity or severity that has been observed; or, if an investigator brochure is not required or available, is not consistent with the risk information described in the general investigational plan or elsewhere in the current application, as amended. For example, under this definition, hepatic necrosis would be unexpected (by virtue of greater severity) if the investigator brochure referred only to elevated hepatic enzymes or hepatitis. Similarly, cerebral thromboembolism and cerebral vasculitis would be unexpected (by virtue of greater specificity) if the investigator brochure listed only cerebral vascular accidents. "Unexpected", as used in this definition, also refers to AEs or suspected adverse reactions that are mentioned in the investigator brochure as occurring with a class of drugs or as anticipated from the pharmacological properties of the drug, but are not specifically mentioned as occurring with the particular drug under investigation (21CFR312.32).

For NDA 15-day expedited reports, there is "implied" causality for spontaneous reports. What this means is that if a healthcare professional or consumer takes the time to report an AE to the manufacturer of the drug or to the FDA, the implication is that the reporter believes that to some degree the drug may have caused the AE. This is not clearly stated in the regulations that require 15-day expedited reports:

> For post-marketing 15-day "Alert reports", the applicant shall report each adverse drug experience that is both serious and unexpected, whether foreign or domestic, as soon as possible but in no case later than 15 calendar days of initial receipt of the information by the applicant" (21CFR314.80(1)(i)).

In the draft, *Guidance for Industry Post-marketing Safety Reporting for Human Drug and Biological Products Including Vaccines* of March 2021, the FDA notes the following:

> For spontaneous reports, the applicant should assume that an adverse experience or fatal outcome was suspected to be due to the suspect drug or biological product (implied causality). For clinical studies, an adverse experience or fatal outcome need not be submitted to the FDA unless the applicant concludes that there is a reasonable possibility that the product caused the adverse experience or fatal outcome (see §§ 310.305(c)(1)(ii), 337.314.80(e)(1), and 600.80(e)(1)).

> Causality Assessment — Determination of whether there is a reasonable possibility that the product is etiologically related to the adverse experience. Causality assessment includes, for example, assessment of temporal relationships, dechallenge/rechallenge information, association with (or lack of association with) underlying disease, presence (or absence) of a more likely cause, and physiologic plausibility.

In the draft, *Guidance for Industry: Good Pharmacovigilance Practices and Pharmacoepidemiologic Assessment* of March 2005, the FDA notes the following:

> For any individual case report, it is rarely possible to know with a high level of certainty whether the event was caused by the product. To date, there are no internationally agreed upon standards or criteria for assessing causality in individual cases, especially for events that often occur spontaneously (e.g., stroke, pulmonary embolism). Rigorous pharmacoepidemiologic studies, such as case-control studies and cohort studies with appropriate follow-up, are usually employed to further examine the potential association between a product and an AE.

The FDA does not recommend any specific categorization of causality, but the categories probable, possible, or unlikely have been used. The WHO uses the following categories: certain, probably/likely, possible, unlikely, conditional/unclassified, and unassessable/unclassifiable. Although the FDA does not advocate a particular categorization system, if a causality assessment is undertaken, the FDA suggests that the causal categories are specified.

In contrast to causality assessment at the individual case level, it may be possible to assess the degree of causality between use of a product and an AE when a sponsor or health authority gathers and evaluates all available safety data in aggregate, including the following:

1. Spontaneously reported and published case reports;
2. Relative risks or odds ratios derived from pharmacoepidemiologic safety studies;
3. Biologic effects observed in pre-clinical studies and pharmacokinetic or pharmacodynamic effects;
4. Safety findings from controlled clinical trials; and
5. General marketing experience with similar products in the class.

FDA concludes: "After the available safety information is presented and interpreted, it may be possible to assess the degree of causality between use of a product and an adverse event".

■ European Union

The EU position on causality is explained in the, "Detailed guidance on the collection, verification and presentation of AE/AR reports arising from clinical trials on medicinal products for human use ('CT-3') (2011/C 172/01/7.2.1 (45))".

> **Causality**: "The definition implies a reasonable possibility of a causal relationship between the event and the IMP. This means that there are facts (evidence) or arguments to suggest a causal relationship". All AEs judged by either the investigator or the sponsor as having a reasonable suspected causal relationship to an investigational medicinal product qualify as adverse reactions. The causality assessment given by the investigator should not be downgraded by the sponsor. If the sponsor disagrees with the investigator's causality assessment, both the opinion of the investigator and the sponsor should be provided with the report.
>
> **Post-registration causality**: Any spontaneous report is considered as having a possible relationship; the EU health authorities actually consider an ICSR would not be reported by a healthcare professional or a patient if this person felt there was a non-drug causal agent.

Since the end of the seventies, the French government has used an "*imputabilité*" decision table based on a combination of chronological criteria (timing, dechallenge, rechallenge), and semi logical criteria (specific laboratory findings, suggestive clinical picture, other explanations likely) leading to a five-degree global score (0, unrelated; 1, doubtful; 2, possible; 3, probable; 4, definite). An additional "bibliographic" score (from never reported to well known) is also considered.[6] The updated method has been published in 2013[7] leading to an increase of the degrees (5–7) for the global score, a new informativeness scale and a clearer scoring for bibliographic assessment. It is legally required to assess all spontaneous case reports occurring in France according to this method. It is not used outside of France.

The French causality method has one very useful aspect which is to help determine the appropriate and useful documentation to be used in a case report. For example, during a phone call this methodology helps the pharmacovigilance specialist determine the most useful and appropriate data to capture for appropriate case analysis. As regards delivering a robust conclusion about causal relationship, experts are still debating...

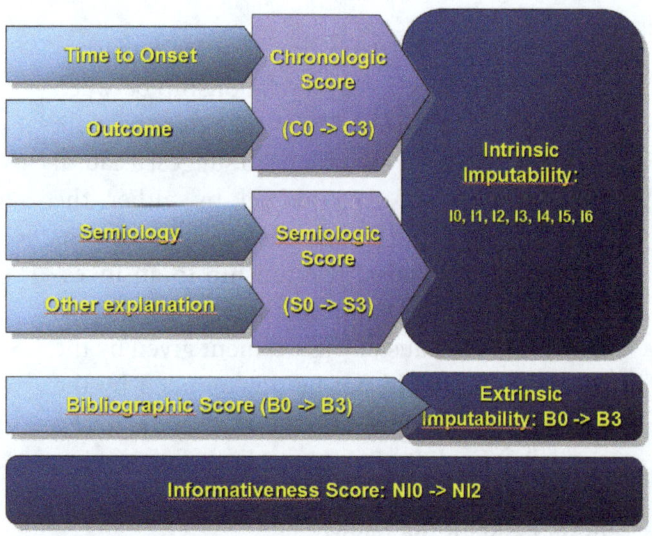

Overall, a frequently used method for post-marketing case reports remains the Naranjo scale or a variant of it. In published case reports, authors frequently use this method which is known worldwide.[8]

[6] Begaud, *Therapie* 1985; 40(2): 111–118.
[7] Arimone, *Therapie* 2013; 68(2): 69–76.
[8] Naranjo CA, *et al.*, A method for estimating the probability of adverse drug reactions, *Clin Pharmacol Ther* 1981; 30(2): 239–245.

CIOMS I Assessment of Causality

It should be emphasized that manufacturers should not separate out those spontaneous reports they receive into those that seem to themselves to be causally related to drug exposure and those they consider not causally related. A physician in making a spontaneous report to a manufacturer is indicating that the observed event may be due to the drug, i.e., the physician suspects that the event is a reaction. In such a case, it would be inappropriate for a manufacturer to impute to the reporting physician an assessment of causality. Thus, all spontaneous reports of serious unlabeled reactions made by medical professionals should be considered as CIOMS reports. However, submission of such a report does not necessarily constitute an acceptance of causality by a manufacturer. That is clearly the position of the US FDA.

Uppsala Monitoring Centre (WHO)

The Uppsala Monitoring Centre uses six categories: (1) certain, (2) probably/likely, (3) possible, (4) unlikely, (5) conditional/unclassified, and (6) unassessable/unclassifiable. They note that these categories are widely used, although not everyone uses all of them. See the chapter in this Manual on the Uppsala Monitoring Centre.

Judgment of Cases When Received Versus at the Time of Periodic Reporting and Signaling

Most of this chapter dealt with judging cases at the time of receipt. For causality, this is primarily for clinical trial cases, but also applies to other types of "solicited" reports. Judgment of seriousness, expectedness, and causality in the acute phase upon receipt is often done with incomplete information and in a "vacuum."

At the time of signaling or PSUR/PBRER preparation, the reviewers now have the benefit of complete (or at least more complete) information on each case, a case series, perhaps a review of animal and other pre-clinical data, a literature review, both interval and cumulative data, and so on. This allows a more nuanced and reasoned judgment. It is not uncommon for causality and the view of the case to change entirely as more data and more cases come in. For example, in the early first in human clinical trials, every AE is unexpected and new. It is very hard to judge causality. With hindsight, later on and with more data, the judgment may be easier. It is highly unlikely that the first case of valvular heart disease seen with Fen-Phen was felt to be due to the drugs. Only when several occurred did this SAE appear to be linked causally to the drug. For cases where there is a high background incidence, assessment of causality may take years and major epidemiological studies to make a valid judgment.

■ Summary and Comments

For IND or clinical trial ICSRs, a binary causality assessment (related versus not related) is needed in order to comply with current regulations.

For post-marketing/post-registration case reports, it is considered that if a reporter takes the trouble to send the ICSR, there is an implied/inferred link between drug intake and AE occurrence. There is no official method accepted worldwide. One single country (France) requests that all spontaneous domestic cases are assessed according to the French Causality Assessment method. As regards causal relationship conclusions, none of the published methods is strongly useful on a case-by-case basis. In addition, pharmacoepidemiology methods are today often considered to be more valid to assess causal relationship for a suspected signal rather than combining "possibly/probably related" case reports. Getting a clear and robust conclusion about drug-induced causal relationship for each case report remains a dream!

Combining seriousness, expectedness and causal relationship on a case-by-case basis allows the drug safety specialist to prioritize case management and reporting to health authorities for pre-registration as well as for post-registration case reports.

But for signal detection purposes, thanks to the current IT systems and the use of AI (artificial intelligence) methodology, considering only the serious unexpected and causally related case reports does not make sense. For example, case reports assessed as non-serious, expected and causally related can generate a signal if these cases together mean an AE frequency increase. By putting aside such case reports, we would miss safety signals. It is clear that many case reports are either expected and/or not related; these reports generate background noise which is useless for signal identification; but they are useful for pharmacoepidemiologic studies among others (case control studies, for example).

Even if PV regulations have similar objectives in different jurisdictions, many countries have their specific requirements. Thus, the EU and US, for example, have slight differences regarding the seriousness or expectedness definitions. However, each Agency requires that their definitions apply to all ICSRs (i.e., domestic and foreign) submitted to them. Moreover, labeledness must be assessed according to the local reference safety information (US PI and EU SmPC), even for foreign ICSRs submitted to them. Unfortunately, the content of both documents can vary for many reasons. As a result, some companies expedite all spontaneous cases that are categorized as serious, without regard to labeledness.

The system for determining seriousness, expectedness, and causality is, to say the least, messy and complicated. One thing that seems to have become clear over the years is that judging causality, particularly for a new drug or for an AE with any drug in an indication or patient population for which there is a high background rate of that AE, is exceedingly difficult on a case-by-case basis. Some drugs in this category take years, millions of patients exposed, and multiple trials and meta-analyses (e.g., Avandia® and cardiac AEs) before an understanding of whether the drug produced a particular AE or group of AEs. Even so, experts may arrive at somewhat differing interpretations of the same data and regulatory actions may be implemented or constrained based on available regulatory tools. The authors' view is that a simpler system, which separates reporting to health authorities from causality judgment, should be considered in a consensus forum.

In this setting, all SAEs or the subgroup of unexpected SAEs should be reported rapidly (say, within 21 days), all deaths and life-threatening SAEs in 7-days and all non-serious AEs every (say) 90 days (current EU Regulation for spontaneous reports). When electronic medical records come into full and effective use for safety assessment on a global basis, then all (validated one hopes) SAEs and AEs would (theoretically) be reported immediately in real time. Or, in fact, the data will be "pulled" by the health agency from the "big data" database for analysis. No need to report ("push") cases to the health agency. This will probably not happen for many years as the technology has a long way to go to make the interoperability of multiple international systems and standards compatible. And then there are detailed technical aspects of coding conventions, etc.

As displayed on the scheme below, drug safety officers can only impact the expected criteria by including new adverse reactions in the labeling documents. For both Seriousness and causal relationship, the assessment is "fixed" thanks to their definition.

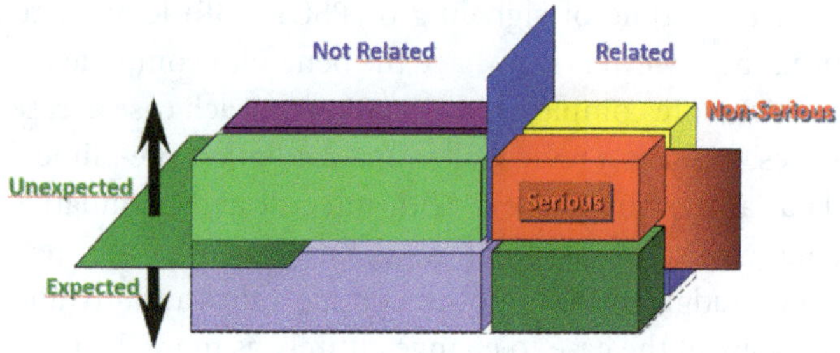

Seriousness, expectedness and causal relationship have mainly been used until now to triage the large volume of ICSRs to be handled as quickly as possible, to identify signals and then protect public health. Thanks to the performance of current IT systems, to automated data entry processes and also to AI, such criteria, will become less and less important.

Then, at various points in time, seriousness, expectedness, causality judgments, and relationships to the drug or drug combinations would be made by the companies, health agencies, and perhaps outside experts from the big data at the same time and perhaps independently. This would hopefully remove "political" judgments from reporting requirements. Maybe someday.

CHAPTER

16

Coding of Adverse Events and Drug Names

As pharmacovigilance becomes more mechanized and computerized, the need for standard terminologies, formats, dictionaries, narratives, and abbreviations grows. The first major standardized areas are the medical coding of adverse reactions/adverse events (ARs/AEs) and medical history and the coding of drug names. Medical coding has become standardized in the world of pharmacovigilance with the use of the Medical Dictionary for Regulatory Activities (MedDRA®).

■ Introduction

Several other coding systems have been used. Two prominent ones are COSTART©, which the US Food and Drug Administration (FDA) used for AE coding until transitioning to MedDRA in late 1998, and WHO-ART®, from the Uppsala Monitoring Centre (UMC). During decades, many pharmaceutical companies used their own internal AE coding dictionary. A dwindling number of organizations still use WHO-ART, which is available from WHO to Regulators (only) and it is no longer kept up to date. Thus, whether required in regulation or not, MedDRA is now the requested standard for coding adverse reactions/adverse events (ARs/AEs), device-related events, product quality issues, medication errors, exposures, medical history, social history, investigations, misuse and abuse, off label use, and indications. MedDRA's structure allows for aggregation of those reported terms in medically meaningful groupings to facilitate analysis of safety data. Some older drug labels in the United States and elsewhere still have non-MedDRA terms (e.g., COSTART or CTCAE, etc.) but most sections of newer labeling have been converted to the MedDRA terminology. An exception in newer US package inserts is clinical information coded with the Clinical Observations Recordings and Encoding (CORE) Problem List Subset of Snomed CT. These terms are included in the "Highlights" section of US package inserts that are formatted according to the Physician Labeling Rule (PLR). In the detailed safety section of PLR format inserts, MedDRA terms are generally included at the PT level stratified by System Organ Class (SOC). In some instances, similar MedDRA terms can be combined without losing meaning for prescribers (e.g., sedation, somnolence, drowsiness can be grouped together in labeling). This can reduce confusion on the part of prescribers. However, it is not always possible and principles for MedDRA Labeling Groupings (MLGs) are being developed. Note that Common Terminology for Adverse Events (CTCAE), with only a few hundred terms, is not as granular as MedDRA, but has "grades" to specify severity of the suspected AR. CTCAE is used for many oncology studies, particularly those sponsored/conducted by the US National Cancer Institute (NCI), the European Organization for Research and Treatment of Cancer (EORTC), and others. Various versions of the CTCAE are available from the NCI website at no charge. See below. Coding is done so that companies, regulators, and others can communicate using the same medical language. ARs/AEs are coded so that similar cases are described (i.e., classified) in the same consistent way and so that they can easily be retrieved, analyzed, and compared. A standard terminology and consistency in its use is invaluable for safety signal detection and analysis.

■ AR/AE Coding

MedDRA

MedDRA was developed by the International Council for Harmonization of Technical Requirements for Pharmaceuticals for Human Use (ICH), based on earlier work by the United Kingdom health authority and others. It was owned by the International Federation of Pharmaceutical Manufacturers and Associations, acting as trustee for the ICH Steering Committee. When ICH became a legal entity under Swiss law, MedDRA ownership was transferred to ICH. A service organization known as the Maintenance and Support Services Organization (MSSO) serves as the repository, maintainer, and distributor of MedDRA and the source for information on MedDRA. The MSSO manages a formal process for Change Requests made by subscribers. A mirror organization, the Japanese Maintenance Organization (JMO), functions in a similar role for the Japanese version of MedDRA (MedDRA/J). Detailed information is available from the MSSO and JMO websites. See https://www.meddra.org/.

- MedDRA is a terminology developed for drugs, vaccines, and medical devices used for standardized coding of medical concepts (but not product names). It is hierarchical, which means that it has multiple levels (five), ranging from the most general to very specific. MedDRA is currently available in 18 languages (Chinese, Czech, Dutch, English, Estonian, French, German, Greek, Hungarian, Italian, Japanese, Latvian, Polish, Brazilian Portuguese, Portugal Portuguese, Russian, Swedish and Spanish). The base language is English and all translations of a medical concept have the same 8-digit code.

Regulatory Status

European Union: MedDRA use is obligatory in the European Union. All suspected adverse reaction reports must be submitted electronically using the most granular MedDRA codes, i.e., the Lowest Level Term (LLT). MedDRA is to be used for the reporting of suspected, unexpected, serious adverse reactions (SUSARs) to the EudraVigilance clinical trial module. In the post-marketing phase, suspected ARs and other relevant data must be coded with MedDRA in both serious and non-serious case reports. Periodic Safety Update Report (PSURs) must also have the AR/AE terms coded in MedDRA, but they are analyzed and displayed at the

Preferred Term (PT) level. Product labeling, the Summary of Product Characteristics (SmPC), and Risk Management Plans should also use MedDRA.

"Standardized MedDRA Queries" (SMQs) are referenced in GVP Module VII as a potential tool in the signal evaluation process. The structure intrinsic in the hierarchy of MedDRA also supports searches, since terms are arranged in logical groupings.

The EudraVigilance Expert Working Group has created a list of Important Medical Event (IME) terms to assist with the classification and assessment of suspected ARs/AEs and aggregate data analysis. Use of the IME list is voluntary. It is updated with each new version of MedDRA and published on the EudraVigilance website. Some companies use the terms on the IME list as "always serious" AEs, though not everyone agrees with this.

United States: FDA has not mandated the use of MedDRA for reporting AEs. s. It has been implemented on a voluntary basis by FDA, regulated medical product manufacturers/distributors, and other stakeholders. US legislation or regulation does not require use of MedDRA by either FDA or Sponsors/Applicants/others; there is no legally-enforceable mandate. However, FDA issued a final rule on June 10, 2014 (effective June 10, 2015), that requires industry to submit individual post-marketing safety reports in an electronic format that FDA can process, review, and archive (not all in ICH E2B format). However, the ICH E2B(R2) electronic case report format specifies use of MedDRA and the associated technical specifications indicate FDA's expectation for MedDRA in post-marketing ICSRs for drugs and biologic products. **So, in practice, MedDRA should be used for all reporting of AEs/ARs**.

For clinical trials, FDA also requires submissions that the agency can review, process, and archive. CDER and CBER submissions with study data must use the standards specified in the Catalog posted to the FDA's Study Data Standards Resources Web page. Controlled terminologies currently supported by FDA include MedDRA. MedDRA is the default terminology for coding adverse events in clinical trial data.

In summary, MedDRA is the *de facto* coding standard in the US for relevant FDA-regulated products intended for use in humans and nearly all mandatory compliance data are currently pre-coded in MedDRA by Sponsors/Applicants. FDA has the expectation that MedDRA will be used by Sponsors/Applicants as they themselves use it in their review of the safety data.

Safety reporting for medical devices requires separate non-MedDRA codes for Event Problem reporting to FDA.

MedDRA is used in most AE reporting to FDA. In practice, as MedDRA is obligatory for the European Union, Japan, and elsewhere and has no widely used competing regulatory terminology, it is wise to use MedDRA consistently for AE reporting.

Note that Snomed CT, ICD, and other terminologies are often used for observational studies when electronic medical records are the data source. See the MSSO website for updates and further regulatory information.

MedDRA is updated twice yearly (April 1st and October 1st), and, in general, users update their own computer systems on the first Monday of the second month following release of each new version by the MSSO. Users may request the addition of new codes to future versions of MedDRA by applying to the MSSO, which then reviews each request. Codes also may be moved, changed, demoted, made non-current, or promoted by the MSSO in the updates. The version number "bumps up" twice a year.

MedDRA terms cover diseases, diagnoses, signs and symptoms, therapeutic indications, medical and surgical procedures, and medical, social, and family histories. MedDRA does not cover drug and device names, study design, patient demographic terms, population qualifiers (e.g., rare, frequent), and descriptions of severity or numbers. It does not give definitions of AEs.

Originally, MedDRA was developed for post-marketing AEs, but it is now used widely for clinical trial AEs. This has produced complex issues with regard to long trials that might run a year or more and go through one or more MedDRA upgrades. When and how to update the codes in an ongoing trial is complex and has multiple solutions. Generally, however, the most current version is used in individual expedited reports. This is the case even when aggregate data from a long-term study might be coded with a single version in a clinical study report. Methodology should be clearly described in the study report and integrated summaries.

MedDRA in Practice

The primary purpose of coding data into a standardized terminology is to analyze it. "A key benefit of MedDRA is its support of straightforward and sophisticated analyses. MedDRA can therefore be used to analyze individual medical events (e.g., "Influenza") or issues involving a system, organ or etiology (e.g., infections) using its hierarchical structure. MedDRA should also be used for signal detection and monitoring of clinical syndromes whose symptoms encompass numerous systems or organs using its multiaxial hierarchy or through the special feature of Standardized MedDRA Queries (SMQs)".

As of September 2023, MedDRA version 26 has more than 80,000 terms arranged into five hierarchical categories (total number of LLTs includes PTs, as each PT is represented at the LLT level. This includes current and non-current terms) The numbers listed below were current at the time of publishing and provided to illustrate the breadth and depth of the number of classified and categorized medical terminology. One can imagine, based on the number of terms systematically coded, that the logical method used to classify these terms:

- System organ classes (SOCs): 29
- Higher-level group terms (HLGTs): >337
- Higher-level terms (HLTs): >1,738
- Preferred terms (PTs): 25,916
- Lowest-level terms (LLTs): 86,714

An example of coding:

- SOC: Cardiac disorders
- HLGT: Cardiac arrhythmias
- HLT: Supraventricular arrhythmias
- PT: Sinus bradycardia
- LLT: Bradycardia sinus, sinus bradycardia
- Verbatims: Slow heart rate, sinus bradycardia, slow pulse, and so forth

Verbatim terms are not MedDRA terms but rather the terms used by reporters, patients, and investigators. They may be medical, lay, or slang terms. Many companies create verbatim dictionaries in which they map the verbatim terms to MedDRA LLT-level terms. Note that in this example, "sinus bradycardia" is a verbatim, LLT, and PT at the same time. Note also that all PTs are LLTs (but not vice versa).

Each term in MedDRA has a unique eight-digit code. This unique number is the same for each translated term in all the MedDRA languages. That is, for example, "nausea" has a unique eight-digit number no matter what language "nausea" is coded in.

Browsers: Because there are so many terms, it is necessary to search for a needed term by computer rather than reading through a printed version of the terminology. For this, the MSSO and other companies have developed software, called "browsers", to allow a user to find the terms he or she needs. The MSSO makes available a downloadable browser to all subscribers.

Commercial browsers are also available. With the browser, one or more words (e.g., pain in the leg) are typed in, and the browser software determines whether there is a direct word-for-word match at one or more of the hierarchical levels. If so, it gives the direct "hit" along with the hierarchical tree; that is, if the direct hit is an LLT, it will display the PT, HLT, HLGT, and SOC (both primary and secondary if more than one exists). If not, most browsers suggest choices for the user to pick from. The choices are often automatically based on previous coding selections. Some browsers do "autoencoding" where one may type in a narrative (prose paragraphs), and the browser will extract and code all medical-sounding terms for the user to examine and accept or reject. Machine learning has been harnessed to gradually improve fidelity and efficiency of autoencoding. We may see further advances artificial intelligence (AI) over the next few years.

The actual coding of AEs is a very complex subject and cannot be fully covered here, but some general thoughts and issues on coding are addressed. The goal of coding is to create one or more AE codes that capture the essence of the problems that the patient experienced. There should not be too many or too few terms but just enough. That is, we should follow the "Goldilocks Principle" and use codes that are "just right", or as Albert Einstein put it: "Everything should be made as simple as possible, but not simpler." Defining "just enough", however, is difficult. ICH provides guidance that coding should ordinarily be at the LLT level. Further, a term(s) should be selected that most accurately reflects the reported verbatim information.

There are many complexities that one encounters when coding:

- Should one be "a lumper or a splitter"? That is, should one code "flu-like syndrome" (the lumper) or "fever", "malaise", "fatigue", "muscle aches", "headache", "chills", and "runny nose" (the splitter)? This may be evident to the reader for a term such as "flu-like syndrome" but less clear for the "Hermansky-Pudlak syndrome" (albinism, visual problems, platelet defects with bleeding, lung disease, and often kidney and gastrointestinal disease).
- When a unifying diagnosis with characteristic signs and symptoms is reported, however, ICH recommends selecting a term for the diagnosis only as a preferred option. No reported information should be excluded and, likewise, information should not be added. For example, a term for a diagnosis should not be selected if only signs or symptoms are reported. When a diagnosis is reported along with terms that are not consistent with the typical presentation of that diagnosis, ICH indicates that the outlying terms should be coded as well as the diagnosis.
- Should one code "cascade effects" or "secondary effects"? For example, if a patient becomes dizzy and falls, breaking his or her shoulder and abrading his or her skin, the primary event is dizziness (and should be coded) but should the other terms — the fall, shoulder fracture, skin abrasions — also be coded and thus considered as AEs associated with the drug in question in the database and future labeling?
- Should provisional or "rule out" diagnoses be coded? ICH recommends that provisional diagnoses as well as reported signs and symptoms should be coded until a diagnosis can be confirmed by the primary reporter. Signs and symptoms do not change whereas a provisional diagnosis might. An alternative would be to code only signs and symptoms. The organization's approach should be documented in a coding conventions document to facilitate consistency across coders and over time.
- In our experience, coding a large number of "rule out" diagnoses is not done and is not a good idea. For example, hypercalcemia (elevated calcium) has a dozen causes. It is not a good idea to code all of these or, depending on the case, any of the causes until there is some evidence to suspect one or more of the diagnoses (causes).
- Should one code "low blood glucose" or "hypoglycemia"? "Low blood glucose" would code to LLT Blood glucose decreased, which is a laboratory test result and links to SOC Investigations. "Hypoglycemia" is a medical condition and would be coded to LLT Hypoglycemia, which links to PT Hypoglycaemia and SOC Metabolism and nutrition disorders. One must understand the nuances of MedDRA to code accurately and consistently. Should laboratory abnormalities be coded as AEs? In the past, this was sometimes done in an arbitrary and inconsistent manner. It has been a problem in clinical study reports or dossiers for Marketing Authorization (MA) when the number of AEs of hypertension did not equal the number of subjects whose recorded blood pressure on physical exams went up, clearly demonstrating that not all elevations in blood pressure were considered to be reportable or codable by the investigator or company as AEs. Some companies code lab abnormalities as a lab test only in the SOC Investigations. Only if there are clinical signs or symptoms do they also code another non-lab term as an AE.
- Coding should not be done at a less specific level, sometimes referred to as "downcoding". For example, coding "edema" instead of "facial edema" or "lung disease NOS (not otherwise specified)" instead of a more specific diagnosis (e.g., pneumococcal pneumonia). This type of "lumping" can mask or hide certain AEs or problems.
- Coding consistency and variability is often a problem, especially when there are multiple coders or coding is done over time (e.g., in a long clinical trial). One might see "elevated liver enzymes", "abnormal liver enzymes", "elevated ALT", or "elevated AST", all of which are capturing the same condition in different patients at different times. This poses problems when one is attempting to retrieve

all the potential cases of liver injury for safety signaling (see section on "Standardized MedDRA Queries") or aggregate AE tables.

- Having too many codes for a particular case makes it hard to understand what the primary or major issues were. In practice, many users try to limit the number of codes in each case to six or eight at most. However, some business partners may require full coding of all reported terms.
- Cultural differences may affect coding across countries or regions. In addition, language issues may alter coding, especially if people are coding in a language (English) that is not their primary language. Further, because of language nuances and cultural aspects, complete translation of every English MedDRA term to all other languages is not possible.

There is, in many cases, no single correct answer to a coding question. Rather it is necessary that coders agree on certain standards, or "conventions", that define (sometimes arbitrarily) how to code. The ICH has published several versions of its coding suggestions entitled "MedDRA® Term Selection: Points to Consider, ICH-Endorsed Guide for MedDRA Users. Application to Adverse Drug Reactions/Adverse Events & Medical and Social History & Indications". A copy is freely available for no charge at the MedDRA website.

The FDA, in its *Guidance for Industry Premarketing Risk Assessment* of March 2005, has commented on coding:

1. "Sponsors should explore the accuracy of the coding process with respect to both investigators and the persons who code AEs."
2. "Investigators may sometimes choose verbatim terms that do not accurately communicate the adverse event that occurred."
3. "The severity or magnitude of an event may be inappropriately exaggerated (e.g., if an investigator terms a case of isolated elevated transaminases acute liver failure despite the absence of evidence of associated hyperbilirubinemia, coagulopathy, or encephalopathy, which are components of the standard definition of acute liver failure)."
4. "Conversely, the significance or existence of an event may be masked (e.g., if an investigator uses a term that is non-specific and possibly unimportant to describe a subject's discontinuation from a study when the discontinuation is due to a serious adverse event)."
5. "Sponsors should strive to identify obvious coding mistakes as well as any instances when a potentially serious verbatim term may have been inappropriately mapped to a more benign coding term, thus minimizing the potential severity of an adverse event. One example is coding the verbatim term facial edema (suggesting an allergic reaction) as the non-specific term edema; another is coding the verbatim term suicidal ideation as the more benign term emotional lability."
6. "Prior to analyzing a product's safety database, sponsors should ensure that adverse events were coded with minimal variability across studies, time, and individual coders."

To limit variability, some companies establish a central coding group that either does all AE coding or performs quality checks to verify that coding done by others is consistent and correct.

Standardized MedDRA Queries (SMQs)

Standardized MedDRA Queries (SMQs) are groupings of terms from one or more MedDRA SOCs that relate to a defined medical condition or area of interest. They help in retrieving cases. This implies they were coded correctly on data entry/input of the cases. The included terms may relate to signs, symptoms, diagnoses, syndromes, physical findings, and laboratory and other physiologic test data. Examples of SMQs that were developed and tested by CIOMS include cardiac arrhythmias, cardiac failure, cardiomyopathy, hepatic disorders, hostility/aggression, hyperglycemia/new onset diabetes mellitus, malignancies, and over 100 more, including subqueries. See the current list at the MSSO website.

A newly developing initiative at the FDA is the development of "FMQs" or "FDA Medical Queries".

These are standard groupings of adverse event terms designed by FDA to help identify potential safety issues during review of clinical trial adverse event data. The FDA announced the release of the FDA Medical Query (FMQ) and Algorithmic FDA Medical Queries (AFMQ) at a Duke Margolis-FDA Workshop: Advancing Premarket Safety Analytics1 on Sept 14, 2022. The description of FMQ and AFMQ can be found in this FDA presentation: Advancing Premarket Safety Analytics. Traditional medical SMQs focus primarily on MedDRA preferred terms, which clinical trial sponsors used to classify adverse events that occur during the clinical trial. The basis is that MedDRA PTs are highly granular with >24000 PTs and each grouping represents a medical concept. The FMQ consists of groupings of these terms that correlate to specific broader medical conditions. For example, the FMQ for "Dizziness" consists of 31 different MedDRA preferred terms. Any trial subject that experiences one or more of these adverse events would be captured as experiencing "Dizziness". The FMQ version 2.1 has over 100 of these groupings and the most recent version is available publicly online.

The goal of the FMQ is to improve safety signal detection in clinical trial datasets and create a standardized approach to increase efficiency and consistency. This is a newly developing concept at the FDA and their current list of FMQs is available to the public for viewing and implementation if desired. One would think... if the FDA is looking at the data this way, shouldn't we also?

Training

Safety departments, regulatory authorities, data entry personnel, and others need to establish detailed coding standards, preferably using accepted (ICH) conventions, and to train the staff on their use. Because employees come and go and because MedDRA is updated twice a year, training coders is usually an ongoing process. The MSSO and several vendors provide basic training courses on MedDRA coding, usually running from 1/2 day to 2 or 3 days. Nevertheless, periodic trainings (internal or external) remain expected by inspectors for both new comers in the PV business as well as for experienced PV employees.

Systematized Nomenclature of Medicine — Clinical Terms

Systematized Nomenclature of Medicine — Clinical Terms (SNOMED® CT) is a comprehensive dictionary of clinical healthcare terminology that was created by combining terms created by the College of American Pathologists and the United Kingdom National Health Service. The main purpose of SNOMED CT is to encode terms used in health informatics and to support the effective clinical recording of data. It is designed for use in clinical documentation in electronic health records (EHRs). A SNOMED CT to ICD-10-CM map was developed by the US National Library of Medicine to support semi-automated generation of ICD-10-CM codes from clinical data encoded in SNOMED CT for reimbursement and statistical purposes. The terminology is owned, maintained, and distributed by the International Health Terminology Standards Development Organization (IHTSDO), a non-profit in Denmark. IHTSDO acquires, owns, and administers the rights to SNOMED CT. It is the primary medical terminology in electronic health records used for decision-support, record-keeping, and certain billing activities. Concepts can be combined at different levels of detail to permit various levels of hierarchical precision. The nature of hierarchies allows information to be selectively retrieved to meet different requirements at various levels of generalization. SNOMED CT supports not only clinical decision-making, but also supports reuse of clinical data for research purposes and epidemiology, etc. Various countries including the United Kingdom, Spain, Australia, Canada, Sweden, the United States, and the Netherlands have joined and are in various stages of implementing SNOMED in their countries. Countries are linked through their National Release Centers and translations are available in at least seven languages. SNOMED CT can be adapted to each country's local requirements via extensions.

It is the most comprehensive clinical vocabulary available and has been designated by the US government for electronic exchange of clinical data to include electronic medical records provider order entry, including e-prescribing, laboratory order entry, remote intensive care unit monitoring, lab reporting, emergency room charting, cancer reporting, genetic databases, pharmaceutical use, and more. It will be or is being used by certain US federal agencies for exchanging clinical information for lab result contents, non-lab interventions and procedures, anatomy, diagnoses and problems, and nursing terms. Other governments, particularly in the European Union, may adopt it.

AE Severity Coding

A common problem for coders is judging the severity (mild, moderate, severe) of an AE. This is, of course, different from the regulatory definitions of "serious" and "non-serious", which may be inconsistent, in a sense, with severity. For example, mild chest pain that is perceived by the patient as mild but which is due to a myocardial infarction and results in hospitalization may be classified as mild or moderate pain. But in fact, the AE was serious according to the regulatory definition because of hospitalization (and "medical importance"). Severity is, perhaps, best assessed by the experienced practitioner who sees the patient first-hand.

Grades

Grade refers to the severity of the AE. The CTCAE displays Grades 1 through 5 with unique clinical descriptions of severity for each AE based on this general guideline:

Grade 1 Mild; asymptomatic or mild symptoms; clinical or diagnostic observations only; intervention not indicated.
Grade 2 Moderate; minimal, local or noninvasive intervention indicated; limiting ageappropriate instrumental ADL*.
Grade 3 Severe or medically significant but not immediately life-threatening; hospitalization or prolongation of hospitalization indicated; disabling; limiting self care ADL**.
Grade 4 Life-threatening consequences; urgent intervention indicated.
Grade 5 Death related to AE.

Most reviewers will make a subjective clinical judgment on severity based on the data supplied and their subjective conclusion about the AE or cases. There exists one objective classification system developed by the US National Cancer Institute for use in its protocols. It is to some degree oncology related but can be useful for other indications and trials. It is called the "Common Terminology Criteria for Adverse Events (CTCAE)". New versions are released periodically. For example, version 4.0 was released in June 2010 and version 5.0 was released in November 2017. Version 6.0 was in progress as of early 2024, but had not yet been released. The grading scale is 1 (mildest) to 5 (most severe, usually an outcome of death). Information is available free and in the public domain at NCI's website, and the actual files, in several formats, with background

Drug Names and Drug Dictionaries

Another requirement in the pharmacovigilance world is a consistent and up-to-date drug dictionary. Ideally, such a dictionary would have all the names of all the drugs sold throughout the world. Unfortunately, this is not a simple task. It is far harder than developing an AE dictionary:

- Each drug may have multiple names (see below).
- Drug names change.
- Drug formulations change: the excipients, the active ingredient, or both;
- A drug with the same trade name may have different formulations or strengths in different countries;
- Generic brand names (when applicable) for the same product differ;
- Spelling varies, and some languages have different alphabets and special characters that are not in the English language;
- Combination drugs have multiple names.
- Drugs may be very similar, varying only in the salt. They may have the same names or totally different names.

■ Multiple Names and Name Changes

In January 2006, the FDA issued a warning to consumers against filling US prescriptions abroad because drugs with same or similar names may contain different active ingredients from those sold in the United States and may thus pose health risks. They gave two examples:

For example, in the United States, "Flomax" is a brand name for tamsulosin, a treatment for an enlarged prostate, while in Italy, the active ingredient in the product called "Flomax" is morniflumate, an anti-inflammatory drug. In the United States, "Norpramin" is the brand name for an anti-depression drug containing desipramine but, in Spain, the same brand name, "Norpramin", is used for a drug that contains omeprazole, a treatment for stomach ulcers.

A drug, even a "simple" drug, usually has multiple names. For example, here is a list of some of the names for the drug cimetidine that are used around the world: Eureceptor, Gastromet, SKF 92334, Tagamet, Tametin, Tratul, Ulcedine, Ulcimet, Ulcomet, Acibilin, Acinil, Cimal, Cimetag, Cimetum, Dyspamet, Edalene, Peptol, Ulcedin, Ulcerfen, Ulcofalk, Ulcomedina, Ulhys, *N*-cyano-*N*-methyl-*N*-((E)-2-([(5-methyl-1H-imidazol-4-yl) methyl]sulfanyl)ethyl)guanidine,1-cyano-2-methyl-3-(2-(((5-methyl-4-imidazolyl)methyl)thio)ethyl)guanidine, 2-cyano-1-methyl-3-(2-(((5-methylimidazol-4-yl) methyl)thio)ethyl)guanidine, Acibilin, Acinil, Cimetag, Cimetum, Dyspamet, Edalene, Eureceptor, Gastromet, Metracin, and Brumetidina.

As noted above, brand names may change. Omeprazole was originally sold in the United States as Losec, but the name was changed to Prilosec at the request of the FDA because of possible confusion with Lasix.

In the United States, the US Adopted Names Council (USAN), which is officially sponsored by the American Medical Association, the US Pharmacopeial Convention, and the American Pharmacists Association, assigns generic names that are unique and non-proprietary. The USAN works closely with the International Non-proprietary Name (INN) Program of the World Health Organization (WHO), which assigns international "generic" names. Different countries or regions may also use different generic names for exactly the same drug: "acetaminophen" is used in the United States and "paracetamol" in the EU and elsewhere. Recently, the H2 blocker ranitidine was withdrawn from the US market. It was sold for many years as Zantac®. The name Zantac360® is now used in the US for famotidine (another H2 blocker).

Much attention has been paid in the last several years to medication errors that are felt to be "low-hanging fruit" in the world of drug safety, as errors in naming, prescribing, and handwriting should be more easily rectified than finding the rare SAE. In the FDA, the review of proposed proprietary names is conducted by the Division of Medication Error Prevention and Analysis (DMEPA) in CDER's Office of Surveillance and Epidemiology (OSE). DMEPA, in consultation with the Office of Prescription Drug Promotion (OPDP) reviews proposed names before approval of an IND, NDA, BLA, and ANDA. FDA does not review proprietary names of products marketed under an over-the-counter (OTC) monograph or those of a distributor or repacker. Similar systems exist in most other countries. See, for example, Health Canada's Guidance for Industry: Drug Name Review: Look-alike Sound-alike (LA/SA) Health Product Names, the United Kingdom MHRA Guideline on Naming Medicines, and the European Union's guideline on naming.

This is obviously a very complex situation. So, in the example above, cimetidine is the "generic" (and the INN and USAN, see below) name of the compound that has a chemical name of *N*-cyano-*N*-methyl-*N*-[2-[[(5-methyl-1H-imidazol-4-yl)methyl]thio]ethyl]guanidine, which has the trade names of Tagamet, Peptol, Nu-Cimet, Apo-Cimetidine, Novo-Cimetidine, and others.

See the website of the Institute for Safe Medication Practices (https://www.ismp.org/) for an excellent discussion of all aspects of medication prescribing and medication errors, including name issues. They publish a list of Confused Drug Names.

In the drug safety world, during the preparation of individual case safety reports and aggregate reports (PSURs, NDA Periodic Reports, etc.), co-medications are frequently encountered that have not been seen before. Because co-medications can play a major role in safety reports, it is critical to know what medications (both prescription, OTC, nutraceuticals, herbal preparations, etc.) a patient has taken. Often, however, a strange name is encountered and much time is spent tracking it down to understand what it is chemically. It is far more practical to maintain a drug dictionary with all drug names and formulations that one can refer to as needed.

As with an AE dictionary, it is critical to enter data in a correct and consistent fashion to retrieve it properly. Inconsistent coding produces incomplete searches during signaling or preparing safety reports. Creating and maintaining a drug dictionary, unlike an AE dictionary, is far harder and more complex. With an AE dictionary, the vocabulary is controlled and relatively finite. Few "new" medical terms or diseases occur. Many of the changes to MedDRA represent refinements to the current terms. MedDRA is reaching, to a degree, steady state, with changes each year in the hundreds rather than in the thousands when MedDRA was first released.

Drug dictionaries are quite different. New drugs are developed almost weekly. New drugs, line extensions, "rebranding", new formulations, and new trade names are developed, approved, and launched somewhere in the world every day, and old drugs are withdrawn. To track the names, formulations, and formulas of all these products in more than 150 countries is an impossible task. Whereas MedDRA is updated twice yearly, a drug dictionary, if it is meant to be complete, would need to be updated daily to weekly to remain current. When a drug name is encountered that is not found in the drug dictionary normally used, or if it is reported from a country or source that is not usually seen, it is worth doing an Internet search to verify what the drug is or contains. Similarly, drugs that are not written in the English alphabet (e.g., Latin, Arabic, Chinese traditional medicines, etc.) should be carefully checked.

■ WHO Drug Global

The most useful drug dictionary available is WHO Drug Global, which evolved from the WHO Drug Dictionary Enhanced and is a product of the Uppsala Monitoring Centre (UMC). See https://who-umc.org/whodrug/whodrug-global=. It covers 171 countries and claims to cover nearly all of the marketed OTC and prescription products used in these countries, as well as many herbal remedies. This broad reach was enabled through collaboration with IMS Health (part of IQVIA from 2017). The UMC-IMS Health collaboration dramatically expanded the WHO Drug Dictionary into a separate dictionary type, WHO Drug Dictionary Enhanced. Biotech and blood products, diagnostic substances, and contrast media are also entered when reported. See the above-mentioned UMC website for further information.

It is required for use in clinical trials by the FDA as of 2019. This dictionary, maintained and published on a twice a year basis by the UMC, contained more than 620,000 unique names as of end 2023. It is updated quarterly. It contains products registered by the FDA, the European Medicines Agency (EMA), EU member states, WHO member states, and elsewhere.

The "Anatomical, Therapeutic, Chemical" (ATC) classification is used in this dictionary to categorize active ingredients according to the body system on which they act and their therapeutic, pharmacologic, and chemical properties. In this classification system, drugs are divided into five different groups and a numerical code is assigned at each level of the hierarchy:

- First level, anatomical main group: A — alimentary tract and metabolism;
- Second level, therapeutic subgroup: A10 — drugs used in diabetes;
- Third level, pharmacological subgroup: A10B — oral blood glucose-lowering drugs;
- Fourth level, chemical subgroup: A10BA — biguanides;
- Fifth level, chemical substance: A10BA02 — metformin;

The coding system is complex. Basically, each product has a unique identifier characterized by the following:

- Medicinal product name
- Name specifier

- Drug code
- Market authorization holder
- Country
- Pharmaceutical form
- Strength available, quantity, and unit of active ingredient.

Companies and other users have handled the dictionary in various ways. Some simply subscribe to the dictionary and use the UMC-issued updates as is. Other companies use the WHODrug Global as a base and add on to it as new drugs are encountered during their regular handling of individual case safety reports each day. This dictionary may then "grow" separately from the official WHO dictionary into a proprietary company dictionary. This would pose reconciliation problems when the new update of the WHO dictionary is issued, and thus some companies may choose not to use the WHO upgrades but rather maintain their own home-grown version. The logic behind this is reasonable in that companies often sell limited lines of drugs and may only rarely encounter other drugs or classes of drugs. A company that makes primarily diabetic drugs needs to have the latest information on all diabetic co-medications arriving on the market but may be less concerned about oncology and asthma drugs, for example. They thus have their dictionary group focus on the drugs they encounter more frequently. The downside is that each company has a different drug dictionary and cannot easily communicate with other companies for licensing arrangements (or mergers) and with health authorities, especially during electronic transmissions, as they have different dictionaries. From the safety officer's point of view, it is necessary to know what drug dictionary is being used and how coding is done, especially in complicated situations and foreign cases.

EudraVigilance Medicinal Product Dictionary

This is a product dictionary developed by the EMA for the European Economic Area for authorized and investigational products. It has standardized terminology for active ingredients, excipients, pharmaceutical forms, routes of administrations, concentration ranges and units, country codes, MAH, and Sponsor data. It is hierarchical and multiaxial in structure and uses a standardized XML schema. EU post-marketing legislation issued in 2010 and EudraLex Volume 10 require all MAHs and sponsors to enter into the dictionary each medicinal product authorized in the EU or used in clinical trials. Unlike the WHO dictionary, the EudraVigilance Medicinal Product Dictionary (EVMPD) uses a broader "multilingual approach" to accommodate the many European languages used. The EVMPD was upgraded to the Extended EVMPD or xEVMPD. As with the EVMPD, each MAH must populate the xEVMPD dictionary with its approved and investigational medicinal products. This is the so-called "Article 57 Database". It is, thus, an EU-centric dictionary and is used primarily by the European Union health agencies for signaling, drug identification, and so forth.

Future

ICH issued a document, M5, entitled *Data Elements and Standards for Drug Dictionaries* in 2005. Five international standards for a new drug dictionary have been developed by ISO called the "International Marketed Medicinal Products" Drug Dictionary (IDMP). This is expected to replace the xEVMPD and to be adopted elsewhere. The xEVMPD has over 500,000 records on medicinal products used in the EU. General Remarks Medical coding is both a science and an art that affects clinical outcome reports throughout the product development life-cycle. Without a thorough understanding of its history, origin, and purpose, we would end up with very messy and incoherent datasets. Individuals who are responsible for the coding of terms, medications, tests and procedures should be trained in MedDRA and its practices. Individuals who are responsible for the consistency review of coding, such as medical monitors or safety review physicians, should also be trained and familiar with these concepts. It's shocking at how many individuals are tasked with the responsibility to code events and yet who do not have the foundational and up-to-date knowledge of the basic principles and theory of medical coding, which is something we all wish to change. MedDRA and WHO Drug training is widely available for free on their websites and companies may also pay for in-person and direct training to their employees. The costs are relatively low in comparison to the unrealized cost of not conducting these activities correctly the first time. Companies should invest in this training and implement it in their employees training requirements, else why even have such methods and standards in the first place.

■ Frequently Asked Question

Q: What is your recommendation if cases recorded in the PV database are to be updated to use MedDRA Coding (e.g., wrong chosen code or new MedDRA term more accurate)?

A: There is not one single possible answer to this question, but a company policy to be defined. If the MedDRA codes previously chosen are inaccurate, an impact analysis should be conducted (impacted case reports, cases already reported to at least one HA (expedited case reports, within aggregate reports (DSURs, PSURs/PBRERs, PADERs), within NDA or CTD, etc.), cases included in previous safety analysis (signal detection, within B-R analysis reports, etc.) to determine the extent of the changes needed. Depending on the outcome of the impact analysis and the medical importance of the codes to be updated, a decision would be made on how to implement the corrective actions keep detailed documentation.

Keep in mind that whichever dictionary(ies) are used, they must be well integrated into the IT system used for pharmacovigilance. Updates are expected to be uploaded within a few weeks of their issuance and any potential changes in old cases due to changed or archived terms must be done rapidly. Most of the commercial database systems for PV are able to do this.

CHAPTER

17

Spontaneous Post-marketing Adverse Events

When a new product reaches the market, a wider population is exposed than in clinical trials and spontaneous case reports play a pivotal and irreplaceable role in providing safety information.

■ Introduction

The adverse events and safety data arising from clinical trials are only a snapshot of data within a very tightly controlled environment. Regulations are in place that require the ongoing evaluation and reporting of adverse events after a product has been approved whether or not it is then marketed (as most approved products are) or not to ensure it continues to show efficacy and remains safe in the public. Therefore, case reports received after approval, otherwise known as post-marketing reports, many of which are reported spontaneously. AEs or ICSRs, continue to be a critical component of the life-cycle management of the safety profile of a product.

■ Why is Post-Market Data Different from Clinical Data?

Before a drug comes to market, it is studied in animals and participants in clinical trials that aim to show the efficacy of the product for a particular selected disease in a highly selected sample of the population. The clinical trials may be large, covering up to 10,000 patients, or very small, covering dozens to hundreds patients (e.g., for orphan drugs or rare diseases). The clinical trials also aim to define the safety profile of the drug, at least in this selected population with this selected disease.

These studies, which are (usually) carried out with rigorous and highly regulated methodology are statistically powered to demonstrate efficacy, but have significant limitations in defining the safety profile. They generally only find frequently occurring adverse events (AEs). For example, if in studying 10,000 patients not a single patient has a particular AE, such as a heart attack, we can be only 95% confident that the chance of having a heart attack based on the data from this trial is less than 1 in 3,333 (per the Rule of Three). If we raise the safety threshold to be 99% confident that a heart attack has an incidence of only 1 in 10,000 with this drug, we would need to have no heart attacks in 46,000 patients studied. In other words, studying even 5,000 or 10,000 patients does not give enough evidence that the major or rare safety issues have been identified before the drug goes on the market for large-scale use in patients with a wide range of disease severity, co-morbidities or co-medications, etc.

This means that the uncommon AEs and even the fairly common AEs (e.g., an incidence of 1 in 500) may not be identified until the drug is extensively used in the general population after marketing. When, say, a million people start using a new drug in the months after a product launch, a "rare" AE with a 1 in 10,000 incidence rate could be expected in about 100 patients. Should the AE in question be dramatic and rapidly discovered, such as *torsades de pointes*, aplastic anemia, or rhabdomyolysis (a severe skeletal muscle injury), there will be a torrent of recriminations about why this was not discovered earlier during the clinical testing. The correct response is that the testing of only 5,000 to 10,000 patients could not pick up such a rare event because this is the way the drug approval system is designed.

Also, of note is that clinical trials are often done in a narrow group of patients. For example, an antihistamine may be tested in otherwise healthy adults between 18 and 60 years of age with allergies. Even if the drug is only approved for use in this population, physicians in most jurisdictions have the right (which they freely exercise) to prescribe the drug for anyone and for any disease. Thus, many people with other diseases and at the extremes of the age range (the very old and young) receive the drug and may have AEs that the healthy 18- to 60-year-old study population did not experience in the clinical trials. The elderly, for example, are particularly sensitive to certain AEs (e.g., swallowing disorders) or to certain classes of psychotropic drugs and they often are taking multiple medications.

Polypharmacy and drug interactions, among other things, cannot be adequately studied in the preapproval setting. Although food interaction studies and some drug interaction studies are done before approval, it is not possible to study "real world" patients (often elderly) who take many drugs and have peculiar or irregular eating and drinking habits. Even after marketing, it is difficult or even impossible to predict or know how the use of three, four, or more drugs given at the same time will act or interact.

Hence, particular attention must be paid to the time just after a product is first marketed to fully understand the drug's safety profile and minimize risks. In a sense, the first 500,000 to 1,000,000 patients who are prescribed the drug after launch are doing the large-scale safety testing. And, outside of clinical trials, the reporting of safety information by healthcare practitioners and other members of the public to manufacturers and drug regulators is nearly always voluntary.

What this means then is that the entire edifice of the drug safety system as it now stands, depends on the good will and energy of nurses, pharmacists, physicians, dentists, and consumers to report AEs. Without them, no one would know of the AEs that are appearing as individual cases in isolated areas around the country or the world. These people must take time out of their day to report such events. The report will inevitably lead to a request for supplementary data (laboratory reports, cardiograms, hospital records, etc.) that are time- and effort-consuming. There is no evident or immediate gain to the reporter. The gain rather is to society at large, which is largely unaware of this noble effort.

Health authorities and regulators well understand the weakness of this system. Major efforts are now under way to look at how the spontaneous reporting system has worked in the past. That is, although we think it is useful and appropriate to rely on this system, did it, in fact, lead to early pick-up of serious problems, leading to a change in the product labeling and its use in clinical practice?

Various health agencies, particularly in North America and Europe, are looking at this question and novel approaches to supplement the existing system.

There is a lot more digital data, sitting in the cloud, on drug safety that is not being looked at in a systematic manner. Obtaining these data on an ongoing basis and using them for safety analysis is an obvious way to identify a drug's safety profile. However, the devil is in the details. The databases around the world must be identified and the data extracted in a valid and consistent way. This is a very difficult task since data collection is not yet standardized and there is little true interoperability across IT systems. It is also important to remember that safety generally represents a secondary use of these datasets. Multiple efforts (both nationally and globally) are under way to standardize and normalize data so that they are easily collected, databased, retrieved, and analyzed in a useful, valid, and rapid manner. If every encounter a patient has with the healthcare system is digitalized, we should be able to retrieve excellent safety data rapidly. This, however, will take years to achieve on a national level, let alone a global level. When this does occur, the spontaneous reporting system may then decrease in importance. The fundamental system now in place to discover AEs with marketed products remains the spontaneous reporting system. This system is used, in one form or another, in many countries around the world; examples include the US, Canada, China, the EU, Japan, South Korea, Australia, New Zealand, South Africa, and many other countries around the world. The WHO and the Uppsala Monitoring Centre actively work with more than 150 countries to set up pharmacovigilance (PV) systems and increase capacity.

The principles of the Spontaneous Reporting System (SRS) are simple. All healthcare professionals (and consumers in most countries, including the US, the EU, and Canada) are encouraged (and sometimes required by post-marketing requirement, such as US REMS or registry studies) to spontaneously report AEs to either the manufacturer or the governmental healthcare agency or a third party. Standardized forms have been developed (the MedWatch form in the United States, the CIOMS I form elsewhere) specifically for this purpose and are available online, in publications (e.g., the *Physicians' Desk Reference* in the United States), as apps on the iPhone and other smartphones, and elsewhere. The form can be folded up and mailed (postage-free), faxed, or filled in online and uploaded to the healthcare agencies. Phone, on-line reports and faxes to the manufacturer and most health agencies are also possible. However, many jurisdictions require companies to use an electronic format (viz. E2B) to transmit safety reports to regulators

In the US, the United Kingdom, and other countries, information submitted spontaneously to the health authority is available for free or for a small fee to anyone in the public under Freedom of Information Acts. The cases are redacted before being released by the health agency to avoid identifying the patient or reporter In the US, in 2022 over 76.000 individual reports were sent directly to FDA (3%) with the remaining 2.3 million sent to the manufacturers who then forwarded these cases to the FDA. Redacted case report data held by FDA in the FAERS database are publicly available over the Internet by using an FDA-supplied public dashboard. Google FAERS public dashboard to examine the data yourself. In 2022, the breakdown of the sources of reports was equally divided by health care professionals and consumers.

Timelines for Post-Marketing Reporting

The requirements for AE reporting have largely been standardized through the International Council for Harmonization (ICH). Reporting for healthcare professionals (and consumers in most places) is usually voluntary and is highly encouraged by regulatory agencies, although there is some skepticism about the utility and value of consumer reports, particularly those for OTC products and those not validated by a healthcare professional.

There is no time frame for reporting by a consumer or healthcare professional after the occurrence of the AE, but obviously rapid reporting is preferred for public health reasons; in some cases, it may save lives. For manufacturers, reporting is obligatory in almost all jurisdictions, and typically within a 15-day (calendar) timeframe, although there are slight differences depending on the region and type of event (domestic or foreign). Any AE that comes into a company, whether through sales representatives, phone calls, Internet and e-mail, literature reports (which must be actively searched for by the company), patient support programs, or other media must be rapidly forwarded to the Drug Safety Unit and reviewed by qualified medical personnel.

For marketed drugs in most countries, all **serious AEs that are unexpected** (i.e., that do not appear in the regulator-approved product labeling) **and possibly related must be r**eported to the health authority by the company within 15 calendar days. In the US, most of the remaining serious and non-serious cases must be reported to the FDA in NDA periodic reports (PADERs) or PSURs/PBRERs (quarterly for newer drugs and yearly for older drugs). In some countries aggregate periodic reporting is done as PSURs/PBRERs, which are prepared according to a schedule, depending on the age of the drug and the country receiving the report. In the EU, PSURs (in PBRER format) periodicity is established by regulators. A regulator may also request a periodic report at any time.

These reports contain line listings of various cuts of the data as well as medical analyses prepared by the company's medical team, usually headed by a physician. They look at AEs that are expected and unexpected and indicate which need to be added to the drug labeling as new ADRs, warnings, precautions, and so forth, and which AEs/ADRs need to be watched with heightened vigilance. These reports are then scrutinized by the regulatory agencies who may agree or disagree with the company analysis and who decide on changes to the drug labeling, conditions of marketing of the drug, and so forth. There is usually dialogue between the health agency and the company before an action is taken, though health authorities are empowered to act immediately and unilaterally if the public health is at risk. At the health agency, the data are then entered into a database and reviewed. Analysis of individual AE cases and of aggregates of AE cases is done.

Specifically, regarding spontaneous reports, a company must set up a failure-proof system to receive, process, report, and analyze AEs. Time is of the essence, because some of the reports must be sent to the health authorities within 15 days. The clock for reporting starts counting down from the moment the first person anywhere in the company (or a partner, co-marketer, etc.) learns about a "valid" AE. This is Day Zero for the report.

■ Sources of Spontaneous AEs

Once a product has been marketed, safety information can be received via a variety of different means and sources, each one needing its own process and procedure to ensure accurate and timely communication of the information. After marketing, a company can receive safety data via:

- Phone, fax, email, mail
- Websites and web forms (with open text fields)
- Social Media accounts (any account that can receive a message from the public, such as LinkedIn, Facebook, Instagram, X, etc.)
- Sales Representatives, Medical Science Liaison (any company representative having direct engagement with healthcare professionals)
- Marketing firms
- Medical Affairs teams and Medical Information Call Centers (MICC)
- Customer Service representatives
- Administrative positions, such as front office staff
- Lawsuits

For phone reports, this means that **any phone number in the company is a potential source of AE reports**, and anyone who answers the phone in the company must be instructed what to do if an AE report comes into a place where it is not normally expected. A rapid and painless (to the caller) transfer system must be set up if the information is not immediately written down by the company employee first answering the call. No one wants to be kept on hold or to repeat the same story for the third or fourth time. It is not acceptable to lose even one AE, so The call must be handled properly. Because some AEs may need to be reported to one or more healthcare agencies within 15 days, time cannot be lost. The company must be ready to accept calls 24 hours a day, 7 days a week (including holidays) and in multiple languages if that is the normal custom in the country. Many companies do not maintain 24-hour coverage in their company, preferring to outsource this function to private companies (sometimes abroad, often in India or Costa Rica). Many companies, even those maintaining a call center during business hours, outsource after-hours calls to poison control centers or private companies. Many companies also use this number (e.g., a toll-free number) for other functions, including product information, queries, and marketing.

Similarly, any e-mail or website or social media site in which an outsider can send a message or key in free text is a potential source of AEs. Many companies, much to their chagrin, receive complaints and AEs on job-posting websites, free sample websites, survey websites, smartphone apps, customer engagement programs, and so forth.

Sales representatives must also be aware that a physician, pharmacist, or other healthcare worker they call on may be the source of an AE. Even innocuous off-the-cuff remarks about a possible AE ("Oh, by the way one of my patients took your other drug XXXX and had a heart attack the next day") made to a company representative constitute a report to the company that must be acted on. Even offhand remarks over the barbecue on a Sunday afternoon in which a neighbor casually relates an AE to a company employee must be reported to the drug safety department! Some pharma companies include a specific sentence in the employees contract which specifies that, should he/she be informed of an ADR with a company's drug, he/she must report this information to the drug safety department within a certain timeframe. Most companies also have this noted in their SOPs and training materials. Many companies require annual training (with documentation of successful and timely completion).

Some companies have media services that review transcripts of newspapers, television shows, websites, blogs, and so forth, looking for anything about their products. Should AEs be noted, they must be sent to the safety department. There is no obligation to scan the web trawling for AEs, but anything found on a company-sponsored website or merely discovered in the course of surfing is a reportable AE.

Lawsuits often represent the point of entry of AEs. The legal department must be aware that they must also report the AE noted in the suit to the safety department usually within 48 hours.

Some people still write "snail mail" letters, and the company mail room or mail screeners must be aware that AEs received in the mail are to be sent to the drug safety group immediately (usually by PDF/e-mail or fax and not interoffice mail).

One of the more complex problems companies face is the phone call or letter that notes a product complaint ("the pill was the wrong color"), an AE ("and then I took it and had violent stomach pains"), and then requests restitution ("I want my money back now!"). These cases must be handled by three or more departments in the company: (1) the drug safety group to get details and report the AE, (2) the manufacturing or quality group to see why the pill was the wrong color, and (3) the marketing/sales group to refund (or not refund) the money. Companies must set up systems to handle this.

■ United States Regulations

The United States reporting requirements for spontaneous reporting are found in 21CFR314.80. Serious, unlabeled (US Package Insert), spontaneous, and literature events, whether felt to be causally related or not, must be reported within 15 calendar days (plus day 0) when the four minimum validity criteria are met. Reports from FDA, either from the MedWatch to Manufacturer Program or FOI, do not have to be sent to FDA but may need to be sent to other HAs.

■ European Union Requirements

The EU regulations are far more complex in terms of sponsor and applicant reporting. Some go to the health authority at the national or provincial level and some go to a non-health-authority-designated agency. All cases should go to EudraVigilance. Reporting depends on whether the case comes from an EU Member State or from outside the European Union. See the extensive descriptions in Good Pharmacovigilance Practice (GVP) module VI (Collection, management and submission of reports of suspected adverse reactions to medicinal products) at the EMA website (Google EMA Good pharmacovigilance practices).

The GVP modules are updated from time to time; local updates from Member States should also be tracked in case of changes in the requirements.

Other Regions

Many countries follow the ICH/CIOMS criteria for reporting valid cases (four criteria: suspect drug, AE, patient, reporter) from spontaneous sources. It is important to triage every case immediately. If it is a serious AE and unlabeled, most jurisdictions require reporting to the health authority within 15 calendar days of first awareness. Some countries have different requirements which often revolve around receiving all domestic SAEs (whether labeled or not) but only some (SAEs that are unlabeled) non-domestic cases. Some countries do not want any non-domestic cases. Some non-English speaking countries require cases to be in the local language, particularly domestic cases.

Australia: Interestingly, Australia only requires Australian SAEs to be reported within 15 calendar days, whether expected or not, using their "blue card" system (the official Australian system to capture AEs is akin to the US MedWatch program and the United Kingdom Yellow Card system) as of this writing. In addition to the "blue card" reporting form (electronic web-form and on paper), the Therapeutic Goods Administration (TGA) accepts E2B ICSRs. Non-serious Australian AEs should be reported as line listings in the PSUR. For post-marketing studies done in Australia, similarly, all SAEs are to be reported in 15 calendar days and the non-serious AEs at the end of the study. Non-Australian cases do not have to be reported. Rather "any significant safety issue or action which has arisen from any analysis of foreign reports, or which has been taken by a foreign regulatory agency, including the basis for such action" should be reported to the health authority (TGA) within 72 hours (www.tga.gov.au).

Canada: Health Canada requires all domestic reports of serious ARs and "unusual failure in efficacy for new drugs" be reported within 15 calendar days. Foreign unexpected serious adverse reactions must be reported in 15 calendar days.

There is now a transition by companies reporting serious AEs to health agencies from paper or fax reporting of paper forms (CIOMS I) to electronic reporting using a standardized electronic format and transmission known generically as "E2B transmissions" after the ICH document of that name. This reporting is either through the Internet (using an electronic gateway or direct entry online into the database). In theory, electronic case transmission of a case is the same to all agencies around the world and simplifies the multiple reporting obligations now in force from country to country. This has not turned out to be entirely the case, however, as various countries (notably the US, Japan, and China) want special or additional information and data in the electronic transmission. Further, the EMA has created a new paper form for output of E2B(R3) ICSRs. Note that most of the local customization relates to administrative detail and not the medical case.

Process Issues

There is also a trend toward reporting from standardized lists of drug names, medical and surgical history, AE codes, laboratory data, and demographic codes. This allows people to document AE cases in a standardized language and format that is easily translated by the computer into any other language. The only area proving resistant to this computerization is the medical narrative, where a case is summarized in prose in a few paragraphs such that the reader can get an understanding of what happened to the patient. Whether a computer-derived narrative (or no narrative at all) will prove to be as useful as a narrative prepared by a safety-trained healthcare professional remains to be seen. Harnessing artificial intelligence and machine learning may facilitate this.

Interestingly, English has become the international language of AE reporting for most countries. PSURs and E2B transmissions are written in English. Some countries require translation of some or all sections, but this is becoming less prevalent as short time frames and international harmonization are requiring that English be the language of drug safety — at least for 15-day expedited reporting and periodic reporting. Sometimes AEs occurring in a particular country must be reported to the national health authority in the language of that country rather than or in addition to English.

After the report is received or uploaded to the database in a company's safety department, it must be logged in and a unique number assigned (either before or after a search for duplicate cases). How this is done depends on whether the case arrives electronically or has to be manually entered into the safety database. A rapid determination must be made by a medical professional to see whether it is an "expedited" or "alert" report that must be sent to the health authorities within 15 calendar days of first arrival. The data must be entered into the database (if not already uploaded), coded, medically reviewed, quality-checked, and dispatched outside the company to the appropriate health authorities, subsidiaries, and business partners, as well as to others inside the company such as clinical research physicians who follow the safety profile of the drug in question. Any horrific AEs that might produce immediate regulatory or public health problems must also be identified and acted on urgently.

From a more general point of view, the wisdom of relying on spontaneous reporting of AEs, and thus trusting the goodwill and timely reporting of the healthcare community and patients, has been seriously questioned in the past few years. As several drugs have been withdrawn from the market or have had urgent labeling changes made following the reports of severe toxicity, the search for a more efficient method of rapidly identifying new safety issues is under way in many quarters. The FDA and EU continue to examine its spontaneous reporting system for efficiency and other health agencies around the world are also examining better mechanisms to capture SAEs.

It is highly likely that electronic healthcare records will in time supplant the spontaneous AE reporting systems now in place. With the electronic tracking of all patients' encounters with the healthcare system (prescriptions given and filled, doctor visits, hospital stays, complaints and diagnoses recorded in standardized forms, etc.), it is likely that health agencies and possibly companies will be able to "mine" the information using complex search algorithms and artificial intelligence tools to do real-time SAE tracking. Prospective use and epidemiology studies will become feasible. Adding genomic data, health economic information, and other data will transform the drug safety surveillance system. This is not likely to happen soon and there will surely be false starts and dead ends in the quest to obtain drug safety data, but there is little doubt that this will occur to everyone's (presumed) benefit. Note also that the regulations for the handling and reporting of post-marketing AEs are not static in spite of "harmonization".

■ Frequently Asked Questions

Q: Is it really worthwhile reporting another penicillin rash or some other clearly well-described adverse event? Isn't this a waste of time, money, and resources that could be better used elsewhere?

A: Yes, that is probably true. Known reactions for old drugs in the approved patient populations using the approved formulation, dose, and route of administration do not really add much to the general knowledge of drug safety. It probably is better to use limited resources looking at newer drugs or patient groups where safety is less well characterized.

This is not what most health agencies (officially) say for the understandable reason that, once they ask healthcare professionals and consumers to start making judgments about what is worth reporting and what is not, they begin the slide down the slippery slope. Their reasoning is that it is better to over report, even known AEs on old drugs, than under report and risk missing something. After many years on the market, even old drugs can have new data found on AEs and in particular drug interactions. Whether enough resources will remain available for this remains to be seen. Regardless, companies must follow the regulations, regardless of the "age" of the product. Perhaps someday if AI includes pharmacovigilance data on AEs, algorithms and software may be able to streamline this process.

Q: Does a doctor or other healthcare professional have the right to report a patient's medical and health information to a private company without the consent of the patient?

A: A good and difficult question. In many jurisdictions (including the US), drug safety reporting by healthcare professionals to companies and the health agency is both legal and encouraged even without the patient's consent. Disease registries have been in place for decades (e.g., for syphilis) in which physicians and hospitals must report cases to the authorities. In other countries, however, the laws can be complex, and some level of consent may be required, particularly if lab tests, X-rays or scans, or other complementary data are also to be sent. The healthcare professional should check on the requirements and limitations in his or her country. In the EU, a major change in data security and privacy has been implemented and the regulation touches all aspects of life, not just drug safety.

Q: Are consumer reports really worth collecting?

A: Clearly, the information collected from consumers is less useful and less able to be acted on than information healthcare professionals supply. Many reasons account for this: imprecise terminology, lack of complete data, misunderstanding by the patient of complex medical issues, and so forth. This is particularly true for OTC products where there is no healthcare professional intervention in most cases, as the patients self-diagnose and self-treat. Having said all that, useful information can still be obtained that will lead to a signal and further investigation. This is probably not an efficient way to do this, however. In addition, companies handling consumer information, particularly via telephone calls, note that it is time-consuming and requires great diplomatic skills from call center workers. Consumers tend to be more talkative, less precise, and more available than medical personnel who want to report the information and get on to their next patient. Again, it is hoped that electronic health records will make this system obsolete in the future.

CHAPTER 18

Generics, Excipients, Placebos, and Counterfeits

Are some adverse events (AEs) more "equal" than others? Are some AEs more important than others? Why are AEs with generics and older drugs important? What should we do with other manufacturers' AEs? Why are AEs associated with new chemical entities critically important? Why are AEs due to excipients so hard to pick up? Why are AEs with over-the-counter (OTC) products also important?

■ Introduction

The reporting requirements for adverse events (AEs) and drugs are generally thought of as being critical for the safety evaluation of new chemical entities (NCEs), also called new molecular entities (NMEs), newly approved for marketing. NCEs, by definition, have not been on the market before. Their safety profile is known only from limited laboratory, animal, and human testing under an IND or equivalent. Clearly, AE reporting is critical in this period, and companies and agencies pay particular attention to AE reports received shortly after launch. Sometimes there is a burst of AEs right after launch and this is known as the Weber effect: a large number of AEs/adverse reactions (ADRs) reported just after launch that decreases after some months to a lower, more steady-state number of reports.

Rare AEs that were not seen in the pre-marketing trials are often picked up in the weeks to months after launch in major markets with good AE reporting structures, such as the United States or Europe. Regulations on AE reporting are written with this in mind.

Given the large number of AEs that drugs can produce and given the limited number of resources that health agencies, companies, and healthcare professionals can devote to reporting and processing AEs, there is an ongoing debate about what AEs are most cost-effective and medically important to collect to protect the public health. Much work is under way to either improve or add to the spontaneous reporting systems in use throughout the world using social media, artificial intelligence, electronic medical records and more. The FDA MedWatch program collects safety information about prescription and over-the-counter (OTC) drugs, biologics, medical and radiation-emitting devices, and special nutritional products (e.g., medical foods, dietary supplements, and infant formulas). See the FDA's website for details. Health Canada, the UK, France, Australia, and many other countries have similar systems. These systems used to be primarily paper based but are now online and on smart phone apps, though paper is still usually accepted for voluntary reporting.

■ Generics

Generic drug products have the same active ingredient as an innovator product and are otherwise bioequivalent. In the US, generic drug products are approved for marketing based on FDA review of an Abbreviated New Drug Application (ANDA) and are overseen by The FDA's Office of Generic Drugs (OGD) within the Center for Drug Evaluation (CDER). As with an innovator product approved under a New Drug Application (NDA), any drug approved under an ANDA must meet the AE reporting requirements in 21CFR314.80. This includes generics as well as NCEs. Non-compliance with these requirements may result in suspension of the marketing approval.

In the EU, similar requirements are in place (see Questions and answers on generic medicines [November 22, 2012] and European Medicines Agency procedural advice for users of the centralized procedure for generic/hybrid applications [January 11, 2021]):

> "As for all medicines, the safety of generic medicines continues to be monitored after authorisation. Each company is required to set up systems to monitor the safety of all medicines that it markets. Regulatory authorities may also perform an inspection of these monitoring systems. If specific safety precautions have to be considered when taking the reference medicine, the same precautions will generally also be required for the generic medicine."

GPVP Module V.B.5.1.1. also notes:

> "For generic medicinal products the expectation is that the safety specification is the same as that of the reference product or of other generic product for which an RMP is in place. If discrepancies exist between approved RMPs for such products, then the applicant is expected to propose and justify the most appropriate safety specification for their product.
>
> "Exceptionally, the applicant for a new generic medicinal product may add or remove safety concerns compared with the safety profile of the reference product if this is appropriately justified (for example, when there is a more up to date understanding of the current safety profile or when there are differences in product characteristics compared with the reference product, e.g. there is a risk associated with an excipient present only in some of the products containing the same active substance)."

If the manufacturer of a branded product receives an AE from a generic version of its product, it should database the AE and report it, as appropriate, as an expedited report or in the periodic report, noting that it is the generic and not the company's branded drug. If the manufacturer of the generic is known, the branded company should still database the event for use in signaling and should send a copy of the event to the manufacturer of the generic. However, not all companies handle it this way. Some companies will not database an AE if the manufacturer is clearly known and the case is sent to that manufacturer. Others will not send a copy to the generic manufacturer. Most other countries have similar requirements for generic drug safety reporting.

There has been some controversy in the US regarding whether generic manufacturers can change their labeling for safety issues seen with their product but not put into the labeling of the innovator product. In general, this has not been allowed. However, if the original manufacturer of the innovator product has withdrawn its product, FDA will select another product to maintain the reference label for the products that remain on the market. This may change over time.

In the EU, for centrally authorized generics, the EMA provides the MAH with the exact wording to be implemented following the innovator's Product Information update; a safety variation is then to be submitted by the generic's company to make the labeling change. A similar procedure is to be followed when a safety concern is first identified for a generic medicinal product.

■ Excipients

An excipient is a theoretically inactive ingredient added to a drug to provide bulk or to give it form or consistency. Regarding excipients, there are many types, including binders, fillers, diluents, lubricants, sweeteners, preservatives, flavors, printing inks, colors, and others. The most common ones used in the US include magnesium stearate, lactose, microcrystalline cellulose, silicon dioxide, titanium dioxide, stearic acid, sodium starch glycolate, gelatin, talc, sucrose, povidone, pregelatinized starch, hydroxyl propyl methylcellulose, shellac, calcium phosphate (dibasic), and others. Standards are set by committees of the United States Pharmacopeial Convention and published in the United States Pharmacopeia and the National Formulary.

Excipients became a major issue in the United States when a sulfonamide elixir was diluted in diethylene glycol (automobile antifreeze) and killed about 100 Americans, including children. It led to the 1938 Food, Drug, and Cosmetic Act. An excipient for drugs is approved for use in the United States by one of the three mechanisms as follows:

1. It meets the requirements of being "Generally Recognized as Safe" (GRAS) under 21CFR182, 184, 186.
2. The FDA approves a petition as a food additive under 21CFR171.
3. It is referenced in an approved NDA for a particular function for that drug.

Excipients for OTC products must comply with section 21CFR330.1(e) as "safe in the amounts administered and do not interfere with the effectiveness of the preparation".

Please refer to the excellent website run by the International Pharmaceutical Excipients Council (http://www.ipec.org/) for further information.

The FDA definition of an adverse drug experience refers to "any AE associated with the use of a drug" (21CFR314.80(a)) without indicating whether the event is associated with the active ingredient (moiety) or an excipient. Should the submitter have some reason to suspect an excipient to be the cause of the AE, this should be noted in the report and the appropriate investigations and follow-up done.

The ICH document Q8 describes in detail how excipients are handled in pharmaceuticals. See ICH's website for the document (www.ich.org).

In the EU, a "Guideline on excipients in the dossier for application for MA of a medicinal product" was published by the EMA in 2008. In addition, the EMA published Q&A documents on the main excipients; they are updated as needed and posted on the EMA website. As with the US, most of the information on excipients is dealt with in the Quality and Manufacturing sections of the regulations. The EU has ongoing new efforts to better characterize and label excipients regarding safety. In general, most countries require Quality Management systems and life cycle risk management for all products. Under this general heading, excipients are included. Thus, if a signal or safety issue should arise regarding an excipient, this is expected to be handled expeditiously. Most regulations require safety reporting for the entire product, not just the active moiety. Thus, adverse events seen with the drug product, whether due presumably to the active ingredient or an excipient, must be handled in the same way as expedited reports or periodic reports as required by regulation and law. The trick is to distinguish an AE due to an excipient rather than the active ingredient. If the former, the problem should be rectifiable, if the latter, then the event is a pharmacologic property of the drug and unlikely to be diminished with manufacturing changes.

It is not uncommon for a quality problem to first enter a company through the safety department and not the manufacturing facility or department. This means that the safety department must have an SOP and strong linkage (and tracking) with manufacturing to deal with such situations.

■ Placebo

As placebos are rarely used explicitly in clinical practice, this refers only to clinical trials. All AEs (whether to active drug, comparator, or placebo) must be captured and databased. The only issue is expedited reporting of placebo events.

In the US, placebo AEs from trials do not generally have to be reported as expedited reports as there is, theoretically, no drug to report. FDA requires that an independent expert committee, a "Safety Assessment Committee" (or equivalent), review all studies in a development program for an overall review of safety on a continuous basis. The investigational product in all expedited reports sent to FDA by study sponsors must be unmasked/unblinded, i.e., the treatment must be identified. In addition, in preparing final study reports, integrated safety sections for NDAs, dossiers for marketing approval in the EU and elsewhere, and comparisons of AEs on active drug and comparator (or placebo) must be reported. Thus, all AEs in a placebo arm of a study should be recorded and tracked in the safety database. See section on "Clinical Trial Unblinding".

In the EU, the standard is reporting of SUSARs. The regulation requires SUSARs to be reported in an expedited manner; but some countries require reporting of all SAEs related to the "biomedical research", not just to taking the active study drug. In this situation, placebo cases need to be reported as expedited reports and in periodic summary reports. The EU Regulation 536/2014 defines an "investigational medicinal product" as "a pharmaceutical form of an active substance or placebo being tested or used in a clinical trial"; therefore, any Serious Unexpected and Related AE is to be reported as expedited reports, even if after unblinding, the concerned product is a comparator or a placebo. This remains quite confusing and different countries handle this in different ways. Hopefully some guidance from the regulators will clarify this.

In regard to reporting of SAEs seen with placebo, Art 42 of regulation 536/2014 (repealing Directive 2001/20 — applicable since May 28, 2016) addresses the reporting requirements specifying that SUSARs with the "investigational medicinal product (IMP)" should be reported. The definition in Article 2 of IMP includes placebo or active comparator. Therefore, all Serious Unexpected and Related ICSRs should be assessed as SUSARs, even if placebo after unblinding.

The common understanding was that unblinding was mandatory to (1) guide the best possible corrective treatment for the concerned subject and also (2) for the company and HA to better understand the risk with the product. But a new debate began with the sentence included in Regulation 536/2014 "22: If following unblinding, an event turns out to be a SUSAR the reporting rules for SUSARs set out in Article 42 and in Section 2 of this Annex shall apply." This seems to mean that for the HA, unblinding is needed to decide if the case is a SUSAR or not. So this has proved somewhat confusing. The common current understanding is to be conservative and to report all Serious Unexpected and Related ICSRs, specifying whether the IMP is the study drug, the comparator or a placebo.

In the United Kingdom, the "Clinical Trials Toolkit" from the United Kingdom Department of Health/Medical Research Council states:

> For blinded trials involving a placebo and an active drug, seriousness, causality, and expectedness should be evaluated as though the patient was on active drug. Cases that are considered serious, unexpected and possibly related (i.e., SUSARs) must be unblinded. Only those events occurring among patients on the active drug (unless thought to be due to the excipient in the placebo) should be considered to be SUSARs requiring reporting to the regulatory authority and ethics committee.

The Good Pharmacovigilance Practice Guide (MHRA Pharmaceutical Press, London, 2009, www.pharmapress. com), from the MHRA, also notes:

> For the purpose of triage of a SAR in a blinded trial, expectedness may be assessed initially

> using the assumption that the test drug has been given. If it is assessed as unexpected against the test drug reference document, it should be unblinded. If, following unblinding, it is seen that the clinical trial subject received the comparator drug, but the event still meets the criteria for a SUSAR, in that it is unexpected according to the comparator reference document (which should be defined in the protocol), then it should be expedited according to the requirements. . . and notified to the company that holds the marketing authorisation for the comparator drug. If, following unblinding, it is discovered that the IMP (investigational medical product) was a placebo, then this event will not require expedited reporting, unless in the opinion of the investigator or sponsor the event was related to a reaction to the placebo, for example an allergic reaction to an excipient (Section 12.3.7, page 140).

In any case, all AEs — whether seen with the study drug, comparator, or placebo — must be recorded in the case report form/EDC system and databased, as they will be used in the final study report to calculate AE occurrence rates for each arm of the study.

Placebo and Breaking the Blind in Clinical Trials

Sponsors should routinely unmask/unblind all serious, unexpected, possibly related AEs (SUSAR) from a trial. If the product in question is placebo, this case is usually not reported to the health agencies on an expedited basis (as the case does not meet the four minimal criteria for a valid case: no drug as well as not being a SUSAR), but kept in the company's database for listing in the final study report. See the section above for more detail. Health authorities in the US and in the EU do not want blinded expedited reports. However, FDA and the EU as well as other health agencies want expedited reports to be unblinded at least to them though perhaps not to the investigators or IRBs. In addition, a Data Safety Monitoring Board (DSMB/DMC), which receives all expedited reports unblinded in real time and determines if there is a safety issue with a specific protocol. The Safety Assessment Committee may also be involved in determining whether an ICSR should be submitted as an expedited report.

In the EU, as a general rule, treatment codes should be broken by the sponsor before reporting a SUSAR to the Competent Authority (Health Agency) and the ethics committee. Once this is done for one region or agency, the case should be reported unblinded to other agencies. As a rule of thumb, all agencies should be told the same thing at the same time.

When an SAE may be a SUSAR and, thus, expeditable, it is recommended that the blind be broken only for that specific patient by the sponsor even if the investigator has not broken the blind. Those responsible for data analysis and interpretation of results at the study's conclusion should be kept blinded.

If the case appears to be a SUSAR and, thus, reportable and expedited, then the blinding should be broken by the safety group or possibly the SAC. Then three possibilities resulting from the procedure of unblinding must be considered as follows:

1. **The patient took the test product:** The case would be reported as a SUSAR to the relevant competent authorities, concerned investigators, and the relevant ethics committees.
2. **The patient took a marketed comparator:** The SAE should be reassessed for expectedness according to the SmPC or labeling for that product. If it is unexpected, then the SUSAR should be reported; otherwise, it is an expected SAR and not reportable on an expedited basis. Not everyone does this, however.
3. **The patient took placebo:** Events associated with placebo will usually not satisfy the criteria for a SAR and therefore are not expeditable in most situations.

In the US, for each AE, a suspect product should be identified. Reports from blinded studies should be submitted only after the code is broken. The blind should always be broken for each patient or subject undergoing a serious, unexpected adverse experience unless arrangements have been made otherwise with the responsible FDA review division. FDA clarified this situation in its final rules, which went into effect in March 2011. They note that serious unexpected suspected adverse reactions should be reported to FDA with the blind broken (unblinded). Placebo reports should not be submitted. The sponsor may propose alternative arrangements before the study starts and write these into the protocol after agreement is reached with FDA.

The FDA also clarified that they do not believe that it is appropriate to report study endpoints as expedited reports for trials that are designed to evaluate the effect of the drug on disease-related mortality or morbidity. However, if a serious and unexpected adverse event occurs for which there is evidence suggesting a causal relationship between the drug and the event (e.g., death from anaphylaxis), the event must be reported as an expedited report even if it is a component of the study endpoint (e.g., all-cause mortality).

■ Picking up AEs Due to Excipients

It is very difficult to pick up AEs due to excipients. The reasons are many. Most drug safety personnel do not pay much attention to excipients and may not even know what excipients are in which drug. Excipients often vary from formulation to formulation of the same drug and may vary in quantity from dose strength to dose strength (e.g., higher doses of the same active ingredient may be larger tablets or capsules and have more fillers and excipients) and may vary from country to country.

Manufacturers change excipients and production methods (with the appropriate Good Manufacturing Practice change control and notification to the regulatory agencies) without telling the drug safety department. Thus, there may be hundreds to hundreds of thousands of individual products with varying excipients manufactured by a large company. These are usually not easily computerized, updated, and searchable. A problem with one excipient in one or only a handful of lots or formulations may go undetected unless there is an obvious and unusual AE and a high level of suspicion on the part of the reviewer.

Manufacturers also often change vendors for excipients, and this, too, may produce issues if product quality or characteristics change. For companies with many products and formulations manufactured in many countries, tracking formulations is a serious challenge for the drug safety group.

One of the authors recalls a product that contained lactose as a filler and that had much more lactose in the United States version than in the Canadian version. When it was discovered that the incidence of diarrhea in the United States was higher than in Canada, the signal investigation revealed the lactose dose difference to be the cause. A very high level of suspicion must be maintained to keep open the possibility of an excipient causing an AE. It is particularly difficult if the AE is common, like diarrhea, or may be caused by the active ingredient itself.

■ Other Manufacturers' Drugs' AEs

For the post-marketing situation, the United States regulations are not clear on this point. There is a section, 21CFR314.80(1)(iii), on how to handle 15-day expedited serious AEs a company receives whose name appears on the product as a packer, distributor, or manufacturer but who is not the applicant (holder of the NDA). This section allows the non-applicant to submit the serious AE to the FDA or to transmit it within 5 calendar days to the applicant, who will then submit it to the FDA. Some have extrapolated from this section to mean that AE reports that are received but are clearly those of another company's product should be sent to the other company. This is a judicious way to handle the matter and represents best (and ethical) practice.

If the drug is a generic version of the innovator product, see the earlier section on how this is handled.

Outside the US, the regulations and guidelines are largely silent on this point. Most companies will immediately send an SAE report to the manufacturer of the drug if the drug and the chemical entity are not theirs. If the drug is a competitor drug with the same chemical entity, the case will be databased usually and transmitted to the other company if known. Some sponsors/applicants will report the case to the HA. In some cases, a concomitant drug is actually felt by the manufacturer to be the cause of the AE. In these cases, many companies will report the case to the HAs and forward a copy of the case to the other manufacturer with a note explaining the situation. The situations and rules are often nebulous, but fortunately, these cases are relatively rare. In the clinical trial setting, as noted, all AEs should be databased and active, and comparator SAEs (when the criteria are met) should be reported as expedited reports. The reporting company may or may not notify the manufacturer of the comparator drug.

In practice, companies collect all AEs that come to them whether the drug in question is their drug, a generic, or a placebo, or whether excipients are suspected. The data are usually handled in the usual way and entered into the database. During the workup, the issues of generic, placebo and so forth are sorted out.

■ Generics

In general, if an AE is reported and the product is identified by the reporter of the AE as a generic and the manufacturer is known, this AE is reported to that manufacturer rather than to the health authority directly. It would be the responsibility of the manufacturer of the product (the generic) to report it to the health authority. Many companies, however, would do both: report the event to the health agencies and to the other manufacturer. If the AE is not known to be from the applicant's drug or from a generic, then the applicant receiving the report must treat it as if it were that company's product and handle it in the usual manner for submission to the authorities. Note in the report that the manufacturer is unknown. This should, nonetheless, be verified in each country where the product is marketed. It is wise to database all cases for the chemical entity no matter the manufacturer, as the data will be used in signaling.

It is obviously important that the correct manufacturer of a drug be identified. Problems might occur with one company's drug and not another's. Causes could relate not just to the active compound but also to manufacturing issues (product quality complaints), different excipients, impurities, supplier issues, and so on. Thus, when a company receives a spontaneous AE for a product it must make a concerted effort to determine the manufacturer, particularly if other versions are marketed, to ensure that the report is attributed to the correct drug.

■ Counterfeit, Impure, and Other Non-standard Products

In recent years, multiple new problems have arisen, leading to increased drug toxicity and adding new challenges to pharmacovigilance:

- **Counterfeits (falsified medicines):** The FDA has become very concerned about counterfeit medications. They have much on the FDA website about this. They state: "Counterfeit medicine is fake medicine. It may be contaminated or contain the wrong or no active ingredient. They could have the right active ingredient but at the wrong dose. Counterfeit drugs are illegal and may be harmful to your health." Counterfeit Fentanyl, BiCNU, Botox, Cialis, Viagra, and weight loss drugs are noted on FDA's website. See https://www.fda.gov/drugs/resourcesforyou/consumers/buyingusingmedicinesafely/counterfeitmedicine/default.htm. FDA has also created a Counterfeit Alert Network (see https://www.fda.gov/drugs/drugsafety/ucm170315.htm which comprises many organizations of physicians, pharmacists, nurses, drugstore chains, and others to aid in rapidly distributing information about counterfeits.

  The EU makes a distinction between falsified and counterfeit medicines (see http://www.ema.europa.eu/ema/index.jsp?curl=pages/special_topics/general/general_content_000186.jsp):

- **Falsified medicines** are fake medicines that are designed to mimic real medicines.
- **Counterfeit medicines** are medicines that do not comply with intellectual-property rights or that infringe trademark law.

The EU issued a directive (DIRECTIVE 2011/62/EU) which came into effect in 2013. It includes measures to protect the public including the following:

- Packaging should have a unique identifier and an anti-tampering device.
- Wholesalers have new responsibilities in protecting the integrity of the supply chain.
- Active substances made outside the EU must be imported with an accompanying written confirmation from the exporting country's regulatory agency.
- A logo must appear on the websites of legally operating online pharmacies and retailers in the EU.

The United Kingdom's MHRA has similarly warned about counterfeits as has Health Canada and other agencies. The World Health Organization has stated that counterfeit medications are now a global problem, affecting both developed and developing countries. The main targets are the most profitable markets where sales and demand are high. Although "lifestyle" medications were some of the first targets of counterfeiters, fake medications are now seen in cancer and cardiac products. Many countries serve as transfer points and not end-user markets.

Online Pharmacies

In the past several years online purchases from pharmacies outside the consumers' countries have proliferated. Many entities and regulatory agencies have warned consumers about fake pharmacies.

Rogue and illegitimate online pharmacies offer potentially dangerous prescription drugs to global consumers. Consumers should protect themselves from substandard, dangerous, and counterfeit drugs by verifying that an online pharmacies is accredited by the National Association of Boards of Pharmacy (NABP). The NABP has several programs such as the "Verified Internet Pharmacy Practice Sites® (VIPPS®) or Veterinary-Verified Internet Pharmacy Practice Sites® (Vet-VIPPS®) that aim to help consumers from potentially harmful and counterfeit products.

A report was released by the NABP in August 2017 on Canadian and other internet and "foreign" pharmacies. See https://nabp.pharmacy/. The NABP is an independent, non-profit organization made up of the boards of pharmacy from all 50 US states, 10 Canadian provinces, Australia and others. The report made several points as follows:

1. They looked at over 100 "pharmacy websites that used "Canada" or "Canadian" in their name or URL or posted a Canadian contact address". They found that three quarters of them (74%), obtained product from outside Canada. Consumers were able to purchase drugs without prescriptions.
2. "Half of the so-called "Canadian" websites sourced drugs from India or a combination of countries where counterfeit products are known to originate.
3. The sourcing countries do not have strict regulations at the level of those in the US or Canada. The danger is that the drugs may be counterfeit, contaminated or subpotent. Quality of products from such sites is not guaranteed.
4. They found that "nearly 96% of these sites were operating illegally, out of compliance with state and federal laws and/or NABP patient safety and pharmacy practice standards".
   - 2,550 were outside the US, 1,557 were inside the US and 6,837 had no location identified.
   - 5,613 sold foreign or non-FDA approved medications.
   - 1,850 of the websites were not secure, thus risking exposure to identity theft and theft of payments.
5. Neither the US or Canadian governments are able to police or regulate these pharmacies.

The WHO has also commented on substandard and falsified medicines as follows:

1. They affect every region of the world.
2. Substandard and falsified medical products from all main therapeutic categories have been reported to WHO, including medicines, vaccines, and in vitro diagnostics.
3. Anti-malarials and antibiotics are amongst the most commonly reported substandard and falsified medical products.

4. Both generic and innovator medicines can be falsified, ranging from very expensive products for cancer to very inexpensive products for treatment of pain.
5. They can be found in illegal street markets, via unregulated websites through to pharmacies, clinics, and hospitals.
6. An estimated 1 in 10 medical products in low- and middle-income countries is substandard or falsified.
7. Substandard and falsified medical products contribute to antimicrobial resistance and drug-resistant infections.

The FDA has issued warning letters informing the website operators that they are engaged in illegal activity in violation of the U.S. Federal Food, Drug, and Cosmetic Act, including:

- offering for sale unapproved prescription drugs of unknown origin, safety, and effectiveness;
- offering prescription drugs without a prescription;
- offering prescription drugs without adequate directions for safe use; and
- offering prescription drugs without FDA-required warnings to consumers about the serious health risks associated with the prescription drug.
- FDA's BeSafeRX campaign is a great way to learn how to buy prescription drugs safely over the internet and a list of warning letters can be found on the FDAs website by searching for "internet pharmacy warning letters".

Authors' Comments for PV Personnel

The counterfeits usually contain a smaller amount of the active moiety or, in some cases, none at all. In the best cases, only fillers are used that should be non-toxic (though the therapeutic benefits of the active entity are non-existent). In the worst case, toxic substitutes are used, and no one has any idea what is in them. Troublesome instances revealed drywall material, antifreeze, or yellow highway paint as the primary ingredient in counterfeit tablets.

The issues here are complex, as various government entities allow, if not encourage, the purchase of medicines for lower prices either online or in jurisdictions out of their legal control ("pharmacies just over the border"). Similarly, reimportation may produce issues if counterfeits enter the supply chain.

One of the interesting and striking observations from experts on counterfeit drugs is that the quality of the packaging must be impeccable, but that the quality and chemicals in the drug product itself is far less important from the point of view of the counterfeiter. Suspicion by the pharmacist or patient of a counterfeit is low if the package appears legitimate, has a real lot number, and is difficult to distinguish from the genuine packaging. Once the user accepts the package as real, the contents are usually not carefully scrutinized. In addition, unlike buying a fake luxury watch or handbag for $3 on the street, where the consumer knows very well he or she is getting a counterfeit ("knock-off") and does not care, the consumer definitely does not want a counterfeit drug product.

This situation is very problematic for pharmacovigilance (PV) and drug safety personnel in government health agencies and companies.

In practice, it is very rare for PV personnel to ask patients or reporters of AEs for the source of the suspected product. The usual questioning revolves around whether the product is branded or generic and not whether it was obtained by mail/Internet or in person at a pharmacy in the US or abroad. In the US, many people obtain their prescription drugs through domestic Pharmacy Benefit Managers or large pharmacy chains' mail order service. This is quite normal and frequent in the US and presents no particular issues or problems as these entities generally maintain very tight control of the supply chain. Nonetheless, counterfeits have been found.

However, if a patient reporting an adverse event or SAE obtained the product from an online pharmacy or from a foreign pharmacy in person, the PV specialist should consider whether there may be an issue with product quality: counterfeit, subpotent, harmful excipients or additives etc. This is above and beyond all the usual issues involved in investigating the SAE such as dosing, drug interactions, etc.

Thus, a PV specialist in the company or health agency may want to attempt to obtain the sourcing information. This may be difficult as the patient may not wish to admit that he or she obtained the product under risky or even illegal (in their eyes) ways.

The PV specialist should also consider the products in question. Some drugs are so cheap and so easily obtained in the US that it is less likely that patients will seek to purchase the drugs online. One pharmacy chain in the southeast of the US offers "free" two week supplies of certain antibiotics and diabetic drugs (with a prescription of course). Many generic drugs are now very inexpensive and hardly worth using an Internet pharmacy. So attention should be paid to sourcing of expensive or hard to get products by the PV specialist moreso than cheaper or generic products though these too have been falsified.

■ Frequently Asked Questions

Q: If resources are limited and demand infinite, should we even bother looking at all generics and excipients? Shouldn't we concentrate on the newest or most used or most dangerous products and concede such things as potential excipient problems in little used products?

A: Yes, you are probably right. It is impossible to track everything. In the US alone, some 4 billion (4×10^9) prescriptions are filled every year. Rather, a triage strategy needs to be developed to make rational use of pharmacovigilance resources and to avoid duplicative work from agency to agency and company to company. Alternatively, the pharmacovigilance of a particular product might be assigned to one national health agency, which would be responsible for worldwide safety surveillance, sort of the way the EU works regarding mutual recognition. One might wish to look at a particular excipient in only, say, five products in five countries periodically to identify safety issues. One must also decide whether to be proactive and do such investigations periodically and in anticipation of potential safety issues or whether to be reactive and start an investigation only after a problem or signal arises. Lots of solutions are possible, but none is on the horizon right now. In general, the authors are pessimistic about this. The ICH attempted to harmonize many aspects of the pharmaceutical business and to a large degree succeeded. However, since the high point of harmonization (the early and mid-2000s) countries and regions are diverging with different requirements (sometimes only mildly different but sufficiently so to increase the overall reporting workload enormously). Broad international agreements on matters such as this are universally agreed in theory but, in practice, are often impossible to put in place.

Q: What about generics? Shouldn't they all be grouped under one marketing authorization or NDA or something like that for AE and signaling purposes?

A: Yes, that is probably a good idea but very difficult to do under the current laws and regulations around the world. Commercial competitiveness also complicates this. Rather, the same result could be attained (and is, in fact, done) at the database level, where data are combined or analyzed over multiple products with the same chemical entity. But this would probably require cooperation among competitors, many of whom are in different countries. Good in theory, not easy in practice.

Q: Do counterfeit products produce more AEs than the branded products?

A: Since counterfeiters of drugs will often put into their products whatever is on hand and cheap, there are many instances of fake drugs that have been found to contain toxic ingredients. The "formulation" may vary from day to day and batch to batch. FDA has frequently reported that various weight-loss products that contained a chemical that could produce high blood pressure, seizures, tachycardia, palpitations, heart attack, or stroke. Similar reports abound. However, some counterfeits will contain no active ingredients and inactive excipients. In this case, the danger is lack of efficacy. So, there is no way, *a priori*, to know or to predict what effects (good or bad) counterfeits produce nor whether they will produce more or fewer AEs than legitimate products.

CHAPTER 19

Artificial Intelligence and Pharmacovigilance

One of the hottest topics in the IT and social media world has been artificial intelligence (AI). AI in the context of product development has been evolving and will continue to evolve. There are now products being developed using an AI model while other products are still being developed the traditional way.

■ Overview

Originally AI was used vaguely to mean "the past of computer science concerned with designing systems that exhibit the characteristics we associate with intelligence in human behaviour". Its use was relatively limited to tasks that humans could not or would not do that could be computerized. These tasks were programmed with various algorithms that were largely static and only did what they were programmed explicitly to do.

A sub-category of AI is "machine learning" which is defined as the field of study that gives computers the ability to learn as humans learn based on data, experience, and algorithms without being explicitly programmed. It was felt by many in the medical and IT worlds that medicine would be an excellent place to use AI. See: *W.B. Schwartz, R.S. Patil, P. Szolovits Artificial intelligence in medicine. Where do we stand? N Engl J Med, 316 (1987), pp. 685–688.* And indeed, AI has been used to develop many systems, software, apps etc. that play a role in medicine and pharmacology.

AI and ML took off in 2022 as a potentially "game-changing big idea" in 2022 with the development of "large language models". These are AI systems that try to mimic human intelligence and analyses. These systems have enormous amounts of data from many sources including books, websites, articles, social media, databases and more.

The system then is trained (and/or trains itself) to see patterns, trends, connections, possible relationships in these data. The bigger the dataset the better the system works as a general rule. It can then generate summaries, reports, charts, graphs, photos, video and audio files etc. from these data in fluent English (or any language it is programmed to know). Some of the systems can enter into a conversation back and forth. Sometimes however, the system makes mistakes, is inaccurate or even misleading. When this occurs, this information is informally called "hallucinations". In 2023 some attorneys used AI to generate a submission to the court which "cited several nonexistent cases, complete with nonexistent quotes and holdings." (Check out Mata v. Avianca (No. 22-cv-01461) for reference).

These systems can be linked to other data sites (e.g. a company's or government agency's data) to improve accuracy and bring new data into the system. FDA has been testing various natural language processing AI systems in drug labeling and causal inference using the FAERS database to review text documents to assess safety. This is currently done largely manually and creating software to enhance these major efforts is the goal. See their BERTox Initiative (https://www.fda.gov/about-fda/nctr-research-focus-areas/bertox-initiative).

■ AI and PV

Much research is now underway using AI in pharmacovigilance. Some of the challenges include finding the appropriate and disparate sources of clinical safety data: FAERS, EudraVigilance, hospital (e.g., electronic medical records), pharmacist and physician challenges, lack of standard terminology and coding conventions, operating systems, software, social media, language and idiomatic phrases, corporate data, quality and validation criteria, etc.

Research is ongoing two broad areas:

1. **AE Case intake and processing.** These areas will replace or assist the manual review of cases to eliminate duplicate cases (particularly nonserious cases and instances of sudden increases in case volume, e.g., during a pandemic, etc.) write case narratives, QA and causality assessments. The first two areas will likely be relatively straightforward to develop but the assessment of clinical causality remains and is likely to remain very difficult to automate efficiently because of the complexity of the variables in causality assessment (incomplete, incorrect or false data, bias in reporting, confounders in data, unreliable reporters, plausibility, etc.). See the chapter in this Manual on causality assessment for further detail.
2. **Signal detection.** Multiple techniques and systems have been available for the last twenty years for signal analysis including Bayesian analysis, Lasso shrinkage regression and many others. These have not proved to be more successful than skilled human clinical analysis by PV experts though they are very useful adjuncts and hypothesis generators for the clinician looking for signals. AI and ML are being used in pharmacoepidemiology and predictive modeling. See the chapter in this Manual on the issues and techniques in such analysis. As a start, FDA launched a transformative national system in May 2008 to explore distributed electronic healthcare datasets. There are several parts: the Sentinel System, Postmarket Rapid Immunization Safety Monitoring (PRISM) system, and Blood Safety Continuous Active Surveillance Network (BloodSCAN). Biologics are included. as part of the Biologics Effectiveness and Safety (BEST) Initiative. To begin to address some of the disparate challenges noted above, a Common Data Model is used for analysis; the System covers more than 10 million lives. AI and ML have been used in "systematic reviews" ("a research technique that attempts to collect all empirical evidence in a particular field, to assess it critically and to obtain conclusions that summarize the research" See https://www.sciencedirect.com/topics/medicine-and-dentistry/systematicreview. Early information suggests that these techniques are more useful than older human methods. As these approaches mature, they may have a greater role in regulatory decision-making.

AI is being looked at in many other areas in pharmacology, transitional medicine and clinical development and product life cycle work.

A useful review of the work in PV by Bate and Stegmann ("Artificial intelligence and pharmacovigilance: What is happening, what could happen and what should happen") from June 2023 can be found at https://www.sciencedirect.com/science/article/pii/S2211883723000217#bib0006

As an example, a recent article confirmed the already added value of AI for both diagnosis and treatment of dermatological disorders (Dermatol Ther (Heidelb), 2022 Dec;12(12):2637–2651. doi: 10.1007/s13555-022-00833-8. Epub 2022 Oct 28. Artificial Intelligence in Dermatology: Challenges and Perspectives, Konstantinos Liopyris, Stamatios Gregoriou, Julia Dias, Alexandros J Stratigos). Nevertheless, the need of an M.D. remains key. For most AI involvements, the expected benefit is linked to rapidity, effectiveness and reliability.

Obviously, this area is developing and it is likely that this summary of AI will be out of date rapidly. Review "AI and PV" in google frequently!

Comments

Are there potential downsides in this area? As with pretty much everything in life, the answer is yes. It is possible that with AI and ML systems easily and cheaply available, the barriers to entry to do PV will fall such that many people and groups will easily do PV. This can lead to people who probably should not be doing PV will come to erroneous, malevolent conclusions. There may simply be too many voices in the field to easily make sound medical judgments. We will need some mechanism of curation to be sure the best and most valid data and judgments are used to make clinical decisions.

Some things are for sure:

- Changes will occur whether we like it or not.
- Tasks that can easily be done by AI will be done by AI, again whether we like it or not.
- Jobs will change, disappear and new ones will open up. Needed skill sets will change.
- There will be multiple players in the field around the world.
- PV will look enormously different in 5 or 10 years perhaps even sooner.
- There will be some nasty and malevolent individuals attempting to subvert, game or manipulate the system due to money, politics etc.
- The criteria for success will initially be such things as number of signals per week. Then, multiple "real" (confirmed) signals identified per week, cost of an identified signal and other measures will be more important. After this wave of measurable operational and processing successes, it will be realized that what really matters will be clinical successes such as time to find a serious signal that leads to product label changes and changes in patient care after a new drug is introduced. Parameters such as number of patient deaths, SAEs, hospitalizations etc. will be the key indicators.
- There will be many more lawsuits (at least in the US).

The initial stages of this development (say the next 5 years or so) will be quite confusing and without clear standards for success. As with most things in the IT world, version 1.0 will be interesting and marginally useful. But down the road, later versions will be the game changers. Right now we are most likely in version 1.2.

CHAPTER

20

Expedited and Aggregate Reporting in Clinical Trials

There are multiple safety reports that pharmaceutical companies and other sponsors must submit to health authorities. This chapter reviews the key reports that are required now by most health authorities.

■ Expedited Reporting

Certain serious adverse events (SAEs) must be reported to health authorities within 7 or 15 calendar days. Most countries use "calendar days" rather than "business or working days", as holidays and working days are not the same everywhere. Some countries still retain different rules for local cases, but by and large, thanks to ICH, CIOMS, and common sense, most countries have standardized on the same timing, format, and content of expedited (also called "alert") reports.

■ Clinical Trial Reporting

Another way to express "clinical trial reporting" is reporting for drugs that are not yet marketed (no Marketing Authorization or New Drug Application (NDA) approval yet). Although this refers primarily to clinical trials, it may also refer to SAEs found in named patient use, compassionate use, solicited SAEs, epidemiologic studies, and other "non-classic" trials and studies.

Most countries require that SAEs, which are unexpected (not labeled), that is, do not appear in the Reference Safety Information (RSI), which is usually the Investigator Brochure, and also that have some possibility (even if small) of being caused by the study drug be reported in 15 calendar days of first awareness by the sponsor. In other words, it must be reported within 15 days from the first notification of anyone in the company (or organization), including its agents, business partners, contractors, distributors, and vendors. This is called a "15-day report", "an expedited report", or "an alert report". In the US, this is referred to as an IND

Safety Report. Note the triple requirement: serious, unlabeled, and possibly related.

A subcategory of this is the "7-day report". In a 7-day report, the patient in question has died or had a life-threatening SAE, which is also unexpected and possibly related (same as above). This report must be sent to the health authorities within 7 calendar days. Note that all 7-day reports are also 15-day reports. Thus, if a report is communicated as a 7-day report, it must also be followed up as a 15-day report, unless full information on the case was provided in the 7-day report. In some jurisdictions, the 7-day "alert" report may be communicated as a phone call, fax, email, or some other less formal communication compared with the more formal 15-day report (on a CIOMS I or MedWatch form, or an E2B electronic transmission). However, many of the key regulators, e.g., the European Medicines Agency (EMA) and the Japanese Pharmaceuticals and Medical Devices Agency (PMDA) require and will only accept structured E2B electronic transmissions from sponsors. If the 7-day report is "informal", then it must be followed up with the usual 15-day "formal" report. If the 7-day report is complete and there are no outstanding follow-up questions, it will cover both 7-day and 15-day requirements. Thus, the 7-day report becomes a 15-day report with the same requirements for follow-up and further reporting, as given in the following sections.

■ United States Requirements for Expedited IND Reports

The Investigational New Drug (IND) obligations are found in 21CFR312. An IND is usually opened and held by a pharmaceutical company, but academics, universities, and individuals may also do so. The term that the FDA uses for the IND holder is generally "the sponsor". The sponsor is obliged to "review and evaluate the evidence relating to the safety and effectiveness of the drug as it is obtained from the investigator" (21CFR312.56(c)). This includes 7- and 15-day expedited reports (21CFR312.32) and annual reports (21CFR312.33). In March 2011, updates to these regulations went into effect.

■ Expedited IND Reports (Alert Reports, 7-Day and 15-Day IND Reports)

Serious, unexpected (unlabeled), AEs from clinical trials for which there is some evidence that the drug caused the event must be reported promptly. Each report identifies all similar case reports, and the sponsor analyzes their significance.

Specifically the FDA regulations state 21CFR312(c)(1): "The sponsor must notify FDA and all participating investigators (i.e., all investigators to whom the sponsor is providing drug under its INDs or under any investigator's IND) in an IND Safety Report of potential serious risks, from clinical trials or any other source, as soon as possible, but in no case later than 15 calendar days after the sponsor determines that the information qualifies for reporting". In each IND Safety Report, the sponsor must identify all safety reports previously received concerning a similar Suspected Adverse Reaction (SAR) and must analyze the significance of the new SAR in light of previous, similar reports or any other relevant information. This analysis should be included in the case narrative.

Unlike much of the rest of the world, in general, a single case will not qualify for expedited reporting to FDA. The regulation, clarified by guidance, expects a sponsor to have the equivalent of an independent panel of experts, a Safety Assessment Committee (SAC), to review all safety data from all studies conducted with a given active moiety. The committee must be composed of qualified experts, who may be employees or non-employees of the sponsor, but must be "independent", i.e., not have direct involvement in the conduct or analysis of any of the studies in the program. The SAC may review both blinded and unblinded data as part of a prospective plan and may also request *ad hoc* analyses. These analyses may include both serious and non-serious AEs. The SAC can make a recommendation to the sponsor regarding submission of IND Safety Reports, but the sponsor alone has responsibility for decisions regarding submission of reports to FDA. Thus, as a practical matter, FDA may receive somewhat different information at different times from other regulators.

The focus is on informative information, which usually requires aggregate analysis, rather than all individual reports on a one-by-one basis.

Expedited reporting must be done for findings from animal studies, epidemiological studies, pooled analysis of multiple studies, or clinical studies, whether or not conducted under an IND and whether or not conducted by the sponsor, that suggest a significant risk in humans exposed to the drug (312.32(c)(1)(ii)). Data from *in vitro* studies (e.g., micro-susceptibility, drug interaction, or genotoxicity) are to be sent as 15-day IND reports if a significant risk to humans is determined (312.32(c) (1)(iii)).

Any clinically important increase in the rate compared to that in the IB or protocol of a serious suspected adverse reaction must be submitted as a 15-day expedited report. Monitoring this is one of the functions of the SAC. The sponsor, in conjunction with the SAC, should assess the "clinical importance". Consideration should be given to the study population, nature and seriousness of the AE, magnitude of the increase, and other relevant factors.

1. The report must be made no later than 15 calendar days after the sponsor's initial receipt of the SAC recommendation to report (which is day 0 and is considered the "clock start date"). Under older regulations the clock start began when the sponsor had sufficient information that the three criteria were met (serious, unexpected, associated) for an expedited report and that the report had the four criteria (reporter, patient, AE, suspect drug) to be valid. This is still the case outside the US. However, FDA has changed these rules as follows:
   - Because the four elements of the minimum dataset are generally readily available in the clinical trial setting, the agency has determined that the definition and the requirement for the minimum dataset are unnecessary and has decided not to require a minimum dataset for IND Safety Reports.
   - The reporting time clock for FDA starts (i.e., day 0) as soon as the SAC informs the sponsor of the recommendation to report to FDA on an expedited basis. However, the SAC should begin work on a new serious report right away to determine the reporting timeframe, within the rest of world clock requirements, not wait for a weekly or monthly meeting. For the rest of the world, day 0 would be the day the sponsor receives the information from the clinical investigator of a serious suspected adverse reaction from a clinical trial. Thus, there may be different day 0s for the US and other countries. These dates must be carefully tracked to avoid late reports.
   - While the IB contains safety information on expectedness, it is the sponsor who makes this determination. Investigators are asked to provide a causality assessment, and this is important outside the US. However, for reporting to FDA, the sponsor alone is responsible for the causality assessment.
   - If any information necessary to evaluate and report the suspected adverse reaction is missing or unknown, the sponsor should actively seek such information.

Thus, when a study site reports any SAE information, the clock starts — even if the information is incomplete or does not meet the minimum requirements. The sponsor must then rapidly obtain the rest of the (minimum) information needed for the expedited report.

If the case has a serious outcome of fatal or life-threatening at presentation (i.e., serious, unexpected, associated, and fatal or life-threatening), the case is to be reported as a telephone or fax report within 7 calendar days of the first receipt. It is important to note that the life-threatening situation is at the encounter, not that it could become life-threatening if it progressed or were more severe. However, there is a nuance here. If the AE presents say as chest pain and is serious but not life-threatening but then evolves over the next few hours into a life-threatening massive myocardial infarction this probably would be life-threatening. This is usually a judgment call, but a rapid evolution of an initially non-life-threatening event would probably qualify.

All 7-day reports are automatically 15-day reports and must then be processed and submitted as expedited reports by day 15 unless the 7-day report was a complete MedWatch or E2B expedited report. Follow-up reports (also expedited reports) are submitted if new information arrives. "Once an expedited report, always an expedited report" (unless nullified).

For expedited reporting, there must be sufficient evidence to suggest a causal relationship between the drug and the SAE, thus creating a Suspected Adverse Reaction (312.32(c)(1)(i)). FDA does not want to receive as expedited reports those cases that are not likely to be related to the drug or otherwise uninformative.

The FDA has clarified that it requires the investigator to report serious AEs rapidly to the sponsor along with a determination of seriousness/life-threatening as well as a determination of causality. However, the sponsor alone is responsible for causality determination under an IND. The sponsor determines expectedness. The most conservative viewpoint ordinarily prevails. That is, in terms of seriousness and causality, if either the investigator or sponsor feels a case is serious, unexpected, and that there is a "reasonable possibility" the SAE was due to the drug, it should be expedited (Table 1).

The events should be submitted in writing, usually on a MedWatch 3500A form (or as E2B transmissions). Reports of safety findings from animal studies and certain other reports (e.g., epidemiology studies) are usually submitted as narratives rather than on MedWatch forms. Most companies do not want to put animal data into their clinical safety database. Non-US cases may be submitted on MedWatch or CIOMS I forms.

All SAEs from bioavailability and bioequivalence studies, whether or not conducted under an IND, must be reported to FDA as expedited reports. From FDA's perspective, reportability does not hinge on whether the event is labeled or not (in the investigator brochure) or whether considered related to the drug (causality) — only on seriousness.

The sponsor must also notify all participating investigators of these reports. The investigators in turn notify the investigational review boards (21CFR312.32(c)(i and ii)). The notification procedure is complex, as not every single individual report goes to the investigators and IRBs (Table 2). Rather important reports or those that alter benefit/risk should be reported. FDA has issued a guidance on this: *Guidance for Clinical Investigators, Sponsors, and IRBs: Adverse Event Reporting — Improving Human Subject Protection* (http://www.fda.gov/downloads/RegulatoryInformation/Guidances/UCM126572.pdf). The sponsor is also required to report information to the FDA from any source, foreign or domestic; clinical, animal, or epidemiologic investigations; commercial marketing experience; literature reports; unpublished papers; and foreign regulatory authorities (21CFR312.32(b)). The FDA retains the right to change the format and frequency of the reports. For marketed drugs, reporting to the IND is not required unless that case is from an IND clinical trial.

Follow-up is required on all safety information received by the sponsor and submitted to FDA as a follow-up to the original (initial) 15-day report. Follow-up information is handled with the same 15-calendar day clock. If a case is received and does not meet the criteria of a 15-day report (e.g., reported as a non-serious case initially) and only later does the receipt of follow-up information show the case to meet the reportability

Table 1. Responsibilities of Investigators and Sponsors in Assessing Serious AEs

Determination	Sponsor	Investigator
Serious/Life-Threatening	Yes	Yes
Causality (Responsible Possibility)	Yes	Yes
Expectedness (Labeled/Unlabeled)	Yes	No

Table 2. Impact of Investigator and Sponsor Causality Assessment on Causality Assessment for Regulatory Reporting Purposes in the EU and the US

	Investigator Causality	Sponsor Causality	Regulatory Causality
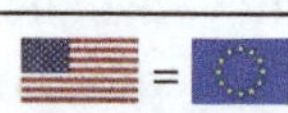	Not related	Not related	Not related
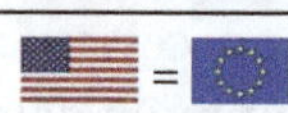	Related	Related	Related
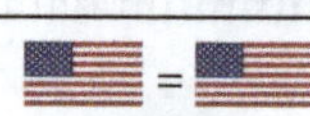	Not related	Related	Related
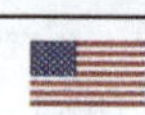	Related	Not related	Not related
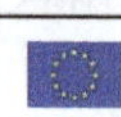	Related	Not related	Related

criteria, the clock starts when the follow-up information is received, and the SAC makes a recommendation to expedite. If a case becomes non-expedited on receipt of follow-up information, the sponsor should submit this new information as a follow-up 15-day report and indicate that the case no longer meets the criteria for expediting.

Other information the sponsor receives that does not quite fall into these categories but which the sponsor wishes to report should be reported as an information amendment or in the annual report. The FDA notes that reporting of a case by the sponsor does not mean that the FDA or the sponsor believes that the report was necessarily due to the drug. This point may prove to be important in any potential litigation in which the sponsor might become involved (21CFR312.32(c)(3,4)). Post-marketing trials should be submitted to the IND (whether conducted under an IND or not) only if the case meets the three criteria (serious, unexpected, possibly related) as determined by the sponsor.

The FDA also notes that in some trials, the sponsor and FDA may reach an agreement to be noted in the protocol whereby certain study endpoints (e.g., a particular SAE such as a myocardial infarction or death) which would normally be considered serious and, thus, trigger expedited reporting will not be reported as 7-day or 15-day reports but rather periodically or at the end of the trial. This type of arrangement would be typical for survival endpoints in oncology studies. In all instances, this must be prospectively customized for each situation. FDA and IRBs, etc. must agree to it. Expedited reports should be unblinded and placebo cases should not be reported on an expedited basis. The SAC will have access to the unblinded cases.

In summary, the sponsor (whether an individual, institution, or company) has full responsibility for determining whether to submit 15-day expedited reports to FDA for clinical trial AEs that are serious, unexpected (not in the Reference Safety Information (RSI)), and for which there is "evidence" of a causal relationship to study drug. The RSI is the Investigator Brochure or Package Insert, depending on which one is used: Investigator Brochure for non-marketed drugs or new indications of marketed drugs and the US Package Insert — usually — for marketed drugs and post-marketing studies. The SAC plays a key role in providing objective advice to the sponsor regarding pan-program safety assessment.

Outside the US, the criteria for a causal relationship are generally softer, i.e., a "reasonable possibility" of association with the study drug rather than a requirement for "evidence". As noted above, epidemiologic, animal, and other studies may also trigger expedited reporting. If the case is a death or is life-threatening at presentation, a 7-day report (phone or fax) must also be made in addition to the 15-day report.

Note that the submission of such reports has become much more complex as divergences have developed from the original consensus documents. Sponsors must be very careful in tracking SAEs which may now be expedited in one country and not expedited in another. In addition, day 0 may not be the same. We are deharmonizing.

IND Annual Reports

In addition to the 7-day and 15-day safety reports, the IND holder must also submit annual reports (21CFR312.33). In lieu of the annual report to the IND, FDA accepts the Developmental Safety Update Report (DSUR) that CIOMS and ICH have developed, as long as the appendices required in the IND regulations are provided. A waiver is not required to substitute a DSUR for the IND Annual Report, but all time periods must be continuously covered without interruption.

For the IND Annual Report, a brief summary of the progress of the investigation(s) must be submitted within 60 days of the anniversary date of the IND. This summary must include the following:

1. Individual study information: A brief summary of the status of each study in progress and each study completed during the previous year:
   - The title and number of the study, its purpose, a brief statement identifying the patient population, and a statement as to whether the study is ongoing or completed.
   - The total number of subjects initially planned for inclusion in the study; the

number entered into the study to date, tabulated by age group, gender, and race; the number whose participation in the study was completed as planned; and the number who dropped out of the study for any reason.

- If the study has been completed, or if interim results are known, provide a brief description of any available study results.
- Summary information obtained during the previous year's clinical and non-clinical investigations.

2. A narrative or tabular summary showing the most frequent and most serious adverse experiences by body system;
3. A summary of all IND 15-day safety reports submitted during the past year;
4. A list of subjects who died during the investigation, with the cause of death for each subject;
5. A list of subjects who dropped out during the investigation in association with any adverse experience, whether or not it is thought to be drug related;
6. A brief description of what, if anything, was obtained that is pertinent for understanding the drug's actions, including, for example, information about dose response, information from controlled trials, and information about bio-availability;
7. A list of the pre-clinical studies (including animal studies) completed or in progress during the past year and a summary of the major pre-clinical findings;
8. A summary of any significant manufacturing or microbiologic changes made during the past year;
9. A description of the general investigational plan for the coming year to replace that submitted one year earlier;
10. If the Investigator Brochure has been revised, a description of the revision and a copy of the new brochure;
11. A description of any significant phase I protocol modifications made during the previous year and not previously reported to the IND in a protocol amendment;
12. A brief summary of significant foreign marketing developments with the drug during the past year, such as approval of marketing in any country or withdrawal or suspension from marketing in any country.

If the sponsor wishes, it may transfer some or all duties for clinical trials (including safety) to a third party, such as another company or a clinical research organization. In that case, the transfer of obligations must be described in detail and in writing to the FDA (21CFR312.52(a)). However, the sponsor retains ultimate accountability.

Other Clinical Trial (IND) Reporting Issues

Reporting the same 15-day alert case to the IND and the New Drug Application (NDA):

This issue arises when there is an open IND and an approved NDA for the same drug. Normally in simple situations, before NDA approval and while the IND is open, all 15-day reports are sent to the IND. After the NDA is approved, reporting should now, in general, be to the NDA. There is one situation where there must be reporting of the same case to both the IND and the NDA.

Double reporting is required if the serious AE meets the three IND reporting criteria (serious, unexpected, possibly related) and is from an IND study. In this case the 15-day report must be sent to both the IND and the NDA.

If the serious AE report is from a non-IND study, then it is reported to the NDA only. Ordinarily the SAC or equivalent would recommend IND reporting, whereas NDA reporting would be independent of the SAC.

Reporting serious AEs to comparator drugs and placebos:

Some countries have been requiring the reporting of placebo and comparator serious AEs. In the US, FDA has made it clear that placebo cases usually do not meet the four-element criteria (patient, reporter, drug, AE) because there is no "drug" and so are not reported. The EU also, in general, does not want placebo cases submitted as expedited reports. However, placebos usually do have excipients and often "benign" compounds, such as lactose, that can produce AEs. In addition, in any placebo-controlled trial, there are usually large numbers of AEs seen with placebos. These are reported at the end of the study in the final study report.

The sponsor of the trial, especially if the trial is a multinational trial, must ensure that all regulatory reporting requirements are met in each country where there is a clinical trial site. These requirements are often different from US/EU/ICH requirements and may also require local language reporting for certain serious AEs with different timelines.

Blinding and unblinding 7-day and 15-day alert reports:

FDA clarified the issue of unblinding in its rewrite of the clinical trial reporting rules. They want all expedited reports submitted to them to be unblinded.

They have stated as follows (Federal Register/Vol. 75, No. 188/Wednesday, September 29, 2010/Rules and Regulations. 59947):

"The agency does not believe that unblinding single or small numbers of informative cases will compromise the integrity of the study. However, if patient safety can be assured without breaking the blind, the agency encourages the sponsor to discuss alternative reporting arrangements with the appropriate FDA review division. Any anticipated alternative arrangements to maintain the blind would need to be described in the protocol, including identification of the serious AEs that will not be reported on an individual basis and the plan for monitoring and reporting results to FDA."

The EU and the member states generally require that cases be unblinded before submission:

The ICH E2A guideline, which the FDA also references and wishes to follow, notes that when possible and appropriate, the blind should be maintained for those persons, such as biometrics (statistics) personnel, who are responsible for data analysis. In large companies, this often turns out to be difficult to do in practice. Although statisticians may be blinded, in most instances when the blind is broken, a MedWatch/CIOMS I form/E2B file is created, in which case it is noted to be the study drug or control. Usually, serious AE reports are routinely widely dispersed: to the clinical trial physicians, monitors, others in the company, the investigators and the investigational review boards, subsidiaries, clinical research organizations, and data safety monitoring boards. "Leaks" occur and the code is inadvertently revealed to those who are attempting to remain blinded. Thus, maintaining a "partial" unblinding is difficult.

Note: Some companies, especially those making ophthalmology products, do not like to use the word "blinded" and prefer to use the word "masked".

Serious AE reporting after the end of the trial:

There are no clear rules in the US for the duration of time that serious AEs should be collected and reported in the study report and to the FDA as expedited reports after a trial ends. Many use an arbitrary 30-day period after the patient's last dose. This may come from the long-standing clinical medicine tradition of ascribing post-operative deaths to the surgery if the death occurred within 30 days of the operation. Clearly, if a drug has a very short or very long terminal half-life (e.g., depot formulations), one may use a different time period.

Survival studies (where all patients are followed until death, such as in cancer trials) present different issues. Here again, many use a 30-day limit after the last dose for collection of serious

AEs. All deaths, however, should be collected by the sponsor and sent to the authorities, if it is believed they meet the criteria for a 7-day or 15-day report. The issue in survival studies is that periodic follow-up to see whether the patients are still alive, one often has serious AEs reported "in passing". What to do with these is an unresolved issue. There is no consensus on this. Some companies collect and report them. Others do not.

European Union Requirements

Expedited Reporting in Clinical Trials

The expedited reporting in clinical trials is covered in the Clinical Trials Regulation 536/2014 repealing the Directive 2001/20/EC. Specifically, the "Detailed guidance on the collection, verification and presentation of adverse reaction reports arising from clinical trials on medicinal products for human use" (2011/C 172/01) covers the subject in great detail. Unlike the situation in the EU for expedited reporting of post-marketing SAEs, which is largely harmonized, clinical trial reporting may still vary somewhat from country to country in the EEA.

Key points from the above guidance include the following:

1. Reportable cases are SUSARs (suspected, unexpected, serious adverse reactions).
2. The sponsor and investigator should both make an independent judgment of causality: "Having a reasonable suspected causal relationship to an investigational medicinal product." (In contrast to the US, where the sponsor alone is responsible for assessing causality, either the investigator or sponsor assessment is used, see Table 2.)
3. Expectedness should be determined using the Investigator Brochure for non-authorized (non-MA) products, and the SmPC for authorized ones.
4. In the concerned trial, SUSARs should be reported for the investigational medicinal product (study drug, comparators or placebo). For SUSARs in other trials, refer to the guidance, as the rules are rather complex and depend on whether there is a Marketing Authorization (MA) in a member state.
5. For comparators, the case should be transmitted to the MA holder of the comparator.
6. Placebo cases normally do not meet the criteria for expedited reporting unless it is possible the reaction is due to an excipient or impurity.
7. The ethics committee in some countries may only receive ICSRs for SUSARs in the concerned trial in that member state. If so, it is recommended that SUSARs from other member states and third countries be reported to the ethics committee (and health authority) at least every 6 months as a line listing and a summary of the main points. The Executive Summary from the DSUR may be used as the summary for ethics committees. Changes in patient risk and new safety issues as well as changes in the conduct of the trial should be reported in 15 days to the committee.
   - Codes should be broken by the sponsor in blinded trials before reporting to the ethics committee and the health authorities. If the blind break shows the product administered was the test drug, then it should be an expedited report; if a comparator, it should be assessed for expectedness against the SmPC and if unexpected, it should be reported; if placebo, such events normally don't satisfy the requirements for expedited reporting, but "where after unblinding SUSARs are associated with placebo, it is the sponsor's responsibility to report such cases."
   - In trials with high morbidity/mortality with many potential expedited reports, the sponsor may reach an agreement in advance with the concerned health agencies concerning SAEs that are treated as disease-related and not handled as expedited reports. The agreed-on system should be noted in the protocol, and it is recommended that a Data Safety Monitoring Committee be used.

Note 1: Even if harmonized at the EU level (see Regulation 536/2014) with SUSARs, expedited reporting for clinical trials can be more requiring in some EU countries. They actually request, depending on the clinical development phase or not, the reporting of all SARs.
Note 2: The rules for reporting expedited reports in the EU depend on the source of information. For medicinal products being approved in the EU but still with ongoing clinical trials, post-marketing SAEs will follow the Post-approval regulation when clinical trials SAEs will follow the clinical development regulation. The same rules apply for aggregate reports: PSURS are due after the first approval and DSURs are to be delivered as long as clinical trials are ongoing.

Development Safety Update Reports

In the EU, sponsors must submit a safety report annually while a clinical trial is under way. The report should concisely describe the safety information for one or more trials. It is known as the Development Safety Update Report (DSUR) and is loosely based on the Periodic Safety Update Report (PSUR) that is used for aggregate reporting in the post-marketing phase. The DSUR was developed by CIOMS (Report of Working Group VII) and ICH (E2F Guideline). These two documents outline the recommended content, format, and considerations for a DSUR. In some instances there may be overlap in content between the PSUR and the DSUR, but each should be prepared as a comprehensive standalone document.

The DSUR is intended to provide a common standard for an annual aggregate summary report for drugs in development (pre-marketing and line extensions). Analysis of safety information on a periodic basis is essential to protection of subjects enrolled in clinical trials. It is also critical to inform regulators and other stakeholders (e.g., ethics committees) at regular intervals about the evolving safety experience with the investigational product. This is particularly important if actions are contemplated to address safety concerns. The main focus of the DSUR is on safety data and the interpretation of those data. Each DSUR should be concise while at the same time it should give assurance to stakeholders that the investigational program is being conducted properly.

Note, however, that while all safety issues discovered during the reporting period should be reviewed, the DSUR should not be the vehicle used to first convey important new safety information or significant new safety concerns.

In addition to standardized presentation of safety information, the DSUR also describes the status of ongoing individual investigations, manufacturing changes, and overall development status and plans.

The main purpose of the DSUR is to provide a summary to regulators on an annual basis. It may also be appropriate to provide a copy to co-development partners or a copy of the Executive Summary (perhaps supplemented with line listings of serious adverse reactions) to ethics committees or other stakeholders.

See the guidance noted above under EU expedited reporting for additional details.

The DSUR has four main sections as follows:

1. **Introduction**
   - 1.1. Background
   - 1.2. Objectives
   - 1.3. Scope of the DSUR
   - 1.4. Relation of the DSUR to the periodic safety update report
   - 1.5. Recipients of the DSUR
2. **General principles**
   - 2.1. Single DSUR for an active substance
   - 2.2. Periodicity and DSUR data lock point
   - 2.3. Duration of DSUR submissions
   - 2.4. Responsibilities for preparing and submitting a DSUR
   - 2.5. DSURs for combination therapies
   - 2.6. Reference safety information
   - 2.7. Format and presentation of DSUR

     The recommended table of contents:

     Title page

     Executive Summary

     Table of Contents

     1. Introduction
     2. Worldwide Marketing Approval Status

3. Actions Taken in the Reporting Period for Safety Reasons
4. Changes to Reference Safety Information
5. Inventory of Clinical Trials Ongoing and Completed during the Reporting Period
6. Estimated Cumulative Exposure
   - 6.1 Cumulative Subject Exposure in the Development Programme
   - 6.2 Patient Exposure from Marketing Experience
7. Data in Line Listings and Summary Tabulations
   - 7.1 Reference Information
   - 7.2 Line Listings of Serious Adverse Reactions during the Reporting Period
   - 7.3 Cumulative Summary Tabulations of Serious AEs
8. Significant Findings from Clinical Trials during the Reporting Period
   - 8.1 Completed Clinical Trials
   - 8.2 Ongoing Clinical Trials
   - 8.3 Long-term Follow-up
   - 8.4 Other Therapeutic Use of Investigational Drug
   - 8.5 New Safety Data Related to Combination Therapies
9. Safety Findings from Non-interventional Studies
10. Other Clinical Trial/Study Safety Information
11. Safety Findings from Marketing Experience
12. Non-clinical Data
13. Literature
14. Other DSURs
15. Lack of Efficacy
16. Region-Specific Information
17. Late-Breaking Information
18. Overall Safety Assessment
    - 18.1 Evaluation of the Risks
    - 18.2 Benefit–Risk Considerations
19. Summary of Important Risks
20. Conclusions Appendices to the DSUR

3. Guidance on contents of DSUR

All sections should be completed; when no information is available, this should be stated.

Title page

The title page of the DSUR should include the following information:

- DSUR number (reports should be numbered sequentially);
- Investigational drug(s);
- Reporting period;
- Date of the report;
- Sponsor(s) name(s) and address(es);
- Statement on the confidentiality of the information included in the DSUR;
- A cautionary statement that the DSUR includes unblinded information, if applicable.

Executive Summary

This section should provide a concise summary of the important information contained in the report. Together with the title page, it can serve as a "stand-alone" document suitable for submission to ethics committees and other stakeholders, if required by national or regional laws or regulations. The following information should be included in the Executive Summary:

- Introduction — report number and reporting period;
- Investigational drug(s) — mode(s) of action, therapeutic class(es), indication(s), dose(s), route(s) of administration, formulation(s);
- Estimated cumulative exposure of clinical trial subjects;
- Marketing approval(s)? (yes/no) — If yes, number of countries;
- Summary of overall safety assessment (based on section 18 of the DSUR);
- Summary of important risks (based on section 19 of the DSUR);
- Actions taken for safety reasons including significant changes to IB;
- Conclusions.
- Table of Contents

4. **Appendices to this guideline**

APPENDIX A — Glossary

APPENDIX B — Examples of tables and table headings for clinical trial listings

APPENDIX C — Examples of the summary of important risks.

The DSUR should be submitted on the anniversary of the first authorization in any member state and within 60 days of the data lockpoint. If there is also an MA for the product, the Periodic Safety Update Report (PSUR) and DSUR dates may be harmonized.

Investigators should be informed in writing with a line listing of SUSARs and a summary of any safety issues that could adversely affect study subjects.

Each member state in the EU may add more requirements in terms of aggregate reporting.

When to Start Collecting Serious AEs in Trials

Safety data collection starts as soon as the informed consent is signed and includes the waiting period or washout period (if there is one), when no study drug is administered. This concept was particularly noteworthy in France, where any safety issue that occurred during the "biomedical research" was reportable. This included placebo AEs, complications of medical procedures, auto accidents on the way to the hospital, and so forth. The idea is that the AEs occurred in regard to the study and not just the study drug.

In regard to FDA reporting, a serious AE that occurred before the drug was administered is generally not related to the study drug and thus does not qualify for a 15-day report. There is at least one situation, however, where this might not always be the case. Anticipatory nausea and vomiting before cancer chemotherapy in patients who have already had therapy is rather common, with an approximate 29% and 11% incidence, respectively. See the National Cancer Institute review of this phenomenon at its website (www.cancer.gov). Thus, one may consider that these serious AEs, which may be due to classic Pavlovian conditioning, are possibly related to the study or treatment drug even though it has not yet been taken.

Canadian Requirements

The sponsor of a clinical trial conducted in Canada is required to notify Health Canada of any serious, unexpected, ADR in an expedited manner. Expedited reporting in Canada follows the 7-day and 15-day clinical trial requirements for reporting, whether the case occurred inside or outside Canada. Each ADR that qualifies for expedited reporting must be sent to Health Canada individually.

For causality, the conclusion of either the investigator or the sponsor that there is a "reasonable causal relationship to the medicinal product" is considered valid.

Follow-up reports of fatal or life-threatening suspected ADRs must include an assessment of the findings. The assessment must include an analysis of relevant previous experience with the same or similar drugs and also the sponsor position on the importance and implication of the report.

In addition, Health Canada may request that a sponsor submit other safety information at any time while a clinical trial is ongoing. Such an *ad hoc* request may include, for example, a line listing of all serious events, expected or not.

There may be additional situations that require rapid sponsor communication with Health Canada on a safety concern. For example, important new data that could impact the benefit–risk assessment or that would lead to protocol changes,

The sponsor must record all AEs in the study (occurring inside or outside Canada), including information that specifies the indication and dosage form at the time of the AE.

Currently, there is no specific timing in the regulations for the ethics committee (called a Research Ethics Board in Canada) to receive periodic aggregate reports. Requirements are thus usually set out by the individual board in its charter or Standard Operating Procedures (SOPs). This is undergoing much discussion in Canada.

Since 2015, Health Canada has required an annual safety review in the format of the ICH DSUR and consistent with the electronic Common Technical Document. The DSUR (and the DSUR Checklist) must be submitted to Health Canada on request. DSURs may also be provided voluntarily by sponsors when justified by important new safety information. In addition, the updated Investigator Brochure must be submitted on an annual basis. This allows Health Canada to get an overview of the drug and trial.

■ Elsewhere

The requirements for expedited and periodic reporting vary significantly from country to country, even within the EU, and sponsors should check locally and frequently about reporting requirements, particularly if there is a study site in that country. It is not uncommon to have local requirements for annexes that supplement the "core" DSUR. Also, requirements and submissions may not always be in written in English. This differs somewhat from the existing situation for post-marketing reporting, which is largely harmonized.

■ Bottom Line

Safety reporting, particularly for expedited reports, has become exceedingly complex and differs from country to country in many cases. The regulations and requirements are continually changing, and it is likely they will continue to do so. PV personnel must carefully track the reporting requirements in all the regions where the product is being used, studied, developed, approved, sold, etc.

■ Q&A

Q: What if during an annual reporting period there was very little patient data received, or no data received? Do we still have to submit an annual progress report such as a DSUR or IND ASR?

A: Some companies wonder if they are allowed to skip a reporting period if little to no information has been received during the reporting period. This could be due to slow enrollment, delayed clinical trial initiation, funding, and many other reasons. However, the lack of, or minimal data, does not absolve a company from sending in an annual report to the authorities. Additionally, there are still other components of the annual report that will change regardless of enrollment data such as literature and pre-clinical data — so to truly have "nothing to report" is actually a lazy way to get out of reporting obligations. It is still required and better to report the null, or absence of data, than not to report at all. If a company however wishes to challenge this requirement, it is in their best interest to communicate this with the appropriate agencies and potentially deal with the outcome later.

Q: What if we miss a report? What if the report is late?

A: Own it. We are all human and even AI will eventually get it wrong. There will be late reports, there will be non-compliance, that is known. To an extent, late reports are generally known to occur and are acceptable within a specific threshold as long as a company acknowledges the deficiency and employs continuous improvement activities. However, how you deal with it is most important. Once a company has identified that a report has been distributed late, either to the authorities, sites, DSMB, Ethics Committee/IRB, or Investigator, start documenting it and the steps you take to remedy the situation. This process is generally referred to as Deviation and Corrective Action and Preventative Action (CAPA) activities. You will miss a report, or the report will be sent late, or within the wrong reporting period — make certain you have operations in place to identify the error and correct then, then own that there was a mistake and simply move on.

CHAPTER

21

Post-marketing Spontaneous ICSR/SAE Reporting

Post-marketing spontaneous reporting of Individual Case Safety Reports (ICSRs) is the mainstay of drug safety at this time, although active surveillance and other approaches are being refined and will have an increasingly important role in protecting patient safety.

■ General Principles

This chapter focuses on ICSRs that arise after a product is approved by a regulator for marketing. In this context, the terms *post-marketing*, *post-approval*, *post-authorization*, and *post-registration* should be considered synonyms. The requirements for reporting revolve around various subsets of adverse events and then the periodic aggregate reporting of the remaining cases (and some ICSRs already reported) with some degree of medical analysis. This system, on its face, is quite extraordinary as it relies on the good will and beneficence of the following:

- Healthcare professionals to voluntarily report untoward events observed with drugs that they have prescribed or administered, and who are not compensated for their efforts;
- Patients and consumers;
- Caregivers and patient advocates; and
- Other stakeholders.

This situation is likely to change over the years for many reasons, including cost and better technology. The regulations governing post-marketing reporting are complex, scattered, and only partially harmonized across regulatory jurisdictions. Various updates and guidances are published frequently, often changing the rules significantly in a single jurisdiction. There is no single source that proactively tracks all changes. The changes are often, but not always, published in English.

(Why countries with their own national languages should publish their internal rules in English is another discussion entirely.) When not published in English, precision, nuances, and cultural context are often lost in translation.

Post-marketing ICSRs versus Clinical Trial ICSRs

Although post-marketing New Drug Application (NDA) or Marketing Authorization Application (MAA) reporting of SAE cases are conceptually quite similar to pre-marketing clinical investigation SAE reports (e.g., IND studies), there are important differences. The sources and reporters of the events are varied as reports are not just coming from trained clinical trial investigators. Lay language is often used in reports from patients/consumers/caregivers. Further, handling and reporting to health agencies are also somewhat different in different countries. These challenges are addressed later in this chapter.

As with clinical trial reporting, there is an obligation for safety reporting after approval of the NDA or MAA. Post-marketing reporting is usually obligatory after approval whether or not the drug is actually marketed (some companies delay marketing for operational or seasonal reasons). In clinical trials, AEs are reported by investigators who are health professionals and usually have a relationship with the company (e.g., sponsored trials). Thus, cooperation and complete medical reports from a healthcare professional are usually ensured, particularly for SAEs in clinical trials. Under governmental regulations, safety reporting is obligatory for the investigator and the sponsor.

The post-marketing period, however, is quite different. Reports may come from many sources, including patients, families of patients, healthcare professionals, sales representatives, literature reports, news reports, health authorities, the Internet, blogs, social media, poison control centers, other pharmaceutical companies, lawyers, and more. Products may be used off label. In most instances, reporting is voluntary for everyone except pharmaceutical companies and rests on the goodwill of the reporters. However, sometimes, patients who report AEs are upset that the AE happened at all. They may assume that drugs are safe and this AE should not have happened. At least in the United States, they often want their money back and, in fact, may have called the company not to report the AE but rather to get a refund or discount coupon.

Healthcare professionals often contact the health agency or the pharmaceutical company to report an AE and are not quite aware that the company, obliged to follow-up and report the case to the authorities, will do extensive follow-up and request copies of reports from the physician's office, the hospital, the laboratory, and even the ambulance service. Busy pharmacists, nurses, or physicians often do not realize what they are getting into when they simply called to do their duty by making a "quick" report of an AE. They did not want to get burdened down with pulling records (perhaps from multiple sources), protecting patient privacy, and sending them to the company.

Report quality is also an issue compared with clinical trial reports, as the quality of the post-marketing reports is quite variable, especially when reported by non-medical people. Consumer reports should have follow-up attempted with the treating physician where possible. The problem is more difficult if the patient used a self-prescribed over-the-counter (OTC) product or herbal preparation; there may be no physician or pharmacist involved at all.

The four elements or criteria for a valid ICSR (sometimes called the minimal dataset for reportability) are as follows:

1. An identifiable patient;
2. An identifiable reporter;
3. A suspect drug(s); and
4. An AE (or fatal outcome if no AE is reported other than "found dead").

If these four elements are present, then the case is considered valid and reportable to Health Authorities (e.g., Food and Drug Administration, European Medicines Agency, Health Canada, Pharmaceuticals and Medical Devices Agency in Japan, etc.). If they are not, the company should make due diligence efforts to obtain the missing data. The data should be stored in a secure, electronic database.

An identifiable patient usually means one or more identifiers are present: age, sex, initials, name, date of birth, and so on. Vague reports such as "I heard there was a patient or two upstate who took drug X and had a stroke" or "a few people had strokes" are not specific enough to meet the criteria for identifiable patient. "A man" or "a young girl" or "six men had strokes" are sufficient to be considered identifiable. Some people feel that AE with an occurrence date, indirectly means an identifiable patient.

An identifiable reporter is usually clearer. It may be the patient or a family member. As a rule of thumb, an identifiable reporter should be one who can be contacted. Thus, an e-mail AE report where there is no information on the sender other than the properly formatted e-mail address would be a valid reporter because one can respond to the e-mail and get follow-up. However, procedures should be developed to determine patient and reporter identifiability and requirements, including for posts on company-sponsored websites.

The suspect drug is also usually not a problem. However, issues do occur as follows:

1. Occasionally, someone will send in an AE report and make the comment, "I don't think this is due to your drug but thought I should report it anyway, just in case." This should still be considered the suspect drug (unless another one is noted) and the reporter's comment noted in the narrative.
2. If it is clear that the drug is the product of another company (e.g., same chemical entity but different manufacturer, whether branded or generic), the case should be sent within 5 days to that manufacturer or company if it is located in the United States. Elsewhere rules vary, but in general, the case should go to the manufacturer/MAH (a PV department policy on how and when to inform competitors can be useful — triage of clinical trial and post-marketing reports to competitors may be different.) If, however, it is unclear whether it is the company's marketed product or another manufacturer's product, then the company must process it as if it were clearly its own product. The lack of clear "ownership" and product identification should be noted in the report.
3. Different formulations of the same active moiety must be entered into the database and reported, as appropriate, unless the product is clearly found to be from another company. Thus, a topical version of a company's product made by another company (but unclear which one) needs to be reported.
4. Combination products that contain the active moiety should also be reported.
5. An audit trail should be kept for all ICSRs triaged to competitors.

The identifiable AE is also usually clear and relates to any untoward event or "bad thing". The AE could include signs, laboratory abnormalities, symptoms, or diseases. More general terms like *experienced unspecified injury* or *irreparable damages* should be excluded, but follow-up should be attempted. Fatal outcome with no AE should be considered reportable ("found dead in bed"). This is the only instance in which an outcome is considered an AE. Death is an outcome and not an AE unless there is no other AE reported.

One should also be sure to distinguish medication errors and product quality issues. Sometimes two or more things may occur in the same report, as in this scenario: "The tablet was blue instead of green and smelled funny; I took two instead of one and then had a bad headache. And I want my money back and I have a question." The product quality, medication error, AE, question, and refund issues should each be handled by the appropriate personnel in the company.

In most countries, the company ("applicant", "sponsor", or MAH, IND holder, NDA holder) must report each AE that is serious and unexpected (i.e., not included in the regulator-approved labeling (= Package Insert for the United States or the product monograph in many other countries, etc.), whether domestic or foreign, within 15 calendar days of initial receipt of the information. For the EU, all serious reports should be expedited to EudraVigilance. Note that this is different from the criteria used for clinical trial reporting, which, in most countries, requires three criteria (serious, unexpected, possibly related to the drug).

Post-marketing reporting only requires two (serious, unexpected) because it is believed that spontaneous reports have "implied" causality or suspicion. The reporter would not have contacted the health agency or the company to report the case if he or she did not believe there was some level of causal relationship between the drug and the AE. As noted above, for reporting to EudraVigilance, the single database in the EU, all serious cases are reported regardless of labeledness because nationally-approved SmPCs may list different suspected reactions.

The company must promptly investigate all SAEs that produce 15-day alert reports and must submit follow-up reports within 15 calendar days of receipt of new information or as requested by the health agency. The number of follow-up reports is not limited. Any new additional information must be recorded and analyzed and then reported to Health Authorities (mainly medically-relevant new information). If additional information is not obtainable, records of the attempts taken to seek additional information should be maintained.

The company selling or making the drug is not the only one obliged to report AEs. This requirement also applies to any person or entity whose name appears on the label of an approved drug product as a manufacturer, packer, or distributor. By extension, this applies also to any agent, business partner, co-marketer, and distributor etc. That is, anyone or any company or entity that may receive an AE and with which the company has a relationship must track and report AEs, usually to the other company but sometimes to the health authority.

Solicited safety information from customer engagement programs, i.e., programs where collection of safety information is not the primary objective, but there is the possibility of two-way communication and, thus, capture of information relevant to safety, should be treated as if it were a post-marketing study. Examples of such programs are patient out-reach programs or disease management or patient support programs, etc. The four case validity criteria must be applied and the three clinical trial reporting criteria must also be applied. That is, the criteria are not those of the post-marketing situation (serious, unexpected), but of the clinical trial situation. However, there are no 7-day reports or reports categorized as "SUSARs" in the post-marketing setting, even though the three clinical trial reporting criteria are applied.

■ Sources of AEs

Post-marketing AEs may come from many sources: sales representatives; the regulatory, quality, compliance, or telephone operator departments and other company employees (such as the chief executive officer's secretary/administrative assistant or human resources); lawyers and lawsuits; individual patients, consumers, family/caregivers, or patient advocacy groups; pharmacists; nurses; physicians, nurses, or other healthcare professionals; health agencies; company subsidiaries; associated business partners or contractors (not part of the company); websites; e-mail; social media; newspapers; the medical literature; poison control centers, late night TV, and radio. Company employees may learn of AEs in informal social settings. The company must set up the appropriate internal procedures (standard operating procedures) to ensure that AEs arriving anywhere in the company reach the drug safety group in a timely manner (usually no more than one or two working days).

Unlike clinical trial reports, where the reporters are usually clinical investigators or their staff who have been trained by the sponsor, many post-marketing reports arrive by telephone from unhappy patients or harried medical professionals. The company needs to establish a careful triage process to identify those contacts that are product-related and ensure they are sent to a medical professional within the company quickly after the operator answers, so that AEs and other product issues are not missed. It is not wise to bounce the call to multiple departments until the right one is found. Voice response systems may fail to elicit the problem ("Press one to get your money back. Press two to reach the medical affairs department. Press three to report an AE ....").

A rather special skill set on the part of the company staff (whether medical professionals or not) who receive these calls is required. The caller, especially a patient, usually wants something quickly (often money or replacement drug) and may be angry and hostile. The call center responder must be cool and calm and obtain the needed medical and demographic information while maintaining empathy and sympathy. Often the caller has contacted the company with a question ("Can drug X cause heart attacks?"), not realizing that the company will explore to see whether there is an AE there. Thus, the call is transformed from a request for information to supplying information that may anger the caller. Sometimes the call is not the first, which often creates unnecessary angst on the part of the reporter. The call center responder should write down (on paper or directly into a database) the caller's information, using direct quotes where possible without admitting that the drug necessarily caused any AEs or produced problems. When the call is from a consumer, an attempt should always be made to obtain the contact information of the patient's physician or other contactable healthcare provider to "medically validate" the report. If follow-up is needed with the caller (e.g., after obtaining medical records), another contact should be arranged.

Literature and Publications

Formal and frequent searches of the published literature using a computerized system (commercial services) that searches large numbers of publications and databases for publications on the company's products (both by trade name and generic name) is required. If the search reveals a citation, article, or abstract that contains a case report or clinical trial with information that meets the four validity criteria and alert criteria, a 15-day post-marketing report must be sent to relevant health agencies, along with a copy of the article (in English usually, in most countries.) This is handled like any other 15-day report, with follow-up sought. If an article describes multiple cases, then a separate report should be filed for each one (for the US, see 21CFR314.80(d)(1,2)). Note that such literature searches are required *weekly* for drugs marketed in the EU and are included in PSURs. The EU requirements for reporting literature are very specific in terms of style ("the Vancouver Style"). Member states may request translation of the article into their national language, though English may be used in an ICSR submitted as an expedited report.

A Medical Literature Monitoring (MLM) service has been set up at the EMA: Case reports are recorded within EudraVigilance by the Agency (see Regulation (EC) No. 726/2004). The list of active substances and literature being monitored are periodically updated and published on the EMA website. MAHs are required to monitor the MLM-identified cases but should not re-report cases to EudraVigilance that have already been identified by the MLM service.

The issue of translation arises periodically. If a publication title suggests that the article contains reportable safety information and if the article and the abstract are in a language that no one on staff is able to read (or even minimally decipher), then the article should be translated to determine whether there is a valid case. This may be very costly for certain languages. Fortunately, most cases are published in English or one of the other major medical languages. There are free Internet tools that will do rough (usually very rough) computer translations of text that may give an idea of whether the article contains safety information and a possibly reportable case. It is unlikely that an agency would consider this translation sufficient. Use of such a service could avoid delays and costs, but at the expense of a possibly faulty translation. Check with the local health agency.

The regulatory reporting clock starts when the four elements of a valid case are identifiable. This may mean the clock starts only when the translation is received if the abstract did not supply the four elements. Companies are expected to search local journals not tracked in the major computer literature databases (e.g., Embase, PubMed), if the company sells in that language market. There are now several companies that offer this service to NDA and MA holders.

For multinational companies with offices around the world, responsibility for journal searches should be addressed early on and up front to avoid duplication of efforts. The international offices are usually useful for obtaining follow-up from faraway reporters and non-English-speakers. However, it is usually not productive to have each international office search its country's journals for AEs unless they are not tracked in the major computerized literature database. This is best done through the central database search.

Other Sources of Reports

Periodically, certain large organizations (such as poison control centers and teratology centers) publish summary or review articles detailing dozens to thousands of reports of AEs with associated drug names. Often there is insufficient information to create individual cases, but occasionally there is a minimal dataset (patient identifier, poison control center as reporter, a suspect drug, and an AE). This may pose a problem in regard to reporting. Usually, follow-up is impossible or impractical. In such cases, it is worth communicating with the health authority(ies) on the best way to proceed. No agency wants to receive 5,000 ICSRs, each with minimal data, any more than the company wants to generate them. A summary letter or a single report covering multiple patients may be acceptable.

Follow-Up

Follow-up on all SAEs should be done to obtain "significant" information, i.e., information that supports further scientific evaluation of the case. There are no absolute rules on what is sufficient in terms of due diligence, but a common rule of thumb in the industry is two or three follow-up requests (registered letters, voice mail messages, or contacts with physician's staff, emails with acknowledgement of receipt and reading, etc.) for "routine" SAEs are sufficient. New, dramatic, unexpected, fatal, or life-threatening SAEs may require many more attempts to obtain adequate data to make sense of the case (the true goal of all these efforts). This means information that provides new medical insight (or even administrative information) that could impact the assessment or management of a case or could change its seriousness criteria. Follow-up information that is considered "non-significant" includes items such as updated comments from the case assessor or corrections of typographical errors. Many in the industry have "war stories" of flying to far-off sites or doing various maneuvers to try to obtain follow-up information on critical cases. All follow-up attempts should be documented.

Follow-up on non-serious expected cases is often not done or expected by regulatory agencies, especially if the AE is already in the labeling. Follow-up on non-serious unexpected cases is, however, generally a good idea and is obligatory in some countries. Efforts are usually limited to one or two follow-up letters, e-mails, or calls.

Notes on United States Requirements for Post-marketing NDA Reporting of SAEs

The US regulations are found in 21CFR314.80 and basically state that the NDA holder has an obligation to promptly review all adverse drug experience information received from any source, "foreign or domestic including information derived from commercial marketing experience, post-marketing clinical investigations, post-marketing epidemiological/surveillance studies, reports in the scientific literature, and unpublished scientific papers" (21CFR314.80(b)). Companies do not have to resubmit to the FDA reports received from the FDA.

There are multiple, scattered guidances, draft guidances, and other documents that cover reporting requirements. They are, unfortunately, incomplete, vague, and in many cases non-specific. The FDA has various pages available on its website with instructions for industry, including the following:

- Post-market Drug Safety Information for Patients and Providers (Regulations and Policies and Procedures for Post-marketing Surveillance Programs;
- Guidances (Drugs);
- Guidance, Compliance & Regulatory Information (Biologics);
- Potential Signals of Serious Risks/New Safety Information Identified from the Adverse Event Reporting System (FAERS);
- MedWatch;
- Questions & Answers on Adverse Event Reporting System (FAERS);
- OTC Related Federal Register Notices, Ingredient References, and other Regulatory Information;

- For small molecules, if it is a foreign-originated report with the same active ingredient (active moiety), then the case should be entered into the database and reported, if the reporting criteria are met:
  - The FDA's 2001 post-marketing AE draft guidance states the following for foreign literature: "Reports of serious, unexpected adverse experiences described in the scientific literature should be submitted for products that have the same active moiety as a product marketed in the United States. This is true even if the excipient, dosage forms, strengths, routes of administration, and indications vary."
  - In regard to the definition of an active moiety, "An active moiety means the molecule or ion, excluding those appended portions of the molecule that cause the drug to be an ester, salt (including a salt with hydrogen or coordination bonds), or other non-covalent derivative (such as a complex, chelate, or clathrate) of the molecule, responsible for the physiological or pharmacological action of the drug substance." From the FDA's "Frequently Asked Questions for New Drug Product Exclusivity". If a company holds more than one NDA for the same chemical entity, the 15-day report should be addressed to the oldest (original) approved NDA if the actual product or formulation is not known or specified.
  - If a company has more than one of its products listed in the report, the case should be sent to the NDA for the first listed product on the report, which is usually the "more" or "most" suspect drug.

The URLs for these documents seem to change frequently at FDA and the best way to find them is to do a search on the FDA website.

MedWatch to Manufacturer Program

The FDA established the MedWatch to Manufacturer Program, in which serious spontaneous AEs reported directly to the FDA are sent by FDA to the manufacturer. Participation must be requested, i.e., eligible applicants (MAHs) must send an enrollment request letter to FDA for each eligible new product. Products are eligible for inclusion for a period that will range from three to 4 years and no reports received by FDA prior to enrollment approval will be sent. Reports will be sent for the balance of the year of program approval plus the next three full calendar years. Products are deleted once a year, at the end of December. The reports contain the reporter's name and address, permitting the manufacturer to do follow-up. The reporter must consent to this. The original report received from the FDA should not be re-sent to the FDA (see 21CFR3.14.80(b)), but any follow-up information should be. Other reports may be received from the FDA under the Drug Quality Reporting System that the FDA established for reporting and receiving quality issues on products analogous to the MedWatch Program.

Reports from the FDA via the Freedom of Information Act

This is a system that allows anyone to obtain information from the US government that is not classified or proprietary (commercial secrets). For a nominal fee, it is possible to obtain from the FDA case reports for any drug (one's own or competitors'). It is a one- or two-step process (however, see below). The initial request produces a standardized printout or CD/DVD with a line listing of AEs. Any specific case may be obtained by then requesting it using its identification number (accession number). The cases received are anonymous in regard to the patient and reporter, thus preventing follow-up. Unfortunately, some follow-up reports are not tied or referenced to the initial reports. If one goes through Freedom of Information (FOI) for information, the request itself is public information and can be found out (by a company's competitors, for example). Thus, there are commercial ventures that perform the search for a company and make the search anonymous.

Note that the FDA has put the cases in FAERS online. The basic information in the case (excluding the narrative though) is now available immediately online using the moderately friendly search engine provided by FDA. Importantly, the FDA case number is given, and this may be used to obtain further information by FOI. This should expedite the process somewhat.

There are reasons both for and against obtaining cases on one's own drugs from FDA:

1. **Pros**
   - The company will know what the FDA knows and will have as complete a dataset as possible. There should be no "surprises", such as communications from FDA about safety matters the company does not know about.
   - The company will be better able to look for signals and perform signal analysis (including data mining) with a complete database.
2. **Cons**
   - No follow-up is possible on a case. What you have is what you have.
   - It may not always be possible to determine whether a case is a duplicate (e.g., it was reported to the FDA in addition to the company, perhaps by a different reporter). As the reporter and patient identifiers are removed, it may be hard to ascertain whether the case is a duplicate.
   - Coding and case handling (e.g., narrative style and content) may be different. At this point, a decision on whether to recode must be made.

Most people nowadays feel that it is wise and ethically appropriate to obtain the FDA reports and any other safety reports available from other health agencies (e.g., drug analysis profiles (iDAPs) from the United Kingdom MHRA or periodic searches online of Health Canada's safety database). The large majority of cases in the FDA database come through the company, so, in theory, there should be few cases received directly by FDA. Some companies obtain competitor safety information in this way. Such data, however, are not permitted to be used in marketing or sales.

Similar FOI systems exist already or are being developed in other countries. Again, issues arise such as duplication, consistency, language, and follow-up when obtaining case reports. Many multinational companies have their local offices obtain these cases where possible. The Uppsala Monitoring Centre in Sweden maintains the largest worldwide safety database, with cases obtained from national health agencies. However, the data are usually only line listings and may be difficult to use to identify new or important cases.

Instructions on Filling Out the MedWatch Form

There are very detailed instructions on the FDA's MedWatch website on how to fill out the MedWatch form (3500A form for manufacturers), and for healthcare professionals (3500 form for all others). Note however, that manufacturers must now submit electronically using E2B rather than MedWatch forms. Companies should review the instructions and put them into place. For electronic submission (E2B) of ICSRs with and without attachments, detailed information is available on FDA website.

European Union Regulations

The European Union regulations and requirements for medicinal products (defined broadly to include drugs, biologics, herbals, etc.) can be found in many documents (Regulation, Directive, Guidances, etc.): the most accurate for this Chapter's purpose are the Directive 2010/84/EU and the GVP Module VI: "Collection, management and submission of reports of suspected adverse reactions to medicinal products (Rev 2)". Other documents would repeat the same information. The sections of the GVP Module VI include:

- Collection of individual safety reports
  - Unsolicited reports
    - Spontaneous reports
    - Literature reports
    - Reports from non-medical sources
    - Information on suspected adverse reactions from the internet or digital media
  - Solicited reports
- Validation of reports

- Follow-up of reports
- Data management
- Quality management
- Special situations
  - Use of a medicinal product during pregnancy or breastfeeding
  - Use of a medicinal product in a pediatric or elderly population
  - Reports of overdose, abuse, misuse, medication error or occupational exposure
  - Lack of therapeutic efficacy
- Submission of individual case safety reports (ICSRs)
  - Submission time frames of ICSRs
  - Report nullification
  - Report amendment
- Modalities for submission of individual case safety reports (ICSRs).

Comments

EU requirements are based on ICH Guidelines. Several points should be highlighted as follows:

- As for many countries, the 15-day report rules apply in the EU for serious ICSRs, i.e.,
  - Expected & unexpected;
  - Related & not related;
  - EU & non-EU;
  - Initial & follow-up;
- Non-serious ICSRs are to be reported within 90 calendar days (initial & follow-up);
- All ICSRs are to be reported to the EMA in Eudra-Vigilance (electronic transfer or direct data entry);
- The clock for ICSR submission starts as soon as the information containing the minimum criteria has been brought to the attention of the MAH (any MAH member or agent or contractor); this date is day 0;
- Requests can be submitted to the EMA to get outputs from the EudraVigilance database.

General Comments

Thanks to the CIOMS and ICH Working Groups, there are high level documents for reporting post-marketing ICSRs. These are not laws or regulations however and some countries either deviate or have their own additional requirements. This can generate confusion and/or difficulties for compliance.

Frequently Asked Questions

Q: This is rather messy, it seems. Would this not be an ideal situation for full harmonization, since the rules are fairly similar already?

A: Yes, indeed. However, the devil is always in the details. It is possible we will get there as data standards for format, contents, and transmission develop. Of course, there will likely be multiple standards and languages, and then we will have to standardize the standards. The issue of language will not be resolved until adequate computer translation abilities are developed. The logical (albeit utopian) outcome of all of this is the reporting of each AE in the reporter's native language to a single global repository from which anyone can obtain complete information and seamlessly go from one language to any other. Perhaps this will go even one step further if electronic medical records become a practical reality. In this setting, it would be possible to "pull" the AEs and the complete medical records from this mega-database (or linked databases/warehouses) without requiring active submission by reporters. If the early promises of artificial intelligence (AI) turn out to be feasible, it is quite possible that many steps in this process can be standardized and harmonized.

Q: Working in a corporate PV department, how can we deal with various local requirements and ensure we are compliant in all countries where our products are registered?

A: This question raises the difficulties corporate PV department face as regards compliance.

1. The first point is to ensure you have a clear and exhaustive view on the PV requirements in all countries where your products are registered.
2. Second, the corporate PV Policy must comply with the most strict/demanding PV requirement for each topic (SAE reporting, non-SAE reporting, timeframes, etc.).

3. Third, this Policy must be shared with all local PV departments to ensure everyone realizes their duty is not only to be locally compliant. They actually must follow the internal corporate rules in order to allow other countries to be compliant.
4. Fourth, a periodic check/audit of the local adherence to the PV Policy should be conducted as part of the quality management system and appropriate measures must be put in place in case of deviations.

CHAPTER

22

Post-marketing Aggregate Safety Reporting

Most countries now accept and usually require the submission of Periodic Safety Update Reports (PSURs) for post-marketing aggregate safety reporting. The US Food and Drug Administration (FDA) accepts PSURs (requiring a waiver though). The older format, the NDA Periodic Report), also called the Periodic Adverse Drug Experience Report (PADER), are still required according to the regulations (unless there is the PSUR waiver), though FDA will still require the Appendices specified in the PADER rule and guidance. The EMA requires the Periodic Benefit Risk Evaluation Report (PBRER) format (even if still using the acronym PSUR for historical reasons).

Introduction

In addition to the 15-day alert reports, FDA requires the submission of New Drug Application (NDA), Abbreviated NDA, and Biologic License Application (BLA) periodic reports. The regulations covering this are found in 21CFR§314.80(c)(2)(I, II). FDA also requires a US Orphan Drug Designation (ODD) Annual Report for products FDA classifies as orphan drugs. We are seeing global efforts to harmonize the expectations between regions regarding the reporting requirements in the post-market setting, so it is likely that this area will continue to evolve over the next decade. Until then, make certain you and your company are kept apprised of the most recent thinking from the agencies regarding this topic, so you aren't in a position of non-compliance.

NDA Periodic Reports

As with Investigational New Drug application (IND) regulations, there are updates scattered in various other FDA documents. Some are arguably specific to pre-marketing settings (e.g., drug-induced liver injury), but should be kept in mind with post-marketing aggregate reporting, too. The list of the relevant FDA documents are as follows:

- Post-marketing Reporting of Adverse Drug Experiences (March 1992);
- Guideline for Adverse Experience Reporting for Licensed Biological Products (October 1993);
- Post-marketing Adverse Experience Reporting for Human Drug and Licensed Biological Products: Clarification of What to Report (August 27, 1997);
- Post-marketing Safety Reporting for Human Drugs and Biological Products Including Vaccines (March 2001);
- Conducting a Clinical Safety Review of a New Product Application and Preparing a Report on the Review (February 2005);
- Drug-Induced Liver Injury: Pre-marketing Clinical Evaluation (July 2009);
- Drug Safety Information — FDA's Communication to the Public (March 2007);
- Format and Content of Proposed Risk Evaluation and Mitigation Strategies (REMS), REMS Assessments, and Proposed REMS Modifications (March 2009);
- Post-marketing Studies and Clinical Trials — Implementation of Section 505(o) of the Federal Food, Drug, and Cosmetic Act (July 2009);
- Providing Post-marketing Periodic Safety Reports in the ICH E2C(R2) Format (Periodic Benefit–Risk Evaluation Report) Guidance for Industry (November 2016); and
- FDA Compliance Program Guidance Manual (for FDA staff). Program 7353.001. Chapter 53 — Post-marketing Surveillance and Epidemiology: Human Drug and Therapeutic Biological Products (December 2015).

See FDA's guidance pages (http://www.fda.gov/Drugs/GuidanceComplianceRegulatoryInformation/Guidances/default.htm). The basic regulations state the following (21CFR§314.80(c)(2)(I,II)):

All "adverse drug experiences" (the FDA term "adverse experience" is synonymous with "adverse event") not submitted as 15-day alert reports must be submitted in the periodic report. A periodic report for each NDA must be submitted quarterly (every 3 months) for the first 3 years after the approval of the NDA. After the 3-year period is over, the reporting frequency is then yearly unless the FDA requests otherwise.

Each report must be submitted 30 days after the close of the quarter for quarterly reports and 60 days after the close of the anniversary date for yearly reports. Thus, the company has 30 or 60 days to prepare the report. The FDA may alter this schedule if they wish to continue quarterly reporting after the 3-year period is over. A supplement or line extension may be a reason for FDA to request more frequent periodic reports after the first 3 years, i.e., a return to quarterly reporting upon approval of a major efficacy supplement.

Each periodic report is required to contain the following:

- A narrative summary and analysis of the information in the report and an analysis of the 15-day alert reports submitted during the reporting interval (all 15-day alert reports must appropriately reference the applicant's patient identification number, adverse reaction term(s), and date of submission to the FDA);
- Separate submission of an electronic ICSR (E2B for drugs and biologics) is required for each adverse drug experience not reported as a 15-day expedited report (with an index consisting of a line listing of the applicant's patient identification number and adverse reaction term(s));
- A history of actions taken since the last report because of adverse drug experiences (e.g., labeling changes or studies initiated because of safety concerns);
- Periodic reporting, except for information regarding 15-day alert reports, does not apply to adverse drug experience information obtained from post-marketing studies (whether or not they were conducted under an Investigational New Drug Application),

from reports in the scientific literature, or from foreign marketing experience;

- Follow-up information to adverse drug experiences submitted in a periodic report may be submitted in the next periodic report.

In August 1997, the FDA published a guidance encouraging NDA holders to submit requests to waive the requirements to submit MedWatch forms for non-serious labeled AEs. Since the requirement for electronic case reporting became effective in 2015, FDA has disallowed these waivers.

The March 2001 Guidance explains the requirements for a periodic report and is officially in effect even though it remains a draft a decade after being published. It is summarized below in the following section.

PSURs to the FDA

The March 2001 Guidance describes the mechanism to obtain a waiver to submit PSURs using the ICH E2C requirements instead of NDA Periodic Reports:

- If all dosage forms and formulations for the active substance, as well as indications, are combined in one PSUR, this information should be separated into specific sections of the report when such separation is appropriate to portray accurately the safety profile of the specific dosage forms. For example, one should not combine information from ophthalmic drop dosage forms and solid oral dosage forms.
- Relevant ICSRs required by the regulations must be sent electronically to FAERS, FDA's primary post-marketing safety database.
- A summary tabulation should be included as an appendix listing all spontaneously reported US ICSRs from consumers if such cases are not already included in the PSUR. Summary tabulations should be presented by MedDRA® SOC of all adverse experience terms and counts of occurrences and should be segregated by type (i.e., serious/unexpected; serious/expected; non-serious/unexpected; and non-serious/expected).
- A narrative should be included as an appendix that references the changes, if any, to the approved US labeling for the dosage forms covered by the PSUR based on new information in the PSUR. A copy of the most recently approved US labeling for the product(s) covered by the PSUR should be included.
- Submission Date and Frequency for PSURs. Applicants can request a waiver to submit PSURs to the FDA based on the month and day of the international birth date of the product instead of the month and day of the anniversary date of US approval of the product. The waiver request should specify that these PSURs would be submitted to the FDA within 60 calendar days of the data lock point (i.e., month and day of the international birth date of the product or any other day agreed on by the applicant and the FDA). Applicants can also request a waiver to submit PSURs to the FDA at a frequency other than those required by regulation. However, there should be no gaps in the timeframe covered.

Note that the FDA, the EU, and other jurisdictions have mechanisms in place to harmonize submission dates. However, if the PRAC specifies a time interval for a product in the EEA with a well-established (and well-behaved) safety profile, it may be challenging to harmonize submission dates for periodic reports. An international birth date (usually the first approval anywhere in the world) can be established with the health agencies, allowing the company to prepare and submit all reports based on this date. Harmonization of periodicity is not always possible using addenda reports to get all the PSURs into synchronization. Thus, reports may need to go into some agencies every 6 months, yearly, 3 yearly, etc., but at least they are all prepared on the same anniversary date each year (e.g., if February 1st is established as the international birth date, then reports would go in with a data lock point of February 1st for yearly or multi-year reports and February 1st and August 1st for 6-month reports).

Post-marketing Periodic Reports

The information contained within a classic NDA Periodic Report (PADER) should be divided into four sections in the following order and each section should be clearly separated by an identifying tab. If information for one of these sections is not included, the applicant should explain why the information is not provided.

Note that if a company prefers to submit PSURs rather than PADERs, it must get a waiver to do this and must add sections to the PSUR that cover all the requirements that are in the regulations for PADERs but not in the PSUR contents. See the PSUR section.

Section 1: Narrative Summary and Analysis

A narrative summary and analysis of the information in the post-marketing periodic report and an analysis of the 15-day reports (i.e., serious, unexpected, adverse experiences) submitted during the reporting period must be provided and should include the following:

1. The number of non-15-day initial adverse experience reports and the number of non-15-day follow-up reports contained in this periodic report and the time period covered by the periodic report (no gaps in time are permitted);
2. A line listing of the 15-day reports submitted during the reporting period. This line listing should include the manufacturer report number, adverse experience term(s), and the date the 15-day report was sent to the FDA;
3. A summary tabulation by the 27 MedDRA SOCs (e.g., Blood and lymphatic system disorders, Cardiac disorders, Congenital, familial and genetic disorders, etc.) of all adverse experience terms and counts of occurrences submitted during the reporting period. The information should be taken from:
   - 15-day reports submitted to the FDA;
   - Non-15-day reports submitted in the periodic report;
   - Reports forwarded to the applicant by the FDA; and
   - Formerly, any non-serious, expected, adverse experiences not submitted to the FDA but maintained on file by the applicant (all valid reports must be submitted).

   For the adverse experience term *product interaction*, the interacting products should be identified in the tabulation.

- A summary listing of the adverse experience reports in which the drug or biologic product was listed as one of the suspect products, but the report was filed to another NDA, Abbreviated NDA, or BLA held by the applicant;
- A narrative discussion of the clinical significance of the 15-day reports submitted during the reporting period and of any increased reporting frequency of serious, expected, adverse experiences when, in the judgment of the applicant, it is believed the data reflect a clinically meaningful change in adverse experience occurrence. This narrative should assess clinical significance by type of adverse experience, MedDRA SOC, and overall product safety, relating the new information received during this reporting period to what was already known about the product. The narrative should also state what further actions, if any, the applicant plans to undertake based on the information gained during the reporting period and include the time period for completing the actions (i.e., when the applicant plans to start and finish the action and submit the information to the agency).
- The narrative discussion should indicate, based on the information learned during the reporting period, whether the applicant believes either that (1) no change in the product's current approved labeling is warranted or (2) there are safety-related issues that need to be addressed in the approved product labeling. If the FDA is considering changes in the approved product labeling, the applicant should state in the narrative the date and number of the supplemental application submitted to address the labeling changes.

Section 2: Narrative Discussion of Actions Taken

A narrative discussion of actions taken must be provided, including any labeling changes and studies initiated since the last periodic report. This section should include:

- A copy of current US product labeling;
- A list of any labeling changes made during the reporting period;
- A list of studies initiated;
- A summary of important foreign regulatory actions (e.g., new warnings, limitations in the indications, and use of the product); and
- Any communication of new safety information (e.g., a Dear Doctor letter).

Section 3: Index Line Listing

An index line listing of ICSRs included in Section 4 of the periodic report must be provided. The line listing for each ICSR submitted should include:

- Manufacturer report number;
- Adverse experience term(s); and
- Identification of interacting products for any product interaction listed as an adverse experience.

Section 4: ICSRs

ICSRs must be provided electronically for the following spontaneously reported adverse experiences that occurred in the US during the reporting period:

- Serious and expected:
- Non-serious and unexpected; and
- Non-serious and expected.

Applicants are no longer encouraged to request a waiver of the requirement to submit ICSRs for non-serious, expected, adverse experiences for drugs and certain biologic products. Adverse experiences due to a failure to produce the expected pharmacologic action (i.e., lack of effect) should also be included in this section.

For ICSRs for serious, expected, adverse experiences, the FDA encourages applicants to include relevant hospital discharge summaries and autopsy reports (or death certificates), as well as lists of other relevant documents that support 15-day reports of serious, unexpected, adverse experiences.

Initial non-15-day reports should be listed in the periodic report in a separate section from non-15-day follow-up reports. All initial and follow-up information obtained for an adverse experience within a given periodic reporting period should be combined and submitted in the periodic report as one initial non-15-day report (i.e., an initial non-15-day report and a non-15-day follow-up report describing the same adverse experience should not be submitted in the same periodic report). Serious, unexpected, adverse experiences should not be included in a periodic report because these should have been previously submitted to the FDA as 15-day reports in E2B format.

If no adverse experiences were identified for the human drug or biologic product for the time period involved and no regulatory actions concerning safety were taken anywhere in the world where the product is marketed, the periodic report should simply state this and be submitted to the FDA along with a copy of the current US labeling. The FDA has encouraged the use of PSURs in place of periodic reports (PADERs).

Other Reports

The FDA requires other reports for "NDA maintenance" as follows:

1. Distribution reports (21CFR600.810): This is a 6-month report requiring the submission of all information about the quantity of product distributed under licensing agreements. It does not touch drug safety.
2. Annual reports (21CFR314.81(b)(2)): This is a yearly report requiring the submission of information from the previous year that might affect safety, efficacy, or labeling as well as information on labeling changes, distribution, chemistry, manufacturing and controls changes, non-clinical laboratory studies, clinical trial data, and pediatric data.

■ Periodic Safety Update Reports

The PSUR is now the basic post-marketing aggregate report submitted around the world. As noted, it was "created" as the ICH E2C guideline and an addendum and the entire document was revised as ICH E2C(R2), the Periodic Benefit–Risk Evaluation Report (PBRER). In the EU, Good Pharmacovigilance Practice (GVP) module VII covers PSURs in about 70 pages. Even though the document is referred to as the PSUR, GVP module VII references the ICH PBRER as the required format (see below). Those who prepare PSURs should refer to both the ICH and GVP documents, as well as any local requirements in other countries.

The PSUR (like the NDA Periodic Report) is the major document for aggregate safety analyses by the authorities. Lateness, poor quality, incompleteness, and errors will be noted and will precipitate inspections and punishment ranging from chastisement to more severe sanctions. In the EU, the EU Qualified Person for Pharmacovigilance has personal responsibility and liability for the report and its contents.

The PSUR serves multiple purposes, including the maintenance and requirements for the authorization, product use, the benefit–risk analyses, the (MAH's views on the product, and the safety issues for the reporting period and, for the whole history of the drug. In contrast to the earlier PSUR requirements, the PSUR in PBRER format contains both interval data and cumulative data. The PSUR is used for signal communication but should not be the sole mechanism used for signaling.

The periodicity of the PSUR/PBRER in the EU and certain other countries is not at fixed intervals; the PRAC determines and publishes the periodicity of PSURs for each product on a "risk proportionate" basis. Note that the periodicity of the PADER in the US is fixed, so that needs to be considered when requesting a waiver to submit PSURs to FDA in lieu of PADERs. In some situations, the authorities may request that the schedule be modified or an *ad hoc* report can be requested at any time. Most countries allow harmonization with the first approval anywhere (International Birth Date, or IBD), and the report in E2C(R1) format is due no later than 60 days after the end of the reporting period. For the E2C(R2)/PBRER format, which has an expanded scope compared with the E2C(R1) format, the ordinary time interval between data lock point and submission varies. In general, a PSUR/PBRER that covers 6 or 12 months must be submitted within 70 calendar days of the data lock. PSURS/PBRERs that cover more than 1 year or *ad hoc* PBRERs must be submitted within 90 calendar days. Some regulators have devised other schedules, so consultation with the MAH with the authority may be needed.

For drugs with significant sales or complicated patient populations, the document can be very large and time-consuming to prepare. It is usually a multidisciplinary effort (Drug Safety, Regulatory, Clinical, Epidemiology, Signaling, Quality, etc.). A written Standard Operating Procedure (SOP) or guideline or manual should exist on PSUR preparation. The previous PSURs and regulatory responses to them for the product should always be consulted before preparing the current PSUR as there are commitments, requests, special analyses, and so forth, that may be required on a continuing basis and should not be discontinued until the commitment is completed or the health agencies agree. The appropriate labeling should be used. It is usually the Company Core Safety Information (CCSI), but it may be the Summary of Product Characteristics (SmPC) if no CCSI exists.

The contents, in brief, include the following:

1. Executive Summary: Brief overview of the key information;
2. Introduction with product characteristics, period covered, and PSUR number (e.g., third);
3. Marketing authorizations in a table with countries and dates, including disapprovals and withdrawals;
4. Update on health agency actions taken for safety reasons;
5. Patient exposure;
6. Presentation of Individual Case Histories (by MedDRA SOC);
   - Brief description of criteria used for cases shown;

- Description and analysis of selected cases:
    - Including fatal cases;
    - New and relevant safety information;
- Line listing of ICSRs (submitted as E2B files);
- Serious suspected ADRs and non-serious unlisted ADRs from spontaneous sources;
- Serious ADRs available from post-approval commitments and studies and named patient and compassionate use;
- Serious ADRs from regulatory authorities;
- Serious ADRs and non-serious unlisted ADRs from the medical literature;
- Other listings as specially required (e.g., consumer reports not validated);
- Studies and Trials:
    - Studies completed during the PSUR reporting period that provide relevant safety information, including epidemiology studies;
- Other important information;
- Any information provided after the data lock point for the PSUR;
- Risk management plans and changes to them;

7. Overall Safety Evaluation:
    - Key new information on serious and non-serious ADRs;
    - Drug interactions, overdose, pregnancy exposures (with outcomes), etc.;
    - Epidemiology, signal and trends, white papers, class effects, etc.
8. Conclusion:
    - Overall risk–benefit analysis;
    - Differences with the current reference labeling document (CCSI or SmPC);
    - Actions to be taken or initiated;
    - Changes to reference labeling documents;
9. Risk Management activities, particularly when non-routine interventions are required to ensure benefits outweigh a product's risks; and
10. Appendices.

Note that individual countries may require additional information and reports or summaries in the local language. The US requires certain additional sections (see below). Some countries may require additional sections in the local language.

PSUR in ICH E2C(R2) Format: The Periodic Benefit–Risk Evaluation Report

The November 2016 FDA guidance describes how applicants can use an alternative reporting format, the ICH E2C(R2) Periodic Benefit–Risk Evaluation Report (PBRER), in place of the PADER, PAER, or ICH E2C(R1) Periodic Safety Update Report (PSUR), to satisfy the periodic post-marketing safety reporting requirements in §314.80(c)(2) and 600.80(c)(2) (21CFR314.80(c)(2) and 600.80(c)(2)). This guidance also describes the procedures applicants should follow if they wish to submit a PBRER in place of a PADER, PAER, or PSUR. The process is different, depending on whether or not the applicant has an approved waiver already in place to substitute the E2C(R1) PSUR for the PADER/PAER. Further, from an operational viewpoint, the timing of US submissions to FDA are the same as the PADER, not the EU schedule. The EMA requires the PBRER format (see Good Vigilance Practice Module VII).

The main changes versus the "classical" PSUR are intended to achieve the following:

- Put the safety data in perspective with efficacy and therefore to re-assess the benefit–risk balance: it is therefore required to include new available efficacy data and to reassess the benefit–risk balance for authorized indications, considering the new/ongoing identified safety signals;
- Be less descriptive on ICSRs but to provide the agencies with analyzed safety data;
- Provide the PBRER assessor with an updated information on:
    - New, ongoing and closed safety signals during the reference period;
    - Risk management and minimization effectiveness.

Note: With such an updated requirement, the regulator considers the PSUR/PBRER and the RMP as complementary tools for a better safety signal and risk management strategy.

■ Frequently Asked Question

Q: So, should we start to do PSURs/PBRERs for the FDA now?

A: Yes that would be a good idea. FDA reviewers prefer the more analytical PSUR/PBRER document. If the company is already preparing PSURs/PBRERs for other health authorities, the move to US PSURs/PBRERs should be relatively doable, even though US-specific appendices are required, and the periodicity may not be aligned. If the company has no experience in doing PSURs/PBRERs at all, now would be a good time to start.

One thing to keep in mind though is that by submitting a PBRER the company is voluntarily giving more information to the FDA (i.e., efficacy, signaling) than is required by regulations. Nothing wrong with this, of course, but it is more than required. Nevertheless, it is considered good practice to inform all regulators of the same thing at the same time, so, if the PBRER is being given to other regulators it makes sense to provide it to FDA. This was a concept in the Report of the CIOMS Working Group II (1992); it was reiterated in the CIOMS V Report (2001). And it might help protect patient safety.

CHAPTER

23

The Mathematics of Adverse Events

This chapter is not intended to be a reference on statistics, epidemiology, or the technical aspects of mathematical data analysis. Rather, it is meant to give a brief and selective overview of some of the "numbers" and quantitative methods used in pharmacovigilance and to show what can be learned from them as well as limitations in the data and the methodologies. This discussion is separate from safety data quality, i.e., "wooliness" of spontaneous reporting information that can confound interpretation of the data.

Introduction

Why is mathematics important or relevant to Pharmacovigilance? During the process of pharmacovigilance, there are some questions that we often ask ourselves that cannot be answered without doing some computations.

- How often will a particular event happen?
- What is the likelihood that this event will reoccur?
- Was this event due to the product?
- Is this event clinically important (i.e. if it occurs how will it impact the life of the patient)?
- Are there identifiable subgroups of individuals who may be at greater risk than others?

A company's safety database consists of serious adverse event cases from clinical trials as well as adverse event cases voluntarily or spontaneously reported to the company by a variety of reporters including healthcare professionals, pharmacists, consumers, and lawyers, among others. The company is required by global regulators to review the safety database to look for new and important safety issues that were not observed in the preapproval time period. Issues important to both the regulators and the manufacturer include whether the signal is a true risk, or is the result of some other factor, how frequently does the event occur, how serious was the event, and whether there are identifiable subgroups who may be at greater risk. Because of the limitations of the spontaneously reported AE data, causality cannot generally be determined. Instead, potential signals identified usually need to be evaluated through other means such as pharmacoepidemiology. See the signaling chapter in this Manual.

In the following example, suppose that one or two spontaneous reports of liver injury with drug X are received at the company safety department or the health authority shortly after the introduction of the drug to the market. A number of factors need to be considered when determining whether the liver cases reflect a true risk of the drug. Considerations include whether there is a reasonable possibility of causality between the liver issue and the suspect drug in those reports; what other compounds, both prescription and non-prescription, was the patient taking; what other concomitant illnesses did the patient have; or whether the liver issue was related to the underlying disease. Other factors to be considered include the temporal association between use of the drug and the event and time to onset. For example, if the patient takes a product for the first time and is diagnosed with cancer within the week, the cancer is unlikely to have been caused by the drug. Also, consideration should be given to other external factors that could cause liver issues such as alcohol consumption, and infection such as hepatitis. If possible, the underlying background rate of liver dysfunction in the treatment population should be determined for comparison. According to these and other diagnostic criteria, the investigator (or independent data committee) will roughly categorize causality as definite, probable, possible, or unlikely or some other causality grading system. Note that for regulatory reporting purposes causality is binary, i.e., a judgement must be made as to whether or not the product had a reasonable possibility of a causal relationship to the AE: yes or no, even in the face of incomplete information. With greater completeness of the report, the greater confidence in the causality assessment. For spontaneous reports it is generally accepted practice to assume a suspected causal relationship, as the reporter had some reason to suspect a relationship as impetus to report the case. Various techniques described elsewhere in this Manual are used to judge whether this is a strong enough signal worth communicating or, if weaker, requiring only continued surveillance.

Note: Many causal relationship methods have been published over the last decades. One interesting reference was published by an epidemiologist in 1965, which is a classic article which has formed the basis for many other methods of assessing whether an event has an association or causal relation to the product.[1]

The next consideration is the frequency of occurrence of this reported AE with use of the drug. By definition, clinical trials can determine the incidence of frequently occurring adverse events in both the study population and the comparison population. Certain epidemiologic methods can also be used to determine incidence primarily with the cohort design. The strengths and limitations of the cohort design are discussed in greater detail in Chapter 6. Another measurement found useful in evaluating drug safety is the "Number Needed to Harm" meaning how many people would need to be treated in order to observe a case of liver dysfunction. Chapter 6 reviews the strengths and limitations of clinical trials and formal epidemiologic study designs, while discussion of drawing inferences from spontaneous reporting data will be outlined below.

It is necessary to differentiate between AE reports received in interventional clinical trials (experimental) or epidemiologic studies (observational) and those received spontaneously or in a solicited manner (surveillance or monitoring systems). The use of statistics is well-described and defined for data generated in formal clinical trials. The patient populations are largely under the control of the investigator or researcher and the methodology for efficacy and safety analysis is well

[1] Hill, Austin Bradford, The environment and disease: Association or causation?, *Proc Roy Soc Med* 1965; 58(5): 295–300.

understood. Placebo- and comparator-controlled trials give clear pictures of occurrence rates of AEs, and significance values and confidence intervals can be determined and used to draw conclusions (at least for efficacy criteria). Clinical trials are usually not designed with sufficient statistical power to make safety judgments using statistics beyond descriptive statistics, that is, no p values.

The safety and efficacy data in clinical trials are typically solid because of strongly controlled data integrity and the sponsor is obligated to monitor documentation according to Good Clinical Practice. In addition, the data collected are more complete in that investigators can be queried for more detailed information. As patients are seen by the investigator at periodic intervals and as the investigator and his or her staff question the patient on AEs, it is believed that few AEs are missed, particularly those that are serious or dramatic in nature. Incidence rates of AEs calculated from these data are held to be valid and useful.

Spontaneous reports received from routine healthcare practice are markedly different from reports identified through clinical trials or epidemiologic studies. These "real world" data are typically voluntarily reported by healthcare professionals, consumers, and lawyers, among others. In addition, certain activities such as patient support programs may generate reports that are referred to as solicited reports.

Spontaneous reports are typically limited because follow-up for additional information is variable, source documents (e.g., laboratory reports, office and hospital records, autopsy reports) are not always available because of privacy issues, busy physicians or pharmacists unable to supply records from multiple sources, and patients do not want to disclose more information. If a healthcare professional was not involved with the reporting such as when a patient uses an OTC product, the information provided usually cannot be verified. Hence, the data integrity of individual spontaneous reports is variable and inconsistent. Often there are duplicate reports of the same case if more than one person reports the case unbeknownst to the others. These duplicate cases are included in regulatory safety databases and may need to be identified and taken into consideration when evaluating an AE.

Case Report or Individual Case Safety Report

A case report, also called an "Individual Case Safety Report" (ICSR), is a clinical observation of a patient who received a drug and experienced one or more AEs during the course of a clinical trial, a pharmacoepidemiologic study, or as a spontaneous report. ICSRs may be sent into regulators by patients, sponsors, or healthcare providers, in paper format via a MedWatch form (US) or by a CIOMS I form (EU). The electronic equivalent of the ICSR is the E2B report, which is an electronic file transmitted to a health authority or company or elsewhere with all the elements of the ICSR. Sometimes cases are published as short reports in medical journals, some of which have been previously reported to health authorities and some not. These cases are picked up in the periodic review of the medical literature conducted by the manufacturer (in the EEA the EMA supervises literature reviews for a discrete list of generic products to minimize duplication). Regardless of the format, each of these case reports has two general categories of information: medical/clinical relating to the patient and the AE and administrative, for example, relating to whether the case is new or follow-up, what country was it reported from and when.

Aggregate Reports

Periodic aggregate reports are reports required by regulators that provide descriptions, or compilations and analyses, of a group of patients exposed to a drug (or sometimes more than one drug, e.g., combination products). In addition to AEs, these aggregate reports include information on other safety issues, such as medication errors or quality issues. There are multiple aggregate report formats such as the Periodic Benefit Risk Evaluation Report (PBRER)[2] which is an important report

[2] PSUR (Periodic Safety Update Report) remains a frequently used acronym; nevertheless, the abbreviation which should be currently used is PBRER (Periodic Benefit Risk Evaluation Report) which provides a safety analysis but also a benefit — risk evaluation

for drugs that have been approved for marketing and is required in the EU. In the US, the equivalent report is called the Periodic Adverse Drug Experience Report (PADERS) while the basis for these 2 reports, the Periodic Safety Update Report (PSUR[3]) is used in the rest of the world (ROW). Whatever the aggregate reports are called, companies are obliged to prepare them in a serious and careful manner and to submit them on time to concerned health authorities. Some jurisdictions may also require customized formats and local language.

Spontaneous Reports

As mentioned previously, there are multiple biases and limitations involved in the quantitative analyses of spontaneously reported data that can result in findings and trends that may not truly represent the real safety profile of the drug. Various factors may act on spontaneously reported data and are worth discussion: where the drug is in its product life cycle, impact of media attention on the reporting rate, regulatory or legal action impacts on reporting rate, the length of time from drug initiation that the AE occurs, and defining the denominator for example.

(1) **Weber Effect:** The Weber effect, also called the product life cycle effect, describes the phenomenon of increased voluntary reporting *sometimes* observed after the initial launch of a new drug. The usefulness of the Weber Effect as a true description of reporting rates over time for new drugs has become somewhat less useful and the Weber Effect is no longer part of drug safety parlance. Although described in previous versions of this Manual, it will not be further discussed here.

(2) **Secular Effects Impacting the Reporting of Spontaneous Reports:** A number of external factors can influence whether a particular adverse event is reported. One of these factors is media attention. Occasionally, there is a particular adverse event reported with a specific drug that may receive a lot of media attention in the lay press due to the nature of the adverse event (death, suicidality), or a public figure has had a particular adverse event. In each case, the greater awareness of that adverse event with a specific drug may increase the likelihood that additional cases are reported for that event and drug, thus skewing the reporting numerator. Anecdotal reports of spectacular efficacy or harm with a particular drug can likewise skew the numerator. This phenomenon is also called *temporal reporting bias* and reflects an increase in AE reporting for a drug or class of drugs after increased media attention or rumor, or use of a medication by a well-known person. This phenomenon can be a regulatory action or a warning from a health agency, social media comments, publicized legal action on a drug are examples. There are many multipliers of this effect, particularly if the event is widely reported or goes "viral" on social media. "Overall adverse drug reaction reporting rates can be increased several times by external factors such as a change in a reporting system or an increased level of publicity attending a given drug or adverse reaction".[4]

The influence of external factors on reporting rates is complex and one example is the still on-going discussion of vaccines and their potential for increasing the risk for autism. Ultimately, it was concluded by the US CDC and others that there was no evidence to suggest a link between vaccines (in particular, those containing thimerosal as preservative) and the risk of autism.

Wakefield and 10 of the original 12 authors describing a link retracted their interpretation of the original data. According to the retraction, "no causal link was established between MMR vaccine and autism as the data were insufficient". An additional factor which questions the validity of the original finding was the lack of disclosure of certain financial conflicts by Wakefield as he was funded by lawyers suing vaccine companies.[5] The medical and media reports and comments on this are extensive. A good place to start is the comment by the CDC "Vaccines Do Not Cause Autism".

[3] PSUR (Periodic Safety Update Report) remains a frequently used acronym; nevertheless, the abbreviation which should be currently used is PBRER (Periodic Benefit Risk Evaluation Report) which provides a safety analysis but also a benefit — risk evaluation

[4] Sachs and Bortnichak, *Am J Med.* 1986; 81(suppl 5B): 49.

[5] Murch SH, Anthony A, Casson DH, Malik M, Berelowitz M, Dhillon AP *et al.*, Retraction of an interpretation, *Lancet*. 2004; 363: 750.

■ Reporting Rates versus Risk

Perhaps the biggest limitation of spontaneous and stimulated ADR reporting and inherent to its nature of surveillance, is incomplete data which can prevent the accurate quantitative estimation of risk.

In a perfect world, how would a reporting rate based on adverse events in the real world be calculated? Ideally, one would calculate the probability for the occurrence of a particular AE in the patients receiving a specific drug and then compare it to the occurrence of that particular AE in patients receiving a different drug or to the general population.

Numerator calculations

Numerator data are almost always incomplete. The number of AEs reported is less than the true number of AEs that actually occur because not all AEs are reported during the post-marketing phase of the drug. As a result, the true number of patients with the AE and the percentage of cases that are not reported are not known. There are many publications describing the underreporting of AE data, but few actually measure the true rate of underreporting ("a known unknown"). It was estimated (about 30 years ago) that in the United Kingdom only 10% of serious ADRs and 2–4% of non-serious ADRs that occur are reported.[6] In the United States, the FDA estimated (about 35 years ago) that only 1% of serious suspected ADRs were reported.[7] In France, it was estimated (about 20 years ago) that "no more than 5% of serious ADRs" are actually reported.[8] Whether these data persist in today's world is unclear. In the future it may be possible to harness point-of-care electronic medical records to automatically obtain more complete digital safety information in near real time. This capability is currently unavailable.

Denominator calculations

For different reasons, complete denominator data are also unavailable. Unless the drug is dispensed through a specialty pharmacy that tracks the individual patients taking that drug, the actual number of patients taking a drug is relatively unknown, or extremely difficult to accurately define. Although one can obtain prescription data and know how many tablets, capsules, or tubes were sold, it is not possible to extrapolate this information to know how many consumers actually took the product in the manner and for the length of time prescribed.

Ideally, denominator data would be reported in a number of ways including patients exposed (for risk estimates), patient-time exposed (number of patients times the length of time each patient took the drug such as patient-months or patient-years) for incidence rates estimates. But instead of accurate denominator figures, the only known data are total number of tablets sold, kilograms manufactured, and prescriptions written or dispensed.

By obtaining these raw data elements, crude reporting rates can be calculated by dividing the number of ADR reports by a quantitative denominator; however, the resulting reporting rates are not easy to interpret.

As an example, in one study, 12 cardiac arrhythmia reports were received for one widely used antihistamine for what was calculated to be 9 billion (9,000,000,000) patient-years of exposure. The resulting reporting rate is 12/9,000,000,000 or a rate of 0.0000000013 cardiac arrhythmia events/patient-years of exposure, which is not a meaningful number. In fact, this number is so low that it is below the naturally occurring incidence of cardiac arrhythmias in the population, meaning marked under-reporting of the AEs may have occurred. Using a different interpretation of these data, one could argue that the drug in question actually *prevents* cardiac arrhythmias, which is clearly not the case. This number is useless to a clinician who needs to make a decision on whether a particular cardiac patient should be given this drug.

Potential sources of denominator data such as kilograms manufactured are available from the company producing the product. Other sources such as number of prescriptions and other potential patient exposure data can be obtained from various third party entities that have access to large databases containing sales/claims data or electronic medical records. Potential confounding factors that can also impact the interpretation

[6] Rawlins, *J R Coll Phys Lond.* 1995; 29: 41–49.

[7] Scott, Rosenbaum, Waters *et al.*, *R I Med J.* 1987; 70: 311–316.

[8] Bégaud B, Martin K, Haramburu F *et al.*, Rates of spontaneous reporting of adverse drug reactions in France, *J Am Med Assoc.* 2002; 288: 1588.

of the reporting rate include the use of generic products that may not be included in the denominator, but for which reported AEs are included in the numerator, as well as counterfeit drugs where the denominator and numerator are compromised. Despite these limitations, drug utilization data can be stratified by gender, age, and other demographic characteristics. Trends over time in usage can be observed.

In summary, as Dr. David Goldsmith has said "The numerator is bad, the denominator is worse, and the ratio is meaningless." *Hence, one cannot calculate quantitative measures of risk for a particular AE based on spontaneous data, only reportingfrequencies. Period.*

■ Quantitative Signal Detection Methods

Although limited in how the data can be interpreted, the large repositories of spontaneous reporting data such as the FDA's FAERS, WHO's VigiBase, and the EU's EVDAS, can be used to monitor certain unexpected patterns of reporting through innovative quantitative techniques looking at proportional reporting. Referred to as *signal detection*, these metrics include the proportional reporting ratio (PRR), the Gamma Poisson Shrinker (GPS), urn-model algorithm, reporting odds ratio (ROR), Bayesian confidence propagation neural network–information component (BCPNN-IC), and adjusted residual score (ARS), sequential probability ratio test (max-SPRT). The PRR is used as an example of the application of quantitative disproportionality method and is described below.[9]

Disproportionality analyses:

There are various methods for conduction signal detection through the use of disproportionality analyses. These methods to some degree employ the concept of expected proportional reporting and calculate an observed versus expected statistic for that particular database. Using the example of calculating the PRR, the measure is most accurate when using large databases such as the large spontaneous reporting databases mentioned above.

This basic PRR is simple to calculate and uses a 2 × 2 table:

	Drug of Interest	**All Other Drugs in database**
AE of Interest	A	B
All Other AEs in database	C	D

Note: PRR = A(A + C)/B(B + C).

For example:

_Drug X	**Drug of Interest**	**All Other Drugs in database**
AE of Interest	345	291
All Other AEs	6901	14556

Note: PRR = 345/6901 (345 + 6901)/291 (291 + 14556) = 1.67.

In words, the proportion of a particular AE divided by all AEs seen with the drug of interest is divided by the proportion of this AE divided by all AEs seen with all drugs in the database. In the previous example, if 3.28% of all AEs seen with drug X are chest pain and 1.96% of all AEs seen with all the other drugs in the database (excluding drug X and its AEs) are chest pain, then the PRR is 3.278%/1.96% or 1.67. This means that there are (dis)proportionately more chest pain AEs with drug X compared with all the other drugs in the database, and this is noteworthy as a possible signal of disproportionality that should be evaluated further.

When the PRR is calculated for all AEs in the database, every PRR will either be below 1.0 or above 1.0. In theory, disproportionality values above 1.0 would suggest that an AE is more frequently reported for drug X than for other drugs in the database. It is important to remember that a signal of disproportionality does not

[9] On these methods, the following references can be looked up: (a) Evans SJ, Waller PC, Davis S, Use of proportional reporting ratios (PRRs) for signal generation from spontaneous adverse drug reaction reports, *Pharmacoepidemiology Drug Safety* 2001; 10(6): 483–486. (b) DuMouchel W, Bayesian data mining in large frequency tables, with an application to the FDA spontaneous reporting system (with discussion), *Am Stat.* 1999; 53(3): 177–222. (c) van Puijenbroek E, Diemont W, van Grootheest K, Application of quantitative signal detection in the Dutch spontaneous reporting system for adverse drug reactions, *Drug Safety* 2003; 26(5): 293–301. (d) Bate A, Lindquist M, Edwards IR, Olsson S, Orre R, Lansner A *et al.*, A Bayesian neural network method for adverse drug reaction signal generation, *Eur J Clin Pharmacol.* 1998; 54(4): 315–321.

equate with risk. There are a number of reasons why events may be presented as disproportionate. For example, the event may already be on the product label, the event may be related to the underlying disease being treated, the event may more likely be related to a concomitant condition or medication, or there may be duplicate reporting of the same case. Although there are more than 80,000 terms in MedDRA, disproportionality analyses are usually conducted at the Preferred Term (PT), Higher Level Term (HLT), the Higher Level Group Term (HLGT) levels, or using SMQs (Standard MedDRA Queries) as well as MedDRA developed adverse event term groupings. Typically, predetermined thresholds are used to put guiderails around the utility of a PRR estimate. A threshold often used with the PRR is based on parameters where the PRR is 2 or higher, the corresponding Chi-Square is 4 or higher, and the minimum number of cases for the drug/event combination is 3 or higher. The higher the PRR, the greater the specificity but the lower the sensitivity of the estimate. Alternatively, one might simply take the 10 or 20 highest PRRs and evaluate those regardless of how high the PRR is above 1.0.

There are other issues with using disproportionality estimates. When the database is small or inappropriate, the estimates may lack validity. Some examples of problems are listed below:

1. For serious and rare AEs adding or subtracting one case can markedly alter the PRR results. For example, if there is one myocardial infarct (MI) in the four- patient database of drug X, this gives an incidence of 1/4 or 25%. Taking away the one case or adding one more MI would change the rate to 0% (0/3) or 40% (2/5). If the database had 1,000/4,000 cases, adding one or taking one away would have a negligible effect.
2. If the database is incomplete, meaning is doesn't contain "all" of the product safety data, or captures criteria differently per protocol, it may not be appropriate to compare the reporting frequency of a particular AE in the population treated with drug X against the frequency of that AE in the whole AE database. If the treatment for drug X is for, say, breast cancer, and is given only to elderly women, then comparing the frequency of an AE in the elderly female population versus the whole database in which elderly women are not predominant may give misleading results.
3. Another issue may occur if drug X is frequently prescribed with drug Y and drug Y ("bystander") is known to produce a particular AE. Unless this is accounted for, it may appear in a simple PRR that drug X caused the AE when it was probably due to drug Y.

Finally, if the safety database used for the denominator of the PRR is small or has a high proportion of a particular type of patient or disease this may also produce flawed PRRs. If one has a sufficiently large database, the PRR can be programmed to run periodically (e.g., monthly or quarterly) using the appropriate filters to generate possible signals. This method will be less useful if MedDRA coding is not crisp and correct. As always, the issue here is generating too many signals with too many false positives for the personnel available to review the signals.

■ Other Data Mining Methods

Although the disproportionality method is commonly used by companies and health agencies to screen and detect signals, other methods have been developed to compensate for some of these above-mentioned problems. Some of the other methods are found in the broad category of "Bayesian approaches". These methods account for the number of cases (cell sizes) and decrease the sensitivity of the PRR score if the cell sizes are small. One method, the Bayesian confidence propagation neural network (BCPNN), was developed by the Uppsala Monitoring Centre and is used for signal detection in their database. Other methods, such as the Gamma Poisson Shrinker (GPS) and the Multi-item Gamma Poisson Shrinker (MGPS), are also used in an attempt to make the PRR more useful. These methods have been used by various health agencies, including the Food and Drug Administration (FDA), the European Medicines Agency (EMA), and the Medicines and Healthcare Products Regulatory Agency (MHRA) which is the British pharmaceuticao regulator. Treatment of these methodologies in detail is beyond the scope of this book, and the reader is referred to the standard textbooks of pharmacoepidemiology. A good, approachable summary of the field is available in GVP Module IX Addendum I — Methodological aspects of signal detection from spontaneous reports of suspected adverse reactions (EMA Good PV Practices Web page).[10]

A brief note on other terms you may run across:

Event rate — The number of subjects experiencing an *AE* as a proportion of the number of people in the population at risk over a specific period of time. For example, 5 per 1,000 person-days.

Absolute risk — The probability of occurrence of an AE in patients exposed to a drug. For example, one may say the absolute risk of a myocardial infarction with drug X is 5%. Obviously, this value is often hard or impossible to obtain and is one reason that pharmacovigilance exists.

Absolute risk reduction — The arithmetic difference between two absolute risk rates. For example, the absolute risk of a myocardial infarction with drug X is 5% and with drug Y 2%. The risk reduction is 5% – 2% = 3%.

Relative risk (or risk ratio) — In a clinical trial or in an observational cohort study, the ratio between the rate of an adverse outcome (e.g., an AE) in a group exposed to a treatment and the rate in a control group. For example, the rate of myocardial infarction in the drug X group is 5% and in the control group 2.5%. The ratio (relative risk) is 5%/2% = 2.5%.

Relative risk reduction — The difference in event rates between two groups, expressed as a proportion of the event rate in the untreated group.

Odds ratio — Also known as estimated (or approximate) relative risk. In case-control studies concerning drug safety, the ratio between the rate of exposure to a suspect drug in a group of cases (with the AE) and the rate of exposure in a group of non-cases (i.e., controls without the AE). Like relative risk from cohort studies, the odds ratio is a useful estimation of the strength of potential cause–effect relationships. This parameter is often used in systematic reviews and meta-analyses.

Risk difference or attributable risk — The difference between the rate of an adverse outcome (e.g., an AE) in a group exposed to an experimental drug and the rate in a control group.

Number needed to harm (NNH) — Also called number needed to harm one. The NNH is the number of patients that must be exposed to a drug to produce an AE/ADR in one patient. Exposure may, for example, be one course or 1 year of treatment. For example, one could calculate based on a study that the number needed to produce one case of rhabdomyolysis with a particular statin is 3,500 patients.

Number needed to benefit (NNB) — A similar concept to the NNH, but reflects the number needed to receive a positive effect from the drug. For example, one might need to treat three patients with a particular statin to get a positive effect (e.g., cholesterol reduction).

Benefit–risk ratio — Various techniques have been developed using such data as NNH and NNB to calculate an actual number for the benefit–risk ratio. Although a number of quantitative approaches have been investigated, it is not possible to calculate an accurate "ratio" using estimates; however, if one can calculate the NNH and the NNB for the particular drug one can calculate a benefit–risk ratio. This is rarely done, however, as the data are incomplete and inaccurate.

Confidence intervals — Most studies are based on samples, not entire populations, which adds an element of uncertainty and unreliability to the results because the entire population was not studied. Thus, we cannot be certain that the 15% of the study population that had serious AEs represents the true value for the whole population rather than just for the smaller sample. The confidence interval represents the range of the correct or true value for the whole population and gives an idea of the reliability of the data and of the estimate. One can calculate various levels of "assurance", 90%, 95%, 99%, 99.9%, and so on, for the confidence interval. Usually, the 95% level is used. The narrower or smaller the distance between the upper and lower values of the confidence interval (called the confidence limits), the more accurate the estimate. The more patients in the study usually produce a narrower (better) confidence interval.

[10] See also "Practical Aspects of Signal Detection in Pharmacovigilance," Report of the CIOMS Working Group VIII. Counsel for the International Organizations of Medical Sciences, Geneva, 2010. See also http://www.ema.europa.eu/docs/en_GB/document_library/Scientific_guideline/2017/10/WC500236405.pdf.

CHAPTER

24

Pharmacoepidemiology: Its Practical Use in the World of Drug Safety

This chapter is not meant to be an introduction to epidemiology or pharmacoepidemiology. There are many excellent textbooks and references in those fields. Rather, this chapter attempts, briefly, to place pharmacoepidemiology in the context of its use in the practical world of drug safety.

Introduction

- *Epidemiology* is the study of the distribution and determinants of diseases in populations. Basically, epidemiology is a discipline that provides tools for assessing diseases and/or exposures within a defined population. Epidemiology studies may provide simple, descriptive statistics such as disease incidence and prevalence as determined in a natural history of disease study or may use more analytic methods to compare disease rates between two groups of individuals and can be hypothesis testing or hypothesis generating in nature. Associations that have been identified through epidemiologic techniques include smoking and lung cancer, high blood pressure and heart disease, increasing maternal age and risk of trisomy 3 in the baby.
- *Pharmacoepidemiology* is a subset of the broader discipline of epidemiology. As defined by the International Society of Pharmacoepidemiology (ISPE), pharmacoepidemiology is the study of the utilization and effects of drugs in defined populations. Pharmacoepidemiology is an important tool in in assessing drug safety when used in conjunction with information from clinical trials and from the spontaneous reporting system which is a database of voluntary reports of adverse events in patients receiving various drugs. Unlike the randomized double-blind clinical trial which is the main study design submitted to regulators for drug approval,

pharmacoepidemiology plays a critical role in understanding both risks and unintended benefits of drugs, can identify subgroups of patients at higher risk of an adverse event, and can provide key supporting information about risks to patients in a real world setting that may keep a drug on the market despite a serious identified risk.

Pharmacoepidemiology as a discipline is population-based rather than based on individuals or patients. Broadly, it can be used to describe treatment patterns or drug utilization within a specific disease or therapeutic area. Other uses include determining the number of new cases of a specific condition in a defined population (such as geographic region, or special populations such as neonates, children, elderly, during pregnancy). More specifically, analytic epidemiologic methods can be used to assess risk such as determining the risk of a specific outcome in patients exposed to a specific drug compared to background risk or compared to patients exposed to a different therapeutic agent. Analytic methods can also be used to determine factors that can contribute to risk or comparative risk (risk factors) or can identify factors that are driving the risk rather than the exposure of interest (confounding factors) which may superficially ascribe an outcome to a particular exposure, when it was actually related to the confounding factor. Sophisticated modelling analytics can be used to examine the individual and shared contributions of individual risk factors or interactions between risk factors.

Pharmacoepidemiology is an important tool in the evaluation of drug safety. It complements the experimental and interventional randomized clinical trial which tests the safety and efficacy of drug products between defined groups of participants. Well-run clinical trials can provide greater rigor and confidence in the study findings, but are generally too small to identify rare risks, risks with long latency periods, or small increased risks added to a large background risk. Pharmacoepidemiologic studies evaluate risks as the drug products would be used in the real world rather than in the tightly controlled confines of a clinical trial.

At the other end of the drug safety spectrum is the spontaneous reporting system which consists of voluntarily reported adverse events that occur once a drug is approved. Signals of rarely occurring adverse events can be identified through spontaneous reports as well as signals or events occurring after long latency periods such as cancer and events that occur during pregnancy. Because spontaneous reports do not have an underlying defined population and may include co-morbidities that were excluded from clinical trials, they cannot be used to determine incidence or to describe comparative risks quantitatively. Pharmacoepidemiology bridges the gap between the signal-generating use of the spontaneous reporting system, and the controlled, experimental hypothesis testing of the clinical trial. These three methodologic tools together provide a more complete understanding of drug-related risks than can be provided by any of these tools alone. In the heavily regulated arena of pharmaceutical safety, pharmacoepidemiology can be used to identify potential and real risks relating to serious adverse events (SAEs) through signal detection techniques. Other methods can then be used to confirm and quantify the risk associated with the signal or to rule it out. Such studies can rarely answer questions about causality but rather give information on probabilities and statistical associations.

Pharmacoepidemiology continues to grow in value as a drug safety tool as automated tools are developed, Real World Evidence (RWE) databases such as insurance claims data and Electronic Medical Records (EHR) become increasingly available, and regulatory expectations as to the manufacturer's role and responsibility for assessing the benefits and risks of their products continues to expand.

Tools for Evaluating Drug Safety

The Randomized Controlled Clinical Trial

To understand the role that pharmacoepidemiology and observational methodologies play in evaluating drug safety, it is important to understand the strengths and limitations of the randomized clinical trial. The randomized controlled clinical trial (RCT) is the design method that is required by global regulators to demonstrate the efficacy and safety of a drug product to support product approval. Participants in RCTs are selected by randomization to receive one compound (experimental) to another (comparative compound or routine practice for example). The randomization component of RCTs controls for factors other than treatment (including both known and unknown bias) that may alter or explain the drug effects so that the efficacy and safety findings are most likely to result from differences between the treatments themselves. RCTs have detailed protocols which provide outline purpose and objectives, inclusion and exclusion criteria, patient drop out, definitions of outcomes, measurement tools, pre-identified analytic methods, length of follow up, and identification of treatment emergent adverse events among many other factors. Because restrictions of who within a disease area are included in the RCT as well as restrictions on other exposures or concomitant medications, the RCT overall, does not and is not intended to reflect how the drug would be used in general practice.

In addition to randomization, another important component of the RCT is the degree to which the trial is blinded. Blinding refers to the extent to which study participants or investigators and their teams are ignorant as to which study compound the participants are receiving. Blinding increases the rigor of the study by eliminating certain factors other than the drugs being tested that may alter or explain any observed differences between treatment groups. The trial may be single-blind (the subject does not know what treatment has been received) or double-blind (neither the subject nor the investigator knows what treatment has been received).

Randomized double-blind clinical trials are complex and resource-intensive to implement and are considered the gold standard of clinical research. RCT studies are conducted primarily during phases II and III of drug development and the results are sufficiently powered to describe the efficacy of the drug. Although safety is also an important outcome examined during the clinical trial, the relatively low number of participants studied and the short period of follow-up only allows for the identification of more commonly occurring adverse events that occur within a short period of time after drug administration.

Pharmacoepidemiologic Study Designs

As previously mentioned, pharmacoepidemiology studies are observational by design. There are three major types of pharmacoepidemiology studies: cohort studies, case-control studies, and cross-sectional studies. The first two study types are most commonly used in pharmacoepidemiology and will be discussed in greater detail. Each study type has distinct strengths and limitations which factor in as to what inferences can be drawn from each study design.

The Cohort Study

The cohort study is the strongest of the three epidemiologic study designs. A cohort study with a single cohort, or a group that is comprised of a common factor such as having a particular disease, is typically used to conduct natural history of disease studies. An example would be following a group of individuals with schizophrenia in anticipation of a new drug for schizophrenia being approved. By understanding the characteristics and disease components of the target population, the pharmacoepidemiologist will see what types of conditions occur in that population that occur outside of exposure to the new drug. In single cohort studies, there is no comparison group and follow up is observational in nature. The occurrence rate or background incidence rate can be calculated such that the background rate for sudden death, for suicidality, or for liver failure can be determined. This is useful information to have early (before approval) to compare to information on adverse events that start being reported once a drug is approved in order to put those events in context.

A comparative cohort study is a study where two groups of individuals with a different study factor, such as one group with a drug exposure of interest and the other group with no exposure, are followed prospectively over time to identify outcomes of interest such as the occurrence of adverse events. The comparative cohort study can be conducted in real time, by identifying the cohorts now and following them into the future, or the study can be a historical cohort study where the cohorts were identified and followed over time in the past. With both designs, incidence rates can be calculated as well as comparing the incidence rate from one group to the other group through the relative risk.

The following tables show an example of calculating relative risk.

Calculating Relative Risk and Absolute Risk			
	Outcome		
	yes	**no**	**Total**
Took the Drug			
Cohort 1: yes	a	b	a+b
Cohort 2: no	c	d	c+d
Relative risk = [a/(a + b)] ÷ [c/(c + d)] or the rate in exposed divided by the rate in the unexposed.			
Absolute risk = [a/(a + b)] – [c/(c + d)] or rate in exposed minus rate in unexposed.			

Example of Calculating Relative Risk and Absolute Risk				
	Experienced bleeding			
	yes	**no**	**Total**	**Rate**
Took aspirin				
Cohort 1: yes	500	10,000	10500	0.048
Cohort 2: no	150	10,000	10150	0.015
Relative risk = [500/(10500)] ÷ [150/(10150)] or 0.024÷0.015=3.2 or those who took aspirin had 3.2 times the risk of bleed compared to those not taking aspirin				
Absolute risk = [500/(10500)] – [150/(10150)] or rate in exposed minus rate in unexposed. 0.048–0.015 = –0.033				

In this example, we have 20,650 study subjects that were divided between 2 cohorts. Cohort 1 was comprised of 10.500 subjects who took aspirin regularly and Cohort 2 with 10,150 subjects who did not take aspirin. The 2 cohorts were followed over time to see who developed bleeding. At the end of the follow up period, 500 subjects in Cohort 1 developed bleeding while 150 in Cohort 2 experienced bleeding. As seen in Table 2, the relative risk was 3.2 in the aspirin group compared to the non-aspirin group indicating that those taking aspirin were 3.2 times more likely to experience bleeding than those not taking aspirin. A relative risk of 1 indicates that the likelihood of getting the adverse event is the same in the treatment group and in the non-treatment group, while a relative risk finding less than 1 would indicate that the treatment group had LESS of a chance of experiencing the outcome of interest than the non-treatment group. The absolute risk shows the absolute risk of bleeding with aspirin use controlling for the underlying risk of bleeding in the unexposed population.

Strengths of the cohort design include the ability to calculate incidence rates and comparative incidence rates (relative risk) which is very important in drug safety, particularly when comparing incidence of an adverse outcome in subjects taking one drug compared to those taking another drug. Another strength is the lack of recall bias which is bias which results when subjects at one point in time to recall events or exposures that occurred in the past and there is differential recall between groups. This will be discussed more fully in the case-control design. Limitations of the cohort design are that they can be costly, labor-intensive, and lengthy to conduct (over several years) if set up as a *de novo* study where, for example, the study is set up at drug approval and the study subjects are followed going forward in time. This limitation can be reduced if using historical data where the cohorts have been identified at some point in time and then medical records which have already been collected are examined going forward from that point in time. Cohort studies can also require large numbers of study subjects if the outcome of interest is rare.

The Case-Control Study

While conceptually cohort studies are prospective in that the design is based on going forward in collecting information from the point of drug exposure, with case-control studies, the design is retrospective in that both drug exposure and outcome of interest have already occurred. Typically, two groups of subjects, with or without an outcome of interest, are identified, and either the subjects are interviewed and/or medical records are examined. to look for what proportion of subjects in each outcome group had the exposure of interest. Put another way, case-control studies determine the chance ("odds" or "probability") of having taken the suspect drug in a group of subjects already suffering from an adverse event and compares that with the odds of having taken the drug in a group of subjects who did not have the event. Large, automated databases such as administrative medical claims data or electronic medical record databases are sometimes used for this study design.

When setting up a case-control study, it is advantageous to select groups of cases (with the event) and non-cases (without the event) that are relatively comparable by matching the two groups by various potential confounding factors such as age, gender, race, concomitant conditions among other factors so that the groups are identical in all other aspects other than the exposure to the drug of interest. Both groups should have the same opportunity to receive the drug.

For example, if a hospital database is used as the basis of the case-control study, the drug of interest should have been on the pharmacy formulary for the entire time period examined in the study. The subjects' medical histories are then examined to see which subjects in each group used the drug in question. The simplified data are then organized into a 2 × 2 table as depicted in Table 3.

	Example of Calculating the Odds Ratio		
	Myocardial Infarction yes	**Myocardial Infarction no**	**Total**
Cox-2 inhibitor yes	10	5	unknown
Cox-2 inhibitor no	50,000	50,000	unknown
Odds Ratio = (0.0002) ÷ (0.0001) = 2 or the those with myocardial infarction were twice as likely to have taken a cox-2 inhibitor that those without myocardial infarction			

An odds ratio value of greater than 1.0 is suggestive of an association between the drug and the outcome of interest. Generally, an odds ratio value of greater than 2.0 is believed to be fairly strong and supports an association. In our example, the odds ratio value of 2 is suggestive of an association and further studies may be needed to confirm or reject an association.

Advantages of case-control studies are that the design is useful for studying very rare adverse events because the investigator seeks out a data source where this outcome is found in a sufficient number of subjects. For rare outcomes, the odds ratio can be considered approximate to the relative risk or risk ratio of a conceptual cohort study. Higher order statistical techniques can be applied such as logistic regression for the adjustment of covariates and risk factors that may confound the association, e.g., severity of the disease treated, or concomitant medications, and possible interactions between drugs.

Case-control studies are fast and relatively inexpensive; however, they are potentially liable to significant bias both in the selection of the subjects for the two groups and in the amount and quality of the drug exposure and medical history data.

The Nested Case-Control Study

Nested case-control studies are studies of case-control design that are nested (or conducted within) a cohort study or a clinical trial. In both situations, the nested case-control study is conducted within one cohort or one treatment arm of a trial. This study design is useful to examine whether there are predictors for a certain outcome in a group of subjects with a similar exposure. One example where a nested case-control study can be used before approval is when a clinical trial identifies a particular risk in the experimental treatment group. It would be useful to understand if this risk applies to all study subjects in that group, or if there are factors that could predict who may be a greater risk of that finding. For example, a particular trial finding is that of excessive weight gain in the experimental drug group. A nested case-control study is then conducted in that study group to see if there are other factors that could predict who may be at greater risk of excessive weight gain. These factors can include age, gender, race, family history, concomitant conditions or medications among other factors. If a subgroup of patients is identified with greater risk such as increased age, that finding could be added into the product information as a precaution.

Confidence Intervals

An important part of any experimental or observation study is whether a finding meets statistical significance. Many studies rely on the p-value to determine statistical significance, but another tool that brings additional information to the significance finding is the use of confidence intervals. The confidence interval reflects the uncertainty of the study finding in that particular sample of study subjects.

If a particular study finds that 15% of the users of drug A had a serious adverse event, the confidence intervals can help determine the certainty that this finding is correct. The confidence interval describes the upper bound and lower bound of where the "true" value is with a pre-determined degree of certainty. Typically, 95% confidence intervals are used. An example is that a study finds that a measure of risk is 3.3 and the 95% confidence intervals are 2.4 and 4.1. A number of conclusions can be drawn from examining the confidence intervals. First, the finding that the lower bound of the confidence interval is greater than 1 indicates that the finding is statistically significant. The values of the confidence intervals demonstrate that there is 95% certainty that the real value of the association is between 2.4 and 4.1 and the finding that the lower bound is greater than 2 indicates that the finding may be substantive. Wider confidence intervals indicate greater uncertainty in the finding which is typically seen with small numbers of subjects. If the confidence intervals include the value of 1, the finding has not reached statistical significance but the distance of the value from 1 can suggest that the finding either does or does not approach significance. If both values of the confidence intervals are below one, the finding is statistically significant and in the opposite direction of the null hypothesis.

■ Conclusions

With the arrival of formal risk management as an integral part of the development and life span of all drugs, the fields of pharmacoepidemiology and drug safety are now more tightly linked than ever.

Health authorities require epidemiologic safety studies, particularly as post-marketing commitments or requirements. Large databases and practitioners who know how to conduct these studies have become more and more available and the methodology has become more refined and automated. Many pharmaceutical companies now have risk management/pharmacoepidemiology departments to handle these studies.

Indeed, the role of pharmacoepidemiology in risk assessment and signal detection has become more prominent as risk management programs become increasingly active over the entire life cycle of products.

■ Frequently Asked Questions

Q: I never was particularly gifted with math and numbers. Do I really have to learn this stuff? Do I really need it in drug safety?

A: Yes, you really need it to interpret and make informed decisions. As electronic medical records become more widespread and large databases are used for epidemiology and observational safety studies, data mining, Bayesian analysis, and other statistical techniques, numerical literacy — as it is called — will be very useful and probably obligatory at some point. Further, as regulatory agencies have embraced epidemiological principles and methods, other stakeholders will increasingly need to understand principles and practices of pharmacoepidemiology as applied to drug safety.

Q: Do regulators accept the findings of pharmacoepidemiology studies?

A: Not only do regulators accept the findings of well-conducted pharmacoepidemiology, these studies are often mandated by regulators to be conducted after the drug is marketed as a condition of approval as part of the post approval commitments.

Q: Are the findings of pharmacoepidemiology studies more decisive than clinical trials in assigning causality?

A: Clinical trials have the more scientifically rigorous study design for formally testing certain aspects of causality; however, pharmacoepidemiology studies may complement and support clinical trial findings and can also suggest potential areas of risk that clinical trials are too small or too short in duration to identify.

Q: This seems like a much bigger topic. Are there experts on this topic out there?

A: Yes... a few pages on this subject won't make you an expert of course! There are advanced graduate degrees in pharmacoepidemiology and many experts in this field. It's important to have someone with this skill set within an organization or available as a consultant or contractor.

CHAPTER

25

Signals and Signaling in the Context of Risk Management

Enormous efforts are made, in terms of people, time, cost, and technology, to collect adverse event (AE) data in companies, governments, and elsewhere. The collection of vast amounts of data is meaningless in and of itself. It is only when these data are organized and analyzed for new safety issues (which are then acted on in the context of risk management) that the true value of this effort becomes apparent. The hunt for meaning is known as "signaling".

■ The Signal — Definition

The Uppsala Monitoring Centre defines a safety signal as follows:

> "Reported information on a possible causal relationship between an adverse event and a drug, the relationship being unknown or incompletely documented previously. Usually more than a single report is required to generate a signal, depending upon the seriousness of the event and the quality of the information."
>
> They comment further:
>
> "This describes the first alert of a problem with a drug. By its nature a signal cannot be regarded

> as definitive but indicates the need for further enquiry or action. On the other hand, it is prudent to avoid a multiplicity of signals based on single case reports since follow-up of all such would be impractical and time consuming. The definition allows for some flexibility in approach to a signal based on the characteristics of individual problems. Some would like a "signal" to include new information on positive drug effects, but this is outside the scope of a drug safety Programme."[1]

Note, however, that there may be instances when a single, well-characterized report with high attributability to drug exposure, e.g., Stevens-Johnson syndrome, may be useful in alerting to a new adverse reaction (see below). A refined definition has been proposed and is being used by experts:

> "Information that arises from one or multiple sources (including observations and experiments), which suggests a new potentially causal association, or a new aspect of a known association, between an intervention and an event or set of related events, either adverse or beneficial, which would command regulatory, societal or clinical attention, and is judged to be of sufficient likelihood to justify verificatory and, when necessary, remedial actions."[2]

The EMA delivered a definition based on the previous publication in Regulation No. 520/2012, which has been included in guidance on Signals (GVP Module IX — Signal Management — 2012 updated in 2017) with the following definition:

> "For the purposes of this chapter, 'signal' means information arising from one or multiple sources, including observations and experiments, which suggests a new potentially causal association, or a new aspect of a known association between an intervention and an event or set of related events, either adverse or beneficial, which is judged to be of sufficient likelihood to justify verificatory action."
>
> "For the purpose of monitoring data in the Eudravigilance database, only signals related to an adverse reaction shall be considered."

Not everyone agrees that all signals based on single cases should not be pursued. Sometimes, however, rare events are picked up after a single case, and certain AEs are almost always due to drugs, e.g., Stevens–Johnson Syndrome, skin fixed drug reactions. Thus, a single case can be a signal, as indicated above. More common problems, e.g., myocardial infarctions, might not be worth pursuing as a signal if there is only a single case in a middle-aged diabetic smoker. But in a 22-year-old, it is worth pursuing.

Signals may be "qualitative" (based on spontaneously reported data) or "quantitative" (based on data mining, epidemiologic data, or trial data). The signal may be a new issue never seen with this product, or it may be the worsening or changing of a known AE or problem, e.g., a previously unaffected patient group is experiencing this problem, or the incidence has increased, or it is now fatal in those it attacks, whereas before it was not. As noted above, qualitative signals may be based on one single striking case or on a collection of cases. In addition, qualitative signals may also be based on pre-clinical findings; experience with other similar products in the class ("class signals"); new drug or food interactions; confusion with a product's name, packaging, or use; counterfeiting issues; quality problems; and more. Thus, the meaning of "signal" is being expanded.

"Signal" is primarily used to refer to marketed products, although the term is occasionally used for new issues in clinical trials. Some people use the term *potential signal* to indicate an issue with minimal data (e.g., only one case report), whereas others use the term *weak signal*. However, these are not consensus terms.

Some signals are very difficult if not impossible to pick up. Signals with very long latencies (onset well after the drug use has ended) or which even skip a generation (e.g., diethylstilbestrol and vaginal cancer) require exceedingly astute observers or great luck to be found.

[1] Delamothe, *Br Med J* 1992; 304: 465.

[2] Hauben A, Defining "signal" and its subtypes, *Drug Safety* 2009; 32(2): 99–100.

Identifying signals, however, is not enough. The signal must be further investigated by doing what is variously called a "signal workup", a "signal inquiry", or a "pharmacovigilance investigation". The ultimate goal and true *raison d'être* of signal discovery and investigation is to determine whether the newly identified concern is indeed due to the drug, and is of sufficient severity and frequency (and clinical importance) in relation to the benefit, to require alerting physicians, nurses, pharmacists, and patients via a change in the product labeling, restricting distribution, television, internet, social media, and other announcements or, in more severe cases, recalling of the product or stopping a clinical trial. It is quite difficult to confirm causality with any degree of certainty and these latter extreme steps should only be considered when there is a high level of confidence that such interventions will positively impact public health.

Signaling is not passive. It is proactive. No longer does one wait for AEs or SUSARs before acting. Rather an active signaling effort must be conducted throughout a product's life cycle. The goal is to detect signals as early as possible to anticipate, evaluate, and minimize problems, not to react to them after the fact.

Notes: When the first PV rules and organizations were set up many years ago, PV people were spending most of their time on case management (AE collection, analysis, data entry, etc.) and very little time on safety signals and risk management. In recent years, this trend has been reversed: most of the PV skills, resources and time are now directed toward signal detection, validation, prioritization, assessment, and benefit-risk management.

Also note that when you do searches the US spelling of signaling and the UK spelling of signalling differ.

Signal Sources and Generation

Signals are looked for in multiple ways. The oldest method is essentially passive and relies on the collection by pharmaceutical companies, government health authorities, or third-party organizations (academic centers, medical registries) of spontaneous AE reports and aggregate analyses of these reports plus any others picked up from other sources, such as solicited cases, compassionate use, surveys, etc. They are then reviewed individually and in aggregate, looking for "striking", "unusual", or "unexpected" AEs or safety issues and trends. Medically qualified people (physicians, nurses, pharmacists) examine large quantities of data, attempting to find the proverbial needle in the haystack, and either discuss within the organization the "potential signals" found or post them publicly (see FDA's potential signal website: https://www.fda.gov/Drugs/GuidanceComplianceRegulatoryInformation/Surveillance/AdverseDrugEffects/ucm082196.htm). This technique is elegantly known as "global introspection". It is quite time-consuming and laborious, but in the hands of astute and insightful clinicians does indeed pick up major problems and still remains, in many respects, the cornerstone of signal generation and identification around the world. A "similar case analysis", which entails review of additional cases that may shed light on the condition of interest, is often very helpful in understanding the medical importance of a newly emerging signal. Global introspection obviously relies on the good will and perspicacity of the reporting physicians, nurses, pharmacists, and patients to send AE reports into the companies or health authorities (without remuneration) and on the goodwill and competence of the data analysts.

It is most sensitive in the following instances:

- The signal is very unusual and rarely seen in general, e.g., aplastic anemia;
- The signal is rarely seen with that drug class (pulmonary fibrosis with beta-blockers, e.g., practolol);
- The signal is rarely seen in that cohort of patients, e.g., cataracts in young non-diabetic patients;
- The signal is fatal, particularly in patient groups who classically do not have high mortality rates, e.g., deaths in 20-year-olds;
- The signal is expected to be seen because it has been reported in other drugs in the same class, e.g., rhabdomyolysis with a new statin;
- The signal is expected because it is due to an exaggeration of the drug's pharmacologic effect, e.g., syncope in patients taking an antihypertensive;

- The AE in question is seen almost exclusively with drugs, e.g., fixed drug reaction;
- The causality is crystal clear, e.g., the tablet is large and sticky and gets stuck in the oral pharynx, producing obstruction; or when immediate swelling and itching is seen at the site of a drug being injected;
- No other drugs, OTC products, neutraceuticals are being taken by the patient(s) in question;
- The drug is being taken for a short time, and there are no or few confounders;
- The patients are otherwise healthy and have no other medical problems beyond the one being treated with the drug in question;
- There is a positive rechallenge, i.e., reaction reappears upon drug reintroduction after a positive dechallenge; same pharmaceutical form and same dosage);
- The AE is different from the signs, symptoms, and problems seen with the disease being treated and would not be confused with the disease itself.

It is less sensitive when:

- The signal has a high background incidence in the general population, e.g., headaches, fatigue;
- The signal has a high background incidence in the population being treated, e.g., myocardial infarctions in middle aged hypertensive smokers;
- The signal represents a worsening of the problem being treated, e.g., fialuridine's effect, producing worsening and fatal hepatitis in patients being treated for hepatitis;
- The patients are taking multiple drugs, e.g., polypharmacy, intensive care unit;
- The patients have major underlying medical problems producing disease, signs, and symptoms, e.g., oncology patients;
- The drug is taken chronically, and many intercurrent illnesses and problems occur over time, i.e., confounders interfere with interpretation;
- There is a negative dechallenge, i.e., the reaction continues even after stopping drug, or the drug in question is not stopped in the patient and the AE disappears by itself anyway.

Increased Frequency

This is a technique that has been on-again, off-again. It has been in favor and out of favor. It basically relies on a statistical calculation of reporting frequency in the current period versus a previous period (e.g., 1Q2020 versus 1Q2019) to see if there is an increase in reporting of a particular AE. The technique is easy to do, and can be computerized and run for all reported AEs in the database for a drug. It has, in practice, turned out to be not very useful. Although signals are, by definition, generated by this process (some AEs go up, i.e., are more frequent and, thus, represent a signal, some go down, and some remain the same). However, increased frequency calculations have, in general, turned out to be false alarms or meaningless, or were easily picked up by other means. Note that some potential confounders, e.g., certain background events such as symptoms of seasonal allergies, may vary over time and could impact assessments of increased (or decreased) frequency.

Nonetheless, it is recommended that frequency analyses be done in PSURs. See: EU GVP Module VII, which indicates that examples of new signals would include an "identified risk for which a higher frequency or severity of the risk is newly found (e.g., in an indicated subpopulation)". The US Food and Drug Administration (FDA) also required frequency analysis until 1997 in its NDA periodic reports, but ended that because it was found to be of little practical use. The FDA has, however, in the draft post-marketing regulations published in 2003 ("The Tome"), FDA proposed reinstating its use. The FDA has also recently asked that frequency analyses be done in clinical trials to see whether an SAE's occurrence (incidence) is rising.

Data Mining

This term is used, sometimes somewhat pejoratively, to describe various automated or semi-automated techniques that generate signals from existing, large, post-marketing databases. These techniques use raw case report data and arrays of drug-AE combinations to calculate "expected" versus "observed" numbers or reporting rates (not frequencies), and use observations of excess reporting as signals. Various techniques exist, including proportional reporting rate (PRR), gamma poisson shrinker (GPS), urn-model algorithm, reporting odds ratio (ROR), Bayesian confidence propagation neural network-information component (BCPNN-IC), adjusted residual score (ARS), and others. These techniques attempt to extract signals that are not obvious using global introspection. Some feel that this is a largely futile exercise since spontaneous reports are "dirty" data with unknown and unknowable numerators and denominators and one cannot "make a silk purse out of a sow's ear".

However, much work is being done on making better use of "dirty" data. One example of a success is called fractional or proportional reporting rates (PRR), also known as "disproportion" reporting rates or "signals of disproportionate reporting (SDRs)":

For each AE, the calculation of the proportion of that AE as a function of all AEs reported for a drug is calculated and compared with the proportion of that AE for all other drugs in the database. This essentially involves running large numbers of 2 × 2 tables, organized as just described (see Table 1).

For example, liver failure for drug X was reported 95 times out of the 1,418 total AEs for drug X. For the entire AE database of all drugs (except drug X), the score of liver failure was, for example, found to be 2,243/41,540 = 0.054.

So, liver failure with drug X is seen with a proportion (or "score", "statistic", "disproportion", or PRR) of 1.24 (that is, 24% more liver failure with drug X compared to the rest of the drugs in the database).

Table 1. Calculation of a Signal of Disproportionate Reporting for Liver Failure Demonstrated Using Mock Data.

	Drug X	All Other Drugs
Liver Failure	95	2,243
All Other AEs	1,418	41,540

Calculation
(95/1418) / (2243/41540) = 1.24
0.067/0.054 = 1.24

Is this a signal? In theory it is, since the proportion is higher than for other drugs. But at only 24%, this is somewhat small if other AEs show a proportion of 200% or 400%. If the proportion of the AE for the drug in question was the same as the proportion for the whole database, the number would be 1.00. This means that the same reporting rate for liver failure is seen with drug X and the rest of the drugs in the database. If there were proportionally fewer liver cases with drug X, the score would be <1.00. Does this mean that drug X actually protects against this AE? In theory, this is the logical extension of this line of reasoning, but it would take much more than this to think there is a therapeutic effect (of sorts) to prevent this AE.

The level at which one considers a signal to be generated could be chosen as anything >1.00, although this will probably produce many false positives. In practice, one might take a high score above, say, 2.0 or more before one starts considering these to be signals. If one does this for all 80,000 or so MedDRA® terms, then one might expect about 40,000 signals (values >1.0) if the distribution was random. This is obviously not practical. Alternatively, one might look at the top 10 or 20 scores. Nevertheless, such an option is strongly debatable as we could miss or not assess signals which could also be important. The purpose is actually to manage all signals and not a predetermined number of signals. Another technique would be to use more complicated filters such as a PRR >3 and a chi-squared test >5 and more than three cases with the drug in question. Whatever approach is used, it should be documented and results should be archived along with the interpretation and disposition.

It is also useful to look at the scores periodically to see whether a particular AE is increasing. That is, it is becoming more disproportionate over time and, thus, may represent a stronger signal. However, there may be other explanations, such as media stimulation of reporting.

To be useful, the database must be reasonably large (though it is hard to say how large). If additional cases are needed to expand the database, it is possible to review redacted cases from the FDA FAERS database, the Health Canada safety database, the MHRA interactive Drug Analysis Profiles (iDAP, formerly Drug

Analysis Prints) reports, and the EMA EudraVigilance database (required by legislation). There may be significant logistical issues in uploading or manually entering cases from these databases into another database. There are many other issues that may make this technique less useful. The other drugs, patients, diseases, and characteristics of the rest of the database should be similar to that of the drug in question. An extreme example would be studying injection site reactions for drug X compared to the rest of the drugs in the database, none of which is given by injection. There would be no injection site reactions for tablets. Or more subtly, if the drug in question is given mainly to elderly diabetics, comparing it to the AE pattern of other drugs given to children would similarly not be very meaningful.

Even if these data mining methods become part of the signal detection process, it should be kept in mind that a statistical link on reported ICSRs does not mean there is a drug-induced causal relationship.[3]

Various data mining techniques are also described in FDA's 2005 Guidance on Good Pharmacovigilance Practices (see below). A comprehensive assessment of various techniques is in "Practical Aspects of Signal Detection in Pharmacovigilance", Report of the CIOMS Working Group VIII (2010, CIOMS, Geneva. ISBN: 9290360828).

As in other areas of drug development, it is expected that AI will introduce changes and (hopefully) improvements in signaling. Generative AI uses extremely large databases and may aid in signal analysis. However, not all Generative AI systems are attached to the internet meaning that the databases are not using new data. It is also not clear if adverse event data are being included in the large databases. Since we are in the very early stages of AI applications, pharmacovigilance personnel should pay attention to new developments and tools being developed in the AI world.

[3]For further details, see Evans, Waller, Davis, Use of proportional reporting ratios for signal generation from spontaneous adverse drug reaction reports, *Pharmacoepidemiol Drug Safety* 2001; 10: 483–486. A comparison of different techniques and thresholds is found in Hochberg, Hauben M, Pearson RK, *et al.*, An evaluation of three signal-detection algorithms using a highly inclusive reference event database, *Drug Safety* 2009; 32(6): 509–525; Deshpande, Gogolak, Weiss Smith, Data mining in drug safety: review of published threshold criteria for defining signals of disproportionate reporting, *Pharm Med* 2010; 24(1): 37–43.

■ Other Sources of Signal Data

Information should be obtained, as appropriate, from sources other than spontaneous reports. Other sources include non-clinical study data, such as *in vitro*, toxicology and pharmacology data, including animal data, the medical and scientific literature, clinical trial data (not all of which may be found in the drug safety data base — non-serious trial AEs are not routinely kept in drug safety's database), external databases (FDA, UMC, etc.), product quality complaints and manufacturing deviations, regulatory authority comments in PSURs or direct communications to the company, and so on. If a Risk Management Plan (RMP) or REMS is in place, signaling should be done with this in mind.

■ Putting It All Together

After data have been found from all the sources noted above (ICSRs, aggregate data, data mining, solicited cases, etc.), the results should be tabulated, reviewed, and "triaged" to determine which findings deserve further consideration now and which go into a "holding box" waiting for more data. This is highly dependent on experience and medical judgment, i.e., there is no precise formula to determine which signals should be investigated rapidly and aggressively and which can sit. Some factors to consider include whether the drug is widely used, whether the signal in question is serious/severe or not, whether the patients are seriously ill, whether the problem is reversible, whether the investigation is easily done, whether the outcome of the investigation can be known in a shortish time rather than years, whether there is health authority or other external pressure (e.g., publicity, Internet activity), and (probably unfortunately) monetary cost.

Organizational Team

Each organization, both drug companies and health authorities, needs to have a formal team with the remit of evaluating safety data and managing safety signals. This is usually a multidisciplinary team that reviews, analyzes, and may also make recommendations on signals. It may be empowered to make decisions or it may function to deliver data and multiple action choices to more senior management personnel. Members include physicians and healthcare personnel from drug safety, epidemiology, clinical research/development, regulatory affairs, biostatistics, quality, risk management, legal (sometimes), pharmacology/toxicology (sometimes), manufacturing (sometimes), and others as needed, including external subject-matter experts. Marketers and sales personnel should not be on the team.

This team should be led by a PV representative and must deliver output against goals, specifying how they will be achieved. Strong safety signal governance is essential because a periodic update on signal management is required in each PSUR/PBRER. To do so, specific tools, means, and processes must be developed; *ad hoc* expertise and skills must also be included in this team.

Signal Workup

Once the signal list has been prepared, the list needs to be prioritized for workup according to the criticality of the signals, i.e., potential to impact the benefit–risk assessment, and the resources available. Of course, lack of resources is never an acceptable excuse for not working up a signal that is important to the public health. This will be an unacceptable reason with the HA (or in court!) for incomplete, inadequate, or slow signal workup, which jeopardizes public health. But realistically speaking, resources will play a role in prioritizing.

Prioritize

There are many ways to prioritize signals. Red, yellow, green is one way, or numerical priorities on a 1–5 scale are also used. Whatever method is chosen, though, it should be documented end-to-end and consistently used. Exceptions will not be well looked upon by inspectors.

Do an initial priority assessment. Highest priority should go to drugs that are new, where the AEs are serious or severe, where there are tampering or counterfeiting issues, where the patient population is ill or apparently at high risk, where the drug is known to be toxic (or has a narrow therapeutic window), where many people use the drug, and to black triangle drugs (the designation in the EU labeling for a product that is subject to additional monitoring), etc. If a medicine is labelled with the black triangle, this is generally because there is less information available on it than on other medicines because it is new to the market or there is limited data on its long-term use. It does not mean that the medicine is unsafe. For better or worse, other issues also enter into prioritization, ones that are less related to public health, such as politics, sales volume, need to "protect" the drug, adverse publicity, showing due diligence in tracking, and others.

Conversely, drugs whose AE profile is mild and where few adverse consequences on the public health are seen or expected would have lower priority. Minor AEs of toxic drugs would probably fall somewhere in the middle of prioritization.

Although difficult to do, efficacy should also be taken into some account when deciding on initial prioritization. Drugs with minimal efficacy with potential new, severe AEs should have a higher priority. To put it another way, if the drug in question was "placebo" such that no efficacy was expected (forgetting placebo effects for the moment), then no AEs at all should be tolerated, and this drug would get a high priority for signal workup.

The CIOMS VIII Working Group suggests the following points to consider in prioritizing signals: medical significance (serious, irreversible, etc.), increasing PRR scores, an important public health impact, easily retrievable data elements, and temporal clustering. See "Practical Aspects of Signal Detection in Pharmacovigilance", Report of the CIOMS Working Group VIII (2010, CIOMS, Geneva. ISBN: 9290360828).

Arrange and Review

Next, the drugs in question should be arranged on a spreadsheet or put into a database. There are various ways to do this. Some suggestions are made here.

One may create an overall summary signaling spreadsheet and then a daughter spreadsheet for each drug/signal combination, e.g., one sheet for Drug X and elevated liver tests or another sheet for Drug Y and atrial arrhythmias. Cases or case series should be arranged on the sheet using a simple or augmented CIOMS II line-listing format, with "augmented" referring to adding additional data to the line listing, such as a brief narrative, clinical course, or causality (see below). Cases may be arranged by date, by seriousness, or by some other factor. Various software programs are available for useful and creative displays of the data (see below).

Next, it is often useful to do causality assessments. In many cases, this should be done again at the time of signal evaluation, even if the cases have an earlier causality from the investigator, reporter, company, or patient. Note that many companies do not do causality assessments on spontaneous reports on intake, as they are presumed to be possibly related by convention. Thus, causality on these cases should be done now. Hindsight, time, and new data may change the original causality determinations. There is no uniformly accepted international classification. Choose a system and stick to it, e.g., related, possibly related, weakly related, unrelated, insufficient information/unknown. Such categories are more useful for assessing serious reports from clinical trials, but, regardless, a yes or no determination must be made at the case level to factor into regulatory reporting: Either related or not related. Causality in signaling is much more nuanced.

Causality should be assigned to individual cases and to the group of cases as a whole. In a case series, no single case may be clearly due to the drug, but the weight of the evidence of the sum of the cases may strongly suggest a likely signal. FDA takes the position that, for clinical trials, it is usually not possible to assign causality on a single case, but rather a case series is required.

The signal should be assessed in terms of the following:

- Magnitude and seriousness of the reaction — public health risk;
- Demographics — age, gender, ethnic background, weight;
- Effect of exposure — duration and dose — changes in risk over time;
- Concomitant medications;
- Drug interactions;
- Comorbid conditions and other confounders;
- Biological plausibility;
- Available alternative treatments and therapies;
- Other issues, e.g., HA request for workup, publicity.

Next, each drug/signal combination should be assigned a signal level based on review of the cases and causalities. Be reasonable in terms of what constitutes a signal. Always keep in mind the benefit–risk balance: not all risks can be eliminated. One such classification is as follows:

- **Strong:** A series of well-documented cases with no alternative causes and ideally with at least one positive rechallenge, i.e., rechallenge criterion not applicable in, for example, irreversible adverse events, hepatotoxicity, etc.
- **Fairly strong:** A series of generally well-documented cases with few alternative causes and ideally at least one positive dechallenge.
- **Average:** A series of cases of variable quality.
- **Fairly weak:** A series of cases that have significant limitations regarding plausible temporal associations or for which there are likely alternative explanations.
- **Weak:** A series of cases that are generally incompletely documented, lack plausible temporal associations, or are generally explainable by alternative causes or similarly.

And then assign an action:

- A signal warranting immediate action to protect public health. These actions may be temporary (if the signal is ultimately determined to be unfounded) or permanent;
- Signal warranting intensive follow-up and further investigation in the form of a clinical trial, an epidemiologic trial, outside consultation, and so on;
- Signal warranting further investigation and follow-up of the current cases, e.g., for outcomes or to be reexamined in, e.g., 60 days;
- Weak signal: continue watching, i.e., no further action at this time;
- Not a signal: no further investigation needed.

The Workup

At this stage, the signals that have been chosen for workup should be so designated and the workup begun. Various steps that can be done include the following:

- Search for additional cases using the appropriate MedDRA terms (or SMQs) in the clinical trial database if some cases, e.g., non-serious clinical trial AEs, are also found in or have not been entered into the safety database;
- Search for similar or additional cases in external databases such as EMA's EudraVigilance database, Health Canada's database, FDA's FAERS database, and the FDA Potential Signals of Serious Risks listing:
  - Consider other databases that can be used for epidemiologic studies in addition to the spontaneous reporting databases noted in the previous bullet. These include Prescription Event Monitoring Databases (Drug Safety Research Unit in the United Kingdom), Linked Administrative Databases (US private healthcare databases), United Kingdom General Practice Research Database (GPRD), as well as specialized databases, such as teratology databases or disease-specific databases, e.g., cystic fibrosis, and governmental databases, e.g., Canadian provinces. The Organization Bridge to Data has a compilation of more than 90 worldwide databases with descriptions of their characteristics, allowing the user to find databases that may suit the signal workup. It may be useful to engage an expert in pharmacoepidemiology at this point to find the right databases and assist in designing the appropriate study.
  - Search out additional literature cases using PubMed, Google Scholar, or other search engines and databases. See if the signal is listed on FDA's potential signal database.
  - Consider reviewing the AE profiles and class effects of similar drugs in that class.
  - Consider more complex, time-consuming, and expensive procedures to validate, strengthen, or refute a signal, such as epidemiologic (observational) studies in large databases (e.g., claims databases), to detect or find rare AEs and obtain information in large patient populations (e.g., tens of millions of patients), targeted clinical trials, and large simple safety studies (LSSS).

The Conclusions and Next Steps

The reviewers should come to a conclusion or conclusions for recommendation to the decision maker or safety committee (see below). As noted, many classifications are available; pick one and stick to it. The conclusions classifications may be simpler perhaps along the lines of the following:

- **Red Signal–High Priority**: SAE previously unknown or unlabeled or inadequately labeled. Quality issues such as adulteration or contamination. This may be accompanied by media attention and public scrutiny despite having only weak or incompletely documented cases. If confirmed, will lead to a reevaluation of the benefit–risk analysis and likely a change in labeling, product withdrawal, and so on.
- **Yellow Signal–Medium Priority**: Further evaluation of the signal is required but the criteria of the Red category are not met. If confirmed, these signals are expected to lead to a change in the risk–benefit analysis and, thus, will require changes in the labeling/packaging in the AE section and possibly also in the indications, contraindications, warnings, and AE sections.
- **Green Signal–Low Priority**: AEs that are already known or labeled and felt not to be a significant safety problem. Signal investigation at this time may be minimal, deferred, or simply kept on a "watch list" looking for further case reports (if any) before re-evaluation. Workup now would not be a good use of resources.

  Note 1: Most signals can be managed by PV experts, with support from clinical, without support from others such as external consultants.
  Note 2: Signal tracking system: Depending on the number of signals to be managed, an IT tool can

be of added value. For pharmaceutical companies with a large portfolio, the number of signals can easily be in the hundreds. A specific IT system may facilitate periodic overviews for the Safety Committee and may help to manage and track any "open" safety signals. Links to relevant ICSRs can be a time and resource saving tool if available in this IT tool/database.

The Safety Committee

Following the prioritization and workup, a mechanism to conclude and act on the signals is needed. This may be a senior safety/risk management committee or it may be an individual (the chief medical officer, for example). Whatever mechanism is used, there must be a formal written procedure to review and adjudicate signals on a regular basis, as well as documentation of consensus decisions. There should be an empowered decision maker in the form of either a person or a committee. For emergency signals, the committee should be able to meet within 24 hours (or even sooner). In a pharmaceutical company, this could be a senior safety committee composed of the chief medical officer, chief safety officer (if not the same person), and heads or senior people from drug safety/pharmacovigilance, regulatory affairs, labeling, clinical research, the legal department, non-clinical toxicology/pharmacology, risk management, epidemiology, and other corporate subject matter experts as needed (e.g., formulations).

If the product is studied or marketed outside the home country, the needs of these countries must also be represented in the decision and action steps. The marketing and sales and similar departments should not, in general, be represented on this committee, as this must be a medical–public health decision. In occasional instances, outside expert consultants, as neutral as possible, given that they are paid consultants to the company, may be invited to join if appropriate. In a health authority, the committee structure should be constituted in a similar manner, with senior medical, toxicology, pharmacology, labeling, risk management, epidemiology, and legal subject-matter experts as well as any other members needed, depending on the structure of the health authority. Attention should also be paid to actions of other health authorities around the world.

The safety committee needs to come to conclusions about issues presented to it. It should never routinely request more data at successive meetings for a particular problem or use other bureaucratic mechanisms simply to delay a decision. Relevant data should be requested and rapidly obtained and decisions made. These decisions should be documented in minutes and archived.

The outcomes should consider the public health and risk management/minimization and what action steps, if any, need to be taken:

1. Label change, variation, and so forth, for marketed drugs (e.g., new ADR, warning, precaution, contraindication); dear doctor/healthcare professional letter; drug withdrawal and, if so, to what level (consumer, pharmacist, wholesaler); and communication plan to the health authorities, public, and healthcare professionals.
2. Further study and consultation regarding this signal.
3. If in clinical trials, stop or change studies to enhance patient protection, notification of the data monitoring committee and/or IRB, adjudication committee, changes in the investigator brochure, and informed consent.
4. Notification of the applicable health agencies (competent authorities) by phone, e-mail, or letter.
5. Other follow-up actions and further review by the committee latere.
6. Effect on the Risk Management/REMS program in place or, if one is not in place, whether to put one in place rapidly. If non-routine risk minimization tools are required, they should be the least burdensome on the healthcare system that will accomplish the goal of the plan.
7. Mechanisms to handle the public announcement and any issues that might arise from that, including legal actions and adverse publicity.
8. If a REMS or RMP is in place, the signal should be considered in context with the plan. It may be necessary to revise, change, or update the plan in consultation with the relevant health authorities. Metrics on effectiveness of tools should be applied at pre-determined periodicity.

9. Either inside or separate from the plan, it may be necessary to take further risk minimization actions, keeping in mind the potential impact on the healthcare system.
10. Recall, withdrawal, etc.

When the committee is in a health agency, depending on legal responsibilities and regulations, the committee needs to decide on label changes, withdrawal, and study cessation in the same manner as noted above for companies. All stakeholders should be engaged in the process.

For an excellent review of signaling, see *Practical Aspects of Signal Detection in Pharmacovigilance*, Report of the CIOMS Working Group VIII (2010, CIOMS, Geneva. ISBN: 9290360828).

■ Computerized Tools for Signal Detection and Workup

Several companies now produce software or tools that can be used as add-ons to a drug safety or clinical trial database. These programs allow for graphic displays, tables, cross-references, lumping, splitting, and various other ways to look at data. They are useful for large numbers of cases when "eye-balling" the data is not feasible. The programs allow for aggregate charts or displays of data in which hyperlinks allow the reviewer to click on a bar, point, or line and see the cases that lie behind that data point. Thus, one can look at a chart of the most frequent SAEs and then click to see the cases either as a case series or as individual case data. *Ad hoc* queries and analyses can be done, such as analyses by age, sex, comeds, diagnosis, and so forth. One can focus only on outliers or particular AEs. Comparisons over time, with different drugs and other sorts of comparisons, can be made. Obviously, this is data-dependent. If there is little data, no comparative data, or incomplete data, the tool cannot really help.

These systems vary but functions found in these tools include a drug profile portal to document and track issues and potential signals with built-in workflow and using various statistical methods, including empirical Bayesian geometric means, relative ratios, proportional reporting, logistic regression, Bayesian multi-item gamma Poisson shrinker (MGPS), and Kaplan–Meier plots, drill down into the data to the patient level, "what if" scenarios, and so forth. Most can be used for clinical trial data and safety data from different databases. Imports of FDA FAERS and other external database information are also possible in most cases. There are several commercially available products to facilitate this.

■ Key Documents on Signaling and Good PV Practices

FDA Guidance on Good Pharmacovigilance Practices of 3/2005

In March 2005, the FDA (Center for Drug Evaluation and Research and Center for Biologics Evaluation and Research) released a Guidance for Industry entitled, *Good Pharmacovigilance Practices and Pharmacoepidemiologic Assessment*. This is an excellent document (though several years old now) and summarizes the FDA's thinking on the topic. It also, to a large degree, reflects current practices in the industry. It references three guidances initially issued in draft form in May 2004 and finalized in May 2005:

1. Premarketing Risk Assessment;
2. Development and Use of Risk Minimization Plans (RiskMAP Guidance); and
3. Good Pharmacovigilance Practices and Pharmacoepidemiologic Assessment.

Note that many of the items in these guidance documents have been changed or superseded by the 2007 PDUFA/FDAAA, such as the change from RiskMAPs to REMS. Nonetheless, these documents are still well worth reading, as their concepts remain the same. Key parts of good pharmacovigilance practices document concerning signaling are as follows:

- Identifying and describing safety signals: From case report to case series;

- Case reports. The FDA recommends that sponsors make a reasonable attempt to get complete information for case assessment during initial and follow-up contacts. Companies should use trained healthcare practitioners. If the report is from a consumer, consent should be sought for follow-up contact with the healthcare practitioner. The most aggressive efforts should be directed at SAEs, particularly those not previously known to occur with the drug.
- Case series. After an initial post-marketing spontaneous case report is found, additional similar cases should be sought in the sponsor's database, the FDA FAERS database, published literature, and other databases. Cases should be evaluated and followed up for additional information where needed and where possible. Of importance are data that would support or reject a causal association with the drug. Although the FDA notes that there is no internationally agreed-on causality classifications, they do note that probable, possible, and unlikely have been used. Cases with confounders should be analyzed too and not routinely excluded. A grading scale is useful in working up a signal, although for regulatory reporting of Individual cases, the causality decision is binary: either related or not.
- After such a review, the cases that support the signal's further investigation should be summarized in a table or other manner to describe the important clinical characteristics.
- The FDA refers to the use of data-mining techniques, but notes that their use "is not a required part of a signal identification or evaluation".
- The FDA then gives guidance as to which signals should be further evaluated: new unlabeled serious AEs; an apparent increase in the severity of a labeled event; occurrence of serious AEs that are extremely rare in the general population; new drug–drug, drug–food, or drug–dietary supplement interactions; identification of a previously unrecognized at-risk population; confusion about a product name, label, package, or use; concerns about product usage, e.g., use at higher-than-labeled doses; concerns that the current risk management plan is not adequate; or "other".
- Calculation of reporting rates. In a somewhat controversial section, the FDA recommends that the applicant calculate the crude AE reporting rates using the number of reported cases of that signal AE in the United States as the numerator and the estimate of US patient exposure (as patients or patient-time) as the denominator. Where feasible, the reporting rates over time or versus similar products or drug classes or versus estimates of the background rate for this even in the general population may be useful. The FDA does warn, however, that these figures are generally used for exploratory purposes or for hypothesis generation. They note that reporting rates are not incidence rates. In practice, use of these figures is fraught with danger. The numerator is bad because there is always underreporting of an unknown degree; the denominator is worse because it is hard to know how many patients truly took the drug (as opposed to filling the prescription) and for how long. Thus, the ratio is often meaningless. A high reporting rate may suggest that the signal is real, but a low reporting rate does not exonerate the drug.

Investigating a Signal

- **Pharmacoepidemiologic studies are cited by the FDA.** There are various types of non-randomized trials that can be done, including cohort (prospective or retrospective), case-control, nested case-control, and others. They can be done at any time (before or after marketing), although they are often done after a signal has been suggested by post-marketing adverse events. The FDA suggests that bias be minimized and that confounding be accounted for. They also suggest that "it is always prudent to conduct more than one study, in more than one environment and even use different designs".
- **Registries.** The FDA defines a registry as "an organized system for the collection, storage, retrieval, analysis and dissemination of information on individual persons exposed to a specific medical intervention who have either a particular disease, a condition (e.g., a risk factor) that predisposes [them] to the occurrence of a health-related event, or prior exposure to substances (or circumstances)

known or suspected to cause adverse health effects". A control or comparison group should be included where possible.

- **Surveys.** Without clearly defining surveys, the FDA recommends that they be done when information gathering is needed. For pharmacoepidemiologic studies, registries, and surveys, the FDA encourages consultation with the agency before beginning.

Interpreting a Signal

The FDA recommends that the sponsor conduct a case level/case series review, using data mining and calculating reporting rates where feasible. Then the sponsor should consider a further study to establish whether a safety risk exists.

When the applicant believes an important safety risk is possible, a synthesis of all information should be prepared and submitted to the FDA, including the following:

- Cases (spontaneous and literature) with exposure information;
- The background rate for the event in general and the specific patient population(s);
- Relative risks, odds ratios, or other pharmacoepidemiology study results;
- Biologic effects from animal work and pharmacokinetic and dynamic studies;
- Safety data from controlled clinical trials;
- General marketing experience with similar products.

The applicant should provide an assessment of the risk-to-benefit balance for the population as a whole and for at-risk groups (if any). The FDA notes that this is an iterative process, and not all actions described in the guidance are done at all times. Proposals on further steps should also be provided along with risk minimization actions. The FDA then makes its own judgment based on the data.

The FDA recommends that applicants develop and continually reevaluate their risk management plans. In some cases, post-marketing reporting of spontaneous AEs will suffice. In other situations, much more may be needed. The FDA notes it may bring potential safety risks to its Drug Safety and Risk Management Advisory Committee or the specific advisory committee dealing with the product in question.

These actions described above represent a careful, step-by-step, well-planned proposal for investigating a signal that allows a thoughtful and logical response to a signal. In many and probably most situations, especially those for non-serious signals or drugs not in the public eye, this process unfurls as described above. However, for situations that make the public eye, e.g., Vioxx, Fen-Phen, the pressures to act before all the evidence is in or assessed are enormous.

Signal review does not occur in a vacuum. Multiple influences play a role as follows:

- Changes in personnel in the company or the regulator may cause loss of continuity in a signal investigation;
- Publicity from consumer groups, the media, patient advocacy groups, and other companies, some of which may be premature or unnecessarily scary and inflammatory;
- Lawsuits;
- Actions by other health agencies outside your jurisdiction;
- The time needed to prepare and carry out whatever actions are proposed, such as registries, studies, data mining, and surveys;
- Further spontaneous reports or lack thereof during the investigation ("Oh no, we just got another case!");
- Pressures from various areas to continue marketing or to stop marketing;
- Extreme positions based on little data;
- Sponsor marketing and financial pressures (lost market and money);
- Pressures on the regulatory agencies (legislatures, companies, consumer groups, media);
- Pressure to do interim analyses or to stop ongoing trials (often for different indications) of the drug in question, which may jeopardize the integrity of the study;
- Privacy and data protection issues.

In addition, the points of view ("agendas") of the protagonists in the drama are clearly different in many regards, although everyone really does want to protect the public health and not hurt people. The following are the points of view using some of the language each group might use to make its case:

- The company wishes to protect its (enormous) investment in a product that took years to develop and to market and that is paying the salary of hundreds or thousands of employees. A "handful" of not clearly proven cases with causality in doubt should not be made public and should not be allowed to "destroy" the drug before the full scientific and medical investigations are completed. The drug is clearly helping the "vast majority" of the patients using it, and the possible occurrence of AEs (even serious ones) should not deprive the rest of the public of the product. Because the drug has a finite life, i.e., patent expiration, the company believes it must protect it as much as possible. The investigation of the signal should be done in private without release of the "debate" to the public. Even if the drug is totally exonerated after the signal investigation, there is usually lost market share and harm to the product. Within the company, no one wants to be the one to "kill the drug", because this can be a career-ending and a stock price-destroying event. Lawsuits will doubtless follow (often no matter what the result of the signal investigation), and the personal and financial liability can be enormous. When lawsuits occur, employees move into defensive mode, spending more and more time with attorneys. In summary, the company will, of course, do the right thing, but only when the data are in and the science is clear. It will not act prematurely.
- The regulatory authority wishes to protect the public health as its primary goal. It wants to do this as early as possible to minimize the risk to the public. Better to err on the side of patient protection than to allow a toxic product to stay on the market (or remain inadequately labeled) for too long, particularly when therapeutic alternatives are available. The agency cannot appear to be too cavalier with the data or to "be in the pocket of the drug companies". It is also far easier to take the position against the "big bad drug companies". In some sense, the drug should be considered guilty until proven innocent. *Primum non nocere* ("Above all do no harm") is an aphorism originally attributed to the ancient Greek physician Galen, but it more likely arose in the seventeenth century. If something bad happens in the US, the Congress, the Secretary of the Department of Health and Human Services, the media, and the consumer groups will attack the companies and the FDA unmercifully.
- With various watchdogs in action, e.g., www.drugwatch.com, more data (much unconfirmed and incomplete) will be released earlier. This will both help the agency protect itself and get the information before the public, but it will also change the shape of the investigation and diminish the use of the drug, perhaps prematurely.
- Consumers want totally safe and totally effective drugs with no risk (and often for free). When bad things occur (because the companies are suspected of withholding data or did not do their job or the FDA may have acted too quickly and did not do its job), someone is at fault and someone must pay and be punished. All data should be available, and the entire process should be transparent. In general, better to err on the side of stopping the use of the drug than continuing its sale and use. And drugs are, indeed, guilty until proven innocent. However, this calculus may be different for products with much competition versus a truly unique product that treats an otherwise unmet medical need.
- The media are delighted when the spectacle plays out, especially with data dribbling out over time and errors with alleged misdeeds by the company or the FDA surfacing. The more sensational, the more errors or inappropriate or illegal actions, the more individuals hurt, the more stonewalling, the more the story captivates the public, moving into websites, and blogs, paywalls and TV time.
- For competing pharmaceutical companies, there are mixed feelings. Clearly, what is happening to another company could happen closer to home at any time, too, with one of their products. However, the competitors are not unhappy if more patients now switch to their drugs rather than using the competitor product that is undergoing a signal investigation. And finally, there is an element of

Schadenfreude (from the German meaning "pleasure taken from someone else's misfortune") that is common in human nature.

All of this suggests that, rather than thinking of the signal investigation process as a careful, rational, well-planned program done in a timely and deliberate manner, one should rather think of the process, for dramatic or serious issues, as the "fog of war", with multiple pressures (some known and some unknown to each player) acting to force rapid and urgent "action" to protect the public.

The consequences of whatever action is taken may have far-reaching and irreversible effects. Drugs that are withdrawn rarely return to the market even if the signal has subsequently been disproven. Label changes adding a new safety warning, AE, or other are rarely taken out of the label even if disproven. The change in medical practice to the use of different drugs (which may be more or less expensive, available, effective, safe, etc.) is similarly hard to reverse.

EU GVP Module IX — Signal Management (2012: Revision 1, Delivered Nov 2017)

This GVP module:

- Provides general guidance and requirements on scientific and quality aspects of signal management; and
- Describes roles, responsibilities and procedural aspects in the setting of the EU signal management process overseen by the Pharmacovigilance Risk Assessment Committee (PRAC).

> "This module is applicable to medicinal products for human use authorized in the EU irrespective of the authorization procedure (centralized or national procedure, including mutual recognition and decentralized)."
>
> "Unless stated otherwise, the guidance provided in the Module applies to all organizations involved in signal management, i.e., marketing authorization holders, national competent authorities and the European Medicines Agency (the "Agency")."
>
> "Individual organizations may follow alternative signal management processes and terminology but should encompass the general principles outlined in this module."
>
> "An addendum to this module, the GVP Module IX Addendum I, describes methodological aspects of signal detection from spontaneous reports of suspected adverse reactions."

The EU signal management process includes the following activities:

- **Signal detection:** To look for or identify signals from any source (spontaneous and/or clinical trials ICSRs, post-marketing studies, publications, large database analysis such FAERS, EudraVigilance, etc.) and inform concerned competent authorities (a 1-year pilot involving MAH evaluation of EudraVigilance data is conducted starting in 2018);
- **Signal validation:** Process to conclude that the available information to support or refute a new potentially causal association;
- **Signal confirmation:** Endorsement of the signal by the PRAC for further work-up;
- **Signal analysis and prioritization:** Process to identify signals suggesting a potentially important impact on patients or the public health or which may significantly affect a product's risk-benefit balance;
- **Signal assessment:** Further evaluation taking into account all available evidence, to determine new risks or whether known risks have changed;
- **Recommendation for action by the MAH:** May include, but not limited to, Product Information update, additional risk minimization measures, Direct Healthcare Professional Communication (DHPC).

The description of the MAH signal management process must be included in the Pharmacovigilance System Master File. Its performance must be kept under control (KPIs and Governance). Within each MAH organization, the signal detection and management process is under the full responsibility of the EU QPPV; the EMA and/or the PRAC address questions and requests directly to the EU QPPV without involving other teams (Regulatory Affairs, for instance).

The EU QPPV is responsible for ensuring management of emerging safety issues (safety issue considered by the MAH to require urgent attention because of the potential major impact on the risk–benefit balance and/or on patients' or public health, and the potential need for prompt regulatory action and communication to patients and healthcare professionals). Such issues are to be reported to the concerned EU competent authorities on an urgent basis.

Any signal, validated by an EU competent authority or provided to the Agency by the MAH, must be confirmed (or not) within 30 days by the PRAC. It is then entered into the European Pharmacovigilance Issues Tracking Tool (EPITT) and requires further analysis and prioritization by the PRAC.

Depending on the signal, various recommendations can be delivered by the PRAC (non-exhaustive list) are as follows:

- MAH
    - Request for additional data;
    - Review of additional data in the next PSUR/PBRER;
    - Update of the product information (labeling);
    - Submit an RMP or update the RMP;
    - Add risk minimization measures to the current RMP;
    - Sponsor a post-authorization safety study.
- Health Authority
    - Collect further information and/or perform additional analysis (national Agency or EMA);
    - Consult other EMA scientific committees or expert groups;
    - Initiate an MAH inspection.

Note: Figures detailing the process to be followed by each stakeholder (MAH, National Agency, EMA, PRAC, CHMP, CMDh, etc.) are appended to GVP Module IX.

The following documents provide additional guidance relevant to signal management:

- Report of CIOMS Working Group VIII on Practical Aspects of Signal Detection in Pharmacovigilance;
- SCOPE Work Package 5 — Signal Management — Best Practice Guide;
- EMA Questions & Answers on Signal Management;
- Screening for Adverse Reactions in EudraVigilance.

Further expectations for the signal management process have been outlined by EMA in "Questions & answers on signal management" (2016, EMA/261758/2013 Rev 2-Corr 2), Question 3, and are as follows:

> "The signal management process consists of detection, validation, confirmation, analysis and prioritization, assessment and recommendation for action."
>
> "Signal detection is the act of looking for and/or identifying signals using data from any source. Signal detection usually involves a combination of statistical methods and review of individual case safety reports, as well as any relevant source of information (e.g., scientific literature)."
>
> "Signal validation is the process of evaluating the data supporting the detected signal in order to verify that the available documentation contains sufficient evidence demonstrating the existence of a new potentially causal association or a new aspect of a known association, and therefore justifies further analysis. The clinical significance of the signal, its previous awareness, the biological and temporal plausibility and any relevant sources of information supporting the association are taken into consideration. Signals validated by the EMA or Member States are entered in the European Pharmacovigilance Issues Tracking Tool (EPITT). EPITT is a database developed by the EMA to promote the communication of pharmacovigilance and risk management issues between the EMA and Member States. Signals for which the validation

process was not supportive of a new potentially causal association, or a new aspect of a known association, are not entered in EPITT."

"Signal confirmation means communication via EPITT, within 30 days of its receipt by the Rapporteur, the lead Member State or a national competent authority that the validated signal is confirmed or not confirmed. Any confirmed signal should be analyzed and prioritized by the Pharmacovigilance Risk Assessment Committee (PRAC)."

"Signal analysis and prioritization are performed by taking into account the potential impact of the signal on the benefit–risk profile of the involved medicine(s). The prioritization dictates the time frame for the subsequent steps of the evaluation of the signal."

"Signal assessment is the scientific evaluation of all the evidence available, including additional data from MAHs, where applicable."

"The steps of analysis, prioritization and assessment result in a PRAC recommendation."

The EMA Q&A document contains additional stakeholder questions on safety signal management and EMA responses to those questions. The document is based on an earlier Q&A document prepared by MHRA. There is practical information on PRAC evaluation of signals and, in addition to the above-captioned documents, is well worth reading.

These are the questions posed in the EMA Q&A document:

1. What is the legal basis for signal management in the European Union (EU)?
2. What is a safety signal?
3. What are the steps of the signal management process?
4. Who is involved in the signal management process?
5. What should MAHs do if they detect a signal?
6. Which medicinal products can be concerned by a signal?
7. When and how are MAHs informed that a signal for their medicinal product is being investigated by the PRAC?
8. How does the PRAC prioritize signals?
9. What could be the PRAC recommendation?
10. Where are the PRAC recommendations on signals published?
11. When and how are MAHs informed that additional data are requested?
12. Are additional data requested of all MAHs with a marketing authorization for a medicinal product concerned by the signal?
13. Can MAHs submit additional data on a voluntary basis?
14. How and to whom shall MAHs submit their responses?
15. Who is the contact point for MAHs within the regulatory network?
16. What are the timelines for assessment of additional data by the PRAC?
17. Do MAHs receive the assessment report (AR) on the data submitted?
18. What should MAHs do if the PRAC recommends a variation to their marketing authorization?

As noted earlier, it is likely that AI will introduce major changes and (hopefully) improvements in the field of signaling. Watch this space.

Frequently Asked Questions

Q: Again, why would anyone want to work in drug safety for a living?

A: For many reasons. Signal detection, analysis, and management usually present a fascinating exercise requiring medical, investigative, tactical, logical, and political skills. One really is acting to help the public health. Most signals, perhaps the vast majority, are rather unextraordinary and non-serious and can be worked up in a thoughtful and timely manner. In these instances, it is very satisfying. Similarly, even in the dramatic instances, the right thing usually does end up being done, and that also is quite satisfying. The probability of a horror scenario is less likely, but that is the risk one takes in this business. As with signaling (and most of life), it all boils down to a benefit-to-risk analysis.

Q: Should the companies try to find signals before the health authorities? If the FDA or the EMA picks up the signal before the company, isn't that a "failure" on the part of the company?

A: This is not a contest in which the fastest pick-up wins. The goal is bettering the public health. Sometimes the company picks up the signal first; sometimes the agencies do. Often, the health agencies see more data than the companies and often the agencies see the safety profile of similar drugs in that class. Also, when particularly gnarly safety concerns arise, regulators have agreements to share information across jurisdictions and they regularly do so. They may thus, have a broader overview and their case series may be more complete than that of the companies. What may be a weak signal to the company may be seen in many or all of the drugs in the class, making it a much stronger signal. Drug safety is tough enough as it is; don't beat yourself up any more than necessary!

CHAPTER

26

Risk Assessment, Evaluation, Management, Mitigation, & Strategy

Risk is a broad concept and applies to everything in life. We take risks when we drive a car, go to work, eat a meal, walk across the street, or take a drug. Benefit–risk management of drugs continuously evolves as a distinct science and is a very important function that aids the patient and healthcare professional, as well as the health authorities and drug companies, in decision-making. This chapter looks at risk, first from a global perspective, and then as applied to drug therapy in the United States with risk evaluation and mitigation strategies (REMS), and in the European Union with risk management plans (RMPs). We work on the presumption that the ongoing process of benefit-risk assessment will ultimately lead to decreased harm caused by products. This, in fact, remains to be seen. Of course, risks must always be considered in the context of a product's benefits.

■ Introduction

The ultimate goal for any new product when being developed, or already on the market, is to prove (and maintain through close and careful monitoring) that the benefit of the product outweighs the known or potential & perceived risks of that product. The benefit-risk assessment of a product for its proposed indication is a case-specific determination that requires a thorough assessment of the extensive evidence of safety and effectiveness submitted by a sponsor in an NDA or BLA (Biologic License Application)[i]. Broadly speaking, the process of "benefit-risk assessment" is making a judgment as to whether the expected benefits (with their uncertainties) of the product outweigh the potential risks (with their uncertainties and approaches to manage risks) associated with its expected use.

Benefit-Risk Assessment, Risk Assessment, Safety Assessment Planning, are all terms used to describe this life-cycle process and they can be done in a variety of ways depending on 1) the size of the company, 2) profile of the product, and 3) differences in regional expectations and requirements. Yes, that's right, the US proposes "one-way", the EU proposes "another", the Australian TGA "another", and so on. However, one will find that the primary intent and theory of this process is the same: Acknowledge and then monitor the known risks, document the perceived benefits, monitor for the unknown, then assess and report on the outcome and resulting actions to continuously protect the patient.

Finally, sponsors of new products and Marketing Authorization Holders of approved ones, must continously prove the benefits outweigh the risks, or they themselves with risk product refusal or withdrawal.

How is Risk Defined?

The concept of risk can be defined in many ways:

- Exposure to a possibility of loss or damage. The quantitative or qualitative possibility of loss that considers both the probability that something will cause harm and the consequences of that something.
- The probability of an adverse event resulting from the use of a drug in the dose and manner prescribed or labeled, or from its use at a different dose or manner, or in a patient or population for which the drug is not approved.
- The exposure to loss of money as a result of changes in business conditions, the economy, the stock and bond markets, interest rates, foreign currency exchange rates, inflation, natural disasters, and war.

However, a common understanding in the healthcare domain is that risk is a combination of the probability of occurrence of harm and the severity of that harm. We can think of risk as the harm or hazard itself. The US (United States) Food and Drug Administration (FDA) stated (May 1999), "Although marketed medical products are required to be safe, safety does not mean zero risk. A safe product is one that has *reasonable risks*, given the *magnitude of the benefit expected* and the *alternatives* available." In other words, the benefits of a medicine should outweigh its risks under the approved conditions of use.

Under the US FDA FD&C Act, for a new drug to be approved for marketing in the United States, the FDA must determine that the drug is safe and effective for use under the conditions prescribed, recommended, or suggested in the product's labeling.[1] The demonstration of effectiveness under this standard requires substantial evidence that the drug will have the effect it purports or is represented to have.[2,3] Because all products can have adverse effects, the demonstration of safety requires a showing that the benefits of the drug outweigh its risks.

For many years, the pharmaceutical world (as elsewhere) has been thinking about risk assessment, risk management, and risk minimization as important, interrelated disciplines. Several documents on risk management have been produced by various groups. Early documents included the US FDA draft guidances in 2003, the ICH (International Council for Harmonisation) E2E guideline finalized in 2005, and a European Medicines Agency (EMA) risk management guidance, also issued in 2005. The EU (European Union) guidance was followed in 2012 by GVP Module V — risk management systems, as subsequently revised (updated

[1] See section 505(d) of the FD&C Act. Under section 351 of the PHS Act (42 U.S.C. 262) licenses for biological products have been issued only upon a showing that the products are "safe, pure, and potent." Potency has long been interpreted to include effectiveness (21 CFR 600.3(s)). FDA has also generally considered "substantial evidence" of effectiveness to be necessary to support licensure

[2] See section 505(d) of the FD&C Act (21 U.S.C. 355(d)). The "substantial evidence" standard refers to both the quality and the quantity of the evidence that the drug will have benefit. See the May 1998 guidance for industry Providing Clinical Evidence of Effectiveness for Human Drug and Biological Products. The Agency has also published a draft guidance for industry on this topic entitled Demonstrating Substantial Evidence of Effectiveness for Human Drug and Biological Products (December 2019). When final, this guidance will represent the FDA's current thinking on this topic.

[3] Biological products are subject to provisions in both the FD&C Act as well as the PHS Act. Biologics license applications have to meet applicable requirements in the PHS Act to ensure the continued safety, purity, and potency of the product (see section 351 of the PHS Act; see also 21 CFR parts 600, 601, and 610).

in 2017), along with several versions of templates for formal risk management documents. Risk management during the life cycle of products is now the norm and is expected by FDA, EMA, and many other agencies. It is also expected by patients and other stakeholders.

The FDA has looked back on labeling changes in the United States over several years, and a striking finding is that safety label changes occur years and even decades after a drug has been approved as new safety issues are reported. For example, changes can occur at 50 or 60 years after approval even for such a commonly used and "well-known" drug as warfarin. Figure 1 from FDA illustrates label changes occurring after first approval. Note that the bulk of the changes occurred in the first 8 or 9 years but drug interactions, AEs (Adverse events) and other important safety issues can occur up to 60 years after approval.

Why Risk Management?

When a new drug first reaches the market, its safety profile is not well characterized. Why? Relatively few subjects have been studied in the clinical trials (especially with orphan drugs), and those who have been studied are usually patients with no other diseases, no or few co-medications, not too young or old, with stringent inclusion and exclusion criteria, relatively short duration of exposure, exclusion criteria and relatively short duration of exposure. These data are further constrained by statistical concerns associated with looking at multiple outcomes. Thus, "real-world" patients have not taken the drug yet, and rare adverse drug reactions (ADRs) have not been detected. It is only in the post-marketing arena, when large numbers of patients have taken the drug, that the safety profile is better characterized. It is only when data on compliance, use in patients with co-morbid conditions, and multiple other drugs (including over-the-counter, OTC (over the counter)), and diets are examined that the real-world safety profile develops. In addition, data from overdose, suicide attempts, unintended pregnancies, and lactation will add to the profile.

Until recently, the primary way to collect such data was from spontaneous reporting systems and periodic aggregate reports (periodic adverse drug experience reports (PADERs), Periodic Benefit-Risk Evaluation Report (PBRER or PSURs), and their various predecessors), and occasional post-marketing studies. Risk management was guided by regulator-approved labeling, but

Figure 1. **Distribution of 2,645 Changes in the US Package Insert for 1,601 Approved Product Applications, by Year After First FDA Approval (October 2002 to August 2005).[4]**

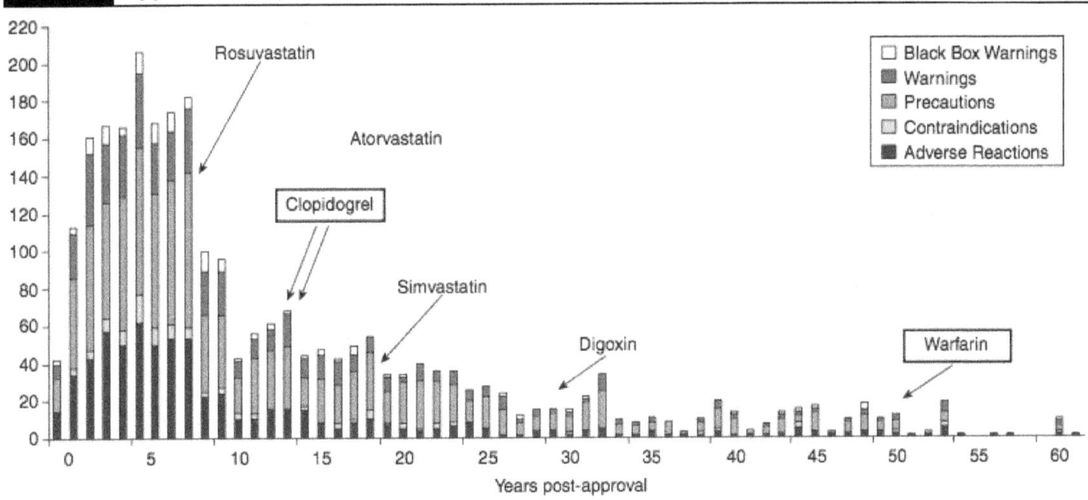

[4] Composition of Safety-Related Labeling for All Drug Products (changes made Oct 2002–Aug 2005, n = 2645 label changes for 1601 NDA/BLA entries)

Source: Modified from T Mullin, CDER (Center for Drug Evaluation and Research), Office of Planning and Analysis, OTS (Office of Translational Sciences) presentation, May 2009 (http//www.fda.gov/downloads/Drugs/DevelopmentApprovalProcess/DevelopmentResources/DrugInteractionsLabeling/UCM205986.pdf).

distinct risk management programs were not done in a formal sense. However, it is now the norm to conduct systematic risk management planning for every innovative product, and some regulatory jurisdictions require specific, detailed RMPs. Social media is now playing a larger and larger role in safety.

Multiple drivers have come into play in pharmacovigilance (PV) and risk management:

- Multiple major safety issues and product withdrawals have occurred: Fen-Phen, Propulsid, Rezulin, Vioxx, Bextra, Tysabri, Zelnorm, ranitidine (Zantac old formulation) and others.
- Rising liability costs from litigation and settlements, particularly in the US.
- The medical community was not happy with drug marketing and drug information.
- ADRs were perceived to be a major health risk, producing death, hospitalization, and significant morbidity. A meta-analysis noted that in 1994 more than 2 million hospitalized patients had serious ADRs and more than 100,000 died, making this the fourth or fifth leading cause of death in the United States.[5] Other publications from around the world noted similar findings.
- A public and media perception that drug companies were villainous, greedy, and cared little for public health and patient safety.
- The Internet, bloggers, social media, and other forums circulating stories, correct or not, on the harm of drugs. Artificial intelligence (AI) is the newest entry in the changes in pharmacovigilance.
- A perception that drug regulators were not doing their job because they allowed harmful drugs to reach the market too quickly.
- A perception that the agencies and industry were too closely aligned.
- Media stories highlighting gifts to physicians, slanted continuing medical education, paid speakers' bureaus, and multiple conflicts of interest.
- In addition, recent economic issues have brought risk management of money, cars, offshore oil wells, pharmaceuticals, Covid and many other activities in daily life into everyone's mind. One result has been that much of the world has become risk-averse (at least for now).

A consensus developed that risk prediction, evaluation, management, and minimization were not well understood and were rarely done and, when done, were done poorly. Better procedures for risk identification (signaling), characterization, mitigation/minimization, tracking, and communication were needed. And this was necessary for the entire life span of the product, not just immediately after marketing. It was thought that companies and health agencies (and in some cases other organizations) needed to be proactive, collect more and better data, put it into electronic databases that were able to "talk to each other", and from which data could easily be extracted for risk evaluation. The benefit–risk analysis (called by the pessimists the risk–benefit analysis) needed to be done in a serious, quantitative, and reproducible manner. It was also understood that the benefit–risk situation will change over the course of a drug's lifecycle and may differ from patient to patient, group to group, indication to indication.

The goals then became the following:

- Early and better detection of ADRs and characterization of the risk in various patients and settings.
- Development and harmonization of data standards and electronic transmission and storage.
- Better communication of known and unknown risks (i.e., important missing information).
- Minimization of morbidity and mortality, i.e., protect patient safety and the public health.

The US FDA

The FDA first published a document on its thinking in May 1999, entitled "Managing the Risks from Medical Product Use and Creating a Risk Management Framework". It addressed pre- and post-marketing risk management and the FDA's role. Further publications have extended and elaborated the FDA's position. However, this topic represents a continuously evolving area of

[5] Lazarou, Pomeranz, Corey, Incidence of ADRs in hospitalized patients, *JAMA* 1998; 279: 1200–1205.

policy and guidance, so stakeholders should review the FDA website on a regular basis for up to date information (www.fda.gov).

The FDA published three guidances for industry on risk management in 2005:

1. Pre-marketing risk assessment.
2. Development and use of risk minimization action plans (RiskMAPs).
3. Good pharmacovigilance practices and pharmacoepidemiologic assessment.

The first guidance, on pre-marketing risk assessment, focuses on measures companies might consider throughout all stages of clinical development of products. For example, a section on special safety considerations describes ways that risk assessment can be tailored for those products intended for use chronically or in children.

General recommended risk assessment strategies include long-term controlled safety studies, enrollment of diversified patient populations, and phase III trials with multiple-dose levels. Some key components of the guidance include the following:

- Providing specific recommendations to industry for improving the assessment and reporting of safety during drug development trials.
- Improving the assessment of important safety issues during registration trials and providing best practices for analyzing and reporting data that are developed as a result of a careful pre-approval safety evaluation.
- Building on (but not superseding) a number of existing FDA and International Council for Harmonization guidelines related to pre-approval safety assessments.

The other two FDA guidances have been superseded but are of historical interest. The RiskMAP guidance describes how industry can address specific risk-related goals and objectives. This guidance also suggests various tools to minimize the risks of drug and biologic products. This guidance has been superseded by the 2007 FDAAA (Food and Drug Administration Amendments Act) legislation that established REMS (see below).

The third guidance, on the post-marketing period, identifies recommended reporting and analytical practices to monitor the safety concerns and risks of medical products in general use.

Concepts espoused by FDA are that all products need full life-cycle risk management, including older and already marketed products. This is ordinarily accomplished by the FDA-approved Package Insert; all products are subject to routine risk minimization. However, some products (both new and old) may need specific risk minimization tools (or REMS) above and beyond routine post-marketing surveillance. The REMS must be tailored to the product and its known important and unknown risks (including missing information); it must be able to minimize a serious risk in a measurable, quantifiable way; and it must be modified if the risks are not minimized. In addition, effective communication methods play a major role in REMS.

From the FDA perspective, each REMS must include a goal to mitigate a specific important risk (or risks), and the tool(s) to accomplish the goal is generally communication of focused information on the specific serious risk(s) and the required non-routine activities, or both. In addition to the applicant and FDA, REMS may involve one or more stakeholders in the healthcare delivery system (e.g., healthcare providers, pharmacists, patients). Considered together, the REMS goal, communications, and other non-routine activities are intended to supplement routine risk minimization activities and make up the safety strategy.

Each REMS is designed to focus on a specific serious safety concern, and it is important to remember that a well-designed REMS is a means by which patients can have access to medications with serious risks that would otherwise not be available to them.

A key part of REMS is communication of the specific serious safety risk(s) that the REMS is intended to mitigate. The communication tools may be directed at healthcare providers or patients or both. Some REMS include requirements for clinical activities that healthcare providers must perform prior to prescribing or dispensing the medication to a patient.

The FDA may require companies submitting new drug applications (NDAs), abbreviated NDAs (ANDAs), and biologics license applications (BLAs) to submit a REMS if FDA "determines that such a strategy is necessary to ensure that the benefits of the drug outweigh the risks of the drug". A company may voluntarily submit a proposed REMS if it believes that a REMS would be necessary to ensure that the benefits of the drug outweigh the risks. New safety information on a serious risk that arises after a product is approved may also trigger a new requirement for a REMS. Also, applicants that had RiskMAPS in place continue with them, with or without modifications, as a "deemed REMS".

The requirement for a REMS is enforceable by law, and if the person responsible for the drug (in the company) fails to comply, the drug is considered misbranded. Penalties of up to $1 million are possible for the first violation and may increase to $10 million for subsequent violations.

The content of a REMS is described in the legislation. There are two major sections: (1) A proposed REMS and (2) A REMS supporting document.

The Proposed REMS from the Applicant/Company

An applicant prepares a proposed REMS to address a serious risk that will appear in the US Package Insert. FDA must approve the REMS and will also assess results of effectiveness assessments of the non-routine interventions. The contents of a proposed REMS are given as follows:

1. Table of contents.
2. **Background:** The REMS should describe the important serious risks (e.g., those seen in clinical and pre-clinical studies), risks seen with similar products or other drugs in the class, and risks expected with the underlying medical problem or disease (e.g., cancer seen with ulcerative colitis). It should also identify subgroups at risk (e.g., certain demographic groups such as the elderly or newborns) and if there are risks seen with similar products (e.g., bleeding with non-steroidal anti-inflammatory drugs [NSAIDs] or rhabdomyolysis with statins).
3. **Goal(s):** The goal(s) and objective(s) of the REMS. The goal is a desired safety-related outcome or understanding by patients and providers. It should be clear and absolute, and aim to achieve maximum risk reduction. It should be pragmatic, specific, and measurable. Following are some examples:
   Patients on *Y* drug should be aware of the risks of rhabdomyolysis (measurable by the number of serious adverse events, or SAEs (Serious adverse events), of rhabdomyolysis).
   Patients on *X* drug should not also be prescribed *Y* drug (measurable by the number of patients receiving both drugs together).
   Fetal exposures to *Z* drug should not occur (measurable by the number of fetal exposures).
4. REMS elements: A REMS may have one or more of the following:
   - Medication guide ("MedGuide") or patient package insert (PPI) — This will be required if patient labeling could prevent SAEs, if the risks relative to the benefits could affect the patient's decision to use or continue using the drug, or if adherence to directions for use is crucial for effectiveness of the drug. Some early REMS were MedGuide only, but MedGuides have been de-coupled from REMS. Some REMS continue to have MedGuides along with other elements. Note that all MedGuides are approved by FDA as part of a drug's labeling, but only a small number of MedGuides are included as a component of a REMS.
   - Communication plan to healthcare providers — This may be variable and include letters to healthcare providers, and information about REMS elements to encourage implementation or to explain certain safety requirements such as periodic laboratory tests.
   - Elements to assure safe use (ETASU) — These will be used if a medication guide and communication plan are not sufficient. ETASUs should not be confused with post-marketing

commitments or requirements (studies or other procedures promised to FDA after NDA approval and as a condition of the approval), which may or may not be part of a REMS. See Table 1 for examples of ETASU.

- Implementation system — If included in the REMS, it should describe the system for implementing, monitoring, and evaluating the intended goals and effects. An implementation system may include a description of the distribution system of the drug, and the REMS may require certification of wholesalers and distributors to ensure they comply. Examples of implementation methods include the maintenance of a validated database to track certified prescribers/dispensers, and periodic audits of pharmacies, practitioners, and others to ensure compliance with ETASUs.
- Timetable for assessments — The assessments should be done no less frequently than at 18 months, 3 years, and 7 years after the REMS is approved by FDA. However, the time required to implement a REMS and for the healthcare system to adopt it should be considered in conducting assessments.

5. REMS assessment plan: What will be done, when it will be done and measured to evaluate whether the goals are achieved, and what the criteria are for success. It is common to measure behaviors of the various factors, which may trigger increased or decreased REMS requirements.
6. Other relevant information.
7. Appendix: Supporting documents are included for each section above.

Other post-marketing actions may be proposed, such as "enhanced surveillance" (often this is ill-defined and turns out to be just a bit more due diligence on spontaneously reported cases), targeted safety studies, large simple safety studies (LSSS), epidemiologic studies (e.g., comparative observational studies), and drug utilization studies.

Table 1. Examples of REMS Requirements that are Considered ETASU; Adapted from www.fda.gov.

ETASU Example	Description
Prescribers must have specific training, experience, or be specially certified	Prescribers may be required to become certified and/or take training prior to prescribing the drug. Prescribers may need to enroll in the REMS and agree to carry out certain activities for safe drug use, e.g., a prescriber may be required to agree to counsel their patients about the particular serious risk, or agree to enroll, and/or monitor patients throughout the treatment course.
Pharmacies, practitioners, or healthcare settings that dispense the drug may need to be specially certified	Pharmacies, practitioners, or other healthcare settings that may dispense REMS medications may be required to take the training, train staff, and oversee all processes and procedures needed to implement the REMS requirements. For example, a pharmacy may need to put a process in place that includes verifying that the prescriber of a REMS drug is certified, patients are enrolled, and that laboratory testing or other certain safe use conditions have been carried out prior to dispensing the drug.
Drug may be dispensed only in certain healthcare settings such as hospitals	The REMS may require that the drug be dispensed or administered only in a particular setting. For example, administration of the drug may be restricted to healthcare settings that have immediate access to supplies or personnel trained to manage a particular adverse event.
Evidence of safe use conditions, such as laboratory test results, may be required before the drug is dispensed or administered	FDA may require that a REMS drug be dispensed only with documentation of safe use conditions. For example, healthcare providers and patients may need to execute a signed patient–prescriber agreement for a teratogenic drug, so they understand the risk and the need to verify a negative pregnancy test for patients who could potentially be pregnant.
Each patient using the drug maybe subject to monitoring	FDA may require that patients using the drug are subject to certain monitoring during and/or after treatment. For example, patients may need periodic vision monitoring if there is a risk of vision loss.
Enrollment in a registry may be required for each patient using the drug	Patients may be required to be enrolled in a patient registry. The patient registry may include all patients or a subset of all enrolled patients that experience the adverse event of concern. The purpose of a patient registry is to follow patients during and in some cases after treatment with the drug.

The Approved REMS

FDA must approve a REMS before implementation. Since the REMS may be a condition of product approval, it is advantageous for the applicant to work with FDA on a possible REMS requirement as early as possible after a serious risk is identified in the regulatory review process.

Design of the REMS is important and, of course, the non-routine tools specified in the REMS should be the least burdensome on the healthcare delivery system, patients, and their caregivers. With FDA's concurrence, the applicant is responsible for ensuring the required assessment plan is appropriately designed, conducted, analyzed, interpreted, and reported. The assessment plan should be designed to assess effectiveness of the REMS, i.e., whether the behaviors of the various factors are consistent with achieving the goal(s) of the REMS. Results of the assessment(s) may trigger increased or decreased REMS requirements. If the desired behavior is sustainable over time, the applicant may be released from the REMS altogether.

Once approved by FDA, REMS are published on REMS@FDA and on the applicant's website for the product. FDA updates REMS@FDA when an approved REMS is revised, modified, or released. In addition, applicants make REMS materials public on product-specific websites hosted by applicants.

Roles of Key REMS Participants

Roles of the various factors in a REMS may be similar across programs, but the specific requirements and risk messages of each REMS are specifically tailored to each medication, the nature of its risks, and the likely setting of the drug's use. Regarding specific requirements for each REMS participant, details are provided in the REMS documents.

1. **Healthcare providers:** Prescribers of medication (e.g., physicians, physician's assistants, nurse practitioners, or other healthcare providers) are important in ensuring that products with REMS are prescribed properly and used safely.

   As with patients, REMS requirements vary by product. One of the more common tools specified in a REMS is communication(s) on serious risks from the manufacturer(s). Providers may have REMS enrollment obligations, training programs, documentation of patient counseling, periodic lab testing or other monitoring, or documentation of safe use conditions, etc.

   Details for each REMS are available at REMS@FDA, in product labeling or on the manufacturer's product websites.
2. **Pharmacists:** Practitioners who dispense medications that have REMS are obligated to dispense as specified and meet other REMS requirements, even though they are not directly regulated by FDA. Requirements will vary from REMS-to-REMS, which may be related to the setting (e.g., inpatient pharmacy versus retail) or requirements for training or certification. Of course, compliance audits for the various requirements will ordinarily be a component. A communication plan for some REMS may include communications directly from the relevant applicant(s).
3. Details about each REMS, including the roles of pharmacies and healthcare settings, can be found at REMS@FDA, in product labeling or on product-specific websites.
4. **Patients and their caregivers:** These roles are important and will vary with the REMS design and requirements. Examples include counseling (e.g., by a prescriber or pharmacist) on an important (serious) risk, what action(s) might be needed to mitigate an important risk, or coaching on how to identify symptoms for consultation with their healthcare provider. Other examples that might be required are pre-treatment (and during treatment) lab testing or enrollment in a registry.
5. For some REMS, documentation must be in order (often monitored real-time by computer) before medication is dispensed.
6. To assist with effectiveness metrics, prescribers, pharmacists, or patients/caregivers may be asked

to participate in various surveys. The results may trigger modification (or elimination) of the REMS tools.

7. **Applicants (manufacturers):** The role of applicants has been codified in legislation. In addition to drug safety obligations required by legislation, FDA has provided various guidance documents on expectations for REMS:

   "Revised Draft Guidance for Industry on Format and Content of a Risk Evaluation and Mitigation Strategy Document"
   This describes a revised REMS document template, designed to improve efficiency of preparing and reviewing REMS documents.

   "Guidance for Industry: Use of a Drug Master File (DMF) for Shared System REMS Submissions"
   This guidance can be helpful if a shared system REMS is required. It permits applicants to share a DMF, which is intended to facilitate coordination submission of shared system REMS-related files.

   "Risk Evaluation and Mitigation Strategies: Modifications and Revisions — Guidance for Industry"
   This guidance provides definitions for "modifications" and "revisions" to approved REMS and how they will be handled by FDA.

   "FDA's Application of Statutory Factors in Determining When a REMS is Necessary"
   This guidance outlines the process FDA uses to comply when applying REMS authorities specified in the 2007 FDAAA legislation. These documents should be sought on the FDA website.

   "Medication Guides — Distribution Requirements and Inclusion in Risk Evaluation and Mitigation Strategies (REMS) Guidance for Industry"
   This guidance clarifies expectations on distribution of MedGuides under various scenarios.

   "Questions and Answers on Draft Guidance for Industry: Medication Guides — Distribution Requirements and Inclusion in REMS"
   This Q&A document provides additional clarification on MedGuide requirements.

   "Development of a Shared System REMS Guidance for Industry" (Draft Guidance)
   This document clarifies aspects of shared system REMS development.

   "Technical Conformance Guide for Shared System REMS Drug Master File Submissions" (the SSR DMF Technical Conformance Guide)
   This is a technical guide for using a shared DMF as part of a shared system REMS.

   "Waivers of the Single, Shared System REMS Requirement Guidance for Industry" (Draft Guidance)
   This provides guidance on the possibility of a waiver from a shared system REMS.

   "Standardizing and Evaluating Risk Evaluation and Mitigation Strategies" (REMS Standardization Report)
   This report outlines four priority projects to standardize REMS, as may be appropriate, and reduce their burden.

   "REMS and Continuing Education for Healthcare Providers — FDA Feasibility Report"
   This describes healthcare professional participation in educational programs that are a part of REMS.

■ Comments

The goals of the REMS are to continually assess the benefit–risk balance and to ensure that it remains positive, if not globally, for all patients treated, then for a subset(s). This may not be clear before marketing, but, where a REMS is required, the best effort must be put into designing a logical and thoughtful REMS, realizing it may change with experience gained after marketing. It should not pose an undue burden on the healthcare system or patients, otherwise unintended consequences, such as diversion to less desirable products, may occur.

Careful thought by a team knowledgeable about the disease and drug in question should work on the REMS.

They need to evaluate the patients and disease to determine whether there are measurable early signs, symptoms, or markers that will allow a risk management intervention to prevent a bad outcome or SAE. This will require review of the data available for the drug and similar products, and an understanding of how the drug will be used in the "real world" and whether different populations from those in the clinical trials will be exposed to the drug. Obviously, much of this may not be known before marketing, making it necessary to change the REMS after marketing starts. The tricky question of off-label use (if anticipated) should be considered and possibly incorporated in the REMS.

Further details and an example of a mock REMS are found in the FDA-revised draft guidance cited above.

Shared System REMS

Beginning in 2009, the FDA began requiring all products in certain classes of drugs to have REMS. The first group in this category was for botulinum toxin products, which had safety issues such as muscle weakness, loss of bladder control, and breathing problems. All such products are mandated to have a MedGuide, communication plan, and a timetable for assessments, but there were no other ETASUs required. Other products with class-wide REMS include testosterone gel drugs and extended-release (ER) oral opioid products. In addition, if a branded product (the "reference-listed drug") has a REMS, the generic versions of the product will also require a REMS. See Table 2. The generic's REMS is the same as that of the branded product, unless otherwise justified and negotiated with FDA. Sometimes all the companies producing a drug may work together on a single REMS. This is usually mandated by FDA rather than a voluntary action by applicants.

The concept behind a shared system is that it would "level the playing field" and reduce the burden for different stakeholders (e.g., applicants, the healthcare delivery system, patients, and regulators). To accomplish this, there is often a single portal to access REMS materials and other information about the program. Efficiencies are also gained by having prescribers, pharmacies, and healthcare settings complete certification and other administrative requirements once rather than for each individual drug. This decreases complexity and bureaucracy for the healthcare system. Such programs also have the potential for cost sharing among participating applicants.

In certain situations, it is possible to obtain a waiver from participating in a shared system REMS. For example, FDA granted a waiver to three ANDA (Abbreviated New Drug Application) applicants for participation

Table 2. Example of Approved Shared System REMS in Effect, as of November 13, 2017.

Products	Number of Applicants	Number of Products	REMS Elements
Alosetron	2	2	ETASU
Buprenorphine transmuscosal products for opioid dependence (BTOD)	13	17	MG, ETASU, IS
Clozapine	11	13	ETASU, IS
Emtricitabine/tenofovir disoproxil fumarate	2	2	ETASU
ER and long-acting (LA) opioids	36	64	MG, ETASU
Isotretinoin iPLEDGE	6	7	MG, ETASU, IS
Mycophenolate	20	33	ETASU
Sodium oxybate (1/3 = one reference-listed drug REMS and another waiver-granted "comparable" REMS for three additional generic products)	1/3	4	MG, ETASU, IS
Transmucosal immediate-release fentanyl (TIRF) products	8	9	MG, ETASU, IS
Vigabatrin	2	3	ETASU, IS

in a single, shared system REMS for sodium oxybate oral solution drug products. Serious risks associated with these products can include central nervous system effects. In granting a waiver to the shared system requirement, FDA found that: (a) the burden of a single shared system would not be easily workable and (b) the ANDA applicants were unable to obtain a license for an aspect of the ETASU that the innovator had patented. Thus, FDA approved a separate shared system REMS for the generic products that was considered "comparable" to the innovator REMS which continued in force. Note that FDA attached a condition that the "comparable" waiver-granted system would be open to future applicants. See Table 2.

■ REMS Template

As noted above, the template is available at "Proposed Risk Evaluation and Mitigation Strategies (REMS), REMS Assessments, and Proposed REMS Modifications".

■ Comments

In theory, a REMS should be short, compact, and not burdensome on patient access or the healthcare delivery system. In practice, many are complex and must be designed with the European Union and other countries' risk requirements in mind. Ideally, a company would like to develop one risk plan for all markets, but the practicalities and requirements for local content have rendered this impossible. Nonetheless, REMS and risk plans will ordinarily focus on a common goal, but the means to achieve the goal may differ in different healthcare settings and jurisdictions. Also, plans need to be thought about across a product's entire life cycle by the appropriate personnel either inside the company or outside as consultants. Review of the publicly available REMS should be done frequently.

There is a continuous and, for now, unresolvable debate that many companies go through when submitting a new drug/biologic application (NDA/BLA). The question is whether one should offer up a REMS voluntarily or let FDA "force" one on the company. The case for a REMS up front and voluntarily is that, if it is good for the public health and the correct thing to do, it should be done without having to be told to do it. It will allow the company to prepare a thoughtful, reasonable, low burden, cost-effective program rather than finding out at the last moment (e.g., just before approval) that the FDA wants a REMS and perhaps an aggressive one that contains more than the company feels appropriate. Negotiations and research on REMS components at the last minute before approval in a pressured atmosphere, where the company may feel obliged to commit to a large program just to get the drug on the market quickly is usually not a good idea. However, some companies are willing to take this risk and not propose a REMS in the hope that the FDA will not require one. This avoids, from their point of view, unnecessary expense and effort. Others argue that the company should propose a REMS but that it should always be minimalist (e.g., just a MedGuide and a communication plan for healthcare providers) to show "good faith" but not to "overcommit". The obvious answer to all of this is that one should do the right thing for patients. It is also hoped that the company's and the Agency's views on what constitutes an appropriate REMS for a serious risk will not differ too much. Unfortunately, the right thing is not always clear, and economics and politics often enter into the decision.

■ European Union RMPs

The fundamental documents establishing PV and RMP (Risk Management Plans) concepts for the European Union are Directive 2001/83/EC (Article 8(3)(ia)), as amended by Directive 2004/27/EC: "The MA (Marketing Authorization) application shall be accompanied by a detailed description of the pharmacovigilance and, where appropriate, of the risk-management system which the applicant will introduce". In addition, Article 9(4)(c) of Regulation EC No. 726/2004, "Requires details of conditions and restrictions on supply or use or with regard to safe and effective use of the medicinal product attached to Opinion..." Detailed requirements are in the EU Good PV Practices (GVP) Module V — Risk management systems, as revised (2017). A CHMP guideline published in 2005 was based, to a large degree, on the ICH E2E guideline. Most of the E2E concepts have since been incorporated into GVP Module V. GVP Module V on risk management introduces the principles of risk minimization and, thus, it should be considered in the context of GVP Module XVI (risk minimization measures: selection of tools and effectiveness indicators) and GVP Module XVI Addendum I (educational materials). Note that all medicinal products must have routine risk minimization measures and only a subset of products has a safety concern(s) that requires additional, non-routine risk minimization measures. Further, due to a variety of reasons, safety concerns that require non-routine measures are not necessarily the same in all parts of the world and neither are the available tools.

All companies must have a PV system (per Article 1 of Directive 2001/83/EC and described in GVP Module I). The PV system that a company maintains is different from the risk management system described in GVP Module V. Per GVP Annex I (Rev. 4), a risk management system is defined as, "A set of pharmacovigilance activities and interventions designed to identify, characterize, prevent or minimize risks relating to a medicinal product, including the assessment of the effectiveness of those activities and interventions [DIR 2001/83/EC Art 1(28b)]." As noted above, for most drugs, the usual "routine" pharmacovigilance activities (spontaneous reporting, PBRER/PSURs, etc.) will suffice. For others, however, certain non-routine conditions or restrictions on supply or use of the product may be appropriate and required (for both centrally and nationally authorized products). The concept is that a product's benefits should outweigh its risks in the target population.

Per GVP Annex I (Rev. 4), an RMP is "A detailed description of the risk management system [DIR 2001/83/EC Art 1(28c)]. The risk management plan established by the marketing authorisation holder shall contain the following elements: (a) an identification or characterisation of the safety profile of the medicinal product(s) concerned; (b) an indication of how to characterise further the safety profile of the medicinal product(s) concerned; (c) a documentation of measures to prevent or minimize the risks associated with the medicinal product, including an assessment of the effectiveness of those interventions; (d) a documentation of post-authorisation obligations that have been imposed as a condition of the marketing authorisation [IR 520/2012 Art 30(1)]."

Bottom line: All drugs need a risk management system, which addresses risk minimization. Routine risk minimization is performed on all products. This is detailed in Parts III & V of the RMP and covers the usual and routine PV activities a company performs. If the applicant and health authorities feel that more actions are needed to control risk for a particular product, then Part III (PV Plan) and/or Part V (Risk Minimization Plan) must be expanded with additional PV and/or minimization measures.

Note 1: A "Safety Concern" in the EU is an important identified risk, an important potential risk or missing information. Early descriptions referred to "important missing information", but reflection resulted in deletion of "important" because if the missing information was so important the product should not have been approved without it.

Note 2: From 20 October 2023, EMA is publishing RMPs (main body and annexes 4 and 6) for all centrally authorized products. This is applicable for initial evaluations (CTD submissions) and for RMP updates as well. From the same date, EMA no longer publishes RMP summaries. The aim is to increase transparency of the safety review process for all centrally authorized products.

■ When is an RMP Needed?

At any point in a drug's life cycle, an RMP may be needed. The health authority and/or the applicant may determine an RMP is needed:

- At the time of application for a new MA or a new active substance;
- For "a similar biological medicinal product";
- For certain generic/hybrid products;
- For an application for pediatric use;
- For a significant change in marketing: new dosage form, new route of administration, new manufacturing

process of a biotech product, significant new indication, new pediatric indication;
- For certain other situations, including fixed combination products;
- In the case of a new (or newly understood) important safety concern for a product without a current RMP (i.e., product was authorized before RMPs were required).

EU RMP Content

The EMA delivered a template (retrievable on the Agency website: EMA/PRAC/613102/2015 Rev.2 accompanying GVP Module V Rev. 2), which is applicable for all medicinal products in the EU. This template provides a detailed table of contents, as for PSURs/PBRERs. For new products, all sections must be completed; for older products, only the applicable sections are required.

Part I: Product(s) Overview (GVP V. B.4)

Part I should provide administrative information on the RMP and an overview of the product(s); the following summary is per GVP V.B.4 (Rev. 2). The information presented in Part I should be "current and accurate in relation to the ongoing application as it is anticipated to appear in the marketing authorization". This should be organized according to the RMP template and the following information must be provided:

- Active substance(s) (INN or common name);
- Pharmacotherapeutic group(s) (ATC Code);
- Name of applicant or marketing authorization holder (expected or actual);
- Invented name(s) in the European economic area (EEA);
- Marketing authorization procedure;
- Brief description of the product and other particulars;
- Hyperlink to the product information;
- Approved and/or proposed Indication(s) in the EEA;
- Dosage (posology) in the EEA;
- Pharmaceutical form(s) and strengths;
- Whether or not the product is expected to be subject to additional monitoring in the EU (at initial marketing authorization application conclusion or with RMP updates).

Part II: Safety Specification (GVP V.B.5)

The purpose of this section of the RMP is to provide the safety profile of the product and discuss the areas that may need non-routine risk minimization activities. Part II includes a summary of the important identified risks, important potential risks, and missing information. Early versions referred to "important" missing information, but, as thinking evolved, if the missing information was really so important, the product should not be approved without it. There is guidance on how this information should be presented.

Part II also addresses at-risk populations, i.e., the populations where the product is likely to be used (including anticipated off-label use) and any outstanding safety questions that need additional data to refine the benefit–risk assessment.

The safety specification consists of eight RMP modules, which correspond to the safety specification headings in the ICH E2E guideline. However, there are additional elements required by the EU (see GVP V.B.5.7, RMP Module SVI, "Additional EU requirements for the safety specification"). This part should also address the potential for misuse for illegal purposes, and, where appropriate, any proposed risk minimization measures, e.g., limited pack size, controlled access program, special medical prescription, etc. (Directive Art 71(2) and GVP V.B.8).

In addition, the following should be addressed in Part II if they could lead to risks related to product use:

- Potential harm from overdose (intentional or accidental);
- Potential for risks resulting from medication errors;
- Potential for transmission of infectious agents;
- Potential for off-label use;
- Evidence that refutes any class-related safety concerns;

- Important risks related to identified and potential pharmacokinetic and pharmacodynamic interactions with other products anticipated for use in the target population;
- Potential risks in pregnancy or lactation, e.g., teratogenic risk (exposure of mother or partner) and effects on fertility;
- Environmental impact, i.e., risks associated with the disposal of the used product;
- Potential risks related to the administration of the product(s);
- Safety concerns specific to special populations, e.g., pediatric or elderly populations;
- For advanced therapy medicinal products, also consider possible specific risks related to such products.

RMP part II should also address risks considered important for inclusion in the list of safety concerns, but also addresses risks not considered important enough for inclusion in the list of safety concerns. This discussion should include a summary of risk seriousness and frequency and their impact on the benefit–risk assessment (by indication).

General considerations for generic products and advanced therapy medicinal products (GVP V.B.5.1)

For generics, the expectation is that the safety specification is the same as that of the reference product or of other generic products for which an RMP is in place. Because of the unique nature of advanced therapy medicinal Products (ATMPs), risks may occur that are not normally a concern with other types of medicinal products. These might include, for example, risks to living donors, risks of germ line transformation, or transmission of vectors. Such risks need to be considered for ATMPs.

Epidemiology of the indication(s) and target population(s) (GVP V.B.5.2 RMP part II Module SI)

This module should include incidence, prevalence, outcome of the (untreated) target disease (i.e., indications), and relevant comorbidities. If appropriate, consideration should be given to demographic stratification (e.g., age, gender, etc.) Disease risk factors and the current standard of care should also be described. The emphasis should be on the situation relevant to the EU. Differences in the epidemiology in different regions should be discussed (where epidemiology varies across regions). This section should also describe the relevant adverse events that would be anticipated in the (untreated) target population in the EU, their frequency, and characteristics. The text should help anticipate potential signals (and possibly facilitate interpretation of them) as well as possibilities for risk minimization. This section should be concise and, as with all parts of the RMP, should be non-promotional. Note that non-EEA data are accepted when considered relevant to the EEA situation.

What else should be included in the epidemiology section? Supplement the above, as appropriate, with the following:

- The natural history of the indicated condition in the untreated population, including mortality and morbidity;
- A discussion on possible stages of disease progression to be treated and applied to the natural history of the indication in the (untreated) population;
- The primary available treatment options with their expected safety profiles (and outcome in the absence of treatment with the medicinal product).

The Non-clinical part of the safety specification (GVP V.B.5.3 RMP part II, Module SII)

This section should include a discussion of findings not adequately addressed by clinical data, such as the following:

- toxicity, including repeat-dose, reproductive and developmental toxicity, nephrotoxicity, hepatotoxicity, genotoxicity, carcinogenicity;
- general pharmacology, including cardiovascular, QT prolongation, nervous system;

- drug interactions;
- discussion of the relevance to drug use in humans.

Clinical trial exposure (GVP V.B.5.4 RMP part II, Module SIII)

This section should start with "limitations". That is, limitations:

- Of the size of the safety database and the patients not studied due to inclusion/exclusion criteria in the clinical trials;
- With regard to patients expected to be exposed to the drug after marketing;
- Regarding the ability to detect infrequent ADRs;
- In regard to finding long-term risks (e.g., cancer); and
- Regarding populations not studied in the pre-marketing period (e.g., pediatric, pregnancy, comorbid conditions, more severe, sub-populations).

Relevant information should be provided in an appropriate format (e.g., tables/graphs) and updated when there is important new information (e.g., new exposure data from line extension studies in a new indication). The content of this section should be assessed for relevance over time and, in the absence of new clinical trial exposure data, does not need to be updated. Tabulated information must be included specifying duration of exposure, age groups, and gender, dose, ethnic origin (overall and per indication for each).

Populations not studied in clinical trials (GVP V.B.5.5 RMP part II, Module SIV)

This section should discuss the populations which have not been studied or have only been studied to a limited degree in the pre-approval phase. This would include populations considered under missing information (e.g., often might include pregnant women, breast-feeding women, patients with renal impairment, hepatic impairment or cardiac impairment, populations with relevant genetic polymorphisms, immuno-compromised patients, and populations of different ethnic origins). The implications of this with respect to predicting the safety of the medicinal product in the marketplace should be explicitly discussed.

Post-authorization experience (GVP V.B.5.6 RMP part II, Module SV)

This section covers clinical post-marketing experience from outside the EU (if any) that is helpful for risk management planning purposes. It should be a concise overview, not a duplication of the PSUR/PBRER. It should discuss exposure data (amount sold, use in special populations, such as children, market research information, etc.), as well as the actual way the drug is prescribed and used (including off-label use) compared with the approved labeling. This section should discuss any new safety concerns and whether any regulatory actions were taken in any jurisdiction for safety matters.

Risks that require further evaluation should be identified and discussed, in particular more frequent or more serious/severe suspected ADRs. The possible mechanism, risk factors, risk groups, reversibility, and estimated frequency should be discussed.

Risk data, where available, should then be presented. This assessment should be based on study or epidemiologic data, which allows for quantitative risk estimation, including excess risk (versus placebo and available comparators), risk by various populations studied, time-to-event data (e.g., survival data), stratification by drug, placebo, age, gender, dose, and so forth.

If pharmacokinetic or pharmacodynamic interactions are suspected, any possible further studies should be detailed.

The impact of the key actual and potential risks should be addressed using strength of evidence, biological plausibility, nature of evidence, potential public health burden, morbidity, and mortality. Special attention should be paid to at-risk, susceptible patient groups. A structured format and classification by exposure, indication, gender, age group, region, dose, time, and risk factors should be used.

Data from indications not authorized in the EU, if any, should also be summarized and implications for the EU should be discussed.

Additional EU requirements for the safety specification (GVP V.B.5.7 RMP part II, Module SVI)

This section must detail the potential for misuse for illegal purposes, if applicable. When appropriate, a pro-active discussion of proposed non-routine risk minimization measures (e.g., limited pack size, controlled access program, special medical prescription, etc.) should be included.

Identified and potential risks (GVP V.B.5.8 RMP part II, Module SVII)

This module should focus on "safety concerns" for the product. This would include details on "important" identified and potential risks, as well as missing information. Non-important risks are also to be listed, even if proposed in the draft EU SmPC (Summaries of Product Characteristics). The reason for not including an identified or potential risk in the list of safety concerns in the RMP should also be justified.

Each important risk (identified or potential) should be detailed; information on nature, severity, outcome, frequency and benefit–risk balance must be provided. For each risk, the following information is to be addressed:

- Evidence source(s) and strength of evidence.
- Characterization of the risk.
- Risk factors and risk groups.
- Preventability.
- Impact on the risk–benefit balance of the product.
- Public health impact.

The impact and measures scheduled in the PV plan and/or risk minimization sections of the RMP are to be detailed in this section. Similar information is to be included for missing information, focusing on risks or populations in need of further characterization or on the anticipated risks or possible consequence(s) of the missing information.

Since RMPs are to be updated according to scheduled milestones, identified important risks, potential important risks, and missing information should be reassessed, according to new information received since the previous version of the RMP. Clear and robust rationales must be provided if the identified or potential risks or missing information sections are modified.

The RMP should also discuss other risks, where appropriate, such as the following:

- Known or suspected class effects;
- Potential for overdose, especially if there is a narrow therapeutic window;
- Potential for transmission of infectious agents;
- Potential for off-label use, particularly use in special populations (e.g., children or the elderly).

Summary of the safety concerns (GVP V.B.5.9 RMP part II, Module SVIII)

A tabulated summary of the safety concerns identified in previous section should be provided per identified risk, potential risk, and missing information. This simplified categorization scheme for safety concerns should be used for the following:

- Important identified risks;
- Important potential risks;
- Missing information.

Part III: PV Plan, Including Post-authorization Safety Studies (GVP V.B.6 RMP part III)

This part of the RMP is intended to present a structured plan for further characterization of safety concerns in the safety specification. It does not include actions intended to reduce, prevent or mitigate risks, which are considered in RMP part V.

Routine PV activities (GVP V.B.6.1 RMP part III)

Routine PV is the primary set of activities required to fulfill the minimum legal requirements for PV in Directive 2001/83/EC and Regulation (EC) No. 726/2004. The purpose in the RMP is not to repeat what is already included in the pharmacovigilance system master file (PSMF) describing these activities.

"Routine" PV activities, not specified in the PSMF, can be as follows, for instance:

- Specific adverse reaction follow-up questionnaires for a safety concerns; purpose and description of the materials used to obtain structured information on reported suspected adverse reactions of special interest; and
- Enhanced passive surveillance high level description, observed versus expected analyses, cumulative reviews of adverse events of interest.

Note that the descriptions of these activities in the PV system master file (PSMF) are not required to be repeated here in the RMP.

Additional PV activities (GVP V.B.6.2 RMP part III)

In this section, the applicant (or marketing authorization holder) should describe additional PV activities such as non-clinical, clinical, or epidemiological (non-interventional or interventional) studies, and explain why they are needed.

For each proposed Post-Authorization Safety Study (PASS), whether committed or imposed, the following should be detailed:

- Study short name and title;
- Rationale and study objectives;
- Study design;
- Study population;
- Milestones.

Studies in the PV plan should be designed and conducted according to legislation and recommendations in GVP Module VIII.

Summary table of additional PV activities (GVP V.B.6.3 RMP part III)

This section should be a complete overview of all on-going and planned safety studies included in the PV Plan, regardless of whether they were designed to assess the safety of the medicinal product, or the effectiveness of the risk minimization measures.

Studies required in jurisdictions outside the EU would not ordinarily be included in the EU RMP, unless they would also be expected to impact an EU safety concern. Of course, safety concerns arising from any such studies should be reported as per the applicable requirements.

Note that for generic products, the PV plan should reflect the outstanding PV needs at the time of their authorization for marketing (not necessarily the full initial plan for the innovator).

Part IV: Plans for Post-authorization Efficacy Studies (GVP V.B.7 RMP part IV)

This section includes a list of the planned and on-going imposed PAES (Post Authorization Efficacy Studies), i.e., studies imposed by an EU competent authority as a condition of marketing authorization, or which are specific obligations in the context of conditional marketing authorization, or marketing authorization under exceptional circumstances. If no such studies are required, RMP Part IV may be left empty.

Part V: Risk Minimization Measures (Including Evaluation of the Effectiveness of Risk Minimization Activities) (GVP V.B.8 RMP part V)

This part should provide details of the risk minimization measures designed to reduce risks associated with the indicated safety concerns. It is applicable for all initial marketing authorization applications, except for generic, hybrid medicinal products, and fixed combination products with no new active substance, where the originator product does not have additional (non-routine) risk minimization activities.

A table listing the routine and additional risk minimization activities, stratified by safety concern, should be provided in this section (i.e., the SmPC section number where the risk appears in the SmPC, the list of educational materials, etc.) A further summary of PV activities should be included, as described in the EMA guidance on format of the RMP in the EU.

Routine risk minimization activities

This section should provide a description of routine risk minimization measures, stratified by safety concern.

Routine risk minimization activities are those which apply to every medicinal product:

- The summary of product characteristics (SmPC);
- Labeling on the inner and outer carton;
- The package leaflet (PL);
- The pack size(s);
- The legal status of the product.

The formulation itself should be described if it is expected to play an important role in minimizing the risk(s) of the product.

SmPC and PL

The SmPC and PL are important tools for risk minimization as they are standardized formats for informing stakeholders about the product. The guideline on the SmPC provides guidance on how information should be organized and presented. Both materials provide routine risk minimization recommendations; however, there are two basic types of messages the SmPC and PL can provide:

(a) Routine risk communication messages (usually found in section 4.8 of the SmPC or Section 4 of the PL).
These communicate undesirable effects to help inform treatment decisions.

(b) Routine risk minimization activities that recommend specific clinical measures to address the risk (usually found in Sections 4.2 and 4.4 of the SmPC, but can also be found in Sections 4.1, 4.3, 4.5, 4.6, 4.7, and 4.9 and Sections 2 and 3 of the PL).
These include specific activities to address the risk(s) of the product. Examples of such activities might be one or more of the following:

- A test before the start of treatment;
- Laboratory monitoring during treatment;
- Clinical monitoring for specific signs and symptoms;
- Dose modification (including discontinuing the medication) related to adverse events laboratory parameters;
- A "wash-out" procedure after treatment interruption;
- Recommendations for contraception;
- Contraindications for use with other medicines;
- Treating or preventing the product's risk factors or harms;
- Recommendations for long-term follow-up.

There are certain other impactful measures that can be considered to minimize potential harms:

Pack size: Since every product has an authorized pack size, planning the number of "dosage units" within each pack and the range of pack sizes available can be considered as a form of routine risk management. Careful planning of pack size could reinforce the need for patients to see a healthcare provider on a regular basis, which could increase the opportunity for testing or another follow-up. A smaller pack size may help address risks of overdose or diversion.

Legal status: In addition to prescription status, government controls may include details of any conditions placed on the supply or use of the product. Approval may restrict by whom the product may be prescribed (e.g., by a specially trained prescriber) or where the product can be used (e.g., in a hospital or in settings with special resuscitation provisions).

Restricted medical prescription: For this option, several factors should be considered (EU Directive Art 71(3)):

- Pharmaceutical characteristics or novelty of the product that should be reserved for a controlled environment;

- Diagnostic procedures require special facilities (follow-up may be carried out elsewhere);
- Very serious adverse reactions (or the possibility of abuse, etc.) can be anticipated that may require special supervision throughout the course of therapy.

Member state customization: It is possible that member states may impose local requirements to adapt to their national situation. The definitions and, therefore, also implementation, may vary in those member states where certain subcategories of risk minimization or their modification are contemplated or are in place.

Additional risk minimization activities: Additional non-routine activities should only be suggested when they would be essential for the safe and effective use of the product. A clear rationale should be provided and these activities should be described in detail. The need for continuing with such measures should also be reviewed on a periodic basis. Where relevant, key messages of any additional activities should be provided in RMP Annex 6 (details of proposed additional risk minimization activities). See GVP Module VIII.

Following are examples of additional measures that might be considered:

- Healthcare professional and patient/carer guide;
- Healthcare professional training material;
- Prescriber checklist;
- Patient diary;
- Patient alert card;
- Pregnancy prevention programs.

For each proposed non-routine risk minimization measure, the following information should be provided:

- Objectives;
- Rationale for the additional risk minimization activity;
- Target audience and planned distribution path;
- Plans to evaluate the effectiveness of the interventions and the criteria for success.

Evaluation of the effectiveness of non-routine risk minimization activities

When the RMP is updated, the risk minimization plan should include the results of any formal assessment(s) of non-routine risk minimization activities when available. Adjustments should be made if a particular strategy proves ineffective or causes an undue burden on patients or the healthcare system.

Summary of risk minimization measures

This section should include all risk minimization measures and PV activities stratified by safety concern.

Part VI: Summary of the RMP (GVP V.B.9 RMP part VI)

This summary must address the following:

- The medicine and what it is used for;
- The risks associated with the medicine and activities to minimize or further characterize the risks:
  - list of important risks and missing information;
  - summary of important risks;
- Post-authorization development plan:
  - Studies which are conditions of the marketing authorization;
  - Other studies in post-authorization development plan.

General Remarks on the EU RMP

The EU RMP can be summarized as follows:

EU RMP Part	Details
Part I: Product(s) overview	Active substance, MAH, MA procedure, product description, indication, dosage, pharmaceutical form(s), and strengths
Part II: Safety specifications	Epidemiology of the indication(s) and target population(s) Non-clinical safety Clinical trial exposure Populations not studied Post-authorization experience Potential for misuse for illegal purposes

(Continued)

(Continued)

EU RMP Part	Details
	Summary of important Identified risks, potential risks, and missing information
Part III: PV plan	PV activities to characterize and quantify clinically relevant risks and to identify new adverse reactions ↳ Routine and additional PV activities (including PASS)
Part IV: Plans for PAES	Planned and on-going PAES that are conditions of the marketing authorization or that are specific obligations
Part V: Risk minimization measures	Actions which will be taken to prevent and/ or minimize risk(s) and results assessment (effectiveness) ↳ Routine and additional minimization activities
Part VI: Summary of the RMP	Product information summary Important risks and missing information Activities to minimize or further characterize risks post-authorization development plan

The RMP should propose non-routine risk minimization actions to take, in addition to usual safety reporting and signal detection:

- If no special concerns are seen, routine PV is sufficient;
- If additional concerns, further activities should be done that can include (note that these are additional surveillance activities and are different from minimization actions (similar to US ETASUs)).
- Safety studies;
- Active surveillance (e.g., formal follow-up of patients filling a prescription for drug *X* with a survey and telephone contact later on);
- Sentinel sites of selected prescribers interviewed and medical record review;
- Intensive monitoring schemes where case data are collected from prescribers or hospitals on a specific drug or problem;
- Prescription event monitoring (especially the United Kingdom). Identify patients electronically and send follow-up questionnaires periodically to find course and outcome;
- Registries by drug, disease/outcome with follow-up questionnaires;
- Epidemiologic studies:
  - Comparative observational studies to validate signals — prospective or retrospective;
  - Cross-sectional studies or surveys to collect data on patients at a single point in time or over an interval regardless of exposure or disease status;
  - Cohort studies of a population on drug *X* at risk for a specific adverse event to be followed over time (prospectively or retrospectively) for the occurrence of that event, allowing the calculation of an incidence rate;
  - Case-control studies where patients with a specific AE already seen are selected and a control group without the AE also chosen. Exposure to the drug is then searched for;
  - Occurrence of disease studies of the specific AE to better characterize the patients at risk, the clinical course, and so forth;
  - Novel designs to be worked out with the health authorities.
- Clinical trials particularly with the subgroups at risk: children, elderly, and so forth;
- LSSS (randomized trial but minimal data collection and follow-up);
- Drug utilization studies of the marketing, prescribing, and use in a population and how this influences outcomes;
- Medication errors should be discussed if there is risk of such a problem.

Next, risk minimization activities (similar to the US REMS ETASUs) should be detailed, and they may include one or more of the following:

- Providing information (SmPC, Patient Leaflet, other);
- Additional educational material for patients, practitioners, and others that could include special training, use of checklists, or guides;
- Restrictions on availability ("legal status change") with use only in hospitals or prescribing only by a specialist;
- Controls at the pharmacy level, e.g., Control of prescription size or time the prescription is valid;
- Informed consent;
- Restricted access;
- Patient registries;

- Special risk communication using other media for key messages.

Direct, periodic measurement of the effectiveness of the activities should be done by looking at metrics, such as the incidence of a particular SAE or outcome such as pregnancy while using the drug in question or a survey of whether leaflets are actually read (and understood).

The PV plan must be a written document covering the safety concerns, objectives and rationale of the proposed actions, monitoring of the plan, and milestones for evaluation. After the HA(s) accept the RMP, periodic updates to the EMA or HAs (Health Authorities) should be done, usually at the same time of the PSURs delivery (if PSUR (Periodic Safety Update Report)/PBRER conclusions raise a need for RMP update) or at pre-defined milestones scheduled in the RMP.

The instructions for the risk management system and plan are found in GVP Module V, as revised. There is a very specific and useful template (revised) that should be followed when preparing the document. The template is referenced in GVP Module V.

Practicalities, Co-ordination, and Other Comments

Risk management strategies in the United States, the European Union, and elsewhere have been in use in their current form for only a relatively short time. US REMS really began in earnest in April 2008 and the 18-month effectiveness assessments are now under way. The instruction documents on risk management are guidance, not regulations, though they are functioning, *de facto*, as obligatory regulations. After periodic review of their effectiveness, modification, i.e., changes in content and requirements have been made for nearly all approved REMS. In the EU, a formal RMP using the EMEA (European Medicines Evaluation Agency) template was first required in 2005; both, requirements and RMP content, evolved over the last 10 years. The role of REMS, RMPs, and post-marketing commitments and requirements is somewhat ill-defined, but will likely be clarified over time.

There are significant differences between risk requirements in the United States and the European Union:

- In the United States, only some products will have a REMS. In the European Union, all new products and old products upon re-approval need some level of a RMP.
- Formats and some content are different in the United States and European Union. The legal requirements are different and are governed by local legislation.
- Attention should be paid to local risks. That is, country- or region-specific risks should be addressed in the European Union and United States.
- In the European Union, the qualified person is clearly identified and has ownership of PV in a company. Ownership is less clear in the United States.

Although there is a large degree of overlap in the goals and content for risk plans in various jurisdictions (the United States, European Union, and Japan in particular), the format, timing, and implementation can be quite different. That is, there is not much harmonization. Companies and agencies are still debating how to use risk plans both strategically and tactically, and, to a degree, companies are debating how much to offer up voluntarily and how long to wait for a mandate from the HA. Evaluation groups are studying risk handling in the agencies in the United States, the European Union, and elsewhere. It is expected that updates and changes will be made in the United States and the European Union requirements. The reader should pay attention to new guidances and regulations from the FDA and European Union and member states, in particular to updates to GVP Module V. The European Union is expected to make changes in the next few years. Subscribing to the FDA's, European Union's, and other agencies' RSS feeds or e-mail alerts is free and a worthwhile adjunct to your other means of keeping current with the changing requirements. Another good RSS feed to subscribe to is that of the European Federation of Pharmaceutical Industries and Associations (EFPIA) at: https://www.efpia.eu/

It is also hoped, perhaps less optimistically, that there will be international coordination and harmonization at some point to avoid duplication of efforts and excess use of limited resources. However, for many reasons, risks in one country may be quite different from those in other countries, and tailored country- or region-specific plans may still be needed.

Risk Management within Pharma Companies

As with most things in life, there is no single best way to do something (or if there is, it is never clear whose way is the best!) Broadly speaking, the fragmentation of risk evaluation at each stage of drug development has changed. For example, in the past it was often common for the clinical team to develop phase I trials based on pre-clinical data without significant input from the group handling later-stage development, marketing, and safety. Now, the tendency is to develop teams with broad cross-functional representation to meet periodically, evaluate the data to date, and outline broad and sometimes specific areas to be examined to evaluate and minimize risk.

In practice, this means several ways of doing business must change:

- There needs to be clear responsibility and governance in risk evaluation, minimization, management, and change management.
- Cross-functional risk teams with clearly delineated responsibilities need to be in place, need to be empowered, and need to act throughout the life cycle of the drug.
- The global players (or stakeholders) include senior management, pharmacology, toxicology, manufacturing, medical research teams, regional/ affiliate/ subsidiary personnel, legal, regulatory, finance, drug safety/ PV, epidemiology, labeling, risk management (in the financial/ insurance sense), marketing, sales, corporate communications, and so forth. That is, at some point, most if not all company groups will be involved in a large or small way. A smaller, practicable working group will usually need to be formed that reports periodically to a senior risk team.
- Tools and processes need to be developed so that each team in the company doing risk does not work "one-off" or *ad hoc*.
- Realistic budgets and personnel must be allocated. Resources will be needed for the team (operational and subject matter experts), not all of whom will do "risk management" in addition to their day job, for data collection from external sources and databases, epidemiologists, surveys and drug utilization studies, post-marketing commitments, external consultants, communication, and so forth.
- From the IT (Information Technology) point of view, it will be necessary for all the data needed for the risk function to be easily accessible. This has broad implications in terms of normalization and standardization of data, timing of data preparation and delivery, accessibility and data security, operational planning, task and responsibility tracking, and planning. There should also be good tools available for signaling and document preparation. The agencies expect this and use these tools themselves.
- Quality management systems are an integral part of risk evaluation and management.
- Understand that for innovative companies and even generic and OTC houses, the old model of spontaneous reporting and PSURs is ending.
- Understand that health agencies talk to one other and that a company cannot say one thing to one agency and another thing (or nothing) to another agency. The world is becoming more risk-averse and more and more will be asked for in terms of risk management.
- Agencies are doing inspections, looking at post-marketing safety commitments and REMS/RMPs in addition to the classic PV inspection. Commitments must be taken seriously.
  - Expect that all safety problems and data will become public rapidly both through the formal outlets (release of data by health agencies) and by the blogosphere and social media.
- The world is flat and global. A core risk plan should be developed that will be moldable and thus useful throughout all jurisdictions.
- We are now in the mid/post-Covid world where risk evaluation and plans have looked at by many more people who otherwise probably would not have thought much about risk/benefit evaluations. This seems widespread and includes the areas of epidemics and pandemics, lockdowns for public health reasons, vaccination, use of new vaccines

and drugs which have not undergone classic testing before approval for public use. Social media and AI are playing larger and larger roles. Where this is heading is unclear as of this writing.
- The world is flat and global. A core risk plan should be developed that will be moldable and thus useful throughout all jurisdictions.

Many of the large multinational pharmaceutical companies and CROs (Clinical Research Organizations) are now investing heavily in setting up large, international structures and teams to handle risk, REMs, RMPs, and the like.

Comments and Suggestions

- Determine whether your company can handle risk management internally. If not, outsource the function but realize that this is not turnkey. The pharma company must maintain clear and continuous oversight and input into the vendor's actions. Delegating a task does not mean transferring the responsibility which remains of the MAH.
- Create a risk function in the company with a designated chief and team. It may not be a full-time task for the participants, but the function is now absolutely necessary.
- Understand that "lack of evidence is not evidence of lack". That is, risks and safety data will accrue over time. The drug's best profile is on the day of launch. It is "downhill" from there.
- Do periodic (e.g., yearly) internal audits of the risk and PV functions.
- Prepare and keep up to date a risk plan using the European Union and US template and E2E principles, which is then tailored as necessary to national or regional requirements. Prepare a PSMF and keep it up to date. This may include a compliance report.
- Appoint and empower a chief safety officer. In the European Union, this is obligatory and is the EU qualified person for PV (EU QPPV). Elsewhere, this role of a "responsible individual person" (and sometimes a deputy to ensure 24/7/365 coverage) is often less clearly defined. Nevertheless, this person should be a medical doctor (or have close access to an empowered MD) with true and real engagement in the company's PV activities. If outsourced, the outsourced QPPV should be an engaged and serious participant in the company's PV activities. Beware of someone who is a QPPV for multiple companies. It's hard enough to do it for one company.
- Create a system of documented internal company communication to be sure of safety and risk issues in faraway (from the home office) areas are carefully followed by a local responsible person (whether in-house or outsourced). This refers to specific drugs as well as regulatory and risk requirements from the local HA. Ensure that all licensing agreements, particularly local contractual obligations, are also covered in all jurisdictions.
- Keep all reference safety information (e.g., US PI, CCSI (Company Core Safety Information), SmPC, investigator brochures, etc.) up-to-date, consistent, and easily available electronically.
- Prepare periodic aggregate reports (e.g., PSURs/PBRERs) for all marketed drugs whether required or not. This, in a sense, forces periodic signaling and safety/risk evaluations (all of which should have an audit trail).
- Ensure adequate resources (not only computer systems and money, but also personnel with appropriate education, training, experience, and other relevant skills, etc.) for risk detection, prioritization, evaluation, and management. Depending on the situation, this may include outsourced functions, epidemiologic studies, and so forth. It will certainly involve integration within the organization's overall PV system.
- Appoint an experienced "point person" to pay attention to risk management, attend national and international meetings, interact with the key players, keep up to date with new requirements, and get "intelligence".

CHAPTER

27

Drug Interactions

Analyzing adverse events (AEs) and ascribing the causality to a particular drug can be quite difficult. This difficulty, however, is magnified when the patient also takes additional drugs. This is sometimes known as "polypharmacy". It is generally believed that the more drugs taken, the greater the risk of AEs and the greater the risk of drug–drug interactions. As the number of different products increases, the ability to ascribe causality to a particular product decreases (or even becomes impossible). There are also other possible interactions with food, herbal products, diseases and alcohol and other foods or beverages.

■ Introduction

Drug–drug interactions: When multiple drugs are taken, it may not be possible to ascribe the adverse event (AE) to one particular drug. In most situations of regulatory reporting, the reporter or the company is generally required to specify one or more "suspect drugs" and, if present, one or more "concomitant drugs". The former are presumed to have a suspected causative role in the AE and the latter not. In clinical trials, the investigator and the sponsor are usually required to specify whether the AE is "related" to the study drug. Study protocols will usually list contraindicated products when known.

Further complicating matters are drug interactions, a situation that occurs when two (or more) drugs are taken that influence each other directly or indirectly. That is, the pharmacokinetics (e.g., blood levels) or pharmacodynamics (effects in the body) of one or all of the drugs may be altered.

For example, the co-administration of desloratadine (Clarinex®) and erythromycin, ketoconazole, azithromycin, or fluoxetine in pharmacology studies produced increased plasma concentrations (Cmax and AUC_{0-24h}) of desloratadine and its major metabolite but did not produce clinically relevant changes in the safety profile. This is an example of a drug–drug interaction producing changes in pharmacokinetics (the plasma levels) but not in the pharmacodynamics (no clinical safety untoward effects or beneficial impact).

A patient may suffer from a pharmacodynamic interaction when taking several products that share the same adverse reaction. For example, when simultaneously taking aspirin and clopidogrel (both reduce the clotting mechanism) plus a non-steroidal anti-inflammatory drug like piroxicam and, unknowingly, another non-steroidal anti-inflammatory drug like ibuprofen (both weaken the gastric lining and promote bleeding), the patient is at great risk of gastrointestinal bleeding.

At the other end of the spectrum is a drug like warfarin, which can be lifesaving, but which has more than 55 potential drug interactions listed by drug class and more than 150 drugs and dozens of botanicals (some of which have anticoagulant properties) by specific name in the US labeling. In addition, several "disease–drug" interactions are listed whereby these specific diseases may produce increases in the Prothrombin Time/International Normalized Ratio (PT/INR). The interactions may produce elevations or decreases in the PT/INR. In some cases, the same drug with warfarin (Coumadin®) may produce an elevation in these levels in one patient and a decrease in another patient. These changes have the potential to produce significant clinical effects by putting the patient at risk for hemorrhage or clotting.

It is impossible, while testing new drugs, to run drug–drug interaction studies against all drugs or even all classes of drugs. At best, sponsors run selected interaction studies against the following:

- The most commonly used drugs that the exposed patients would be likely to take because of their age, diseases, sex, and so on;
- Drugs that might be expected to produce interactions based on pharmacology or *in vitro* data (e.g., cytochrome P450 metabolism) or based on historical data from similar drugs in the class.

These studies tend to be done on healthy patients in short-term clinical pharmacology trials using the study drug and (only) one other drug. Drugs that are suspected of producing interactions but are significantly toxic by themselves (e.g., cancer drugs) generally cannot be studied in this manner because of ethical considerations.

Note that there are enormous numbers of possible interactions. In the US, there are about 1,500 approved drugs (if you define "drugs" narrowly since there are over 19,000 approved drug products in the US including generics, different formulations of the same chemical substance etc.) For these 1,500 drugs, there are 1.1 million combinations of two drugs, 562 million combinations of three drugs and 243 billion combinations of four drugs! Using the larger number of 19,000 there are more than 10^{70} possibilities for two drugs!

It is hoped that one day pharmacogenetics may provide better means of answering drug–drug interaction questions but we are not there yet.

Cytochrome P450

Many data on drug–drug interactions are based on study of the cytochrome P450 (CYP) system. CYP represents a large group of enzymes whose function is primarily to catalyze the oxidation of organic compounds, in particular drugs but also lipids, hormones, and other chemicals. The enzymes are found primarily in mitochondria or endoplasmic reticulum in cells and are distributed throughout the body. The enzymes we are most concerned about are found mainly in the liver and handle the biotransformation/metabolism of drugs in preparation for elimination from the body. Various drugs may increase or decrease the activity of one or more CYP enzymes by inducing the synthesis of the enzyme or inhibiting the enzyme's activity. Thus, if a drug inhibits an enzyme, then another drug that is metabolized by this enzyme may accumulate to toxic (ADR-producing) levels. Conversely, synthesis of more enzyme may increase metabolism of the second drug, lowering its levels and thus producing less efficacy (and perhaps fewer AEs). On the other hand, if the drug absorbed is a prodrug (e.g., codeine, which is metabolized to morphine), an increase in its metabolism may lead to an increase in toxicity, whereas a decrease in metabolism will lead to decreased efficacy This may be unimportant if a drug has a wide therapeutic window but may be life-threatening if the window is small and critical concentrations of the drug are needed for efficacy.

FDA publishes a list of "Drug Development and Drug Interactions: Table of Substrates, Inhibitors and Inducers". See https://www.fda.gov/drugs/development-resources/drug-interactions-labeling.

The EMA provides information on its website as regards to Drug-Drug Interactions (https://www.ema.europa.eu/en/investigation-drug-interactions-scientific-guideline)

Action on the CYP system is not limited to drugs but can be caused by herbals, tobacco use (e.g., smoking), and some foods. A good example is the herbal Saint John's wort, which is a potent inducer of CYP3A4. If Saint John's wort induces more CYP3A4, drugs metabolized by this enzyme (the drugs are referred to as substrates), such as cyclosporine or innadivir, may be cleared more rapidly and have less efficacy. See the Australian TGA's site (https://www.tga.gov.au) on St. John's Wort and the article "St John's wort (*Hypericum perforatum*): drug interactions and clinical outcomes" https://www.ncbi.nlm.nih.gov/pmc/articles/PMC1874438/.

As noted above with warfarin, certain patients who are either debilitated or suffer from certain diseases (e.g., autoimmune disorders, cardiovascular disease, gastrointestinal disease, infection, psychiatric disorders, respiratory disorders, seizure disorders, and others) may be at greater risk for drug interactions, and the more severe the underlying disease, the greater the risk.

Note the marked complexity of the issue here if patients are taking multiple drugs. The tables and measurements, which are usually based on studies done in normal individuals during phase I and are really qualitative. They do not indicate whether the changes (induction or inhibition) will be large or small. This is usually due to the great variability in individuals that is seen in clinical trials.

Add on multiple drugs, some of which may inhibit, some of which may induce, some of which may do either depending on the individual, and it becomes clear that the tables of interactions are at best guides and alerts to pay attention to the possibility of drug interactions. Drug–drug interaction studies of three or more drugs are rarely if ever performed due to the challenges of interpreting results. Thus, it can be said that whenever someone is taking three or more drugs, there is usually no data available on how these drugs may interact. The patient is, in effect, an $n = 1$ experiment. That is, it is not possible to accurately predict how the patient will tolerate the new drug. The prescriber and the patient must pay careful attention to the clinical state of the patient after any new drug is added since there is no good way to predict what may happen.

Drug–Food, Drug–Alcohol, Drug–Disease and Other Interactions

It should also be noted that there are possible drug–food (e.g., grapefruit juice), drug–nutrient, drug–disease, drug–herbal, and drug–alcohol interactions. It is also worth keeping in mind that drug–OTC interactions may be missed if the OTC products a patient is taking are not asked for by the questioner or remembered by the patient. There have been attempts to mine data on large databases, looking for drug interactions. One method uses the disproportionality scores for the two drugs in question for an ADR suspected of worsening by an interaction. Individual scores are calculated and then an "interaction" score is determined. This method has not been too successful or widely used. Other methods calculate confidence intervals for each drug and compare them to a confidence interval for a combined "virtual drug" of the two drugs combined in an attempt to estimate the drug interaction effect.[1]

[1] See Leone, Magro, Moretti, *et al.*, Identifying adverse drug reactions associated with drug-drug interactions: data mining of a spontaneous reporting database in Italy, *Drug Safety* 2010; 33(8): 667–675; and van Manen, Fram, DuMouchel, Signal detection methodologies to support effective safety management, *Expert Opin Drug Safety* 2007; 6(4): 451–464.

The FDA issued a guidance entitled "Clinical Drug Interaction Studies — Cytochrome P450 Enzyme- and Transporter-Mediated Drug Interactions Guidance for Industry" in January 2020. To find this and other relevant drug interaction documents search for "Drug Interactions | Relevant Regulatory Guidance and Policy Documents" on fda.gov. There are also drug interaction "checker" tools of variable quality for drugs, foods, and alcohol freely available on the Internet. Some of the "checkers" occasionally point to incorrect information.

These are primarily aimed at clinical pharmacology and drug development rather than pharmacovigilance. Until better methodology is developed for ascertaining drug–drug interactions before widespread use in patients, we are still at the individual patient level.

■ Frequency

In reality, drug–drug interactions represent a major problem in medicine today that is not well recognized by many clinicians. We may consider some of these to be "medication errors" because known drug interactions where there are significant clinical risks of either lack of efficacy or AEs should not occur. These drugs should not be prescribed or taken together. Electronic prescribing has significantly helped to prevent this somewhat for both prescribers and pharmacists However, the use of bad drug combinations is common.

In a study in Toronto, Canada, 909 elderly patients receiving glyburide were admitted with a diagnosis of hypoglycemia. In the primary analysis, those patients admitted for hypoglycemia were more than six times as likely to have been treated with co-trimoxazole in the previous week. Patients admitted with digoxin toxicity ($n \times 1{,}051$) were about 12 times more likely to have been treated with clarithromycin in the previous week, and patients treated with ACE inhibitors admitted with a diagnosis of hyperkalemia ($n = 523$) were about 20 times more likely to have been treated with a potassium-sparing diuretic in the previous week. The authors concluded that many hospital admissions of elderly patients for drug toxicity occur after administration of a drug known to cause drug–drug interactions and that many of these interactions could have been avoided.[2]

In a database study of 1,600 elderly patients in six European countries, the subjects used on average seven drugs per person; 46% had at least one drug combination possibly leading to a drug–drug interaction. On average, there were 0.83 potential drug–drug interactions per person. Almost 10% of the potential interactions were classified "to be avoided" according to the Swedish interaction classification system, but nearly one third of them were to be avoided only for predisposed patients. The risk of a sub-therapeutic effect as a result of a potential drug–drug interaction was as common as the risk of adverse reactions. Furthermore, differences in the frequency and type of potential interactions were found among the countries.[3]

In the US, it is estimated that 25% of the overall population takes five or more drugs per week. Of those over 65, 50% take five or more and 12% take 10 or more drugs per week.[4]

Another study[5] found the possibility of a drug interaction in 275 older adults with polypharmacy was 80%. The probability of at least one interaction was:

- 50% for persons taking 5–9 drugs,
- 81% with 10–14 drugs,
- 92% with 15–19 drugs, and
- 100% with 20 or more drugs.

Addition of each new drug to a 5-drug regimen increased the risk of an interaction by 12%.

A review of polypharmacy can be found at: Polypharmacy. 2022. Dona Varghese, Cecilia Ishida, Hayas

[2] Juurlink, Mamdani, Kopp, Laupacis, Redelmeier, Drug–drug interactions among elderly patients hospitalized for drug toxicity, *JAMA* 2003; 289: 1652–1658.

[3] Bjorkman, Fastbom, Schmidt, Bernsten, Drug–drug interactions in the elderly, *Ann Pharmacother* 2002; 36: 1675–1681; Bjorkman, Fastbom, Schmidt, *et al.*, *Ann Pharmacother* 2002; 36: 1675–1681. For an excellent review of drug therapy in the elderly, see Bressler, Bahl, Principles of drug therapy for the elderly patient, *Mayo Clin Proc* 2003; 78: 1564–1577.

[4] *Toxicol Int* 2012; 19(1): 68–73.

[5] *Ann Pharmacotherapy* 2013; 47(3): 324–332, doi: 10.1345/aph.1R621. Epub 2013 Mar 12.

Haseer Koya. StatPearls Publishing https://www.ncbi.nlm.nih.gov/books/NBK532953/.

Communication

There is a growing recognition that the mechanism for communicating medical information (in this case drug interaction information) is not adequate and is not achieving its goals. FDA and others have embarked on various newer mechanisms and procedures (including the use of social media, sometimes curated) to better communicate safety information. Interestingly, in the US, the responsibility and liability for drug interaction issues seem to be falling more on the pharmacist than on the prescribing physician, perhaps for the following reasons:

- Colleges of pharmacy in the US include courses in their entry-level degree programs designed to instruct students on aspects of drug interactions, including detection, incidence and significance, types of drug interactions, mechanisms by which interactions occur, and the role of the pharmacist in monitoring drug therapy to either avoid or resolve potential drug interactions.
- Most pharmacies (particularly the large national and regional chains in the United States) and healthcare systems are heavily computerized, allowing pharmacists to screen patient medication profiles for potential drug–drug interactions when processing new and refill prescriptions. Some software automatically flags this for the pharmacist and patient and, in certain instances, can even provide feedback alerts to prescribers. Smartphone "checker" apps provide convenient tools for patients, although the information is not always strictly controlled, However, the *Chicago Tribune* newspaper did a "study" of 255 pharmacies (both chains and independent pharmacies) in which reporters, who did not identify themselves, brought in two prescriptions for drugs that clearly should not be given together (per the drug labeling). The pharmacies missed informing the "patients" that these drugs should not be given together in half the cases. The range was from 30% failure in a large national chain to 72% in independent pharmacies; subsequently some of the pharmacies made changes in response to the expose'. Although one cannot necessarily generalize this to all pharmacies, the message is clearly buyer beware.

The astute "pharmacovigilant" should always be aware of the possibility of interactions and pay attention to other medications being taken as well as OTCs, herbals, nutraceuticals, foods, alcohol, and the patient's diseases for clues to interactions. Not an easy task at all!

CHAPTER

28

The Many Players in the World of Pharmacovigilance

There are many players in the world of pharmacovigilance (PV) — Companies, Governments, Non-governmental Organizations, and Others. The interactions are complex. Alliances are formed and severed as issues or interests change. The groups are active in various causes in the medical and pharmaceutical world, touching not just on safety but on healthcare costs, drug prices, and healthcare availability.

■ Introduction

Patients who take medicines and suffer from adverse events (AEs) are the first and primary group involved in drug safety. Healthcare professionals make up the next category and include those who prescribe, sell, or dispense medications and those who also help deal with the AEs. Other participants in the medical world include pharmaceutical companies, pharmacies, pharmacy/formulation committees (in hospitals and medical groups), insurance companies, drug/pharmacy benefit managers (in the United States), technology assessment groups, and others who decide which medications are made available or reimbursed and which are not.

Patients suffer the consequences of adverse drug reactions directly and personally, sometimes suffering dearly or even dying. Patients and their families are becoming more sophisticated about research drugs and treatments they take or will be willing to take. They use the internet to check social media, websites, apps, support groups, and more. The last or first resort is a Google search or now AI. Some sites and sources, of course, are far more accurate and unbiased than others. Some are misleading or downright wrong.

Yet patient perceptions are quite variable. Sometimes there may be a perception that every AE that occurs is due to the drug, and, at other times, there is not a real awareness or level of suspicion by the patient that a particular problem could be due to one or more drugs. Many patients believe that if the government agency has approved the drug for marketing it is "safe and effective". This is an unfortunate phrase since it implies absolutes — totally safe and always effective — when in fact its meaning is rather more like: *this product has benefits that outweigh the risks (sometimes not by much) when used by the approved patient group, at the approved dosage and route of administration, for the approved length of time for the approved indication(s).* Safety is not absolute or guaranteed and is not (ever) fully known, and some patients may have totally unexpected (idiosyncratic) bad side effects. This concept is hard to convey. And sometimes it is challenging to distinguish an adverse reaction from the progression of the patient's underlying disease.

It is often presumed (sometimes incorrectly) that a drug cannot produce an adverse reaction if it has been taken safely for months or even years by an individual. Drug–drug, drug–food, and drug–alcohol interactions, manufacturing issues, and so on are almost never thought of by patients as explanations of their problem. Patients often do not think of over-the-counter (OTC) products, "health foods", "nutraceuticals", or "herbals" (which may contain drugs or interact with drugs), cosmetics, and illicit drugs as culprits in adverse reactions. Physicians too often forget to ask about them when taking the medical history and investigating medical problems. Many patients who are receiving multiple drugs, particularly the elderly, who are often "polypharmacy" patients, cannot recall the drugs or the doses they take. Moreover, when patients take multiple drugs, it is hard to know or predict drug interactions.

In some societies or cultures, there has been a perception that AEs are the fault of the patient and represent a weakness or a shameful act on the patient's part and that they need to "tough it out". This attitude is changing as the dissemination of information occurs but is still seen in some older patients.

Healthcare practitioners prescribe, dispense, and administer drugs. When AEs or reactions occur, it may not be the same prescriber, dispenser, or administrator who has to deal with the drug's medical consequences. Emergency rooms may not be able to get immediate access to the patient's medical records or drug history, for example, though it is hoped this will change as electronic medical records become widespread and standardized — though privacy laws and regulations may ultimately limit accessibility even if the technology permits it.

■ Pharmaceutical (Biopharmaceutical) Companies

Pharmaceutical companies play a major role in the world of safety. In the United States, most AEs on marketed drugs are reported to the manufacturers — the pharma companies. In other countries, most AEs may be reported to the health agency or other institutions (e.g., medical centers, pharmacies, national or regional pharmacovigilance (PV) centers, etc.) The companies, through trade organizations, e.g., PhRMA, JPMA, and the EFPIA (see below) and the International Council for Harmonization (ICH), have worked with the US Food and Drug Administration (FDA), the European Medicines Agency (EMA), Japanese regulators, and WHO (as well as many other organizations that have joined this effort more recently) to harmonize the safety reporting procedures, requirements, formats, documents, and expectations. This effort has been largely successful because the requirements for reporting certain serious AEs from clinical trials and post-marketing situations are clear, consistent, and quite rigorous (7 or 15 calendar days). Major efforts are under way, with varying degrees of harmonization and cooperation between the industry, government, vendors, and Standards Development Organizations in the areas of electronic transmission and standards (e.g., digital formats for transmission of healthcare documents, laboratory tests, cardiograms), risk management and minimization, clinical trial standardization, machine learning, and more. This operational aspect is, in a sense, the low hanging fruit and, with sophisticated IT resources, many of these operational aspects of data collection and storage run very well. The higher hanging fruit which is harder to reach is the analysis of these data and the detection of "safety signals" and their analysis. The ultimate goal, we should not forget, is to get new, clinically important and trustworthy safety data to prescribers and patients as rapidly as possible. And these data should be presented in meaningful language that is appropriate for the target audience.

These efforts regarding "mechanics and operations" go beyond the pharmaceutical industry as the FDA and the Department of Health and Human Services and many other governmental and private entities standardize the transmission of healthcare data among all stakeholders (hospitals, doctors, pharmacies, laboratories, insurance companies, NGOs, etc.) and produce significant additional benefits for the public. Most dealings between scientific personnel in the industry and the FDA, EMA, and other agencies are cordial and correct, with the goal of protecting the public health and helping each do his or her job more efficiently and more rapidly, given limited resources. Complicating this effort are privacy and safety protections introduced in many countries including the US and EU. In addition, hackers and cybercrime also complicate matters. The data and analytical tools must be safe, secure, and fit-for-purpose with access limited to only those who should have access. This is a major issue now and laws and regulations have only started to address it.

The reverse of this coin, however, is represented by controversies about specific medical products and safety issues. Some people (consumer groups in particular) believe there is too much cordiality and warmth between the regulators and the regulated, allowing the companies to "get away" with many things to increase profit at the expense of public health. However, there is little evidence for this, even though people move from the government to industry (as in other regulated industries) and vice versa. They claim that this may compromise the safety of the public because regulators will be hesitant to cross or oppose a company they may shortly wish to work for. There are clearly professional and medical differences between and within the companies and the industry. Many of these "battles" occur behind closed doors or through written (e-mail) or telephonic communications. Most of these communications are privileged to protect intellectual property and not available to the public.

This came to the fore during the Covid crisis of 2020 and beyond. The flow and trustworthiness of information from FDA, CDC, the White House, academia, EU health agencies, WHO and many others were chaotic, often confusing and even contradictory. The public did not know what to believe in regard to taking the various Covid vaccinations, masking, lockdowns, and proposed therapeutics.

In addition, there has been some bad behavior on the part of the pharmaceutical companies in the Oxycontin/opioid crises, epinephrine pen pricing and the rapid jump in Daraprim pricing from $13.50 to $750 per tablet. Pharmaceutical companies play a major role by promoting their products to healthcare professionals and the public (direct-to-consumer advertising in the United States in particular). Sometimes the promotion is not balanced in the eyes of the FDA, and Warning Letters are sent to companies by the FDA's Office of Prescription Drug Promotion (OPDP). See the Warning Letter section of the FDA's website. FDA and other health agencies are now struggling with social media in which drugs are publicized, criticized, and commented upon by users, providers, and companies on blogs, tweets, and Facebook, Twitter, Instagram and elsewhere without fair balance and often without attribution. Much of the "information" is not curated. It is often hard to know what data are real and what data represent "fake news".

Physicians and other healthcare workers are also "detailed" by pharmaceutical representatives on products for their patients. The detail (the "sales pitch") should contain balanced information and include the ADR profile. The approved prescribing information should also be supplied.

■ Governments

In each country or region, there is, of course, the governmental agency or agencies that regulate medicines (the FDA, the EMA, the Medicines and Healthcare Products Regulatory Agency (MHRA), the Agence Nationale de Sécurité du Médicament et des Produits de Santé (ANSM), etc.) In addition to the agency, its parent organization may exert significant control and pressure (in the United States the Department of Health and Human Services; in other countries the Ministry of Health or Parliament/National Assembly/Congress), and so forth. In the United States, Congress and other federal departments and agencies also provide healthcare and medications (e.g., Veterans Affairs, the Department of Defense (DOD) for the Armed Forces, the Centers for Disease Control and Prevention (CDC), Medicare, Medicaid and others), as do state/provincial and local health departments, including boards of health.

Some countries separate drug safety from drug approval, and some countries, particularly in the European Union, have an overlay at the European level in addition to national- and local-level agencies involved in drug registration, pricing and safety.

Government entities involved directly or indirectly in drug safety are complex. In the United States, at the federal level, the executive cabinet-level (ministry-level) Department of Health and Human Services controls the FDA and other health-related agencies and entities. The US Congress controls the budget for the FDA and has legislative oversight of FDA and other health matters. Other federal-level groups with major interests in healthcare and pharmaceuticals include the Veterans Administration, which maintains hospitals, clinics, and pharmacies; the US armed forces, which also maintain hospitals clinics and pharmacies; and the National Institutes of Health, the National Cancer Institute, and the Centers for Disease Control and Prevention. Similar complexities may be seen in many countries around the world, depending on their level of centralization and federalism. Some countries (France in particular) have tight arrangements with academic medical centers in the world of drug safety.

At the state and local level in the United States, there are state and local health departments, Medicaid offices (the program that supplies healthcare to the indigent and certain others at the state level), and state budget and formulation offices. One of the recent controversies has been the push by state and local governments to aid consumers in importing prescription drugs from outside the United States.

Views on drug safety by all of the players may sometimes be simplistic and polarized, especially if they are conveyed in short sound bites. One may hear that the health authority should approve safe drugs only after careful and thorough study. Side effects, if any, should be mild, reversible, and of limited duration. Some supposedly neutral observers refuse to admit a drug to a formulary for cost reasons rather than for medical reasons and justify this with either lack of efficacy or increased safety concerns. Others believe that there should be no more than two or three products in any particular class of drugs because the me-too drugs add no value to the public health. Others feel that the FDA, the EMA and other agencies have been too slow and too strict in approving new drugs for dying patients or diseases with no adequate treatment currently. Some want drugs approved (or given interim approval) based on early phase II trials which are positive ("right to try"). This is starting to happen. The safety profile will be further explored in the post-marketing setting. Each of these positions has its positives and negatives and there is no consensus yet.

Consumers often believe that, if any really bad side effects occur, someone (somewhere) should be made to pay. At the extreme end, some groups assume malevolence and ill will on the part of the drug companies, whose goal (they say) is only to make money, and helping the ill is a "side effect" of making profit. There are periodic reports of bribery or various illegal actions to get drugs sold, studied, or put on formularies. The FDA encourages whistle-blowers to come forth with information on bad behavior with the inducement of substantial monetary rewards. As rhetoric heats up, the science and clarity disappear.

The controversy and politics tend to cloud some of the very real areas of controversy and concern:

- How much secrecy should be permitted in the competitive area of drug development and drug safety? How much transparency should there be? What happens in emergencies and pandemics?
- What is the role of the industry in patient and healthcare professional education?
- Is direct-to-consumer advertising a good or bad thing for the public and how does it play regarding drug safety?
- Is a single-payer system for drugs a good or bad thing for drug safety, and is it too expensive?
- Are the current drug safety systems in the United States, the European Union, and elsewhere adequate?
- Should the universities be more heavily involved? Should there be a single national formulary?
- Should me-too drugs be limited? Is the WHO Model List of Essential Drugs (http://www.who.

int/medicines/publications/essentialmedicines/en/) a good way to handle pharmaceuticals?

- Should drug safety be separated from the drug agency that approves drugs, as the approvers would be hesitant to "admit" they might have approved a drug with safety issues that appear after marketing?
- As healthcare is finite and demand infinite, how should rationing of care, treatment, medications, etc., be done?
- Should some level of drug imports by consumers from abroad be tolerated or even encouraged to save money? And how will quality be ensured?
- How should OTC drug safety be handled? Are consumer reports without any healthcare professional confirmation worth collecting and how much effort should be expended in their analysis?
- Should cosmetics, "health foods", supplements, etc. be more heavily regulated?
- What role should automation and Artificial Intelligence (AI) play in safety?

One positive outcome of the controversies of the last several years in drug safety is more availability and transparency of safety information by companies and governments in some areas of drug safety. This has been accelerated and enhanced by the expanding domains of digital data, data standards, and analytical abilities. Detailed information on most clinical trials is now available online at governmental websites, such as Clintrials.gov in the US (www.clinicaltrials.gov) and the Clinical Trials Information System (CTIS) in the EEA, as well as pharmaceutical companies' individual clinical trial sites.

Post-marketing AEs are now appearing online or are available as files of variable user-friendliness. The FDA now has a fairly user-friendly system to search the post-marketing safety database known as FAERS. The EEA repository for AEs (pre- and post-marketing) is EudraVigilance. See the Database chapter in this Manual for further information.

Anonymized line listings and individual MedWatch reports are available from the FDA for nominal fees or from private companies (for higher costs but with anonymity of the requester). The data can also be downloaded from the FAERS website. Other countries (France, Canada, the UK, etc.) also have websites with similar search pages.

Much of the older and some of the current clinical trial data are largely proprietary and unavailable to the public or medical profession beyond what is in a drug's labeling, monograph, or presented in summary form at clintrials.gov. The European Union puts summaries of some approvals ("European Public Assessment Reports" or EPARs) online, and the FDA has some Summary Bases of Approval (SBOAs) also available online. Data from many clinical trials are published as peer-reviewed articles. However, the emphasis is usually on efficacy/effectiveness and detailed safety data are often limited.

The EMA, via the Pharmacovigilance Risk Assessment Committee (PRAC) is posting monthly meeting minutes on the website; this highlights transparency on their processes and decisions.

Many countries (United States, United Kingdom, Japan) have Freedom of Information laws that allow anyone to obtain non-classified and non-proprietary data for minimal cost. However, often one must know exactly what one is looking for. "Fishing expeditions" can be hard or not permitted.

The United Kingdom MHRA also has a Freedom of Information act and some safety information is available. Interestingly, unlike the US government's published information, which is not subject to copyright, there is strict copyright control of information released by the UK government:

> "All material created by the Medicines and Healthcare products Regulatory Agency (MHRA) is subject to Crown copyright protection. We control the copyright to our work (which includes all information, database rights, logos and visual images), under a delegation of authority from the Controller of His Majesty's Stationery Office (HMSO)."
>
> "The MHRA authorizes you to make one free copy, by downloading to printer or to electronic, magnetic or optical storage media, of any items featured on this website (excluding Agency logos) for the purposes of private research, study and reference. Any other copy or use of Crown copyright materials featured on this site, in any form or medium is subject to the prior approval of the MHRA."

Further information on the "Crown Copyright" can be found online. One public venue where differences are aired, often with full media coverage, is represented by public meetings of the FDA advisory committees and similar groups in other countries. See the FDA's website Regarding advisory committees, in particular the Drug Safety and Risk Management Advisory Committee. These are standing committees called by the FDA to discuss and recommend courses of action in controversial or unclear areas in which the agency wishes external advice. Members include the FDA and academia, a patient advocate and, sometimes, non-voting industry members. They receive, in advance, data from the FDA and the industry and then meet in public (usually) to discuss the issues involved. The companies are usually well represented in the audience and industry scientists often make presentations. The discussions are usually scientific and technical but can become adversarial and even quite heated. Some sessions may be held behind closed doors and are not open to the public when proprietary information is discussed. Recent FDA practice has been to broadcast the public portions of meetings in real time. Transcripts and presentations of the public sessions are often available shortly afterward on the FDA website. These sessions are often attended by media and Wall Street/Venture Capital types when public companies' products are involved. Comments by the committees often influence stock prices of both the company whose drug is discussed, and competitors' drugs whose sales might be threatened by a new drug. This is a good example of transparency in the world of pharmaceuticals.

Broadly speaking, professionals working in the drug safety area of government and industry tend to be more aligned and better able and motivated to share ideas with each other than are professionals in other areas of the industry (research, marketing, legal, etc.), because they are less constrained by legal restrictions and by competitive issues (e.g., anti-trust concerns). Sharing ideas about "what works" operationally in drug safety, PV, and risk management is common and is seen particularly with operational issues (e.g., drug coding, conventions for the Medical Dictionary for Regulatory Activities (MedDRA) coding of AEs, and, for oncology products, the Common Terminology for Adverse Events (CTCAE)). Proprietary drug-specific safety information is not shared. Such alignment and cooperation is now international and facilitated by the web. Data are now being shared on Facebook, LinkedIn and other social media. Shared databases of anonymized clinical trial data are being assembled by trusted third parties for research purposes. Key regulators, e.g., FDA, EMA, Health Canada, and others, have confidentiality agreements under which they hold virtual meetings on a regular basis to share perspectives.

It is in everyone's interest for AEs to be sent to the FDA and other health authorities in a timely, complete, and correct manner. Companies do, in fact, want their competitors to have well-run and efficient safety departments so that the competition's AEs are sent to the health agencies in a timely and complete manner too!

■ Media

The *media*, including social media, the Internet (blogs, websites, RSS feeds, wikis, customer engagement programs, etc.), and old *media* (television, radio, newspapers), play active roles from all perspectives of the political and medical scene. This field is evolving, with the health agencies struggling to understand how to use the media themselves as well as how to regulate use by industry. The newest addition to this scene is AI which does indeed promise to be yet another "game changer". The agencies use Facebook and many other social media sites and apps and many other modalities on the internet. They are also adapting the old paper-based reporting systems to the Internet (MedWatch, Yellow Cards, Blue Cards, etc.). Nonetheless, agencies must be careful what they put on the Internet and how they use these sites. There is much controversy over Tweets by senior political or medical leaders! The Covid wars of 2020-2022 are a prime example of this. Issues of privacy and hacking are also arising. Data security and privacy are major topics of the big Internet players now. It is likely that data sharing will become more restrictive in the future.

Other aspects of the Internet are now "fake news" and information overload with far too much information available — not all of which is reliable.

■ NGOs and Lobbies

Non-governmental organizations (NGOs) play major roles in healthcare throughout the world, including the World Health Organization (WHO) in drug policies and its affiliate, the Uppsala Monitoring Centre in Sweden (See Chapter 11), in drug safety, pandemics and other public health areas; various foundations that fund healthcare initiatives (e.g., the Gates Foundation); the Drug Safety Research Unit in the United Kingdom; and others.

Lobbies or professional organizations, NGOs from many domains (e.g., Pharmaceutical Research Manufacturers of America [PhRMA], European Federation of Pharmaceutical Industries and Associations (EFPIA), International Society of Pharmacoepidemiology, the Centers for Education and Research on Therapeutics, the American Association of Retired Persons), OTC drug manufacturers, generic manufacturers, hospital groups, vaccine manufacturers, device manufacturers, physician groups, nursing groups, pharmacy groups, consumer groups, disease groups, and advocacy groups, such as Public Citizen (https://www.citizen.org/), also play roles in drug safety. The list is growing.

These groups, which often espouse special interests, petition or file position papers to influence legislation, regulatory decisions, and perceptions at the local, state/provincial, and national levels as well as in litigation and in the media. The groups work from all parts of the spectrum, including some who strive to increase profits, speed up or slow down drug approval, and increase or decrease governmental oversight and regulation.

Some NGOs are now actually functioning as pharmaceutical companies setting up clinical trials in areas of need (particularly in resource-constrained settings) where the pharmaceutical industry does not venture (for many reasons). One example is TB Alliance, a non-profit, which has several new and old drugs under clinical trial for the treatment of tuberculosis.

■ Industry Organizations

The industry organization for pharmaceutical companies in the United States is PhRMA (www.phrma.org), and in Europe it is the European Federation of Pharmaceutical Industries and Associations (EFPIA) (www.efpia.eu). In Japan it is the Japanese Pharmaceutical Manufacturers Association (JPMA). Not all companies are members, especially the smaller companies and those that do not do research. PhRMA, which is based in Washington, DC, has 13 offices, including in China, Japan, and the United Arab Emirates. PhRMA supports multiple functions including lobbying for the industry's position on public issues and legislation, outreach to the public, assisting with patient assistance programs, and representing US industry in the ICH. Its goal is to "encourage discovery of important new medicines for patients by pharmaceutical/biotechnology research companies." This is a highly political and controversial area.

The EFPIA is based in Brussels, with an office in Japan. The EFPIA is an association of associations and includes national industry associations in Europe as well as biopharma companies. Similar organizations exist in other countries and industry associations also exist for vaccines, OTCs, biologics, generics, and cosmetics.

In Canada, the industry association is known as Innovative Medicines (http://innovativemedicines.ca/).

There are multiple other organizations representing OTC manufacturers, generic manufacturers, parenteral drugs, vaccine companies, biologics, device manufacturers, and cosmetics that interact, as well as groups representing physicians (American Medical Association in the United States), hospitals (American Hospital Association in the United States), nurses, insurance companies, and so forth. The permutations and combinations of interactions are many, complex, and growing, as groups sometimes work with one another and sometimes against one another. As attributed to Benjamin Disraeli, "There are no permanent allies, no permanent friends, only permanent interests."

Litigation, Lawyers, and Legalities

Litigation plays a major role in safety decisions made regarding drugs in some countries, particularly the United States. Any significant episode of AEs produces a flurry of lawsuits, often numbering in the thousands. They may take years to resolve, and costs run into the billions of dollars. The issues usually revolve around who in the company and sometimes in the government knew about the drug's toxicity, when it was known, whether it was adequately publicized and labeled, and whether remedial actions were taken in a timely fashion. In the United States (and other countries such as Canada, Italy and France) the phenomenon of "class action lawsuits" often plays a significant role in drug safety litigation. In these lawsuits, a group of people (sometimes a very large group) will sue a company or several companies if their problems are similar. This groups many hundreds or thousands of people into one lawsuit.

To a large degree, litigation and the fear of litigation influence behavior in the drug safety world. Some companies are hesitant to admit in a report sent to the health authorities that their drug might have caused a particularly serious AE. Such reports can be used in court cases against the company or against the reporting physician, nurse, pharmacist, and hospital, even if the report only notes the possibility of a causal relationship with the drug (e.g., "a causal relationship cannot be excluded", "possibly related", "probably related"). The United States is the major country where such issues occur, but hesitancy in commenting on causality may be seen in reports to health authorities outside the United States because these reports may be obtained and used in US courts, especially if the reports are easily available in English (e.g., from the United Kingdom, Canada, Australia, New Zealand, Uppsala Monitoring Centre).

Workers in the field of PV should familiarize themselves with the rules (both written and "unwritten") about how much and what sort of statements and conclusions can be made in reports submitted to governments, kept in computers, or on file, and which are "discoverable" (that is, may be obtained by lawyers for use in court cases). If a drug safety case from a company has entered the legal system via a lawyer or lawsuit, the drug safety group will often have to work through the company's legal department to obtain follow-up information and to do its normal drug safety follow-up and due diligence. Some companies also have a legal review of all reports submitted to health authorities (e.g., expedited reports, PSURs).

Finally, drug safety personnel may be called on to testify in court and to give long and complex depositions either in individual cases that are on trial (e.g., malpractice, unexpected SAEs, or deaths) or in large lawsuits (such as class action suits in the United States), particularly those following major drug withdrawals (Baycol®, Vioxx®, etc.)

Other Groups

Consumer groups, insurance companies, employers paying health insurance, health maintenance organizations, retired persons groups, and others also play roles, sometimes direct and sometimes indirect, in drug safety. Broadly speaking, many or all of these groups favor, to some degree or another, lower-cost (or even "free") drugs, limited formularies ("no need for me-too drugs"), generics, OTC status for many more drugs, and lessening the influence of pharmaceutical companies and increasing the role of regulators, without giving much thought to what this might do (both positively and negatively) to drug safety, or result in other unintended consequences. In the United States, many of these groups have strong lobbies in Washington, DC, and at the state levels. Many similar groups exist outside the United States, but their activities and influence on the political systems do not appear to be as strong as in the United States.

■ Organizations for Drug Safety Personnel

There are several organizations that personnel working in the field of drug safety often join as follows:

- **DIA (formerly the Drug Information Association):** The big international organization covers all areas of the drug world, with academia, industry, government, and others joining. They have annual meetings each year in the United States, Canada, Europe, and Asia. They run training programs, publish a journal, Therapeutic Innovation and Regulatory Science, and have an extensive (though hard-to-navigate) website. Annual membership costs are fairly low, and if one is joining only one organization, this is usually it.
- **International Society for Pharmacoepidemiology (ISPE):** The main organization for pharmacoepidemiology, including PV and risk management. Members are from industry, academia, government agencies, and non-profit and for-profit private organizations. Members have degrees in a number of fields, including epidemiology, biostatistics, medicine, nursing, pharmacology, pharmacy, law, health economics, and journalism. They hold multiple meetings each year and publish the journal Pharmacoepidemiology and Drug Safety.
- **International Society of Pharmacovigilance (IsoP)**, originally formed as the European Society of Pharmacovigilance — An international non-profit scientific organization to foster PV both scientifically and educationally and to enhance all aspects of the safe and proper use of medicines in all countries.
- **Regulatory Affairs Professionals Society (RAPS):** A global organization of regulatory professionals. A bit peripheral to drug safety, as they cover the full range of drug regulatory matters. They offer training and hold meetings and have publications of interest to drug safety personnel.
- **Academy of Physicians in Clinical Research (APCR):** A non-profit membership organization representing physicians (MD, DO, MBBS or equivalent) engaged in or preparing to engage in clinical research within Clinical Practice, Academic Institutions, Specialized Medical Clinics, and Pharmaceutical Industry Researchers.
- **European Programme in Pharmacovigilance and Pharmacoepidemiology (Eu2P):** An organization that is a European private and academic partnership offering training in PV and pharmacoepidemiology for specialists and non-specialists. They work with universities in Spain, Italy, UK, The Netherlands, and Italy.
- **Institute for Safe Medical Practices (ISMP):** A US non-profit organization devoted entirely to medication error prevention and safe medication use (www.ismp.org).

Many PV groups have been created on social networks; as of today, they are not replacing the large, official and well-established organizations. This could change in the next years, mainly for rapid information exchanges.

■ Conclusion and Comments

And, finally, there are the unfortunate patients and sometimes unfortunate individual doctors, pharmacists, and nurses who deal on one-to-one levels and who must wade through the controversy, politics, and unclear and equivocal safety information ("the following AEs have been reported with this drug but causality cannot be determined") to come to good decisions for individual patients. When it comes to specific numbers, it is usually prudent to demur because that number could change tomorrow (or tonight).

The bottom line is: drug safety is a high-stakes, multi-party, politicized, highly controversial affair with multiple players involved with multiple agendas and multiple millions of dollars, euros, yuan, rupees, and so forth. Data are often soft, incomplete, and skewed in one direction or another. One should look at multiple sources for information and keep an open mind on the ultimate outcome of safety issues with drugs. Usually the "truth will out", although it may take a long time.

■ Frequently Asked Question

Q: So then how should the individual in the doctor's office, hospital, drug company, health agency, or elsewhere act? What can the individual do to help sort this out?

A: In general, act as a good scientist and citizen, an honest person, and do not judge until there is a good amount of evidence examined from multiple sources. Trust but verify. A good rule of thumb would be whether you or a loved one would take the product in question.

Company safety personnel should always act with the public health foremost in their mind and the company profits secondary. This may be difficult because there are always pressures to "protect the drug" or "hold off on this signal until the data are stronger". Safety workups and signaling should always be done with due diligence and an open mind. Sometimes those terrible-looking serious AEs really do melt away after all the data are in. When the results are bad for the drug, these data must be conveyed to management and to all involved health authorities in a timely and correct manner. That can be an unpleasant experience, but "always do the right thing."

Practitioners, pharmacists, nurses, and patients should maintain a healthy skepticism regarding data, whether they are from the company, academia, the health authority, or the media — especially during the acute controversy when the "fog of war" is at its height and angry words, images, and charges are flying. They should seek out data from all sides and from neutral authorities (if such exist). Healthcare practitioners must always act in the best interest of the patient.

As a person rises in the company or governmental hierarchy in drug safety, the pressures increase as well. More money, more sales, more lives, more consequences (intended and unintended) are in play. This can clearly influence one's judgment in safety and medical matters even unintentionally. To quote the dictum of Lord Acton: "Power corrupts; absolute power corrupts absolutely". Another useful piece of wisdom is from the late Senator Daniel Patrick Moynihan: "Everyone is entitled to his own opinion, but not his own facts".

Patients should find honest, caring health personnel and trust them to act in their best interest. Nonetheless, verification (looking at the approved drug labeling, looking on the Internet at reliable sites, being treated at major or academic medical centers, etc.) is also well worth doing. Good luck.

CHAPTER

29

Pharmacovigilance System Master File

Companies applying for or holding Marketing Authorizations (MAs) for biopharmaceutical products in the EEA, must have a critical document on file: the Pharmacovigilance System Master File (PSMF). Likewise, in India a company must have in place the PvMF, which is extremely similar to the EU PSMF in format and purpose. Indeed, the India-specific document can be produced from the EU PSMF. These master files required in the EU, India, and elsewhere should not be considered as a static document only but as a dynamic tool that supports active governance of the PV System and undergoes constant revision. It must be kept up to date and details are described in the EU Guideline on Good Pharmacovigilance Practice (GVP) Module II. The master files are prepared and kept in good order by the MAH and provided to the regulator on request (promptly!)

■ Introduction

This document is legally required at the moment of submission of a Marketing Authorization Application (MAA) in the EU. As described in GVP Module II, the content of the PSMF should reflect global availability of safety information for medicinal products authorized in the EU, presenting information on the pharmacovigilance system applied at global, regional, and local levels. The PSMF will be required for pharmacovigilance (PV) inspections by European Union Competent Authorities. Several non-EU countries are now following this concept and require a similar document. It is a wise idea to prepare this document (customized for specific regions that require it) and keep it current. By preparing it, the company will deliver a detailed overview on the status and quality of the company's PV system for government inspectors and other interested parties such as marketing or development partners. According to GVP Module II, the PSMF is required as part of a quality management system.

The EU Pharmacovigilance System Master File (Guideline on Good Pharmacovigilance Practice Module II)

See EU GVP Module II for details

The key parts of the PSMF are as follows:

- **EU Qualified Person for Pharmacovigilance (EU QPPV)**
  - Responsibilities guaranteeing that the EU QPPV has sufficient authority over the PV System;
  - CV with the key information on the role of the EU QPPV (including qualifications and experience specific to PV and proof of EudraVigilance registration);
  - Contact details including back-up arrangements (24/7);
  - Same information for the deputy EU QPPV, if applicable;
  - Copy of the EU QPPV registration dossier (and deputy EU QPPV if applicable; and
  - List of delegated/outsourced tasks:

  Note: Any delegation, backup, commitment, etc., must be in a signed document or contract.

- **Organizational structure of the MAH**
  - Organizational structure of the MAH, showing the position of the EU QPPV;
  - All sites in the world where the PV functions are undertaken with their specific roles and responsibilities; and
  - Delegated/outsourced activities with details on partners references, roles and responsibilities (of note, contracts may be requested by health authorities during inspections or on an ad hoc basis).

- **Sources of safety data**
  - Description of the main units involved with safety data collection, on a global basis, for solicited and spontaneous case collection (products authorized in the EU);
  - List describing the country, nature of the activity and the product(s) and providing a contact point (address, telephone and e-mail) for the site;
  - Detailed information about third parties, including their specific roles and responsibilities; and
  - List of study sources, including any studies, registries, surveillance or support programs sponsored by the MAH through which ICSRs could be reported. The list should describe, on a worldwide basis, the status of each study/program, the applicable country(ies), the product(s) and the main objective.

- **Computerized systems and databases**
  - List and description of the main PV systems and databases;
  - Location, functionality and operational responsibility for computerized systems and databases used to:
    - Receive, collate, record and report safety information;
    - Identify and manage safety signals;
    - Manage PSURs/PBRERs, RMPs (scheduling, production, review, validation and submission);
    - Manage Corrective and Preventive Actions (CAPAs), etc.;
  - Fit-for-purpose assessment of the IT system (increasing dependance on The Cloud presents challenges);
  - Validation status of key aspects of computer system functionality: change control, nature of testing, back-up procedures and electronic data repositories vital to PV compliance; and

- Description (and location) of the available documentation.

- **Pharmacovigilance processes**
  - "Continuous" monitoring of product risk–benefit profile(s);
    - Results of evaluation and the decision-making process for taking appropriate measures;
    - Signal generation, detection, evaluation, and management;
    - Procedures and instructions concerning
    - Safety database outputs;
    - Interactions with clinical departments, etc.;
  - Risk management system(s) and monitoring of the outcome of risk minimization measures;
  - ICSR collection, collation, follow-up, assessment, and reporting (specifying local versus global activities);
  - PSUR/PBRER scheduling, production and submission;
  - Communication of safety concerns to consumers, HCPs, and the competent authorities; and
  - Implementation of safety variations to the SmPC and PIL, considering both internal and external communications.

- **Pharmacovigilance system performance**
  - Targets for the performance of the pharmacovigilance system;
  - Correct reporting of ICSR assessment (with figures/graphs on timeliness for 15-day and 90-day reporting over the past year — within Annexes);
  - Metrics used to monitor the quality of ICSR reporting, PSURs/PBRERs or other submissions;
  - Overview of the timeliness of PSUR/PBRER reporting to competent authorities in the EU;
  - Overview of the methods used to ensure timeliness of safety variation submissions compared to internal and competent authority deadlines; and
  - Overview of adherence to Risk Management Plan (RMP) commitments, or other obligations or conditions of the MAH that are relevant to PV.

- **Quality system**
  - Document and Record Control: description of archiving arrangements;
  - Procedural documents;
    - General description of the types of documents used in PV (standards, operating procedures, work instructions, etc.);
    - Applicability of these documents at global, regional or local level within the organization;
    - Controls that are applied to their accessibility, implementation and maintenance;
    - Information about the documentation systems applied to relevant procedures and documents under the control of third parties, e.g., licensing partners;
    - List of specific procedures and processes related to the PV activities and interfaces with other functions or partners (EU QPPV & backup activities; contractual agreements; collection, processing, data entry, quality control, coding, classification, medical review, and reporting of ICSRs; aggregate reports preparation, validation, delivery & transmission, signal detection & management processes; benefit–risk evaluation processes; internal & external PV communication; interaction between safety issues and product defects; responses to requests for information from regulatory authorities; handling of urgent safety restrictions and safety variations; meeting commitments to agencies, etc.).

- **Training**
  - Description of the training systems and where the training records, CVs, and job descriptions are filed.

- **Auditing**
  - Information about QA assurance auditing of the PV System (audit plan approach, reporting mechanisms and timelines, etc.);
  - List of scheduled and completed audits (five year rolling period), including notes on any changes to plan; and
  - Specific note for any major and/or critical finding with a summary of CAPA(s).

- **Annexes to the PSMF**
  - Annex A
    - Tasks delegated by the EU QPPV;
    - CV of the EU QPPV;
    - EU QPPV contact details;
  - Annex B
    - List of contracts & agreements;
  - Annex C
    - Description of sources of safety data;
  - Annex D
    - Additional information on computerized systems and databases;
  - Annex E
    - Lists of procedural documents;
  - Annex F
    - Lists of Key Performance Indicators (KPI)s;
    - Current results of performance assessment;
  - Annex G
    - Audit schedules (including changes);
    - List of audits conducted and completed;
  - Annex H
    - List(s) of products covered by the PV system;
    - Any notes concerning the MAH per product;
  - Annex I
    - Logbook;
    - Documentation of history of changes for Annex contents.

As you can see, this is an incredibly complete and complex document that can run, with appendices, several hundred pages in a large multi-national pharma company. Keeping this complex document up to date may be a full-time job in some companies.

Comment

Clearly the PSMF has been well thought out by the EMA. It requests information that will show whether a company has control (at least on paper) over each of the key areas in drug safety. Pre-registration PV activities and organizations are not, strictly speaking, within the scope of the PSMF. However, the PSMF must be at the ready when a marketing application is submitted, not only after authorization.

This is a major document (and a legal requirement) with multiple annexes/appendices and contains data that must be obtained from many sources within the company. Much of the data may not be handy or readily available to the PV department. This document should be prepared as a matter of routine, updated periodically, and kept on file. It will be inspected!

Additional comments:

- Companies should view the PSMF as a living document, which should be kept up to date, with a strict versioning process, posted on a secured repository, under the direction and control of the EU QPPV. Someone must "own" it and be responsible for it within the organization. The EU QPPV is that person, even though many of the associated tasks are often delegated.
- It should be considered as a tool to gain assurance that the PV system is compliant and to document information on deviations/deficiencies or risks in the company's PV system.
- The PSMF must be provided to EU Authorities upon request within 7-calendar days, but a request may be made for an immediate response. In practice, this means that the PSMF must be up to date and immediately available. For large companies, it may be quite challenging to prepare this "on the spot" for an audit or inspection.
- It must be registered in the EMA EudraVigilance System (Article 57 database).
- A PSMF is to be available for any company:
  - Having at least one registered medicinal product in one or more EEA country(ies).
  - Regardless of the registration procedure (centralized, national, mutual recognition or decentralized).
- When delegating any activities concerning the PV system and its PSMF, the MAH retains ultimate responsibility for the PV system, for submission of information about the PSMF location, for maintenance and for its provision to competent authorities upon request.

- The PSMF is a global document covering the company's entire PV system. Activities outside the EEA can and do impact the EU PV scope and system.
- One single PSMF by company is simpler but depending on the company's history, organization, products, etc., several PSMFs can be envisaged; but any chosen option must be defensible in front of inspectors. Reasons for more than one PSMF might include split of independent business units within an organization, e.g., one business unit for vaccines and another for traditional chemical medicinal products. Of course, as more jurisdictions outside the EU require an equivalent document for their region, these must be created and maintained.
- The site/country where the PSMF is located in the EU is important and much thought should be given to where the company locates the EU QPPV and PSMF. This is because the Member State where the PSMF is held becomes the supervisory authority handling all relations with the EMA as well as PV inspections. Note that, as a practical matter, most PSMFs are "located" in the "cloud" and the supervisory regulatory authority usually defaults to the country where the EU QPPV operates. If this is not the case, the situation and reasons must be fully explained in writing and be kept on file.
- When preparing a PSMF, it is wise to include more stable information in the main body of the document, i.e., any information which does not change frequently. Examples might be SOPs and computer system information, etc. Other information may change relatively quickly (e.g., contact information) and this should be put into the annexes/appendices. This makes updating the document easier. Updating must, of course be done, formally and under the aegis of the quality system in place.
- The PSMF is an EU document but a local PSMF (at the affiliate level in large companies) can be useful. The purpose is not to duplicate information already included in the EU PSMF but rather add specific local organization, processes, etc. The document is generally in English but "validated" translations may be appropriate.
- Even if the company does not operate in the EU, it might be wise to keep on file a document like the PSMF summarizing how the safety system works in the company. This may be requested if marketing partners in the EU are or become involved. It may be very difficult to prepare this document in a hurry if a new marketing partner is enlisted with little notice to the safety department and anyone else preparing the PSMF.
- Ownership of the PSMF must be clear. It is usually the EU QPPV. However, he/she may not do the actual collection and preparation of all the multiple parts of the document but he/she will be held responsible for it.

In summary, the EU PSMF is a complex, obligatory document that must be carefully and accurately done. It is used as the basic information source for inspections. It should also reflect reality. It is not a theoretical document. The processes and systems described in the PSMF must really exist and be visible to the inspectors when they inspect the company, talk to PV personnel, etc. It must be kept up to date. Likewise, for other jurisdictions that may require similar documents (and they all must be in synch).

CHAPTER

30

The Qualified (Individual) Person(s) Responsible for Pharmacovigilance

This chapter addresses responsibility for a MAH's pharmacovigilance system.

■ Single Point of Responsibility for Post-Marketing Pharmacovigilance

For companies with products registered in the European Union (as well as in certain other territories), Directive 2010/84/EU requires that there be an EU "Qualified Person for Pharmacovigilance" (QPPV). This is a critical role and function within the company. The concept of a QPPV or a "an individual person responsible for pharmacovigilance who is permanently and continuously available to the MAH" is most interesting: a named individual (and backup) takes corporate and personal responsibility for the functioning of drug safety and the pharmacovigilance (PV) system for each company that has a Marketing Authorization (MA) in the respective jurisdiction. In many cases, the responsible person must reside in the covered territory for enforcement purposes For example, the EU QPPV must reside in the EU. In most jurisdictions, if a company does not yet have an MA or a submission and is only doing clinical trials, there is ordinarily no requirement for a responsible person. However, a candidate responsible person must be identified and named at the time of MA submission. In addition, a pharmacovigilance (PV) system that addresses requirements in the post-marketing phase must be in place even if the system is not yet being used. More than 70 jurisdictions, some within the EU, have adopted the role of a qualified or responsible person for pharmacovigilance.

The EU QPPV functions at the EU level. Others operate at the country level. In the EU, all local QPPVs must report to the EU QPPV. The EU QPPV position and requirements are defined in Directive 2010/84/EU and GVP Module I.

The concept of the QPPV originated in the EU. However, this role has since been legislated elsewhere over the years. Examples are: Australia, Belgium, Bulgaria, Croatia, Cyprus, Czech Republic, Denmark, France, Germany (called the Stufenplanbeauftragter), Greece, Hungary, India, Latvia, Lithuania, Luxembourg, Netherlands, Poland, Romania, Russia, Slovakia, Spain, Uganda, United Kingdom, and others. Note that having a requirement on the record does not ensure compliance, particularly when enforcement is not consistent and penalties for non-compliance are variable. Check detailed requirements locally.

The US has yet to require a single qualified person for pharmacovigilance, which can contribute to a lesser degree of understanding of requirements when US-only organizations expand outside the USA

Since there is no direct counterpart for the EU QPPV in the US and Canada the responsibility for a pharmacovigilance system lies at the corporate level. Note that the EU QPPV is not responsible for manufacturing issues; there is a separate QP for manufacturing.

Directive 2010/84/EU and GVP Module I note the following:

- Each company must submit a summary of the applicant's pharmacovigilance system master file (PSMF) which shall include the following elements:
  - Proof that the applicant has at his disposal a Qualified Person Responsible for PharmacoVigilance (QPPV);
  - The Member State(s) in which the qualified person resides and carries out his/her tasks; and
  - The contact details of the QPPV.
- The MAH should have permanently and continuously at his disposal a QPPV residing and operating in the EU or EEA with 24/7 availability.
- One QPPV per PV system in a company is required, but one single QPPV may have oversight of several PV systems. There could be a qualified deputy also residing in the EEA. The name and contact information must be provided to EMA/Member States.
- Some Member States require a named person/national QPPV, too. This person may or may not be the same as the EU QPPV.
- The QPPV should be appropriately qualified, with documented experience in all aspects of pharmacovigilance. If the QPPV is not medically qualified (i.e., an MD), access to a medically qualified person should be available 24/7.
- The EU QPPV has multiple responsibilities:
  - Establishing and maintaining/managing the MAH's pharmacovigilance system;
  - Ensuring that a PSMF is in place and up to date (some jurisdictions also have local requirements for the equivalent of a local or regional PSMF, which must be consistent with the EU PSMF);
  - Ensuring that all ARs (including literature searches) are collected, collated, and accessible at least at one point within the EU;
  - Ensuring preparation, validation and submission of ICSRs and synthesis reports (PSURs/PBRERs, RMPs, benefit–risk assessment, etc.) and company-sponsored post-authorization safety/efficacy studies (PASS & PAES);
  - Evaluating continuously the overall pharmacovigilance system, including in particular, during the post-authorization period;
  - Having oversight of signal detection and risk management, including PASS/PAES and risk minimization measures (routine and non-routine measures); being involved in the review and sign-off of protocols of PASS conducted in the EU or included in the RMP approved in the EU;
  - Being aware of any new information about benefit–risk assessments for all registered drugs;
  - Ensuring that any request from the health agency is answered fully and promptly;
  - Being the contact person for EMA PV inspections as well as inspections by other non-EU agencies and third parties.

Note: GVP Module I specifies that "The QPPV may delegate specific tasks, under supervision, to appropriately qualified and trained individuals, for example, acting as safety experts for certain products, provided that the QPPV maintains system oversight and overview of the safety profiles of all products. Such delegation should be documented." Accountability may not be delegated,

The QPPV should have oversight of the PV system, including and, therefore, "sufficient authority to influence the performance of the quality system and the pharmacovigilance activities and to promote, maintain and improve compliance," i.e., authority over:

- The organization of the Drug Safety department, processes, tools, and performance/compliance;
- The needed measures for signal detection and risk management activities, including benefit–risk assessments;
- The decision to take for variations, urgent safety restrictions, and communication to patients and healthcare professionals;
- Partnerships.

The MAH, as well, has responsibilities to the following:

- Support the QPPV and ensure appropriate processes, resources, communication mechanisms, and access to all sources of relevant information in place for the QPPV.
- Ensure full documentation of all procedures and activities of the QPPV.
- Implement mechanisms for the QPPV to be kept informed of emerging safety and risk–benefit issues including clinical trials and contractual agreements.
- Ensure the QPPV has the authority to implement changes to the MAH's PV system to maintain compliance.
- Ensure the QPPV has input into Risk Management Plans and the preparation of regulatory action in response to emerging safety concerns.
- Ensure the presence of back-up procedures (e.g., in case of non-availability of personnel, AE database failure, failure of other hardware or software with impact on electronic reporting and data analysis).

Note: The MAH may transfer/outsource PV activities to another person or organization. A detailed and clear written contract must be in place documenting such transfers and outsourcing. The contracted person or organization should implement QA/QC and allow auditing by the MAH. It is possible to outsource the EU QPPV function but the ultimate responsibility for all PV obligations always resides with the MAH.

Practicalities

The QPPV is a responsible and very challenging position. The person must be involved and have real influence in the safety system of the company. He or she must be knowledgeable and able to discuss, at least at a high level, particularly during a governmental inspection, the PV system in place globally, including standard operating procedures (SOPs); working documents; quality assessment/quality control (QA/QC); databases in use for drug safety, privacy, and security issues; all products marketed in the EEA and where they are sold outside of Europe; global licensing; distribution; co-marketing; agency commitments; compliance status and key performance indicators (metrics); signal identification; analysis and workup mechanisms in place; specific signals and safety issues pending globally; the risk management system and business continuity/crisis management plans in place; post-marketing trials under way, and new indication trials for marketed drugs; safety training; and issues with health authorities (HAs).

He or she must review and sign Periodic Safety Update Report (PSURs/PBRERs) and other PV documents submitted to HAs. To succeed in this position, communication across the organization is critical! There must be mechanisms in place for the QPPV to send and receive information and data he or she needs on a timely basis to do the job. Good communication skills are also needed to link the QPPV with management, drug safety, the rest of the organization, the European Medicines Agency (EMA) and member state HAs, deputy and national QPPVs, and so forth. There must be a formal job description, and many companies also have a formal, written contract with the QPPV. The person, often a medical doctor (MD), should have senior management's ear.

Many companies, particularly small companies and generic houses, will outsource the QPPV to a Clinical Research Organization (CRO) or consultant. Although this is legal and feasible, the company and the QPPV must take the job seriously, e.g., who covers during holidays and vacations?. Some QPPVs at CROs may be performing this function for 15 or more clients! Whether this is practical and wise is debatable. All delegation, both within the company and outsourced, must be rigidly and carefully documented. The specific delegated functions must be written down and all parties must sign off. Note that all companies with MAs must have a QPPV. This includes generics, over-the-counter products, and so forth. No exceptions. Large companies with many products or marketing partnerships may need to have staff supporting the QPPV in the company, especially if information is needed from other continents or non-EU countries. Sometimes convincing personnel in company divisions abroad who do not normally interact with headquarters may not fully appreciate that they must supply information to support sales in the EU. This can be a challenge, especially if there is frequent turnover in far-away places.

The EU QPPV is not required to be part of the PV team. He/she can have a non-PV position with oversight of the PV organization and performance. In such circumstances, it is best to have the EU QPPV at least at the same hierarchy level of the head global PV.

Note: The CMO or the Head of Global PV can also be the EU QPPV as long as they are appropriately qualified.

Frequent QPPV Inspection Findings by the EMA

- No QPPV or interim measures (change of QPPV, no backup procedures for absence, etc.);
- More than one QPPV per PV System or unclear organization; lack of Local Person for PV (LPPVs) in coutries where the products is licensed but not marketed;
- Not resident or operating in the EEA;
- No job description;
- Failure to notify Competent Authorities of QPPV details;
- Lack of 24/7 coverage;
- Inadequate oversight of the pharmacovigilance system (ICSRs, PSURs/PBRERs, RMPs, PASS, PAES, safety profile of products, audits and inspections, QA & QC, database(s));
- Lack of training or experience (or lack of documentation of same);
- No or inadequate training of drug safety staff;
- Roles and responsibilities not formally defined (especially important if parts of role are delegated); and
- Inadequate access to medically qualified personnel.

Penalties can be severe and can include fines of up to 5% of the MAH's EU sales, with further penalties if the problems are not promptly corrected. Civil and criminal penalties for the MAH and the QPPV are possible.

Frequently Asked Questions

Q: Why would anyone want to do this job?

A: Good question, and we may not have a good answer. Perhaps a combination of responsibility, power, the desire to have a meaningful job that makes an impact, a good salary (though some say they could never be paid enough to do this job), visibility, and the like. For people who like and accept being empowered (and who really are empowered), and who like playing a fascinating role with interactions in all areas and in all levels of the company and with health authorities, this can be a marvelous job. Until something bad happens. Then the stress level rises and it truly becomes a 24/7 job, particularly in the age of the Internet, with instant communications and media knowledge of problems (often incomplete or poorly understood). Word of problems and misbehavior travels quickly.

Q: Why would anyone *not* want to do this job?

A: Good question also! As specified before, such responsibilities could become a 24/7 job with real and stressful roles and responsibilities, particularly if the QPPV does not have the full support of the company. As icing on the cake, two legal consequences must be emphasized: First, even after the EU QPPV transitions to new responsibilities or a different organization, he or she will still be responsible for a safety issue that occurred during his or her tenure as EU QPPV. In addition, any decision/measure, taken (or not taken) during the EU QPPV tenure can be challenged at any time and that individual will be committed "forever". In other words, one can be prosecuted ten, twenty or more years after leaving the EU QPPV post. Second, as an EU QPPV and in case of a major safety issue, you can face criminal charges. In such a situation, it would be too late if you did not, before the issue arises or at the start of your QPPV tenure, secure a commitment of well-financed legal support from the MAH. Many EU QPPVs have tried to include such a protective statement in their contract, but most often, the company is reluctant to accept ... Have fun!

Q: What do I do if I am QPPV but not empowered and cannot get management to act on the appropriate needs, resources, and safety issues?

A: Quit. First, do your utmost to convince management that this is serious business and certain things must be done. You may need to get allies to make the case (e.g., the regulatory and legal colleagues in the company or an outside auditor). Point out the key sections from the EU Regulations. Document fully in writing everything you have done and everyone notified (and when), all items, actions, resources, and so forth, that you have requested, plus the responses. Always do and say the right thing and document it. Give it a reasonable attempt and length of time to get actions and corrections. It helps to have a forceful type-A personality. If all fails, update your CV and get a new job. You'll sleep better and your gastric acid and blood pressure will return to normal.

CHAPTER

31

Product Labeling

Labeling is a general term encompassing many things about a drug. Human drug labeling contains a summary of the essential scientific information needed for the safe and effective use of the drug. Labeling is divided for pharmacovigilance purposes into several different documents. For drugs that are not yet on the market (approved or authorized for sale), the labeling used for adverse events (AE) reporting and all other "official" considerations is the "Investigator Brochure" as prepared by the sponsor and submitted to the health authorities, Institutional Review Boards/Ethics Committees, Data Safety Monitoring Boards, and investigational sites. After a drug is approved for marketing (e.g., New Drug Application or Marketing Authorization granted), the labeling that is used for regulatory reporting of AEs changes to that document prepared by the sponsor and submitted to, negotiated with, and approved by the health authority for that jurisdiction: Prescribing Information, Medication Guides, Patient Package Inserts, and/or Instructions for Use, and/or carton and container labeling, the "Package Insert" (PI) in the United States, and the Summary of Product Characteristics (SmPC or sometimes erroneously referred to as the SPC (Supplementary Protection Certificate; sometimes Single Point of Contact)) in the European Union. The other

key labeling document is the Company Core Safety Information (CCSI). All are discussed in the following sections.

Introduction

Labeling, the creation, maintenance, and updates to, is generally managed and overseen by the Regulatory Affairs and Legal departments as the documents encompassed in these activities are regulatorily controlled and submitted to the agencies, and often to IRBs/ECs and DSMBs. Even though the Regulatory Affairs team should own the process for the creation, maintenance, and updates to these documents, companies with limited resources may outsource the responsibility to vendors, consultants, or CROs, or other functional areas such as Safety & Pharmacovigilance, or Medical Affairs. Regardless of who at the company oversees these activities, there should be standardized procedures in place that are cross-functional and involve the input and involvement from regulatory affairs, safety and pharmacovigilance, clinical development, biostatistics, data management, medical affairs, legal, and ultimately approved by the Chief Medical Officer or Scientific Officer responsible for the scientific data for that product. Final company approver should be an individual (by title in SOPs) rather than a department. The procedures should be label specific, outlining who is responsible for the maintenance and update of each, the timetable for updates (scheduled and variations due to new safety data), as well as the submission and archival responsibilities.

Note that the requirement for labeling and safety reporting begins when the product is approved even if marketing is delayed. Marketing might be delayed for various reasons (e.g. manufacturing scale up, awaiting the onset of the disease being treated such as influenza in the autumn and winter etc.).

Investigator Brochure

The requirements for the Investigator Brochure (IB) are listed in ICH E6 Guidance on Good Clinical Practices, which has been adopted in most jurisdictions, including the FDA which issued a guidance for Industry in 2018, E6(R2) Good Clinical Practice: integrated Addendum to ICH E6(R1) is the IB is a compilation of clinical and non-clinical data on the study product that is relevant to the investigators performing the trial, allowing them to understand the rationale and key features of the drug. Its purpose is to provide the investigators and others involved in the trial with the information to facilitate their understanding of the rationale for, and their compliance with, many key features of the protocol, such as the dose, dose frequency/interval, methods of administration: and safety monitoring procedures.[1] It is the sponsor's responsibility to prepare the IB and keep it up to date. It summarizes the chemical, physical, and pharmacologic properties of the drug; non-clinical studies; effects in humans; including absorption, distribution, metabolism, and excretion (ADME) data, as well as clinical studies in volunteers and patients covering both efficacy and safety. Marketing experience, if available, is also included. There should be a single IB, in English, for global use.

The IB should include a brief summary highlighting the significant physical, chemical, pharmaceutical, pharmacological, toxicological, pharmacokinetic, metabolic, and clinical information available that is relevant to the stage of clinical development of the investigational product. The Summary should be followed by, at a minimum, the following sections: Introduction, Physical, Chemical, and Pharmaceutical Properties and Formulation, Nonclinical Studies, Nonclinical Pharmacology, Pharmacokinetics and Product Metabolism in Animals, Effects in Humans (Pharmacokinetics and Product Metabolism in Humans, Safety and Efficacy, Marketing Experience), Summary of Data and Guidance for the Investigator.

The IB should contain summaries of safety across multiple trials with indications in sub-groups using tabular summaries of Adverse Drug Reactions (ADRs). Important differences in ADR patterns/incidences across indications or sub-groups should be noted if present. The IB should provide a description of the possible risks and ADRs to be anticipated based on prior experiences

[1] FDA E6(R2) Good Clinical Practice: Integrated Addendum to ICH E6(R1) Guidance for Industry March 2018.

with the product and with related products. Any precautions or special monitoring to be done should also be noted. The overall aim of this section is to provide the investigator with a clear understanding of the possible risks and adverse reactions, and of the specific tests, observations, and precautions that may be needed for a clinical trial. This understanding should be based on the available physical, chemical, pharmaceutical, pharmacological, toxicological, and clinical information on the investigational product(s). Guidance should also be provided to the clinical investigator on the recognition and treatment of possible overdose and adverse drug reactions that are based on previous human experience and on the pharmacology of the investigational product. Note: While Overdose is not necessarily an AE, it can lead to AEs or be considered as a product quality defect and should be monitored for safety and outcome of the patient. The IB can be dozens of pages long and should be more inclusive rather than less inclusive. It is not a marketing document and will be reviewed by investigators, Investigational Review Boards/Ethics Committees, and Data Safety Management Committees/Independent Data Monitoring Committees.

The IB should be updated yearly or more often if new, clinically relevant information, particularly about safety, becomes available. This document is used in the preparation of 7- and 15-day expedited (alert) reports to the health authorities, partners, and for investigational new drug annual reports (e.g., Development Safety Update Reports, or DSURs); the criteria "expected" or "unexpected" is assessed according to the IB content.

After a drug is approved for marketing and if it is also in clinical trials, it will have both an IB and post-marketing labeling (e.g., EU SmPC, US PI). Note that a product is not ordinarily approved/launched simultaneously in all markets, so multiple documents (not necessarily fully complementary) may exist.

Company Core Safety Information

The "Core Safety Information" (CSI), or "Company Core Safety Information" (CCSI), which is part of the larger "Company Core Data Sheet" (CCDS), contains the key safety data for the marketed product. This document was defined originally by the CIOMS III and CIOMS V working group reports. The CCSI contains (only) basic safety information that should appear in the safety labeling for the product in all countries where the product is registered/licensed. It should not contain speculation or safety information that might appear in only one country's labeling for some local reason. Thus, the information in the CCSI represents the minimal safety data that should appear globally in all local or national labeling. Additions may be made in local labeling beyond what is in the CCSI if the local health authority or company so chooses (insists?). Marketing considerations should not play a role in preparing the CCSI. AEs due to excipients should be included, but those that have no well-established relationship to the drug should not be included. The CCSI is used to determine which AEs are considered "listed" when preparing Periodic Safety Update Reports (PSURs/PBRERs). It is not used for expedited reporting expectedness (the approved, post-marketing label is used instead).

Other safety documents used in various countries include the Development Core Safety Information (DCSI), the Development Core Data Sheet. They are all like the CCSI and contain key safety information used for clinical trials, periodic reporting, and so forth.

United States Labeling for Marketed Products

The US requirements for labeling are summarized in 21CFR1. The official definition of labeling for a marketed product is 21CFR1.3(a) as follows:

(a) Labeling includes all written, printed, or graphic matter accompanying an article at any time while such article is in interstate commerce or held for sale after shipment or delivery in interstate commerce.

(b) Label means any display of written, printed, or graphic matter on the immediate container of any article, or any such matter affixed to any consumer commodity or affixed to or appearing upon a package containing any consumer commodity.

Thus, in the US, "Labeling" includes the FDA-approved written material describing a drug, such as the Package Insert and the packaging and box that a drug is shipped or sold in. Commonly used terms for the subset of labeling designated "Package Insert" include "professional labeling", "direction circular", "approved labeling", and "package circular" or just plain "labeling." It also includes the FDA-approved patient labeling (called "Medication Guides") where this exists.

In 2003, the FDA introduced the new requirements for the electronic specifications for exchange of Package Inserts, called "Structured Product Labeling" (SPL), using a document markup standard approved by FDA and Health Level 7. All Package Inserts must be submitted in SPL format. See FDA's website for further information on this labeling initiative.

The specific requirements for drug labeling are found in 21CFR201.57. These labeling requirements, include the following:

> Highlights section, drug names, dosage form, route of administration and controlled substance symbol (if such a drug), initial US approval, boxed warning (if any), recent major changes, indications and usage, dosage and administration, dosage forms and strengths, contraindications, warnings and precautions, adverse reactions, interactions, use in specific populations (including pregnancy, teratogenicity, geriatric and pediatric use), patient counseling information, revision date, drug abuse/dependence, overdosage, clinical pharmacology, non-clinical toxicology, clinical studies, references, how supplied, and patient counseling information.

Note that the highlights section is a short summary (1/2 to 2 pages) of the rest of the Package Insert. Labels before 2006 largely have the same sections, though there is no highlights section, and the safety sections are much shorter in many cases.

FDA issued a guidance covering the new requirements in more detail, entitled *Labeling for Human Prescription Drug and Biological Products — Implementing the New Content and Format Requirements.* Several other guidances covering the various sections of the labeling were also issued.

The guidance covering the adverse reaction section will be discussed briefly here as follows:

1. The goal is to include only information useful to practitioners making treatment decisions and monitoring patients. Exhaustive lists of AEs should be avoided.
2. The Adverse Reactions (ARs) section should contain those that occur with the drug itself and ARs from the class, if appropriate, and even if not yet observed with the new product. Clinical trial and spontaneous reports must be listed separately.
3. All serious and otherwise important ARs should be listed and cross-referenced (e.g., Boxed Warning, Warnings and Precautions).
4. ARs that resulted in a significant rate of discontinuation or other clinical intervention, such as dose change in clinical trials.
5. ARs from clinical trials is the major component of the AR section and should include the most commonly occurring ARs (e.g., all ARs >10% and 2 × placebo rate). This section should describe the clinical trial database in terms of exposure, number of patients, demographics, types of studies, doses, and so forth. Data should be presented in a table to allow side-by-side comparisons. The best available data should be used — placebo-controlled and dose response studies.
6. Less common ARs should be presented if clinically important and here is a basis to feel that a causal relationship to the drug exists.
7. Additional information should be given for the most clinically significant ARs (i.e., most common, cause discontinuation, or dose change or require monitoring).
8. Dose response, demographic, and sub-group information should be included if important.
9. If there are multiple indications and/or multiple formulations, a discussion about these issues regarding safety should be included.

10. A separate listing of spontaneous ARs should be included, particularly those that are serious, frequent, or seem to be causally related ARs.
11. When reporting rates are included, all cases of that AE should be used rather than just those the reporter feels are related.
12. Comparative safety claims (frequency, severity, or character of the AR) must be based on data from adequate and well-controlled studies.
13. Negative findings, if convincingly demonstrated in an adequate trial, may be included.
14. Data may be pooled from studies when the studies are appropriate to pool (similar design, populations, etc.).
15. Data should be coded meaningfully and grouped as appropriate (e.g., sedation, somnolence, and drowsiness should be grouped as a single AR). Syndromes should be used where appropriate (e.g., hypersensitivity).
16. ARs should be categorized by body system, by severity (in decreasing frequency), or by a combination of both. An appropriate frequency cutoff may be specified.
17. Quantitative data (e.g., labs, vital signs, ECGs) should be presented as rates of abnormal values, with a cutoff for inclusion (e.g., five times the upper limit of normal) rather than a grading system.
18. If the AR rate is less than it is for the placebo, this information should not be included unless there is a compelling reason to do so.
19. Statistical significance should not be included unless based on an adequately designed and powered study.
20. The label should be reviewed at least annually to be sure all appropriate data are included.

For an example of this labeling, see the Zyprexa (olanzapine) label. The label has historically been 35 pages long, and the Warnings and Precaution section runs about 8 pages and includes 7 tables. The AR section runs 9 pages and contains 14 tables, and the Interactions section runs 2 pages. From a practical point of view, if a practitioner has a question, such as "Does this drug cause headache?" and if it is not listed in the summary, the most expedient way to find this is to load the document onto a computer or handheld device or pull the label from an online database as a PDF file and search for that term. Multiple hits may occur, leading to listings in several tables from which the practitioner can draw his or her conclusions. One might observe that this is not necessarily a quick or practical way to find out whether a specific AE or problem has occurred with the product in question.

In the United States, many, but not all, prescription drug labels are printed in the reference book known as the Physicians' Desk Reference (PDR), published yearly by Thomson. It is about 3000 pages long and has photos of many of the products as well as the product information.

Daily Med (https://dailymed.nlm.nih.gov/dailymed/index.cfm) from the US National Library of Medicine also has the labeling, however the official copies of the drug label remains the responsibility of the company. There are also many other companies (e.g., rxlist.com and drugs.com) and organizations that have drug information available on line that is taken from the approved US labeling. They are often more user-friendly than the labeling itself and are often broken down by sections that are easily navigated. Other countries have the equivalent publications with drug labeling.

Many drug labels and patient information for specific drugs can be found at the FDA website (https://labels.fda.gov/). In addition, most pharmaceutical companies have posted their product labeling on their websites. If the drug is sold in multiple countries, each local company website usually posts the local labeling.

Regardless of where a drug label is posted (see above), the official copy of the drug label remains the responsibility of the company and company employees, safety personnel, etc. should only be referencing approved company drug labels for assessing expectedness; it is considered poor practice for a company to instruct employees to reference a non-company sponsored website (such as Daily Med, Drugs@FDA, RxList, Drugs.com, etc.) as the company does not own or operate those websites and cannot guarantee the accuracy of the data on them.

European Union Safety Labeling for Marketed Products

The requirements for labeling in the European Union (which is called the Summary of Product Characteristics [SmPC or SPC]) is found in EudraLex Volume 2C, which includes the requirements for submitting the dossier for a new product (https://ec.europa.eu/health/documents/eudralex/vol-2_en). The SmPC "sets out the agreed position of the medicinal product as distilled during the course of the assessment process". It cannot be changed without agreement by the health authorities. If a drug is approved centrally in the European Union, or if the labeling is harmonized, then there should only be one SmPC per product (in English), though there may be additional SmPCs for the same chemical entity if there are different forms or strengths. Drugs that are not approved or harmonized may have a different SmPC in each member state. The SmPC will usually be in the local language of the country.

Similar to other country labeling, the SmPC includes the name, strength, pharmaceutical form, composition, indications, dosing (called "posology"), method of administration, special populations (renal, hepatic impairment, elderly, genotype-particular patients, pediatrics), contraindications, special warnings, precautions (including ARs to which healthcare professionals need to be alerted), interactions, fertility, pregnancy and lactation, effects on driving and machine use, undesirable effects (adverse reactions), overdose, pharmacological properties, pre-clinical safety data, pharmaceutical details, including excipients, incompatibilities, shelf life, storage, appropriate container, disposal instructions, and registration and update information.

The adverse reaction section should include all ARs from clinical trials, post-authorization safety studies, and spontaneous reports "for which a causal relationship between the medicinal product and the adverse event is at least a reasonable possibility". ARs should not be listed if there is no suspicion of a causal relationship. The section should contain the following:

- A summary of the safety profile containing information on the most serious and/or most frequent ARs.
- A tabulated list of ARs with frequency. It should be a single table in general though separate tables may be used in exceptional circumstances (e.g., using a product in different indications or dosages). MedDRA® Preferred Terms (PTs) should be used. If appropriate, data from several trials may be pooled.
- A description of selected ARs that "may be useful to prevent, assess or manage the occurrence of an adverse reaction in clinical practice." For further detail, see Volume 2C.

The full information to be included in each section, is specified in the "Guideline on Summary of Product Characteristics". Quality Review of Documents (QRD) templates were developed by the EMA; they give strict recommendations on the format to be used. Package Leaflet guidelines have been updated several times over the past years; the last update is dated June 2023. They can be retrieved on the European Community Website.

Due to the numerous languages used in the EU, the translation part in the process of labeling updates remains tricky. Except for decentralized procedures (where the SmPC is approved in the local language), the SmPC is proposed, discussed and validated in English. Then a translation process is done taking the new English language label and translating it into each local language. Previously, the pharma companies had to provide the EMA with all translated SmPCs within a very short timeframe. Due to significant translation mistakes, the EMA is now, (prospectively and for labeling updates only), preparing the approved updated section in each of the 24 official EU languages.

Other Countries

Most countries of the world have fairly similar registration and approval systems, involving a multidisciplinary review of all the submitted data and labeling based on the submitted data. The approvals may vary significantly from country to country; however, they are based on different data submitted or emphasized, different indications requested, different formulations, different patient populations treated, and local customs. Thus, the labeling may be somewhat different from country to country. In addition, in non-English-speaking countries, the labeling is, of course, in the local language.

Comments about Labeling Content

In the European Union, the approved labeling is known as the Summary of Product Characteristics (SmPC). There is a curious use of terminology by some people. In the United States, the generic term *labeling* (sometimes called the "Package Insert", or "PI") is used to refer to the official FDA-approved US product information. The word "labeling" is also used in the United States for the SmPC when referring to European labeling. Some in the European Union, conversely, use the term "SmPC" when they are referring to their own official labeling or to the US labeling. Thus, one might hear a reference to the US SmPC — a concept that does not really exist in the United States. This refers, in practice, to the US official Package Insert and not the European Union SmPC.

In terms of pharmacovigilance, sections of labeling of most interest include the AEs, warnings, drug interactions, precautions, and pregnancy information. In particular, the labeling is used to determine whether a particular AE that is reported for that product is expected in many but not all countries, if an AE is expected, it does not have to be reported to the health authority as an expedited report. Class labeling of a particular AE/AR is not considered expected or labeled for the purposes of expedited reporting in most jurisdictions.

Changes, additions, removals, "variations", and alterations to product labeling must usually be approved by the health authority concerned. In many jurisdictions, the sponsor (NDA holder, MAH) may change the labeling to add an urgent safety warning without prior approval by the health agency. In the United States, this is known as "Changes Being Effected". Of course, the FDA must be told rapidly. This is permitted.

> "to add or strengthen a contraindication, warning, precaution, or adverse reaction for which the evidence of a causal association satisfies the standard for inclusion in the labeling...to add or strengthen a statement about abuse, dependence, psychological effect, or overdosage...to add or strengthen an instruction about dosage and administration that is intended to increase the safety of the use of the product" (See CFR Title 1).

See, for example, 21CFR601.12 Changes to an approved application for biologics. Similarly, in the European Union, "urgent safety restrictions" are permitted. In such circumstances, the MAH is required to submit a variation within 15 cal. Day and speed up the implementation for both SmPC and PI.

Note that drug labels do not always use MedDRA terms for AEs. Many drugs are quite old and date back many years to pre-MedDRA days. Thus, terms used are from other dictionaries, such as COSTART or WHO-ART, or the terms may be non-standardized. In addition, CIOMS has developed the concept of MedDRA Labeling Groupings that may appear in labels. This can clearly produce issues when one attempts to determine whether a term (e.g., a MedDRA term) is considered labeled or listed if a similar but not quite exactly matching term is found. Semantic interoperability remains aspirational, so other terminologies may continue to be represented in labeling, e.g., Common Terminology Criteria for Adverse Events (CTCAE), with or without severity grades, for some oncology products.

In Canada, the equivalent of the PDR is called the Compendium of Pharmaceuticals and Specialties, available in English and French. In France, it is called the "Vidal" (this website is in French) and in Germany, the "Rote Liste" (this website is in German). In the United Kingdom, SmPCs and Patient Information Leaflets (PILs) are available on the MHRA website.

OTC Labeling in the United States

The labeling for OTC products in the United States is usually different from the labeling of prescription products. With most OTC drugs, labeling is derived from "monographs" (the CFR sections dealing with these products and specifying which products may be sold without an NDA or Abbreviated New Drug Application, ANDA). OTC drugs are used by patients and consumers without a healthcare intermediary (physician, pharmacist, nurse) to explain the product, its use, its adverse events, and so forth. The labeling is what is written on the package (box) in the section marked "Drug Facts". This is a lay version of a Package Insert but is often very skimpy regarding AEs. Sometimes none are listed at all. This is often most surprising because certain products that had extensive lists of AEs (e.g., loratadine, non-steroidal anti-inflammatory drugs, and others) in the Package Insert when they were prescription drugs now have minimal safety information in the OTC Drug Facts. Note that an OTC product in the US may be a prescription product elsewhere.

Some OTC products may be sold under an NDA or ANDA, and these products may have a classic Package Insert. These drugs do not fall under the monographs and were previously prescription drugs with an NDA or ANDA that remains in effect.

Similarly, for food supplements, there is a label marked "Supplement Facts." Many companies that sell OTC products sell supplements, drugs, devices, and sometimes even cosmetics, making for very complicated AE collection and reporting.

This labeling situation complicates AE reporting to the FDA. A product may be an OTC through (usually) one of two mechanisms: (1) an approved NDA or ANDA that was originally for a prescription product that has been switched to OTC status or (2) through the OTC drug monograph process. Safety reporting obligations depend on which route was used. For products with an NDA or ANDA the requirements are the same as for prescription products (e.g., expedited reporting, approved labeling, Periodic Reports/PSURs). Until 2007, there was no obligatory safety reporting for monograph products, though some companies voluntarily submitted safety reports, usually for SAEs. The Dietary Supplement and Non-prescription Drug Consumer Protection Act of 2006 and a subsequent guidance in 2009 clarified the situation. On this matter, an FDA Q&A should also be checked (see FDA Website)

The reporting requirements are as follows:

1. Manufacturer, packer, or distributor whose name is on the label (called the "responsible person") must submit to FDA all SAEs with a copy of the label within 15 business days.
2. All follow-up information received within 1 year of the initial report must be submitted within 15 business days. Note that the law states only 1 year of follow-up, but FDA has indicated that it wants no time limit. That is, report all follow-ups forever.
3. MedWatch (3500A) form or E2B to be used for reporting. Mandatory reporting by applicants must be via E2B.
4. The NDA definitions for minimum criteria, reportability, and so forth, are in effect here:
   - For brand families, it is necessary to know the active ingredient to have a reportable drug;
   - If multiple suspect drugs, submit Individual Case Safety Report (ICSR) to FDA and to other manufacturers.
5. No aggregate reporting requirements.
6. Signaling is required for the NDA/ANDA products but is not specifically stated to be required for monograph products, though it would be wise to do so.

Note: In the European Union, there are no OTC products without MAs, so all prescription drug reporting requirements apply to OTC products. In practice, many companies treat all OTC products the same and do expedited reporting, periodic reporting, and signaling. Some countries have multiple and more complex rules, including "OTC" and "behind-the-counter" products, which do not require prescriptions but which may (in the latter category) require the customer's talking to the pharmacist before being able to purchase the product.

■ Labeling Update Process

When an authorization dossier (e.g., in the US an NDA and in the EU a MAA) is submitted, the company team working on its preparation must, among other things, submit proposed labeling (US PI, EU SmPC & EU PL, etc). Starting from scratch, the team must combine and summarize the often large amounts of data collected during the non-clinical and clinical development. This is submitted in most cases as "annotated" labeling — that is, each statement, claim or fact must be backed up by data referenced in a footnote. The final, approved labeling usually does not have all the annotations and footnotes.

After approval with the product on the market, new information (efficacy, safety, regulatory, etc.) will become known which needs to be included in the Product Information. Such new information generates a labeling update. The scheme below highlights the main steps, milestones and stakeholders involved in this process in the EU. It is similar for US labeling updates.

In large pharma companies, a specific team is devoted to labeling activities, most often within the Regulatory Affairs department. After initial drug approval and marketing, between 80% and 90% of the labeling updates are due to new safety concerns. **This means both the PV and Labeling teams must work closely together.**

The Labeling Committee decision-makers must be senior managers from PV, Reg. Affairs, Med. Affairs and Legal. They usually meet as a committee and approve the content and wording of the labeling updates. This is an iterative process, as regulators and

In many cases, the key document that is updated is the CCDS/CCSI which then serves as the source for updating all other local labeling documents (US PI, EU SmPC, EU PIL, etc). Considering the importance of FDA and EMA at a worldwide level, some companies prefer to update CCDS/CCSI, US PI and EU SmPC at the same time and therefore request the Labeling Committee to approve these three documents.

For labeling updates, in order to ensure consistency across countries, the best approach is to provide the affiliates with a rationale or "package" for any labeling update. Such documents are then submitted to local agencies, supporting the update proposal.

When receiving the CCDS/CCSI update with the scientific rationale, the affiliates prepare the local label update which is then submitted to the local agency. After assessment and potential wording changes, the new label is implemented and therefore made available to patients and healthcare professionals in that country.

Most companies maintain a computerized archive of all labels used in all languages in all affiliates. This would include both the current labeling in use in each country as well as previous versions of the labels which are now out of date. These archived labels may be needed for research, scientific publications, lawsuits, etc.

From beginning to end, this complex process can take months or even years. However, if a label change is urgent or critical, it may need to be done in a matter of days. Companies and health agencies must have a mechanism to do this. In many countries, all label changes must be approved by the health agency. However, for emergencies, some countries allow labels to be changed immediately ("changes being effected" in the US) with approval by the health agency in the next day or two.

Figure 1. Schematic Relationships in Labeling Updates.

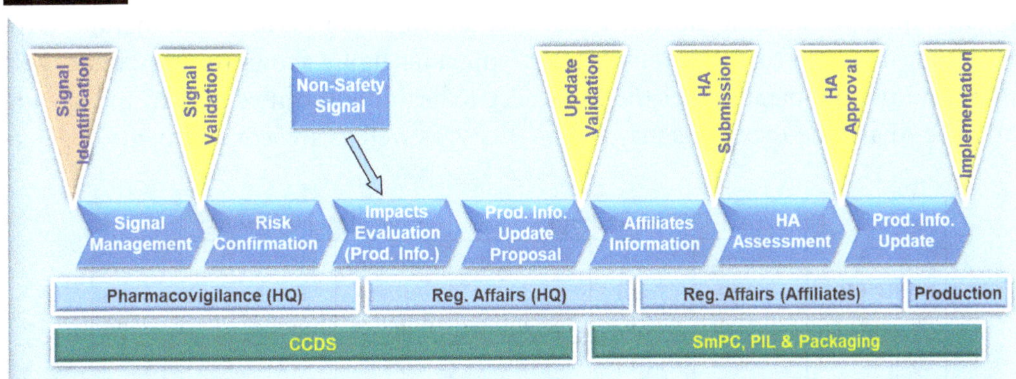

CCDS: Company Core data Sheet HA: Health Authorities HQ: HeadQuarters
PIL: Product Information Leaflet SmPC: Summary of Product Characteristics

In countries with limited Regulations, they usually consider a reference country (EU, USA …) for labeling content; both SmPC and PIL are then copied/pasted from those of the reference country.

Comments

The pharmacovigilance worker in a company or health agency should be sure to receive updated labeling by the group in charge of preparing these documents. Though obvious, this is not always routine. Groups other than those that deal with pharmacovigilance usually prepare labeling, and preparers may not always remember to distribute new labeling to drug safety and other groups that need it.

For pharmacovigilance professionals, knowledge of the labeling for the drugs for which they are responsible is **absolutely necessary**. For drugs with many AEs, it is generally a good idea to prepare a separate table as a reference, listing the AEs, to aid when determining expectedness. These AEs may, in fact, appear in multiple sections and at varying levels of specificity. They should be harvested and grouped appropriately so that a ready reference (known as a "cheat sheet") can be consulted when evaluating and coding AEs. It may be useful to list the corresponding MedDRA terms and level (verbatim, preferred term, lower-level term). Some computer safety databases are able to mechanize the specific MedDRA terms that are considered labeled/listed, obviating the need for such "cheat sheets". All such cheat sheets should be controlled and validated.

Many drugs have multiple labeling documents if there are different preparations (e.g., different labeling for intravenous and oral preparations of the same active ingredient). The AEs in the two labels may differ because some will be route-specific (e.g., injection site reactions or those related to a first-pass effect after oral intake).

Some companies are working on QR code solutions for labeling. A QR code (abbreviated from Quick Response Code) is the trademark for a type of matrix barcode (or two-dimensional barcode) first designed for the automotive industry in Japan. A barcode is a machine-readable optical label that contains information about the item to which it is attached. The goal is to allow one to scan a QR code on a drug package with a smart phone or other device after which the package leaflet/labeling immediately appears (in your native language) on your cell-phone screen. Such a solution would ensure that each patient has the up-to-date drug label. The QR code option for labeling is not likely to be required in the short term but some health authorities are investigating whether such a mechanism should be made mandatory in addition to the current word-rich printed process.

The UK MHRA is one of the health agencies that performs many PV inspections. Their inspections are well known to be thorough and detailed. Each year they publish the most frequent findings identified during routine periodic and special "for cause" inspections. Note that the information for 2021 occurred during the height of the Covid pandemic and lockdowns. Fewer inspections were done and it is not clear that one can ascribe the drop in critical and major findings to improvement in labeling.

In 2014, the most frequent critical findings were due to labeling update (42% of critical findings). This percentage decreased to 17% in 2017 (20% in 2021 — the limited number of critical findings over the past years does not permit meaningful interpretation). The previous figure shows the importance and attention the UK health authorities give to the labeling update process as well as any commitments (e.g., content, format,

	Critical findings			Major findings		
MHRA PV Inspections	Labeling update number	Total number	Percentage	Labeling update number	Total number	Percentage
2014	8	19	42%	21	192	11%
2021	1	5	20%	5	59	8%

timelines) that the company might promise to the health agency. This concern is shared by all health authorities and companies must scrupulously handle label updates and commitments made to each agency (https://www.gov.uk/government/statistics/pharmacovigilance-inspection-metrics-2009-to-present).

Frequently Asked Questions

Q: It seems rather duplicative and wasteful to have each country handle the labels separately. In general, wouldn't the safety profile be the same worldwide? Wouldn't one label be sufficient for a marketed drug?

A: In theory, both questions should be answered with a "yes". However, labeling is quite complicated, and each health authority wants to reserve its right to review and change the labeling. The CCSI is the common worldwide label, and this concept seems to work well and could reasonably be extended to full official labeling. That said, there are situations in which a drug might work differently in one group or region. Thus, regional differences requiring different labels may be justified in some cases. Nonetheless, all differences and sub-groups could still be listed in one single global label. One, two, or perhaps three countries at most could be responsible for a drug and its labeling, safety profile, and updates. This probably is feasible but, given the geopolitical situation in the world, is unlikely to come about anytime soon.

Q: Since the health agency in each country has the ultimate approval authority for all labels, it seems then that they would have the responsibility for label updates. What is the actual responsibility of the pharmaceutical company?

A: In theory, we could consider each health authority to be independent and responsible for the content of the label, as they actually approve the document. In reality though, the scientific and medical data **are** handled primarily by the pharma companies. It is the companies that receive most ADRs and source data on their drugs. The companies prepare ICSRs and aggregate reports (PSURs/PBRERs) and submit them to the agencies with this data. If, by chance, the health agency is the first one to receive new and important information, the agency will often immediately contact the company and send them the data so that both the agency and company can review to it and put in place any changes necessary.

Many health agencies are small and do not have the capacity to review all data on all drugs approved in their country. So it is generally accepted that the responsibility lies with the companies. Most lawyers would agree with this!

More generally, we can describe four different reasons to support the view that labeling is largely pharmaceutical company's responsibility:

- **Scientific and medical:** it is the company's responsibility to include any important and up to date information in the labels to help patients and healthcare professionals to be fully aware of the information for safe prescribing and use.
- **Ethical:** As drugs are products used to treat or prevent diseases/symptoms, it would not be ethical to hide needed information.
- **Regulatory:** The product information documents are heavily regulated and each company must fully comply with all regulations in all the countries where their drugs are authorized.
- **Legal:** Media attention on major drug safety issues can produce or magnify the legal risks and consequences of incomplete or inaccurate labeling. This can lead to lawsuits against companies.

In the US, there is the concept of the "learned intermediary". This doctrine states that a manufacturer (e.g., the pharma company) has fulfilled its duty of care by providing the prescriber (e.g., the physician) of all needed information ("material risks"). It is then the prescriber who informs the patient of risks. This is a complex legal doctrine. Certainly, consult with an attorney knowledgeable in this area for more definitive information.

CHAPTER

32

Business Partners and Exchange of Safety Data

Development costs for a new chemical entity from creation to marketing can cost from $160 million up to $4.5 billion based on 2021 data (https://link.springer.com/article/10.1007/s40273-021-01065-y). In addition, patents are now being challenged and generics are proliferating. Many new products, particularly biologics and oncology products are developed by small, start-up companies who do not have the capacity to do the full development.

One response to these phenomena includes the development and marketing of a product by multiple partner companies; small companies can also sell their products to big pharma at the end of phase I, II or III. The cost for development of a new chemical entity from creation to marketing can be in the billions and require an endless number of legal arrangements between other manufacturers, packers, co-developers, licensees, and even other marketing authorization holders depending on the region. The variety of entities are often referred to as a lump of "business partners" and are an important and critical part of the pharmacovigilance system when considering the safety data that can be known and researched by each entity.

Therefore, when discussing sources of safety data, we must consider the variety of different business partners and entities that have access to important safety data and develop a process for the exchange of that data to remain compliant with regulations and ensure up-to-date information regarding a product at any given time. The activity of organizing the proper arrangements and exchange of safety data in a timely manner for even a small to mid-size pharmaceutical company can often be a full-time job and requires direct and well managed cross-functional engagement with areas such as Legal, Quality, Finance, Marketing, and Clinical Development. It is extremely important to establish and maintain efficient communication between and among all relevant functions, particularly when two or more business entities are partners.

Introduction

A common method used by companies to share costs and reduce risks is partnerships. The goal is to speed up development and use the additive or synergistic strengths of each partner. Co-development may be limited to two partners, but combinations of three or more partners are common, especially when expanding into areas (e.g., Japan, China) where language, laws, and customs are often a challenge for US and European companies or small start-ups. The current trend in the pharmaceutical world is for co-development and co-promotion/marketing of products as expenses skyrocket and simultaneous rather than sequential international development occurs. We are seeing large, small, and midsized companies creating contractual arrangements with one or multiple other pharmaceutical companies, contract research organizations (CROs), and other vendors to handle development, sales, marketing, safety handling, regulatory matters, phone centers, manufacturing, and just about every other possible function except senior management. These contracts may be short-term or long-term and involve companies all over the world. There are many possible combinations; some partners are chosen for expertise in a particular country or region or technical discipline.

Whenever two or more companies join forces for whatever reason, a written contract must be developed between or among them. Normally, these contracts are developed by the "business development" or the "licensing group" with input from the legal department and other groups on a "need-to-know" basis. Often, they are developed under great secrecy (for competitive reasons), and others in the company are not informed of the situation until the last minute, when their input and/or approval is requested, often with a minimal amount of lead time. ("The CEO wants to sign this contract tomorrow morning. Please approve your section now.")

The safety group (unless involved in due diligence) may be one of those groups learning about the agreement at the last minute and asked to review a document with a minimal or even non-existent safety section. Sometimes when the safety section is present, it is incorrect and would not keep the company in compliance with regulations in countries where the partners are working or help protect the company from litigation and other pitfalls. This can be a problem if the CEO wants to sign the agreement immediately (see above).

When such a situation occurs, the immediate acute step is to ask that the safety section, if inadequate, be removed and replaced with one or both of the following:

1. A "generic" or "one-size-fits-all" safety section (see below).
2. A statement that a safety section is needed and will be developed by the safety groups of the respective signatory companies to cover safety data issues within, say, 90 days. It will be appended to the agreement or will act as a stand-alone

agreement (whichever the lawyers prefer). This time frame may need to be shortened if the sales or studies start in a shorter time. Often, however, studies or sales will not begin for several months, giving all parties sufficient time to develop a safety section. One advantage of a stand-alone pharmacovigilance agreement is that it can ordinarily be modified relatively easily if (when) regulations/requirements change during the course of the contract. The parties would then not need to open and renegotiate the entire contract. Sales or development of a drug should not be started by a partner unless a safety section is in place.

Why a Written Safety Exchange Agreement is Needed

Why does a company need a Safety Data Exchange Agreement (SDEA) or Pharmacovigilance Agreement (PVA)? Primarily, it is required by law (e.g., FDA: 21CFR314.80(b); EU: See Good Vigilance Practice, modules I and II). Secondly, these agreements help facilitate the successful and timely exchange of data regarding a product, thus further increasing compliance with safety reporting obligations. Thirdly, if these agreements are tracked and executed properly, it will assess with the overall oversight of the Pharmacovigilance System for any given product, thereby increasing visibility to the EU QPPV via the PSMF and other key safety stakeholders globally.

One may come across individuals in a company that see this activity as a burden of task and an unimportant hindering activity, which can lead to non-compliance and a disruption of the exchange of data. And it adds to the overhead of the partnership! Therefore, it is critical to ensure the applicable functional areas are all trained on the legal basis for these requirements to receive successful buy-in and cooperation.

There are other reasons to have safety agreements in place:

- To give guidance and instructions to all involved parties regarding their responsibilities for drug safety;
- To ensure that all parties receive the safety documents they need to remain in full compliance with all regulatory and legal requirements in their jurisdictions of sale or study;
- To ensure that adequate signaling is done periodically and that a benefit-to-risk analysis incorporates as complete a database as possible;
- To produce the best product labeling possible to enhance proper product use and to protect the public health;
- To have the contract and PV data ready for a corporate audit or health authority inspection; and
- To have data available for litigation should that situation arise.

A general principle to keep in mind during exchanges with the other partner(s) is to try to avoid, as far as possible, duplication of work. Quite often, this is challenging as the other partner refuses any compromise and wants to stick to its internal rules and SOPs. Nevertheless, accepting duplicate tasks means that very often additional prospective periodic quality controls to ensure consistency must be put in place to ensure compliance and data reconciliation to avoid conflicts because of non-compliance/discrepancies/divergences. Duplication also adds to cost. The best option is to share risks and responsibilities in an equitable way based on the skills of each company. For example, a partnership between a big pharma and a small startup company may be worked out such that there is one single safety database under the control of the big pharma with access (either full or limited) by the smaller company. The smaller company may be given other duties (e.g., case follow-up by the small company in its territories).

Telling the Safety Department about a New Contract or Arrangement

The safety department should be informed of any agreement being negotiated early in the process so it can review the document and determine what is needed concerning safety. It is usually prudent to perform a due diligence evaluation of the pharmacovigilance functions of the parties to the contract as early in negotiation as prudent (the due diligence process must also investigate past PV activities to ensure no safety signal has been missed for the concerned product(s)). This approach should be included in company standard operating procedures (SOPs) that address the negotiation of agreements with other parties where drug products (either finished products or components) are involved. Agreements for non-product-related items do not need to be included (e.g., raw chemical products, supplying vending machines, or ordering furniture).

Many types of arrangements must have safety agreements. They include but are not limited to agreements on licensing-in or licensing-out; manufacturing; co-marketing; co-development, including pre-clinical or clinical development; advertising; clinical study research; consultants; contract sales forces; distribution; disease management programs; patient support programs; promotion and co-promotion; speakers bureau consultants; master vendors; other vendors; and other services. These contracts should cover all possible permutations: prescription drugs, over-the-counter drugs, drugs that are prescription in one country and over the counter in another, biologics, vaccines; blood products, devices, nutraceuticals, cosmetics, foods, and combination products (a device with a drug in it, such as a prefilled syringe, a drug-impregnated gauze pad, or two drugs in one tablet, etc.)

■ The Generic, Boilerplate, or Template Agreement

Even before any agreement is on the table, the drug safety and the legal groups (at least) should develop a "boilerplate", "generic", or template agreement approved by management and general enough to be inserted into almost any type of contract anywhere in the world, either in the body of the contract or as an appendix, until a customized agreement is made to replace it. An appendix is usually preferred, as it is easier to change without opening renegotiation of the commercial aspects when pharmacovigilance regulations change. Multiple regional versions and languages might be necessary. The agreement should, at the very least, specify the following:

1. Exchange between the parties of all serious adverse events (SAEs) from clinical trials, spontaneous reporting, solicited reporting, literature, special arrangements (e.g., named patient or compassionate use or patient support initiatives), Internet and social media safety reports and reports from health authorities.

   Cases should be exchanged as E2B files (or on either MedWatch/CIOMS I forms) within a specified time frame from first receipt by anyone in the companies or their agents. Coding conventions, e.g., MedDRA®, should be exchanged and agreed. Reports should be exchanged in sufficient time to meet expedited reporting rules (usually 15 calendar days) so that exchange should, in general, be no later than 3–5 calendar days.

   Deaths and life-threatening SAEs from trials should be exchanged in time to meet 7-day reporting requirements (e.g., 2–3 calendar days) for deaths and life-threatening events. If this is too difficult to distinguish from other SAEs, then all SAEs should be exchanged in 5 or so calendar days.
2. All regulatory submissions (Periodic Safety Update Reports [PSURs/PBRERs], NDA Periodic Reports, Annual Reports, and their local equivalents) should be exchanged between the parties within a specified time (e.g., 1 week) after submission to the health authorities by the responsible partner. If one party wishes to review the document before submission, then this must be specified, and time allotted to perform the review. If separate parties will be performing different, but related functions, e.g., party A handles case processing and party B is responsible for aggregate reports, this should be clearly defined, including a dispute resolution process.
3. In case of Health Authority questions, details must be provided on whether the other partner must be informed only or involved in the drafting of the response (before decision for an option,

estimate the potential number of questions to be managed and therefore, the workload).

4. A formal and detailed safety agreement will be completed by the two (or more) drug safety groups within, say, about three months of the signing of the business contract, if deemed necessary.

The above generic agreement should suffice in almost all cases until the formal safety document is created. Sometimes it may suffice as is. Additions, of course, may be added to the generic agreement if the specific case warrants it and if there is sufficient time to get agreement internally and from the other contractual partner(s). This could include exchange of communications with the health authorities, including safety reviews of PSURs/PBRERs, literature searches, and a data dump (e.g., a paper printout or an electronic file of all AEs in the safety database) from the partner holding the safety database.

■ Developing a Safety Agreement with the Safety Department

As soon as the type of contract is determined and the safety department is brought into the discussions, the area of involvement should be ascertained: geographic territories (e.g., United States or European Union only, United States and the European Union, Canada, Japan, UK etc.), regulatory and marketing status indications (MA/NDA approved, in clinical trials only), labeling, etc. This allows the tailoring of the specific agreement to ensure that all needs are met.

At this point the safety and regulatory departments will be able to determine what is needed. If the drug has never been marketed, for example, there will not be an issue of existing post-marketing spontaneous SAE reports, and this may not need to be included in the agreement (though a clause indicating that the agreement will be revised, say, two months before a marketing request is submitted anywhere in the world. In the EU, the post-authorization PV system must be in place at the time the MAA is submitted). If more than one partner is involved, this also allows the signatories to determine various responsibilities and negotiate any new or altered requirements; if possible, it would then make sense to develop one single PV agreement applicable to all partners rather than separate agreements. This may not always be doable, however.

Again, there is usually no "one-size-fits-all" safety arrangement that can simply be dropped into a contract to take care of everything. Each agreement must be negotiated individually. Usually, face-to-face contacts between the two (or more) safety departments facilitate the successful preparation of a safety agreement.

As always, contrary to the saying, business is personal, and it is always easier to develop a successful working relationship of trust and confidence if personal contact has been established rather than relying only on e-mails, video conferences, and telephone calls. A meeting should be set up at the earliest reasonable time after preliminary negotiations are started to hammer out the final document. The safety department needs to be given sufficient authority to negotiate such an agreement (pending, of course, final management and legal approval on both sides).

The complexity of these agreements increases exponentially if multiple companies, CROs, and territories are involved. In such situations, it is usually worthwhile for one of the companies or partners to take the lead in safety matters. Some agreements, particularly for co-development programs, provide for a joint safety committee that receives regular updates and provides a platform for decision-making on important safety matters. When consensus cannot be reached within the committee, the agreement should specify an escalation process for timely resolution of the issue.

In the EU, the regulations require that Pharmacovigilance Master Files (PSMFs) are cross-referenced between companies. In addition, any link with other PV organizations must be outlined in the PSMF and a list of contractual agreements must be appended. Some countries require local versions of the EU PSMF.

Requirements must be deciphered, and responsibilities agreed. Maintenance of these documents must be specified. See below.

Pharmacovigilance Agreement Database

For companies that make many agreements worldwide, it is imperative that a database containing the key points of the safety agreements and the agreements themselves be maintained. Multi-national companies may have thousands of such agreements, in multiple countries, in multiple languages, often with differing products, durations, responsibilities, and territories. Even if the contract is restricted to a non-English speaking territory and the local language is used in the agreement, an English version should be available (and updated) for audits and inspections (see below).

The agreements will become out of date rapidly as new terms are made, new products launched, new formulations made, new regulations are introduced, and new partners (or distributors or sales forces, etc.) brought in or terminated. These Pharmacovigilance Agreements (PVAs) need to be revisited when regulatory requirements change. A database will help track this. The database may start as a spreadsheet, but it may be necessary to develop or purchase a database to track and report on agreements. The purpose is to have a repository of all PV versioned agreements but also to have a tracking tool with reminders for key milestones/commitments. As always, the database must have the appropriate security, testing, validation, and change control. Note that this is separate from the safety data database, which contains SAEs and AEs, etc., and the clinical trial database.

Historically, the legal and new business departments will not keep sufficiently detailed records to ensure regulatory compliance regarding safety matters (a sad fact). Thus, it falls on the local drug safety department to do its best to ensure that all revisions to agreements are transmitted to the central (or designated) safety department. A dedicated person must be designated as liaison and have the responsibility to track and revise such agreements and changes to them. Any new conditions (new INDs, NDAs, Marketing Authorizations, new products, new regulations, new PSUR/PBRER dates, etc.) must be transmitted to the drug safety groups involved (e.g., the case processing group, the aggregate reports group). In the European Union, the EU QPPV is responsible for ensuring that this occurs. Periodic reports of contracts in force, dates of expiration (where they exist), and obligations should be issued to the parties who need them.

Safety Agreement Contents

Ideally, all agreements should be in English or available in English, especially in companies that work or sell across borders. This is not always the case. If not, they should be translated into English for all parties involved to be able to know and adhere to their obligations. Translation software may be used realizing, however, that the translation may contain errors and is not certified. The contents should cover the following sections:

Regulatory Status

A table by country with approval date, license holder, companies marketing the product, and name (generic and brand) should be included. A copy of the regulatory table in a PSUR/PBRER is usually acceptable. It should contain:

- IND or equivalents;
- MAs, NDAs/BLAs, or equivalents (in the European Union, type of approval: central, mutual recognition, etc.);
- REMS/RMPs in place;
- Other: named patient/compassionate use, restrictions on use, etc.

Regulatory Responsibilities

The regulatory status of the products may not be the same in each territory or country. It may be a marketed product in one and in clinical trials in the other. All this must be tracked. It should be clarified what regulatory status and responsibilities are to be held by each party and in what country (if multiple countries are involved). Particular attention should be paid to assignment of regulatory responsibilities in countries where each contractual party has a regulatory office or physical presence. The actual names and contact information for the responsible parties should be listed in an appendix (allowing easy updating of changes in personnel, phone numbers, e-mail, etc.).

It should be clarified who reports in each country, who makes contact with health authorities, who answers questions (and if consultation with the other party is obtained or not within X number of days, etc.), and how REMS/RMPs or special conditions are handled. A mechanism should be outlined for the obtaining of any waivers or changes to routine procedures that may be desired by the clinical teams, such as reporting certain SAEs monthly or quarterly rather than as expedited reports.

For the European Union, the EU Qualified Person for Pharmacovigilance and contact information must be clearly specified. If there are two (one in each company), duties must be agreed on in writing and the competent authorities so notified. Nevertheless, depending on the registration status and/or on the agreement between partners, one single EU QPPV or several may be nominated. The EU dictates that one pharmacovigilance may have only one QPPV, so if possible, it is best to have only one single EU QPPV. The same consideration, including updates of name and contact information, should be given to other territories that require a person responsible for pharmacovigilance.

■ Regulatory Documents

The owner and maintainer of documents should be specified for the Reference Safety Information (RSI), e.g., Investigator Brochure, the SmPC/PIL, all other labeling (CCSI), the Package Insert (PI), the product monograph, the investigational and clinical core safety documents, and protocols. Any consultation and approval for each should be specified. The timing and format of exchange should be spelled out for all documents. There should be an assurance that the latest documents in force will be sent out to all parties automatically on update or revision.

■ Health Authority Queries and Requests

It should be stated clearly how health authority requests and queries are to be handled. Usually, the company in the country where the request is made must do the physical answering (in the local language), but the content of the response needs to be done by agreed-on methods and must be consistent with the parties' stance elsewhere, particularly if it is a critical medical question involving stopping of studies, drug withdrawal, or labeling change. Case-specific questions of minor import may usually be answered locally, but anything more important should be resolved by the appropriate groups in each company (usually through a joint operating committee).

A method of dispute resolution must be specified so that senior management can make the final determination in the appropriate time frame. This usually involves the regulatory and safety departments as well as the clinical research groups in each company. Any "pass through" situations (e.g., by a CRO to the sponsor) should be spelled out. The mechanism of answering questions and requirements from health agency reviewers of aggregate reports should also be made clear, particularly if questions are received from multiple authorities for each DSUR, PSUR/PBRER, or PADER, RMPs or REMS, etc. The agreement should specify who should be notified (and how and the required timeframe) of queries, requests, responses, and changes (if any). A tracking mechanism should be in place so no query "falls through the cracks."

■ Regulatory Submissions

Who submits which documents in which countries should be clearly noted. This includes individual cases (7- and 15-day cases) whether by paper or E2B. Whether copies of submissions should be exchanged (even though the electronic file or identical MedWatch or CIOMS I form has already been exchanged by the drug safety groups) should be stated. This might be necessary if the other party wishes to know the serial number (in IND submissions) or date of submission. Roles and responsibilities for EudraVigilance submissions should also be clarified. If MedWatch or CIOMS I forms are used for exchange, provision must be made to database those reports that must be rolled into aggregate tables for submission to regulators (or to respond to queries, etc.).

Similarly, all other regulatory submissions (investigator brochures, labeling changes, PSURs/PBRERs, NDA periodic reports, annual reports, IND annual reports, information amendments, desk copies, post-marketing commitments, REMS/RMPs, etc.) should be spelled out and exchange methodology noted. It is critical to specify whether the other parties have review and approval privileges or are merely given information copies of such documents.

■ Investigator and Investigational Review Board/Ethics Committee Notifications: Blinding and Unblinding, Data Monitoring Committees (DMCs/DMSBs/DMSCs), Data Safety Boards

The mechanism and responsibilities for the preparation of the investigator notification of expedited reports (also called the investigator letter), new IB versions, and changes in the benefit–risk analysis need to be detailed. In addition, in those countries where the sponsor must inform the Ethics Committees/Investigational Review Boards, this should be spelled out. It should be clarified whether the same exact letter is to be used worldwide, and if so, whether a mechanism for its preparation (within the same 15-calendar daytime frame required for the alert report) must be specified. The language is usually English, but any requirements for translations must be noted and responsibility specified.

Most regulatory agencies prefer or require that all expedited reports be submitted unblinded (the code broken). If this is done, the companies must agree on a mechanism for unblinding and the transmission of the unblinded cases (or just the unblinding code) to the other party(ies). This can be challenging if companies want to keep the clinical research team and statisticians blinded.

If one or more Data Safety Management Boards (DSBs/DSMBs)/Data Monitoring Committees (DMCs) are involved either in clinical trials or even (as some companies now do) after marketing, the responsibilities of the partners in regard to these committees should be spelled out, including the powers and functions of the boards and the interactions with the various partners.

Similarly, if a DSB/DSMB is created (per FDA guidance or other HA recommendation) to oversee the whole project and all the protocols, the membership, duties, and functioning must be specified. Safety Assessment Committees (SACs), if they exist, must also be agreed upon.

■ Safety Databases

The parties should agree on who will keep and maintain what data in their respective databases. It should be agreed by all parties that one party (often the largest company; the originating company, or the party with the more robust pharmacovigilance function) maintains the "official" database that will be used as the definitive one for preparing all regulatory reports.

It is nearly impossible, if not totally impossible, to maintain up-to-date, fully reconciled databases when each party has its own database. The maintenance of reconciled, separate databases by each company (even if the same brand of commercial database) produces differences between or among the databases. Problems arise if there are different drug dictionaries, different ways of handling data (e.g., laboratory), different coding conventions, different MedDRA versions, different narrative writing styles, and so on. Mechanisms exist where outside parties may have limited access to the official database though the database owner often hesitates to allow this. Also, duplicative databases add to the cost structure.

If agreement cannot be reached on allowing one partner to maintain the official database, all parties should "agree to disagree" and accept that each will maintain a database but that one agreed-on database will be the "official" one for regulatory reporting and audits/inspections. In the European Union, the EU Qualified Person for Pharmacovigilance must be physically present in an EU member state with direct access to the database, making this database the "official" one for the European Union at the very least. The database is supposed to also be situated in the country where the EU QPPV is located. However, this requirement was created when databases remained on individual, physical servers. Now with cloud computing, this point is, to a degree, moot but it is still in place. In any case, the EU QPPV needs immediate access to the data even if access is via an intermediate person (often a technical person).

As an alternative, only one database is maintained by one company with access to the data for the drug in question by the other companies. This has been problematic in the past but newer technologies, with the database located in the "Cloud", can go a long way to resolve this if all parties agree. The major difficulties are usually political and corporate rather than technical or IT.

The parties must agree on whose SOPs, guidelines, manuals, and so forth, apply where, when, and to whom. In some cases, one or more new SOPs will be created for that partnership only. In other cases, each party uses its own SOPs and reconciliations or changes are made as needed.

■ Definitions

Either in the body of the agreement or as an appendix, the parties should agree on the definitions of terms used, including serious, non-serious, medically significant (important), labeling, expedited, expected, unexpected, labeled, unlabeled, listed, unlisted, and causality (relatedness) in clinical trial cases. This may be a contentious issue because there are no international standards for causality, and the parties need to agree on definitions, particularly for ambiguous terms such as *unlikely related*, the four criteria for the minimal dataset, clock start date, and so on. The language of exchange should be specified as well, and how documents not in English will be handled (full translations or not, certified or not). It is quite challenging to agree on text to describe medical judgement.

The clock start date is sometimes an area of controversy. The United States and the European Union largely agree that the clock start day is day zero and it starts when anyone anywhere in any company, agent, distributor, and so forth, receives sufficient detail to make the case a valid ICSR (patient, drug, reporter, AE). Not all countries agree on this, however, and some start the clock at a later date (when the case is received by the company in that country from a foreign source). The most conservative and usually wisest course is to start the clock when the first person anywhere has enough detail for the case to be valid.

■ Data and Mechanisms of Data Exchange

The physical exchange method must be specified as follows:

- Paper copies versus E2B;
- "Push versus pull", that is, does party A send ("push") data to party B or does party B go onto a website or portal to obtain ("pull") it. How are confirmations handled? It is not enough for party A to send a case; party B must actually receive it. This needs to be verified with acknowledgment of receipt mechanism built in, i.e., automatic;
- Mechanism of transmission: e-mail with attached PDF files, etc., source documents; in some exceptional situations faxing is still done;
- Documents in which a signature copy (hand-signed or electronic signature) is needed to be maintained on file;
- Privacy and anonymization issues to ensure data security and privacy.

Documents to be exchanged must be specified. This is particularly critical for individual case reports.

Will an E2B file be exchanged or will the exchange media be MedWatch forms, CIOMS I forms, an SAE data collection form, or source documents? If CIOMS I or MedWatch forms are exchanged, will they be complete or in draft and on what day after clock start? Will all review be done by partners electronically in the database? If source documents are exchanged initially, will finalized MedWatch or CIOMS I forms or final electronic case files also be exchanged? Is it acceptable that each party creates its own narrative and coding, realizing that there will be differences between the two (or more) parties? If reconciliation is desired, how can this be done rapidly so that 7- and 15-day reports are consistent? How are follow-up data requested and handled?

1. In practice, it is common for the party that receives the case to handle the full processing of the case (including follow-up). A completed E2B file (or other agreed medium) is sent to the other partner(s) by a particular calendar day (often 3–4 days after clock start). This will allow the other parties to upload or enter the data into their database (unchanged) and transmit any expedited cases to the health authority, per their obligations under the PVA. This will also allow them time to check the case against local labeling if the product is marketed with different labeling in the recipient company's territories.
2. Once a sufficient volume of cases is attained (suggesting success in the clinical trial or marketing), a "well-oiled machine" must exist to process and transmit SAEs, particularly if the volumes are high. Reconciliation and "discussions" over particular cases must be the exception and not the rule if on-time regulatory reporting is to be maintained. Keep in mind that submission of a case as an expedited report does not admit that the drug caused the event.
3. Seven-day expedited reports from clinical trials must be handled in a much more rapid time frame (usually 2–3 calendar days) to ensure regulatory compliance.
4. Companies should reach agreement that the most conservative call on seriousness, expectedness, and causality carries the day for SAEs. That is, if one company believes a case is unlabeled or possibly related and the other does not, the case is considered unlabeled or possibly related. This may force a company to submit a case as an expedited report that it does not believe to be one because the other company does. If this is the case, management should be made aware of this to avoid possible issues down the road. A mechanism for timely dispute resolution (or default) should be specified.
5. If CROs are involved, the agreement must account for them in terms of timing and exchange method. Written agreements with the CROs are, of course, required. The regulatory agencies must be notified in writing of the duties devolved onto the clinical research organization(s).

   Note that working with multiple CROs (e.g., one or more on each continent or one of the CROs is the "lead CRO") can be very tricky as many of them are competitors. There may be difficulties in getting such competitors to work together to exchange cases, share and review SOPs, etc.
6. In the European Union, if there are several companies and thus, several EU QPPVs, the single "designated" QPPV should be noted and the dealings between and among the other QPPVs clarified. Similar relationships in other territories that require local responsible persons should, likewise, be clarified.
7. Follow-ups are done by the party receiving the original SAE (or non-serious AE if follow-ups are done for these). The other parties may pose questions for the company doing the follow-up but usually follow-up is left to their discretion and medical expertise. It should be specified when it is done and how frequently.

All follow-up information is handled in the same manner as initial information. It should be stated clearly who reviews the worldwide literature for SAEs and NSAEs and how they are handled when found. If the drug is marketed in the European Union, literature for the product should be searched weekly. This includes accessing EMA's Medical Literature

Monitoring database for relevant case reports from the literature. In addition, MAHs with EU MAs must search the EudraVigilance database and perform signal detection.

A method used by many companies is as follows:

- All SAEs are exchanged as E2B files (or CIOMS I/ MedWatch forms) by calendar day 10 at the latest after clock start anywhere in the world at the first company (or agent) and used as-is, without changes to coding or narrative. Much less commonly, the SAE data collection form or source documents (from clinical trials and spontaneous cases) are exchanged by calendar day 5. In this case, each company writes its own narrative and does its own coding based on this "source document" to create an ICSR. Each company submits its own version to the regulatory agencies in its domain. Because these reports are created by each company on their own, they differ and will require reconciliation or default for signaling and aggregate reporting. If some documents are not in English, this should be noted and should not be a surprise to the company receiving untranslated documents.
- All clinical trial deaths or life-threatening SAEs are exchanged within 3 or 4 calendar days. Sometimes this is limited to the subset of unlabeled (unexpected) cases only; this requires that the receiving company trust the judgment of the sending company on labeledness. This covers 7-day expedited cases.
- All non-serious spontaneous cases are exchanged on a monthly basis (or twice monthly if the volume is very large). Computerized line listings or E2B files (or MedWatch/CIOMS I forms) may be used.
- Non-serious clinical trial cases are not exchanged and are kept only in the clinical trial database of the company(ies) doing the trial. Non-serious cases must be periodically reviewed for seriousness (or adverse events of special interest) to ensure all serious cases are identified.
- Follow-up is done for all SAEs, with at least two contacts attempted for spontaneous cases (more if a critical case such as an alert report) and whatever is necessary for clinical trial cases (the investigator should be accessible to give complete follow-up).

Signaling, Safety Reviews, and Risk Management

The agreement should specify how signaling is done by one or more parties and, if so, how disputes are resolved. It is common to form a safety review committee that meets periodically, usually by telephone, webinar, or video conference, to review the logistics and operational issues of safety handling as well as any SAEs and safety signals that arise. All signals must be tracked to resolution.

Usually, the logistics and operations dominate the initial meetings until all glitches are resolved. At that point, with operational issues minimal and with more SAEs arriving, the signal reviewers predominate. Meetings may be weekly to biweekly initially and then at a monthly or quarterly frequency if no safety or signaling issues arrive. Ad hoc meetings should be held, as needed, for urgent issues. It should be clear how risk management is handled and who prepares and approves any RMPs or REMS that might be needed.

Note: A Partnership Management process must be implemented. As specified above, it could be part of the periodic exchanges about signal and risk management. Nevertheless, each party must have active and ongoing oversight of the exchanges and be able to identify any deviation from the contracted agreement in order to alert the partner, if needed.

Audits

A quality system procedure should be in place to ensure that all requirements for safety are in place. Audits of each partner should occur periodically to ensure this. The audits may be done by each company (or a third party) and should look at the contracts to be sure they are adequate and that their provisions are followed by the responsible parties.

■ Other Issues

If not noted elsewhere, mechanisms for dispute resolution should be described in detail.

- Other product-specific issues relating to devices, vaccines, biologics, and nutraceuticals;
- Any specific regulatory requests (e.g., special reporting of certain SAEs or reporting of adverse events of special interest) should be mentioned;
- An agreed-on time to review the safety exchange agreement should be specified. It is usually yearly but may be more or less frequently if circumstances warrant. Any change in regulatory status (e.g., a new trial, indication, MA/NDA approval) or new safety regulations should trigger a review of the safety agreement;
- Agreement on who does medical literature searches, including responsibility for searching the EudraVigilance Medical Literature Monitoring service, should also be noted;
- Risk management agreements and post-marketing commitments/requirements with health agencies should also be exchanged and agreed on;
- Risk management/minimization issues (including measuring effectiveness of any non-routine interventions) and post-marketing commitments and promises;
- Inspections and audits of one another and by third parties (that is, health agencies). How are they handled? Who is present? How are issues resolved?;
- All arrangements must be written down in the Pharmacovigilance System Master File (PSMF) kept by companies with MAAs or MAs in the European Union and in other territories where required;
- Duplicate submissions of cases to the same health authority must be avoided (Who runs duplicate detection?);
- A mechanism to track changes in safety regulations and requirements should be in place and the agreements updated as needed;
- Usual and unusual marketing arrangements and programs must be covered (e.g., patient support programs, local clinical or observational trials);
- If companies merge, acquire, or sell or transfer the MA, the safety responsibilities must still be done and accounted for;
- Any outsourcing or sub-contracting (if permitted) should be agreed by all parties;
- Training, particularly where differences in procedures produce different processes, must be done, coordinated, and documented, as necessary;
- A mechanism to handle crisis management, recalls, withdrawals, and stopping trials must be developed and agreed on;
- Appendices.

The appendices should contain information that may change frequently, including names, addresses, contact information, territories in question, product names, and registration numbers.

■ Soft Points

- Do not underestimate cultural (both national and corporate) differences, language matters, business etiquette, communication, leadership, and logistics. Someone must be in charge and the maximum in diplomacy and goodwill should be used to smooth and resolve the issues that will inevitably arise.
- Keep in mind time zones when partners are on two or more continents. If Asia, North America, and Europe are involved, someone will always be up in the middle of the night for any teleconference! Also, consider differences in national holidays; definition of "weekend" in the US and Saudi Arabia falls on different days of the week.
- Particular difficulties may occur in "big pharma" — "small pharma" agreements. The "big" players should be particularly sensitive not to dictate a "know-it-all" attitude. There must be understanding that some things will be difficult politically and culturally in the other company because of politics, culture, stubbornness, and local legal matters. Small companies may not have the resources of big players and one person may have many responsibilities.
- It is wise to have at least one face-to-face meeting before the contract is in place and then periodically after the contract begins.
- Not everybody speaks, writes, or understands English well. This is particularly an issue between a large company located in a native-English-speaking country and a small firm in a non-English-speaking

country. Not everybody realizes they don't speak or understand English well. Again, sensitivity to such differences should be kept in mind.

- Management should be (where possible) sensitized to the criticality of safety data exchange. Failure to get this right can produce enormously bad consequences for all parties (not to mention the patients!).

Comments

Health authorities and inspectors are now paying particular attention to Pharmacovigilance Agreements (PVAs) as more complexity has been introduced into the pharmaceutical world, with more outsourcing, fragmentation, and specialization of functions.

Inspectors insist that all responsibilities be noted in contracts and agreements so that all PV obligations are fulfilled. In the European Union, the EU QPPV or delegate will be the focal point for this. The inspectors will expect the contracts and documents to be available and the appropriate parts to be in English so that they (and the drug safety department) can evaluate them. Since PVAs can be signed by partners from different countries (or states in the US), it may be useful to specify according to which law they will refer in case of dispute.

Drug Due Diligence

Before buying or licensing in a medicinal product, an assessment of its dossier should be conducted. A dedicated team can be set up to run this Due Diligence (DD). Usually, the following stakeholders are involved: Non-clinical, Clinical, Marketing, Legal, Medical, Regulatory, PV, and manufacturing.

The purpose is to conduct a deep analysis on all available data and then deliver a synthesis report for the Senior Management, which will then take the decision to buy (or not to buy) the product.

For PV data, the challenge is to identify two kinds of difficulties or weaknesses: PV System Robustness and Drug benefit–risk profile, as shown in the following table.

Table 1 Example of Categories of Potential Pharmacovigilance Challenges

The PV System Robustness	The Product Safety Assessment
Quality Assurance system (including previous CAPAs or Inspection findings)	Drug Class Safety profile
Case Management processes	Identified Risks
Regulatory Compliance	Potential Risks
IT System	Missing Information
Partnerships/SDEA	Risk Management Plan
Signal Detection Process	Safety Surveillance during Clin. Devt
Risk Management System	Benefit/Risk Balance
Pharmaco-Epidemiology	
PV Organization	
PV Members Education & Training	

For each item, a deep analysis is to be conducted. Therefore, the DD is usually managed on site in the other company, a list of all needed documents is to be provided to the counterpart at least several days before the face to face DD; each requested document must be provided.

As regards PV System robustness, it is key to identify strengths and weaknesses for each specified item; e.g.: if we identify that the PV team did not manage ICSRs according to the currently accepted standards, this could explain the perhaps overly positive safety profile delivered at the end of the clinical development. On the other hand, if the PV System is assessed as robust enough, it would mean that one can trust the provided safety data. When running the DD for PV, it is also important to check whether any critical changes have impacted the partner organization during the clinical development program; we can imagine for instance that a PV System is robust for two years, but had been weak over the previous years during clinical development.

The second level of assessment is linked to the drug safety profile and then to the benefit-risk balance. This is more classical for PV employees but must be delivered after a careful analysis. In the DD report, PV must actually provide the company's senior management with a PV assessment as well as with proposals if the collected data are raising doubts or unanswered questions. If it is key to assess the available data, it is also key to identify the important missing data, if any.

Even if many stakeholders are involved in the DD process, the PV conclusions are those which can break the deal. The DD PV report must be very clear in the conclusion with a "Yes" or a "No", sometimes specifying reservations leading to a "conditional Yes"; having to face to a significant safety issue soon after contract signature can be very challenging if not anticipated in the DD conclusions.

Sometimes, alas, safety issues can be buried or coded to minimize or even hide them. The authors have seen this unfortunately. In general, trust but verify.

Finally, beware if one or more of the partners want the DD analysis to be delivered orally and not in writing. The assessment should always be documented in writing.

CHAPTER

33

Where Data Reside

Safety data can come from a variety of sources; limited sources during clinical development, expansive sources after market. Much of it is reliable and verified (for example from tightly controlled clinical trials), but much is not. The challenge is obtaining the necessary and relevant data, verifying that it is valid and correct, ensuring that no duplicates occur, getting it into a database accurately, and making valid clinical judgments at the individual patient level and at the aggregate (public health) level. Since data continue to accumulate over time, as with everything else in drug safety, this is a moving target. This chapter will focus mainly on external sources of safety related data.

■ Introduction

Adverse event (AE) data are collected all over the world by many people and groups. There is little standardization in the way they are collected, how they are measured and graded, how they are stored, and how they are used. Some of the data are collected as a matter of public health, and some are collected by pharmaceutical companies, other companies, non-governmental organizations (NGOs), or patient advocacy groups that process the data and make them available or sell them to others. In theory, with the International Council for Harmonization (ICH), the Council for International Organizations of Medical Sciences (CIOMS), the Medical Dictionary for Regulatory Activities (MedDRA®), and work products of other Standards Development Organizations, such as ISO, HL-7, and CDISC, the PV world is moving toward improved standardization and use of these data.

AE data reside in several places. One main resource is the US Food and Drug Administration (FDA).

FDA Adverse Event Reporting System

The FDA has a large amount of data stored in four publicly accessible databases of primarily post-marketing safety data, as well as other proprietary databases containing clinical trial information. The FDA database for all approved drug and therapeutic biologic products, the FDA Adverse Event Reporting System (FAERS), is discussed here.

FAERS (www.fda.gov), like its predecessor, FDA's Adverse Event Reporting System (AERS), is a repository for information about AEs, medication errors, and product problems on marketed drug and therapeutic biologic products. It is ICH E2B compliant and MedDRA® is used for coding.

The FAERS database contains the following:

- Voluntary reports from healthcare professionals and consumers submitted directly to FDA through the MedWatch program;
- Reports from manufacturers required by regulation, stratified as:
  - Expedited reports, which have at least one SAE that is not in the Package Insert;
  - Non-expedited reports, all reports that do not meet the criteria for expedited reports;
- Biological Safety Reports (BSRs), which are a unique type of 15-day reports submitted to FDA until 2005.

AEs for human cells, tissues, and cellular and tissue-based products (also known as HCT/Ps) and blood and blood components are also included in FAERS but are only available through a Freedom of Information (FOI) request (see below).

FDA uses FAERS data to look for new safety concerns, evaluate regulatory compliance of manufacturers, and respond to outside requests for information. If a potential safety concern is discovered, further evaluation is performed. This might involve conducting additional studies, e.g., querying Sentinel data. (FDA's Sentinel System does not actually have a single database, but, rather, is able to query a network of anonymized electronic health records.)

Based on an evaluation of available data and the concern, FDA may take regulatory action(s), such as updating a product's labeling information, restricting the use of the drug, communicating new safety information to healthcare providers and the public, or, in rare cases, removing a product from the market. Of course, in some instances no action is needed.

FAERS data are available to the public in these ways:

- FAERS Public Dashboard which is an interactive web-based tool that supports queries;
- FAERS Quarterly Data Files which has raw data extracts that can be downloaded (searches require familiarity with relational databases); Redacted ICSRs, which can be obtained through Freedom of Information (FOI) requests to FDA https://www.fda.gov/regulatoryinformation/foi/default.htm.

FAERS Public Dashboard

Direct search capability is provided to the public by the FAERS Public Dashboard). The reports in FAERS should not be considered complete and should be interpreted with caution. FDA includes a lengthy disclaimer with the FAERS Public Dashboard. The following is an extract of the disclaimer: "Although these reports are a valuable source of information, this surveillance system has limitations, including the potential submission of incomplete, inaccurate, untimely, unverified information. In addition, the incidence or prevalence of an event cannot be determined from this reporting system alone due to potential under-reporting of events and lack of information about frequency of use. Because of this, FAERS data comprise only one part of the FDA's important post-market surveillance data and the information on this website does not confirm a causal relationship between the drug product and the reported adverse event(s)."

The Public Dashboard is designed to facilitate easy data queries by the public. Data can be displayed in chart format. For example, users can view a summary of AE reports received from 1968 to the most recent quarter for which data are available or for a specific timeframe. Users can also search on a specific product within a specific timeframe and sort by simple demographics. Data updates are made periodically.

Data fields available through the FAERS Public Dashboard are a subset of the data fields available in the FAERS Quarterly Data files. This is subject to change over time. Also, FAERS Public Dashboard data may not be identical to the corresponding data in the FAERS Quarterly Data files due to different data extraction dates. The data may be downloaded into Excel spreadsheets.

FAERS Quarterly Data Files

Quarterly (non-cumulative) data files since January 2004 are available for downloading. Data include information on patient demographics, the drug(s) reported, the adverse reaction(s), patient outcome, and the source of the reports. The actual files can be downloaded directly. The data can be manipulated (though not easily), and various companies offer services that include periodic updates, data searches, or repackaging of the data in a more user-friendly form. The database cannot be searched directly.

There is a variable lag of several months between AEs being reported to the FDA and their making it into the quarterly data files. Should further information be desired after reviewing the data from the quarterly report, the full MedWatch form (anonymized to protect the reporter and patient) can be obtained using the unique identification number assigned to each case by the FDA.

Redacted ICSRs

Individual FAERS reports, with personal identifiers redacted, may be requested via the Freedom of Information (FOI) process.

There are private companies that, for a fee, will make the requests anonymously and some companies use these services to obtain information on their competitors' products while remaining anonymous. An FOI request can be made online. Although getting and using the data can be difficult, it can be rewarding because large amounts of detailed data are available, particularly for newer products. The full MedWatch forms are available, redacted, and the narratives can be read to obtain clinical summaries of the cases.

■ Clinical Trial Data

There are few clinical trial data in the FAERS database. (These are reports for products with an approved NDA that are also being used in an investigational trial under an IND.) The clinical trial data are proprietary and are generally not available, although some advocacy groups would like to see a change in this. The clinical trials registry housed by the National Cancer Institute (NCI) will hold more data (including more safety information) in the next few years as increased compliance with legislative requirements evolves. In early 2018, FDA announced that it is starting a pilot project with the voluntary assistance of several pharmaceutical companies to release some heretofore proprietary data. If this succeeds, expect more data to become available from clinical trials.

Some clinical trial safety data can be found in Summary Basis of Approval documents that the FDA releases when a drug is approved. They are not easily found on the website and need to be searched for using the search box. There are certain cooperative efforts to consolidate clinical trial data, safety and efficacy, for trusted third party guardianship and anonymization so data can be re-purposed for research use. For example, Project Data Sphere (www.projectdatasphere.com), an independent, not-for-profit initiative operates a platform, essentially a free digital library-laboratory that provides one place where the research community can broadly share, integrate and analyze historical, patient-level data from a broad cooperative of academic and industry phase III cancer clinical trials.

Post-market Requirements and Commitments may be searched for at https://www.fda.gov/drugs/guidancecomplianceregulatoryinformation/post-marketingphaseivcommitments/.

Potential Signals of Serious Risks/New Safety Information that FDA has found in FAERS is available at https://www.fda.gov/drugs/guidancecomplianceregulatoryinformation/surveillance/adversedrugeffects/ucm082196.htm.

Approved Risk Evaluation and Mitigation Strategies are available at https://www.fda.gov/drugs/drugsafety/rems/default.htm.

Finally, FDA was required by the Food and Drug (FDAAA) of 2007 to do a periodic review of new drugs (New Molecular Entity Post-marketing Safety Evaluation), looking at all data within 5 years of first approval.

The FDA also has databases containing clinical trial information as well as drug-specific information, including labeling for approved drugs.

The Uppsala Monitoring Centre

The Uppsala Monitoring Centre maintains one safety database and two coding "dictionaries" that safety officers should know about.

VigiBase

VigiBase (https://www.who-umc.org/vigibase/vigibase/) is the AE database that the UMC maintains on behalf of the World Health Organization. The data are supplied by national health authorities. Much of the data is from the US and are supplied by the FDA. The UMC does not review or assess the individual cases put into the database, but it does pharmacovigilance analyses and signaling based on drug-event pairs.

Certain details, such as case narratives, etc., are not available for review. Not all of the supplying countries allow their data to be released. The database does not contain all the data found in the national databases (e.g., FDA's FAERS, EMA's EudraVigilance) but rather contains extracts restricted to domestic data. The UMC notes that the data are "available to anyone with a health professional degree-level education (physician, dentist, nurse, pharmacist)". The database contains information on marketed drugs as well as OTC products and some herbals.

Three types of reports are available. Ad hoc searches can also be done if none of the reports below are suitable. Samples of the output are available. Results can be presented in either WHO-ART or MedDRA, although there is a transition to MedDRA since WHO-ART is no longer being maintained:

- Overview Reports give numbers of reported cases with a specified reaction, a whole organ class, or all reactions listed for individual drugs. The information is grouped by reporting country or by year. Reactions are listed by preferred term. The summary gives the result as the total number of reactions for the criteria specified, listed by preferred term. In the "by year" and "by country" reports, the reactions are sorted by system organ class.
- ADR profiles provide similar information in a graphical and tabular format.
- Detail reports include further details about each individual case (date of report, case number, type of report, reporter, country, seriousness, death outcome, patient demographics, relevant medical history, AEs [MedDRA and WHO-ART terms], causality where available, suspect drugs, and concomitant drugs). Narratives are not provided by the national authorities and are not available. The reports are available as case reports (one case per page or multiple pages if long), CIOMS line listings (.xls format), or spreadsheet (.xls format).
- Customized searches are available. Costs of searches run roughly between $500 and $1200. Requests can be made directly to the UMC by e-mail, fax, or snail mail. Reports are returned electronically usually within a week or two. In addition, the UMC has arrangements with several vendors that provide web access and tools for using the UMC data, as well as FDA FAERS data.

The UMC's coding dictionaries (WHODrug Global and WHO-ART for AE coding) are discussed elsewhere in this manual.

EMA EudraVigilance Database

EudraVigilance is a data-processing network and management system for reporting and storing suspected

ADRs from clinical trials and in the post-marketing setting for products in the European Economic Area (EEA). It was launched in 2001 and has been upgraded many times. For clinical trials, SUSARs only are recorded and all spontaneous reports (non-serious and serious) are recorded for post-marketing ICSRs (since 2010).

EudraVigilance is used for the electronic exchange of AEs among the European Medicines Agency (EMA), member states' health authorities, MA holders, and sponsors of clinical trials in the EEA; detection of possible safety signals; and the continuous monitoring and evaluation of potential safety issues.

There are two modules: The EudraVigilance Clinical Trial Module (EVCTM) and the Post-authorization Module (EVPM). These merely represent partitions with somewhat different business rules, but the external face of EudraVigilance remains a single transactional database.

The database is maintained by the EMA for the European Commission. Aggregate data are available to the public (but see www.adrreports.eu). Companies are required to obtain data on their own products and perform signal detection procedures. Data are received from companies under obligatory reporting requirements and voluntary reports from the public, which are transmitted by member states' health authorities. Analytical tools are available.

Health Canada

Health Canada's drug safety database is available online for immediate searches. See https://www.canada.ca/en/health-canada/services/drugs-health-products/medeffect-canada/adverse-reaction-database.html.

MHRA

The United Kingdom health agency has information from its Yellow Card Scheme available as interactive Drug Analysis Profiles (iDAPs), which replaced Drug Analysis Prints (DAPs). iDAPs contain complete listings of all suspected ADRs from the Yellow Card Scheme, organized by active ingredient, and have potential for use in signal detection. They include healthcare professional and consumer reports for a particular medicine, as well as manufacturer reports. In addition to individual listings of suspected adverse reactions, totals of suspected ADRs, total reports, serious ADRs, and fatalities can be calculated. Suspected reactions can be stratified and displayed as tables or graphs using a series of sorting options. Data can be sorted by demographics and visualized by MedDRA® System Organ Class, High Level Group Term, High Level Term, and Preferred Term. There are various other customizable display options, such as timeframe, etc. The information is updated periodically, although there is a time-lag of about a month from receipt of a suspected ADR by MHRA to availability in the interactive files. In addition to digital displays, output is available through a print function.

In addition, MHRA, along with an independent advisor (the Commission on Human Medicines), produces a monthly Drug Safety Update (PDF newsletter) that contains summary information on new safety concerns for healthcare professionals.

To promote increased awareness of medicine safety and reporting of suspected ADRs by the public, MHRA has run a series of public-facing information campaigns on drug safety. Traditional outlets as well as social media have been used to encourage Yellow Card reporting to facilitate the safe use of prescription and OTC medicines.

See www.gov.uk/drug-analysis-prints for iDAPs.

Teratology Data

The Teratogen Information System (TERIS) and the online version of Shepard's Catalog of Teratogenic Agents are available at http://depts.washington.edu/terisdb/. TERIS is an online database (housed at the University of Washington) containing a series of agent summaries, each of which is based on a systematic, well-developed review and analysis of published clinical and experimental literature. Assessment of teratogenicity is based on reproducibility, consistency, and biological plausibility of available clinical, epidemiological, and experimental data. Summaries may be accessed using either generic or brand names (domestic or foreign). Each summary includes a risk assessment derived by consensus of an advisory board comprising authorities in clinical teratology.

An updated, automated version of Shepard's Catalog of Teratogenic Agents is distributed with TERIS. Users can access both systems simultaneously at the URL above.

■ General Practice Research Database and Clinical Practice Research Datalink

The General Practice Research Database (GPRD), managed by the Health Economics Research Centre (HERC) at the University of Oxford, is a large database of anonymized longitudinal medical records from primary care practitioners that can be linked with other healthcare data via the Clinical Practice Research Datalink (CPRD). Comprehensive observational data have been collected on more than 10 million active patients for research from around 460 primary care practices throughout the United Kingdom.

The Clinical Practice Research Datalink (CPRD) is a governmental, not-for-profit eHealth research service managed by the MHRA, with partial funding from the UK National Health Service. An important aspect of the available services is to provide linkages between datasets. CPRD combines the expertise and activities associated with GPRD with the UK Department of Health's Research Capability Program (RCP).

Together these assets are used for queries and research on drug safety, clinical epidemiology, disease patterns, pharmacoeconomics, and many other subjects in healthcare. Results have led to improvements in drug safety, best practice, and clinical guidelines. In addition to PGRD data, CPRD also uses primary care data from clinical trials.

For GPRD see https://www.herc.ox.ac.uk/downloads/health_datasets/browse-data-sets/general-practice-research-database-gprd.

For CPRD see https://www.cprd.com/Home/.

■ Other Registries and Databases

There are many registries around the world containing safety data related to drugs. It is often quite difficult to find these databases and obtain access to data, especially those that would be useful for obtaining safety data when preparing Risk Management Plans (RMPs) or Risk Evaluation and Mitigation Strategies (REMS). Databases can be located with information on exposure or outcomes, pharmacoepidemiology and pharmacoeconomic studies, as well as other studies of drug safety. A paid subscription is required. See its website for further information (www.bridgetodata.org).

It is likely that drug safety databases will grow explosively in the near future as various efforts in the US, the EU, and Asia to create data warehouses, linked databases, and electronic medical records databases continue to incorporate advances in interoperability of IT systems. The collection, standardization, normalization, transmission, and validation of the data, using approaches developed by Standards Development Organizations, such as HL-7 (www.hl7.org) and CDISC (www.cdisc.org), are moving ahead. When large amounts of good digital data and analytical tools become available, the world of drug safety will change markedly. As of today, the spontaneous reporting system remains the most valuable, but thanks to machine learning and artificial intelligence, the systems/databases specified in this chapter could become, as a first step, an additional tool to detect safety signals. Some additional databases may be found using the various AI search apps.

CHAPTER

34

Information Technology and the Safety Database

Any company that receives more than a handful of adverse events (AEs), whether for marketed products or for products only in clinical trials, needs a database to collect, assemble, and report on these AEs. As the rest of the chapters in this book indicate, the regulations and reporting requirements are voluminous and follow tight standards in terms of content, format, and timing for reports to HAs and contractual partners. It is thus necessary to have an AE database that allows, at the minimum, manual data entry, electronic data entry via E2B or a customized upload and output of required forms and various aggregate data, e.g., for PSURs/PBRERs, IND annual reports, Development Safety Update Reports (DSURs), and NDA periodic reports as well as any other customized or national/local reports. Export capabilities are also necessary as E2B files or other customized exports. Many of the databases used for drug safety also allow for complex analysis and data mining of AEs, such as increased frequency and disproportionality calculations. Machine learning is improving the efficiency of some systems. Some have automated export and import capabilities, e.g., the electronic safety gateway for EudraVigilance.

Introduction

Many databases also have workflow and quality components built in with email and messaging functionality. Some companies customize their databases, though more and more companies are buying one of the standard packages ("shrink-wrapped software" or "commercial off the shelf" systems) available from various vendors. As databases get larger and larger and more and more complex, the ease and ability of transferring data from one database to another database becomes more difficult and costly. Thus, once a company commits to one database, it often will use that database "forever". Mergers and acquisitions of the database vendor can produce significant headaches for the user community if the vendor no longer supports the database or it is upgraded. This is changing somewhat with the use of the "cloud" for data storage and efforts to improve interoperability of systems. This, however, is just the tip of the iceberg. This chapter reviews the issues and specialized needs around safety databases.

Required Safety Database Functionality

The following list represents a high level view of the functions that a safety database must have to meet the needs of a multi-national drug safety department. For smaller single-country departments, the needs may be somewhat less. However, it is wise to consider future business arrangements, wherein your safety department may be involved in co-development or co-marketing with a licensing partner that operates outside your country and you must intercalate into their global PV system. There will surely be other requirements needed now or in the future that are not listed here. Business conditions can change rapidly. Scalability and the ability to change and customize the database as requirements change are critical. Note that there is some duplication and overlap among the following sections as some requirements are common to multiple areas.

Data Entry

- Upload capabilities from other databases, e.g., phone center and clinical research databases, via manual, E2B or other formats;
- Case data entry to include all needed fields to produce a completed MedWatch form, CIOMS I form, other locally required forms, PSUR/PBRER, PADER, CIOMS line listings, E2B transmission, and so forth;
- Tabular entry of laboratory data as well as manual entry (lab data often comes to sponsors electronically);
- Seriousness, expectedness (labeledness), causality at case level and adverse event (AE) level by the investigator, company, CRO, others (that is, multiple entries possible for an AE causality in particular);
- Multiple narratives for the same case, e.g., short narrative, long narrative, non-English narrative, case comments, blinded narrative. Mechanism to handle follow-up information in the narrative (overwrite versus append). Size limitations on the field;
- Ability to handle multiple labels (e.g., Summary of Product Characteristics, US Package Insert) producing different expectedness classification depending on the local label;
- Ability to handle one or more reporters for a single case;
- Versioning, with multiple versions possible for each case, e.g., by country and submission to HAs;
- Tracking of information in and out (case log for audit);
- Support for the Medical Dictionary for Regulatory Activities (MedDRA®) (multiple versions and languages), WHO-Drug Dictionary (and others);
- Tight link to a MedDRA browser to allow easy coding;
- Tight link to the drug database;
- Ability to handle central and computerized lab data imports (uploads) with multiple normal ranges and in different formats;
- Handling of multiple product types such as devices, drugs, biologics, combination products, injectables, medication errors, product quality complaints, blood products as needed;
- Duplicate check for cases using multiple fields, e.g., name, postal code, age;

- Ability to add fields as needed, e.g., new business partner case reference numbers or changes in regulations;
- Ability to close/complete a case and reopen it as needed;
- Ability to have scanned source documents attached or linked to cases;
- Required fields customizable by users (with caution!) and a controlled process to do so;
- Edit checks, e.g., system will not allow entry of data to show that a 50-year-old patient has a birth date of January 12, 2015, or that a male is pregnant;
- Ability to handle clinical trial, spontaneous, solicited/unsolicited, named patient use (NPU), literature, pregnancy, and other types of cases;
- Ability to handle multiple doses of each drug (to account for starting, stopping, restarting, dose change, etc.);
- Spell check in multiple languages;
- Automated case narrative; and
- Ability to handle combination drugs, drug-device combination products, OTC products, and so forth.

Workflow

- Ability to track and move a case through its processing using customized business rules set up by users;
- Communication ability at the user and case level, e.g., a reviewer can electronically ask a question of the person who entered the case data via email, SMS, etc.;
- Version tracking of each case with multiple different versions existing simultaneously for a case, e.g., US version 2, EMA version 3, Japanese version 4;
- Metrics to measure status of groups of cases with groups customized by the user, e.g., each work team has its own metrics and management has aggregate metrics;
- Duplicate checking and ability to duplicate a case or archive a case;
- Ability to process literature reports;
- Ability to handle customized case identification numbering with each case having multiple numbers;
- Multiple clock start dates, which may vary by country;
- Follow-up letter generation to reporter or patient;
- Correspondence tracking and reminders;
- Returned product request and tracking; and
- Ability to use external software tools, bolt-ons, apps.

Administration

- Customized access limits at user, country, group, case, drug level, e.g., France cannot read Germany's cases, team handling drug X cannot see drug Y cases;
- Security and passwords — 21CFR11 & EU compliant;
- Scalability (able to add more users, countries, drugs, business partners easily);
- International use (if needed);
- Multiple language and character set support;
- Tickler (reminder) system;
- Audit trails (full unless there is a clear reason not to have complete audit trails);
- Validation and validation scripts for any upgrades;
- The US Health Insurance Portability and Accountability Act of 1996 (HIPAA), Public Law 104-191, included privacy provisions for electronic healthcare transactions and code sets. Likewise, the EU General Data Protection Regulation (GDPR), 2016/679, is a law on data protection and privacy for all individuals within the EEA. It also addresses the export of personal data outside the EEA. The GDPR is more stringent than HIPPA, so many companies based elsewhere but operate in the EEA have adopted GDPR protections worldwide. Other jurisdictions have local data privacy laws. Taken together, this means that the ability to anonymize a case is quite important because there are penalties for misbehavior;
- Tracking of submissions for expedited and aggregate reports to multiple HAs;
- Case cannot be downgraded (serious to non-serious or unexpected to expected) without senior staff signoff; and
- A Japanese version with the ability to produce the appropriate E2B file ("the J file") in the Japanese language. Other local or regional requirements may emerge that will expand needs in this regard.

Vendor Support and Information Technology Issues

- User groups;
- Support from vendor and internal IT colleagues at home-base and worldwide user sites (ability for load-sharing);
- Ability to customize when new regulations and requirements are put in place;
- IT support capability in-house;
- Secure, off-site physical location, e.g., the Cloud;
- Upgrade policy and support for older versions;
- Hardware needs and compatibility with other hardware and software; and
- Backup system, e.g., every hour, nightly, weekly, with alternate power source, redundancies, and ability to reconstitute database contents within 24 hours (or less) in case of emergency.

Validation

- A fully validated system and validation strategy in place going forward;
- Change control in place; and
- Must be acceptable (including documentation) to United States, European Union, MHRA, and other inspectors.

Labeling Functions

- The database should be able to store the AEs that are labeled/listed for each drug and formulation, and to identify which cases, based on the local labeling, seriousness, and causality (for clinical trial cases), are 7- and 15-day reports to HAs in various countries, which go into PADERs/PSURs/PBRERs, and so forth;
- Labels for multiple countries should be storable and useable in this manner. Strategy on handling labeling in non-English languages.

Reporting Functions

- Draft and final versions of all usual reports: ICSRs (electronic or paper forms), PSUR/PBRER tables, listings, NDA periodic, and IND annual tables, Investigator Letters, cover letters to regulatory agencies in English or other languages with the agency address, case number and drug automatically inserted into the letter;
- Other reports: United Kingdom Yellow Card, French imputability in French, English, and other languages;
- Export to EudraVigilance for both clinical trial and post-marketing cases;
- Ability to identify, based on algorithms that are entered into the database, which cases are 7-day and 15-day reports and which cases go into aggregate reports, e.g., PSURs/PBRERs, NDA periodic reports, including follow-ups. Note that ICSRs included in PBRERs are sent separately from the PBRER in E2B format;
- Ability to import E2B files and data from other database and place into templates, e.g., insert case numbers, drug name, and dates into MS Word documents;
- Ability to query easily, e.g., Query By Example, on all fields to produce queries that can be made into reports without the need of a programmer to develop an SQL query;
- Batch printing, transmission of local forms, or line listings of query or report results in PDF files;
- Ability to save queries and reports at the user level;
- Ability to anonymize reports and queries (e.g., no initials, no reporter names or addresses);
- EudraVigilance reporting and retrieval; and
- Epidemiologic, data-mining, and other reports using internal functions or add-on ("bolt-on") tools.

Data Export and Import

- E2B import with strategy on how to triage, flag, or run edit checks to "accept" a case before adding it to the database, especially if an earlier MedDRA version or different drug dictionary was used;
- E2B export to multiple sources with automated receipt acknowledgment and multiple headers or content changes, e.g., different file for Japan, United States, and European Union for the same case;
- Automated transmission of cases based on business rules to internal and external recipients,

e.g., a particular drug's cases go to licensing company externally and recipients internally 5 days or 10 days after first receipt date; and
- Ability to generate other formats for data export (Excel, PDF, etc.).

Pharmacovigilance Functions

- Note that some or all of these functions may be done by external software or databases separate from the PV/drug safety database, e.g., reconciliation of PV and clinical trial project database. The external operations may or may not be tightly linked to the safety database;
- Ability to produce pharmacovigilance reports and data-mining, both defined in the software and customized by the user;
- Ability to use add-on statistical, epidemiologic, and other tools and reports;
- Drug usage data stored and used in queries and reports;
- Ability to use a third party's software; and
- Signal detection and trend analysis.

Database Support

With a complex safety database in place, the drug safety group will need dedicated support from the technical services within the organization (be it a health agency, a pharmaceutical company, or a service provider). This will usually require one or more people working full-time with the drug safety group. This is critical, as the IT personnel, to better serve, must learn a significant amount about how the safety business runs.

The IT group (either internal or outsourced to a vendor) will serve multiple functions, including administering hardware and software, upgrades, user access and security, ad hoc queries (by the programmers), ongoing maintenance, bug fixes, new reports and projects, audit and inspection support, and validation and change control. In addition, there will be many behind-the-scenes personnel, e.g., database administrators, server maintenance, network personnel, involved in support of the drug safety database. If some or all of these functions are outsourced, an internal IT expert should oversee the operations of the outsourced companies and ensure that all requirements (regulatory, legal, and contractual) are followed and met.

It is usually good for both the drug safety and the IT personnel to have "one-stop shopping". That is, requests for IT support or for new projects should go through one person (or single group) within the drug safety department to one person/group in the IT department to manage the flow of work and requests, track projects, clarify needs, and ensure priorities are met. The IT person will then coordinate the behind-the-scenes actions in the IT department, e.g., network personnel, database administrators, software vendors, etc. Thus, the drug safety personnel should be able to go to one IT person for any computer issues and not have to figure whom to go to in IT: the database coordinator, the software support team, or the hardware support team. And the IT personnel do not have to figure out whom to contact in drug safety.

The database must support all privacy and security requirements from around the world. Changes in requirements may occur over time in various countries and they may involve both changes in the IT system/database and in workflow procedures. Whatever database is used, it must be able to handle multiple and sometimes conflicting privacy and data protection requirements. This may involve storing personal identifier information (names, addresses, reports, etc.) in separate files in separate servers, sometimes within the European Union. These rules are complex and changing. Many companies have dedicated privacy officers who can assist in these issues.

Data Entry

Companies must make strategic, organizational, and operational decisions on where data entry should occur, especially if they are multi-national companies. Single-country companies are able to have their safety data entered centrally in one or at most two facilities. This streamlines operations and allows for standardization across all data entry personnel and for backup data entry if one site should go out of service, e.g., fire, loss of electrical power, etc. Some companies will outsource some or all of the safety functions.

Multi-national companies must deal with issues of multiple languages, the need for follow-up on AE cases by local personnel in the local language, local reporting requirements (again, often in the local language), and the need for consistency and a single message (saying the same thing to all HAs in each AE case or safety issue). Companies respond to these needs in multiple ways, depending on their size, geographical location, number and type of products and indications. Typically one of three models is chosen when determining who will conduct data entry and have ownership of the safety database:

1. Fully In-house model — this is where the company will purchase or license the database themselves, host it directly on their server, and hire employees to conduct the data entry for all cases.
2. Fully outsourced model — this is where the company will hire a CRO or vendor, one or multiple, that will help the company fulfill their obligation for data entry, collection, and reporting. A company may choose to select a vendor to house all of their safety case processing needs or select a few smaller companies to 1) host the database, 2) conduct case processing and assessment, and 3) conduct expedited reporting.
3. Hybrid Model — This is where the company will outsource a lot of the heavy lifting to an external vendor such as the safety database hosting, setup, configuration, and maintenance, but may keep in house the case processing and reporting.

The decision as to which model is right for a company will (as many times stated) depend on the company's size, financial capabilities, and development goals. For example, a company that desires to only develop products through Phase 1 and then divest or sell may choose a fully outsourced model, versus a company that desires to take their product to market may initially chose outsourced (due to limited financing in the early stage of development), then move to hybrid modeling and further to fully in-house model of management.

The critical issues, whichever mechanism is chosen, are as follows:

- Maintaining standards and consistency across multiple and diverse data entry sites, often speaking different languages and working under different conditions and time zones, is always challenging;
- Organizational reporting may also present issues if the safety personnel abroad report only locally and not "dotted line" or directly to the head safety office;
- Training is harder over greater distances even with online and other high-technology training tools;
- Quality is more challenging to measure and maintain;
- IT issues occur in terms of storage, networks, security, data transmission speed, continuous supply of utilities, and other support;
- Data privacy issues may arise if data is shipped from a region with tight data privacy and security rules to areas of less stringent data protection rules (e.g., the United States, in the eyes of the European Union); and
- *Time zones interfere with workflow*: It is almost impossible to arrange a simultaneous teleconference among Asia, the United States/Canada, and Europe due to time differences without pulling somebody out of bed. The International Date Line also presents some dating problems ("This report came into the United States today from Japan, where it was received tomorrow"). In addition, business hours don't overlap: the day crew working in North America will have to interact with the night crew working in Asia. The working day does not overlap either, e.g., Sunday is a normal working day In Saudi Arabia, but not in the UK. The UK has bank holidays that are not recognized elsewhere. If one is aware, careful logistical planning can overcome these seeming impediments.

Data Transmission (E2B)

In this section, the practicalities of setting up E2B for data import and export are discussed. E2B export of individual case safety reports is now obligatory for manufacturers to HAs in Japan, the EU, the US, and certain other countries.

There are several issues in E2B export:

- The E2B file differs somewhat in each of the three major regions due to regional requirements in regulations that pre-date electronic reporting. In particular, a separate file ("the J file") for each case must be prepared for Japanese reporting, as it is required by the Japanese HA in addition to the standard E2B file. The EU and the US also have some differences in requirements that have forced mandatory reporters to prepare three separate files, one each for the United States, Japan, and the European Union. Most of these differences relate to administrative needs and the medical portion of ICSRs is essentially the same for all trading partners.
- The database structure of some old databases or cases is not fully compatible with E2B transmissions. For example, laboratory data may be entered into structured fields or as free text. Some companies have dozens of years of laboratory data stored as free text in their database. It is usually not necessary or worth the effort to reenter the data into structured tables. However, decisions must be made on how these data will be entered moving forward. Electronic data entry or downloading of laboratory data may alleviate much of this problem, although uniform "standards" are not in place amongst various trading partners.
- Technical issues exist on gateways, drug dictionaries, and MedDRA versions.
- A process must be set up within a company to verify that all appropriate reports have been sent to the appropriate HAs (and/or business partners) on a timely basis and that they were received and successfully uploaded into the receivers' database(s). Most of the modern commercially available drug safety databases handle these issues fairly well and companies are now expected by the regulatory agencies to handle these technical differences and submit cases correctly and on time. Outsourcing companies (CROs) are able to do E2B submissions for companies that are not equipped for direct E2B transmission themselves. There are corresponding issues in regard to E2B (or database-to-database) import of files from business partners and other companies. In addition, there are other issues, technical and otherwise, that will not be considered here. All Pharmacovigilance Agreements (PVAs) should take the above points into consideration.
- How to screen and triage a report coming in. Should it be uploaded automatically into the receiver's database or should it be kept in a "holding area" until drug safety personnel are able to perform edit checks and review the file for content and format to ensure that it meets the appropriate criteria for entry into the database?
- How is the file actually reviewed by the staff? Online? Printed out?
- Screening for duplicates may be done in the triage area or after uploading. Duplicates are defined as receipt of the same case containing no new information whatsoever.
- A strategy must be found for identifying, handling, and versioning follow-up reports for cases already in the database.
- Dictionary incompatibility. If the sender has not yet upgraded to the latest version of MedDRA or the drug dictionary and the receiver has, how is the case handled? If different, and possibly incompatible, drug dictionaries are used, how are the data handled? Are business partners synchronized (and employ the same conventions) is there an escalation process for discrepancies?
- How is security handled regarding encryption, viruses, and so on?

E2B(R3)

Things are changing rapidly. ICH has decided that the future versions of E2B will be created in collaboration with "Standards Development Organizations" (SDOs) to widen use around the world, to promote interoperability, and for use by more than pharmaceutical companies and health agencies. Thus, the International Organization for Standards (ISO), Health Level 7 (HL7), the CDISC, the International Health Terminology

Standards Development Organization (IHTSDO), European Committee for Standardization (CEN), and others have implemented a single, common ICSR standard, ISO IS 27953-2:2011: Health informatics — Pharmacovigilance — Individual case safety report — Part 2: Human pharmaceutical reporting requirements for ICSR. This double-badged standard (owned by ISO and HL7), has been developed based on ICH E2B(R3) business requirements. ICH has developed an ICH Implementation Guide as part of an implementation package that is composed of several documents, including Q&A. Founding regulators have issued regional Implementation Guides to supplement the ICH package and have used the entire package for implementation.

ISO has also developed a complex suite of five standards and nine supporting documents for Identification of Medicinal Products (IDMP), intended for use with ICSR exchange. These standards specify data elements and structures to uniquely identify and exchange information across the entire lifecycle of a drug product, i.e., products in development, investigational products, products under evaluation, and approved products:

ISO IS 11238:2012

Health informatics — Identification of medicinal products — Data elements and structures for the unique identification and exchange of regulated information on substances.

ISO IS 11239:2012

Health informatics — Identification of medicinal products — Data elements and structures for the unique identification and exchange of regulated information on pharmaceutical dose forms, units of presentation, routes of administration and packaging.

ISO IS 11240:2012

Health informatics — Identification of medicinal products — Data elements and structures for the unique identification and exchange of units of measurement.

ISO IS 11616:2012

Health informatics — Identification of medicinal products — Data elements and structures for the unique identification and exchange of regulated pharmaceutical product information.

ISO IS 11615:2017

Health informatics — Identification of medicinal products — Data elements and structures for the unique identification and exchange of regulated medicinal product information.

■ Database Migration

At some point, most companies will have to migrate their safety data (often called "the legacy data") to a new or upgraded safety database, or from one vendor to another. Many companies will also, at some point, have to import safety data should they acquire an already marketed product. Sometimes companies merge and combine their safety systems. These situations require the transfer of data from the originator's database into the acquirer's database or vice versa. This data transfer is generally a painful exercise requiring the expertise of the drug safety, IT, regulatory, and other groups. It can be difficult and time-consuming if participant numbers are in the hundreds of thousands to millions, with billions (or more) of data points! However, with most database having E2B capabilities, the transfer of the information from one system to the next is becoming easier. The data will still have to be examined and mapped into the new database and if the previous database had a lot of customizations, this will also create challenges. Although much of the data can be automatically transferred using algorithms, some of the data will need to be examined and transferred manually. This is the case with conversion of E2B(R2) data to conform with the E2B(R3) requirements (and vice versa). The transferring team will find inexplicable data and not be able to trace the "cleaning rules" applied when the data were entered or transferred in the past. Multiple moves of data over the years worsen this problem. This happens to companies, regulators, and service providers.

The migration process can take months to a year for large and complex databases. An internal team, often with outside consultant assistance, should be assembled for this project, with careful project management, quality control, validation, and full documentation of all processes, changes, and alterations. The company should expect an inspection by the concerned health agencies (FDA, EMA, MHRA in particular) after the migration.

When a company makes the determination to migration safety data from one place to another, great care should be taken to ensure accuracy and completeness of the information migrated. The company should put into place a migration plan to document the steps involved for the transfer, how discrepancies will be managed, and how the migration itself will be documented. During a BIMO inspection for example, it is largely assumed that any database migration will be subject to review and scrutiny.

1. Something to consider when preparing for and conducing a safety database migration should be to Create a Data Migration Plan which summarizes and documents:
   a. New and old Safety Database information, such as database names, version information, MedDRA version information, etc.
   b. Date of the migration initiation & target completion dates
   c. Risk Management procedures for delays in the migration and how those risks will be mitigated
   d. Responsible persons/parties involved in the migration and a table outlining roles and responsibilities between each party
   e. Source of incoming data and data type to be transferred (Line listings, MedWatch, CIOMS, E2B .xml files, narratives, source data information, etc.)
   f. How the data will be transferred (electronically or manually, or both)
   g. What steps will be taken to ensure all cases received were successfully migrated, such as a reconciliation step at the end of the migration to ensure case A made it from Database X to Database Y for example
   h. How to handle discrepancies or errors found in the case files during the migration phase
   i. If a clinical trial is ongoing at the time of migration, how incoming cases will be handled (will they go directly into the new system or will initial case processing pause with the new system until all legacy data is transferred?)
   j. What will signify when the migration is complete? Will the company implement a data migration completion form that requires a signature of the owning/responsible parties?
   k. Where will the documents of the transfer be stored

The process of creating such a plan will ultimately improve the outcome of the migration and help when one may have to review the migration activities during an inspection.

Clinical Data Interchange Consortium

CDISC is a global, multi-disciplinary, non-profit "SDOs" that has established electronic data standards to support the acquisition, exchange, submission, and archive of clinical research data and associated metadata (www.cdisc.org). Their goal is to develop and support global, platform-independent data standards that enable information systems to easily exchange data to improve medical research and healthcare.

CDISC standards are vendor-neutral, platform-independent, and freely available.

Systematized Nomenclature of Medicine Clinical Terms

SNOMED is a hierarchical, clinical terminology or dictionary that covers diseases, clinical data, microorganisms, drugs, procedures, adverse events, and more. It has more than 344,000 "concepts". It will encompass MedDRA and much more, although there is not a 1:1 correlation of these two terminologies. It was created by the College of American Pathologists and the UK National Health Service. The US Department of Health and Human Services in 2007 agreed to participate in the development of Systematized Nomenclature of Medicine Clinical Terms (SNOMED CT) for use with electronic health records. It is available free of charge to everyone in the US.

This is a highly complex area that is constantly changing and evolving. Not all efforts are fully harmonized around the world, and it is possible, if not likely, that multiple standards will develop over time. Although these efforts are just beginning to touch drug safety, it is expected that the systems, procedures, business models, IT, and all other aspects of drug safety will change over the years as these standards are put into practice.

■ Frequently Asked Question

Q: This seems incredibly complex and not necessarily understandable by non-IT people doing pharmacovigilance. Is this a problem?

A: Well, it certainly is in some companies and agencies. The bureaucratic, IT, and regulatory complexity is increasing rapidly as we now enter Drug Safety 3.0! More and more jobs are compartmentalized, making it much harder to have a good overview of how PV works. The creation in the EU of the Pharmacovigilance System Master File (PSMF) helps one figure out how the system works at a high level, even if it is very complex. Such a document does not exist in the US. This document, however, may not cover IT in sufficient detail looking at all IT systems (validated and non-validated) in use. Many have pointed out that such complexity may make it easier to hack a system, thus, putting everyone at risk. So yes, this is a problem! We need greater IT literacy and transparency in pharmacovigilance.

CHAPTER 35

Data Privacy and Security

Approximately 30 or so years ago, with the advent of enormous changes in communication, the Internet, personal computers, smart phones and tablets, social media, Artificial Intelligence (AI), etc., it has become clear that personal privacy and data security are major issues in medicine. With the Internet and identity theft, the question of who has access to what data is now in the forefront of people's and governments' minds.

■ Introduction

For many years, medical data were believed to be the property of the treating physician or hospital, and they were kept confidential by those parties. In the United States, Europe, and elsewhere, there was no right to privacy as defined by law, and sometimes patients were denied the right to obtain or even see their own medical records. The law that was in place in the United States was state law, which varied from state to state, offering inconsistent levels of protection. Similarly, in Europe and elsewhere, laws were national or local, such as they were.

That viewpoint has largely changed, and a person's health data are now believed to be owned by that individual. There are now clear limitations on what third parties (physicians, hospitals, companies, and governments) can and cannot do with the data. In the United States, the federal government and local governments have enacted laws on privacy. The European Union now has rules and regulations that cover all member states (some of which have put forth additional and tougher privacy and security protections). There is even an EU Data Protection Supervisor, an independent position appointed by the European Parliament and the Council with responsibility for protection of personal data handled by EU institutions, bodies, and agencies. Canada, Australia, Japan, and other countries have also tightened their privacy protections.

For the purposes of drug safety and pharmacovigilance, two major governmental acts, worth studying in detail, largely represent the state of privacy around the world: the US Health Insurance Portability and Accountability Act (HIPAA) and the European Union (EU) Data Privacy Regulation & Directive and recent changes, including the General Data Protection Regulation (GDPR), which became effective in 2018. They are reviewed here and the implications and effects on drug safety are discussed.

In keeping with the context of this text, this chapter intends to provide a general summary of some of the data privacy laws and regulations that could impact drug development and research, but it by no means provides the complete summary of the topics that should be considered. Relevant to drug safety and pharmacovigilance, the concerns regarding data protection and privacy apply to the collection of source information as it pertains to adverse event data, mainly serious events, and the clinical course of the patient which often requires the attainment of electronic medical records from sources such as physician notes, hospital admission and discharge summaries, surgical records, and post mortem autopsy reports. Since the implementation of laws such as US HIPAA and EU GDPR (https:gdpr.eu), pharmaceutical companies and drug developers have, and continue to, struggle with the fine balance of obtaining relevant clinical data to support the product development, and maintaining patient and data privacy and security. All Marketing Authorization Holders (MAHs) must comply with pre and post-marketing pharmacovigilance requirements, such as reporting of adverse events (AEs), while simultaneously ensuring that personal data are processed only where necessary and only where the parties involved assess this necessity at every stage of the PV process. This is a difficult and overwhelming task to ensure compliance and should be overseen and managed not only by the safety group, but be heavily managed by a Data Protection Officer (DPO) and Compliance Officer.

■ United States Health Insurance Portability and Accountability Act (HIPAA)

Unlike the European Union, the United States does not have one global law for data privacy and security. Rather, different parts, or "sectors," of the country have different approaches. The healthcare sector is covered at the federal level by the Health Insurance Portability and Accountability Act (HIPAA) as well as various other state and local laws, regulations, and court cases. Laws and regulations, which have been revised several times, are arcane and complex.

These regulations cover health plans, healthcare clearinghouses, and those healthcare providers ("covered entities") who handle personal healthcare data and conduct certain financial and administrative transactions on paper or electronically. All medical records and other individually identifiable health information held or disclosed by a covered entity in any form, whether held electronically, on paper, or orally, are covered. Some of the privacy and security features are summarized as follows:

- Providers and health plans must give patients a clear written explanation of how they can use, keep, and disclose their health information.
- Patients must be able to see and get copies of their records and request changes and corrections. Corrections are not required to be made by the document holder, but, if not, the "dissenting opinion" must become a part of the record. In addition, a history of most disclosures must be made accessible to patients on request.
- Patients' authorization to disclose information must be obtained before their medical information is shared. In addition, specific patient consent must be obtained for certain other uses, such as releasing information to financial institutions or drug companies, etc.
- Patient consent to release information must not be coerced.

- Disclosures of personal information must be limited to the minimum necessary to fulfill the intended purpose of the request.

Covered entities must follow these requirements, at a minimum:

- Written privacy procedures must be in place and must include who has access to protected information, how it will be used within the entity, and when the information would or would not be disclosed to others. Covered entities must also take steps to ensure that their business associates, e.g., contractors and vendors, etc., protect the privacy of health information.
- Covered entities must designate a privacy officer and provide sufficient training to staff so that their employees understand and follow the privacy protections and procedures.
- Covered entities must provide a means for patients to make inquiries or complaints regarding the privacy of their records.
- Psychotherapy notes (used only by a psychotherapist) are held to a higher standard of protection because they are not part of the medical record and are never intended to be shared with anyone else.
- Failure to comply may lead to civil or criminal penalties, including fines and imprisonment.

Examples of when personal health information may be released:

- Oversight of the healthcare system, including quality assurance activities;
- Public health research approved by a privacy board or institutional review board;
- Judicial and administrative legal proceedings;
- Certain law enforcement activities;
- Emergency circumstances;
- Identification of the body of a deceased person or the cause of death; or
- Activities related to national defense and security.

The HIPPA requirements clearly have implications for pharmacovigilance. Much discussion occurred and the Food and Drug Administration (FDA) ultimately issued a clarification regarding the appropriate and responsible release of patient-specific information (Manufacturers Sharing Patient Specific Information from Medical Devices with Patients Upon Request: Guidance for Industry and Food and Drug Administration Staff, October 30, 2017).

The FDA fully recognized that pharmaceutical companies are required by law and regulation to maintain databases of adverse events occurring in individuals who have taken their products, reported by health professionals and others. The data identify the person making the report and may or may not identify the individual patient or subject. The data come both from clinical trials of new products and from the post-marketing data of drugs already on the market.

Although in such data there is often no specific patient identification (e.g., name and address), there may be sufficient patient data such that it would be possible in many cases, with only minimal effort, to identify the patient based on the known data (e.g., hospital, dates of hospitalization, age or birth date, patient initials, sex, diagnosis, treatment, and hospital course). These data are often required to be submitted to health authorities and are necessary for clinical and epidemiologic evaluation of the adverse event and safety profile of the drug. It is vitally important to know that certain events occur in special populations (e.g., only in children, females, or the elderly). There is a broad consensus in the industry and in the health authorities that these data are vital for maintaining and protecting public health. Removal of these demographic data would make the data much less useful for safety and epidemiologic analyses. Identification of safety problems occurring with both new and old drugs would suffer if the flow of these data were hindered.

The FDA addressed this in the March 2005 Guidance for Industry: Good Pharmacovigilance Practices and Pharmacoepidemiologic Assessment. The FDA notes: "It is of critical importance to protect patients and their privacy during the generation of safety data and the development of risk minimization action plans. During all risk assessment and risk minimization activities, sponsors must comply with applicable regulatory requirements involving human subjects research and patient privacy."

It is also clear that "covered entities", such as pharmacists, physicians, or hospitals, are permitted to report AEs to the health authorities without problem from HIPAA. The FDA notes: "The Privacy Rule specifically permits covered entities to report adverse events and other information related to the quality, effectiveness, and safety of FDA-regulated products both to manufacturers and directly to FDA (45CFR164.512(b)(1)(i) and (iii), and 45CFR164.512(a)(1))." In 2018 the FDA commented on MedWatch and HIPAA: "The HIPAA Privacy Rule recognizes the legitimate need for public health authorities and others responsible for ensuring public health and safety to have access to protected health information to carry out their public health mission. The Rule also recognizes that public health reports made by covered entities are an important means of identifying threats to the health and safety of the public at large, as well as individuals. Accordingly, the Rule permits covered entities to disclose protected health information without authorization for specified public health purposes." See: https://www.fda.gov/safety/reporting-serious-problems-fda/hipaa-compliance-reporters-fda-medwatch

In various subsequent initiatives and documents, FDA has reiterated its commitment to protecting privacy and there is a broad understanding that drug safety data may be reported to manufacturers (sponsors) and to the FDA in the interest of public health.

■ The European Union and the Privacy Regulation & Directive

The European Union's approach to privacy is somewhat different from that of the United States. The United States does not really have the equivalent of the pan-European protections that exist in the European Union, where a key directive (95/46) covered data protection and privacy. A Regulation (2016/679) and a Directive (2016/680) have been issued in 2016; Regulation repeals the Directive 95/46 since May 28, 2018. Each EU member state was required to transpose the Directive into local legal requirements no later than May 6, 2018. A good summary of the current European Union Privacy Legislation can be found at the website of the European Commission and the website of the EU Data Protection Supervisor.

In October 1995, the European Commission proposed "Directive 95/46/EC on the protection of individuals with regard to the processing of personal data and on the free movement of such data." All member states in the European Union implemented local laws and regulations covering the contents of this directive. These laws and regulations vary from country to country, and some are stronger (more protective of privacy) than the EU regulation itself. It had an impact on drug safety, although less than originally feared.

Regulations and Directives cover all personal data, whether electronic or on paper, and are not limited to health information but broadly cover all other areas of personal data including racial or ethnic origin, political opinions, religious or philosophical beliefs, trade union membership, processing of genetic data, biometric data for the purpose of uniquely identifying a natural person, data concerning a natural person's sex life or sexual orientation, and so forth. The legislation refers to the "processing" of personal data. Processing refers to "any operation ... which is performed ... such as collection, recording, organization, storage, adaptation or alteration, retrieval, consultation, use, disclosure by transmission, dissemination ..."

As a general rule, processing of personal data is *a priori* prohibited in the EEA, except in the following circumstances:

- The person in question has given consent. The processing is necessary for the performance of a contract;
- The processing is necessary to meet a legal obligation;
- The processing is needed to protect the vital interests of the person in question;
- The processing is needed to carry out a task that is in the public interest or is done in exercise of official authority;

- The processing relates to personal data which are obviously made public by the data subject;
- Healthcare
  - "Processing is necessary for the purposes of preventive or occupational medicine, for the assessment of the working capacity of the employee, medical diagnosis, the provision of health or social care or treatment or the management of health or social care systems and services on the basis of Union or Member State law or pursuant to contract with a health professional (...);
  - Processing is necessary for reasons of public interest in the area of public health, such as protecting against serious cross-border threats to health or ensuring high standards of quality and safety of health care and of medicinal products or medical devices, on the basis of Union or Member State law which provides for suitable and specific measures to safeguard the rights and freedoms of the data subject, in particular professional secrecy".

Member States may maintain or introduce more specific provisions to adapt the application of the rules of this Regulation to ensure lawful and fair processing.

Personal data can only be processed for specified explicit and legitimate purposes and may not be processed further in a way incompatible with those purposes. The person (European Union citizen) in question has the right to be informed when his or her data are processed. The person has the right to see all the data processed about him or her as well as the right to changes and corrections to incorrect or incomplete data. The data must be accurate and relevant to the purpose they are collected for, should not contain more information than is necessary, and should not be kept longer than necessary. The person may object at any time to the processing of personal data for direct marketing.

A "right to erasure" (to be forgotten) and a "right to restriction of processing" have been introduced in the EU. This is rather controversial. Any EU citizen may therefore request to:

- Erase personal data when
  - No longer necessary;
  - Consent withdrawal;
  - Data unlawfully processed;
  - Data collected in relation to the offer of information society services;
- Restrict personal data processing when
  - Accuracy of the personal data is contested;
  - Processing is unlawful;
  - Personal data required by the data subject for the establishment, exercise or defence of legal claims;
  - Data subject has objected to processing.

A supervisory authority is to be nominated in each member state. They shall monitor and enforce the actual application of this regulation. All EU supervisory authorities shall cooperate with each other.

Data may not be transferred to a third country where there is an inadequate level of data protection (if personal data are transferred outside the EEA, special safeguards are foreseen to ensure that the protection travels with the data). The United States is not considered to have adequate levels of protection for European Union data. EUGDPR — Information Portal https://eugdpr.org/ "The EU General Data Protection Regulation (GDPR) is an important change that strengthens data privacy; enforcement began on 25 May 2018. Organisations that are not compliant could face heavy penalties, including monetary fines. Additional detailed information is available on the GDPR portal: https://eugdpr.org/."

Data Privacy in Clinical Trials and Product Development

Data privacy in clinical research as well as in the post approval stage of product development is a cumbersome task that involves and touches many aspects of a company's system. In clinical trials, documents such as the Informed Consent and Protocol should have language included that contains statements regarding the collection, handling, processing, reporting, and storing of protected health information such as personal data as well as biological samples. A quick search of local regulations (HHS.gov for the US for example) can provide you with examples, checklists and templates to consider when drafting the consent form and taking into consideration the language required regarding data privacy and protection. ICH E6 (make sure you are referencing the most current version and any addendum published) regarding Good GCP, includes a checklist for declaring what information will be collected, how it will be kept private, and details for how long it will be held. It is important that a company's DPO or Legal officer be a part of the review to ensure compliance with applicable privacy laws.

When it comes to a company's obligation to publish and provide data protection activities, one has to consider all of the inbound and outbound communication channels possible for the collection of sensitive personal and protected health and other information. Systems such as a company website that tracks personal data will most likely now have "Privacy Disclosures" with references to contact their corporate legal group with any further questions.

Other areas to consider where data can be obtained and stored which should have policies in place documenting protection measures include company phone lines, fax, email addresses, corporate databases such as the safety database or Medical Information Call Center (MICC), and online media sources such as product websites and social media pages.

A note on Record Retention:

Companies must implement procedures which document the use and retention of personal drives, network folders, and e-Mailboxes such that it is clear how the network is accessed, by who, and for how long data is retained. There are a variety of laws which required MAHs to retain relevant records pertaining to the development of a product and companies should disclose these obligations to the public as it pertains to the records and maintenance of their data. MAHs must retain PV data for at least 10 years after that product is no longer on the EU market unless stricter local requirements apply. For example, Finland requires that AEs gathered in Finland be kept for 50 years after the marketing authorization expires; this requirement applies to data gathered from Finland and from occurrences that took place in Finland. Different rules apply outside the EU; e.g., Health Canada requires keeping individual reports for 25 years from case creation.

■ Frequently Asked Question

Q: This is rather complex. How should companies handle this?

A: Clearly internal legal and regulatory expertise and communication must be in place to cover and protect data and patients in all jurisdictions involved. If the company cannot handle this internally, external assistance must be used. There is little tolerance, by both governments and individuals, for breaches in data privacy and protection. In addition, attention must be paid to external vendors (e.g., server parks, archiving companies) who also handle the data. Many companies have established a data protection office headed by a Chief Data Privacy Officer.

CHAPTER

36

Children, Elderly, and Other Special (Vulnerable) Groups

Similar to the testing of new drugs in pregnant women, the testing of drugs in special ("vulnerable") groups pose unique challenges. Special groups include children, neonates, and the elderly as well as other groups with specific disease states, genetic conditions, and, sometimes controversially, various ethnic, racial, or religious backgrounds. The question here is whether the presence of the "special" condition alters the effects of the drug and produces more or different adverse events (AEs). The benefit–risk balance of a product may be different in these different groups, particularly if cognitive challenges adversely impact the consent process.

■ The Theory

Children

Children are a special group because they are not simply "small adults" but rather are (depending on age and other factors) biologic beings, who absorb, distribute, metabolize, and excrete drugs differently from adults. This can change over time in an individual as organs mature.

Key documents on pediatric drug development have been developed by the International Council for Harmonization (ICH):

(a) The "E11 Guideline: Clinical Investigation of Medicinal Products in the Pediatric Population" (2000):
(b) The "Addendum to ICH E11: Clinical Investigation of Medicinal Products in the Pediatric Population E11(R1)" (2017) with an associated FDA guidance in 2018
(c) "Pediatric Extrapolation".

These three documents are available at www.ich.org. These guidelines note that understanding safety in the pediatric population presents special challenges because children differ from adults in having still-developing body systems. Additional considerations are described in the ICH guidelines.

Long term studies or surveillance data, either while patients are on chronic therapy or during the post-therapy period, may be needed to determine possible effects on skeletal, behavioral, cognitive, sexual, and immune maturation and development. Usually the pediatric (safety) database is limited at the time of approval. Some regulatory jurisdictions require pediatric studies (or at least a proposed pediatric development plan) prior to initial product approval. Exceptions to such requirements include studies of Alzheimer's Disease in children or other situations where it would be impossible to complete a scientifically valid study. Therefore, post-marketing surveillance is particularly important. In some cases, long-term follow-up studies may provide additional safety and/or efficacy information for subgroups within the pediatric population or additional information for the entire pediatric population.

The ICH guideline also addresses the definition of a "child", noting four possible categories (see Table 1). Also, according to the ICH E11(R1) guideline, the neonatal period for pre-term newborns is the day of birth through the expected date of delivery plus 27 days. However, there are several other schemes, as displayed in Table 1.

Note that for assessment of safety (or efficacy) in children, chronological age alone does not consider many other important aspects. Safety of a drug in the pediatric population may be dependent on physiological development, organ system maturity, and other factors. Stratification of children into age groups is somewhat arbitrary and, in some situations, may not have a scientific basis for understanding safety.

In the United States

In the United States, the FDA and professional societies have been encouraging pediatric pharmaceutical research by companies for many years, but these efforts generally met with little success because of the hesitancy to test new chemical entities in children and babies.

In December 1998, the FDA issued a final rule entitled "Regulations Requiring Manufacturers to Assess the Safety and Effectiveness of New Drugs and Biological Products in Pediatric Patients". This rule required that every new product contain a pediatric assessment or a deferral or waiver of this assessment. It also allowed the FDA to require pediatric studies and required a pediatric section in New Drug Application (NDA) periodic reports.

In September 1999, the FDA issued a Guidance for Industry entitled "Qualifying for Pediatric Exclusivity under Section 505A of the Food, Drug and Cosmetic Act". This guidance allowed the FDA to request, before approval of a drug, that pediatric clinical trials be done. As an industry incentive to do this, a 6-month additional period of "exclusivity" (patent protection) could be granted. This was followed up by additional FDA actions, including a draft guidance in 2000 on pediatric oncology studies, and other guidances on complying with this rule, including one in 2000 on complying with the Pediatric Rule (21CFR314.55(a) and 601.27(a)).

However, major changes occurred with the 2007 PDUFA/FDAAA legislation. Two sections of the FDA

Various Approaches to Classify "Children" by Chronological Age.

Age Group Category	ICH E11 (2000) and ICH E11(R1) (2017)	WHO (2007)	FDA (2014)	EMA (2014)
Term to Newborn/Neonate	0–27 days	0–28 days	Birth to 1 month	0–27 days
Infant/Toddler	28 days to 23 months	>28 days to 23 months	1 month to 2 years	1–23 months
Child	2–11 years	2–11 years	2–12 years	2–11 years
Adolescent	12 to 16–18 years (region dependent)	12 to 16–18 years (region dependent)	12–16 years	12–18 years

Amendments Act (entitled the Pediatric Research Equity Act (PREA) concern children as follows:

- Title IV reaffirmed FDA's authority to require a manufacturer to submit an NDA for a new chemical entity, indication, dosage form, dosing regimen, or route of administration to submit a pediatric assessment. Sponsors may be given waivers from this for appropriate reasons (e.g., no pediatric formulation, disease does not occur in children, etc.).
- Title V allows FDA to give an additional 6 months of marketing exclusivity to a manufacturer of a drug who submits data on pediatric use. These data do not need to result in an approval for safety or efficacy of the product in children, i.e., positive data are not required. An internal FDA review committee was established in 2007 and has been meeting frequently. The committee issues reviews, conducts assessments, and label changes; various studies have been requested. The Pediatric Advisory Committee has issued many product-specific safety reviews. Labeling changes for safety that relate to children are available at www.fda.gov.

  In May 2023, FDA issued two draft guidances for industry entitled, Pediatric Drug Development: Regulatory Considerations — Complying with PREA and Qualifying for Pediatric Exclusivity Under the BPCA and Pediatric Drug Development Under the Pediatric Research Equity Act and the Best Pharmaceuticals for Children Act: Scientific Considerations. Both guidances provide FDA's core thinking on recommendations to support the approval of drugs, biological products, and vaccines under the Pediatric Research Equity Act (PREA) and/or the Best Pharmaceuticals for Children Act (BPCA). The guidance documents revise and replace earlier guidance for industry How to Comply with the Pediatric Research Equity Act.

There has been much discussion and movement regarding pediatric safety and labeling. One major area of controversy revolved around the use of cough and cold products (usually over-the-counter, OTC) in children, especially young children. After much discussion, FDA and the manufacturers agreed on a labeling change, noting that the products should not be used in children younger than 4 years of age. New measuring devices and childproof packaging changes were also introduced.

Another area that has produced and continues to produce controversy is the use of psychiatric drugs in children. In particular, the FDA has issued an advisory about the use of selective serotonin reuptake inhibitors (SSRIs) and suicidality, notably about their use in children and adolescents. A similar advisory was issued by the European Medicines Agency (EMA).

In the European Union

Legislation, Regulation (EC) No. 1901/2006, covering children aged 0–17 years was passed in 2007.

The key elements of the legislation include as follows:

- Creation of a Pediatric Committee in the EMA;
- A requirement for pediatric data based on a Pediatric Investigation Plan (PIP) for new products and certain products already on the market and still under patent. If this is done:
  - An additional 6 months of patent protection may be granted for "regular" products and a 2-year extension for "orphan" products;
  - A new Marketing Authorization (called the pediatric use marketing authorization) may be granted, giving a 10-year period of market protection;
- Provision for a European database of pediatric clinical trials;
- Data from pediatric clinical trials must be submitted to the regulatory authorities;
- A European Pediatric Clinical Trials Network was set up along with new funding for studies with off-patent drugs;
- Use of an identifying symbol on the package of all products approved for children.

EMA also has issued additional guidance): "Guideline on good pharmacovigilance practices (GVP) Product- or Population-Specific Considerations IV: Paediatric population" (2018).

For further information, see the EMA website (www.ema.europa.eu) and the MHRA website. The latter site has extensive information on the history and status of pediatric drug issues as well as drug-specific assessment reports.

Bottom line: Despite aggressive initiatives in the US, the EU and elsewhere, the status, knowledge, and safety of drugs for use in children still remains unsatisfactory and largely unknown. The few studies on the subject show that more than 15 years after implementation of these regulations, the number of publications of pediatric studies remains much lower than the number of publications of studies conducted in adults; moreover, pediatric clinical trials are of lower methodological quality (design, number of included participants, choice of outcomes, etc.[1]). In practice, children are often treated as "small adults" because the initiatives still do not get around the fact that most companies, physicians, and parents are loath to perform clinical trials on children. On the other hand, is it ethical to skip studies in children if the product will be used in that population? Much of the safety data comes from post-marketing reports of AEs seen in children given drugs developed primarily for adults. It is not clear how this situation can be resolved. Similarly, the other key safety issues, such as drug–drug interactions, drug–food interactions, dietary and other safety matters are largely unknown in children, and most recommendations in these areas are based on extrapolations from adult data (much of which is also unsatisfactory). The spectrum of disease, drug use, and dietary variety are different in children of various maturities and, of course, differ from adults.

[1]Cho SM, Serghiou S, Ioannidis JP, Klassen TP, Contopoulos-Ioannidis DG. Large Pediatric Randomized Clinical Trials in ClinicalTrials.gov. Pediatrics. 2021 Sep;148(3):e2020049771. doi: 10.1542/peds.2020-049771

Zhong, Y., Zhang, X., Zhou, L. *et al.* Updated analysis of pediatric clinical studies registered in ClinicalTrials.gov, 2008–2019. BMC Pediatr 21, 212 (2021). https://doi.org/10.1186/s12887-021-02658-4

Groff ML, Offringa M, Emdin A, Mahood Q, Parkin PC, Cohen E. Publication Trends of Pediatric and Adult Randomized Controlled Trials in General Medical Journals, 2005–2018: A Citation Analysis. Children (Basel). 2020 Dec 15;7(12):293. doi: 10.3390/children7120293.

The Elderly

The elderly, like children, also represent a special group in pharmacovigilance for several reasons. For example, functional organ impairment is common, comorbidities are frequent, and there is often a "requirement" for concomitant drug therapy. In addition, life expectancy and quality of life are to be considered. This is a recipe for special challenges in pharmacovigilance.

But who is elderly? Miriam-Webster defines an elderly person as someone who is "rather old, *especially* being past middle age". An important document with a clearer definition is the 1993 ICH E7 guideline, "Studies in Support of Special Populations: Geriatrics" (see www.ich.org). The ICH E7 guideline defines the geriatric population as patients aged 65 years or older. As with children, however, there is a range of function that may impact the pharmacology of drug products without a clear relation to chronological age. Also, there are certain diseases that are seen only or primarily in the elderly (e.g., Alzheimer's Disease or osteoporosis).

The elderly tend to have more diseases than the young, especially those that are related to chronic conditions (hypertension, osteoarthritis, hyperlipidemia, diabetes, etc.) or habits (smoking, alcohol use, obesity). Depending on many factors, the elderly are often slower than young adults in recovering from acute disease. The result is often more drug exposure. As a consequence, the elderly consume more drugs and for longer durations. Hence, the risk of drug–drug interactions may increase, particularly if there is a decrease in renal or hepatic function. Finally, pharmacokinetics and pharmacodynamics may also be altered in the elderly, producing different effects from those that would occur in younger adult patients. Swallowing disorders and dysfunction are often worse in the elderly than in the young. A tablet or other oral preparation that is large, sticky (e.g., having a hydroxycellulose outer layer), or oddly shaped may be difficult to swallow and could even get stuck or cause obstruction in the pharynx or esophagus.

Drug–drug, drug–food, drug–alcohol, and drug–disease interactions also may be different in the elderly, but these areas are largely unexplored. For example, diets of the elderly who do not have teeth would logically be different from their toothed counterparts. What is the potential dietary impact on drug-food interactions? There are many other confounders, particularly in the post-marketing phase. What is the impact of pill splitting (of varying accuracy)? What does administration of a crushed tablet in applesauce or through a naso-gastric feeding tube affect?

The paucity of data here presents challenges for geriatricians in daily practice. FDA has recognized this and has a collaborative "Safe Use Initiative" to reduce preventable harm from medications using specific interventions. Tools include container design, container labeling, drug safety communications, and educational programs, etc.

As long ago as 1996, it was clearly noted that 21.3% of community-dwelling elderly patients in the US received at least 1 of 33 potentially inappropriate medications.[2] This led to the creation of a list of medications that should not be used in the elderly.[3] This is based on the so-called Beers criteria for medication use in the elderly as follows:

- always to be avoided;
- rarely appropriate; and
- sometimes indicated but often misused.

Of course, as new medicines and formulations enter the market, some may be inappropriate for use in the elderly, perhaps due to interactions with other medicines or dietary practices. The Institute for Safe Medication Practices is a good resource for easy-to-use lists of practical, evidence-based recommendations on reduction of medication errors in various situations.

[2] Zhan, Sangl, Bierman, Miller *et al.*, Potentially inappropriate medication use in the community-dwelling elderly. *JAMA* 2001; 286: 2823–2829. Renom-Guiteras A, Meyer G, Thürmann PA. The EU(7)-PIM list: A list of potentially inappropriate medications for older people consented by experts from seven European countries. European Journal of Clinical Pharmacology. 2015;71(7) doi: 10.1007/s00228-015-1860-9 Fick DM, Semla TP, Steinman M, *et al.* American Geriatrics Society 2019 Updated AGS Beers Criteria® for Potentially Inappropriate Medication Use in Older Adults. J Am Geriatr Soc. 2019;67(4) doi: 10.1111/jgs.15767.

[3] See Fick, Cooper, Wade, Waller, Maclean, Beers, Updating the Beers criteria for potentially inappropriate medication use in older adults. *Arch Intern Med* 2003; 163:2716–2724.

FDA and the ICH E7 Guideline

The 1993 ICH E7 guideline, "Studies in Support of Special Populations: Geriatrics" was published by the FDA in August 1994 as FDA guidance. It is directed primarily at drugs expected to have significant use in diseases of the elderly (e.g., Alzheimer's Disease) or at drugs that are used in large numbers by the elderly (e.g., antihypertensives). As noted above, the guideline takes an arbitrary definition of geriatric as 65 years or older but recommends seeking out patients 75 years and older for studies. In general, there should be no upper age limit. Nor should the elderly with concomitant diseases specifically be excluded, because these are frequently the patients that most need to be studied. An ICH Q&A document was created in 2010 to supplement the E7 guideline.

The guideline recommends that geriatric patients be included in phase III and, at the sponsor's option, phase II studies in "meaningful numbers". For diseases "not unique to but present in the elderly", a minimum of 100 patients studied is recommended. For studies of diseases of the elderly, it is obviously expected that most of the patients studied will be elderly.

Pharmacokinetic studies should be done to determine whether the drug is metabolically handled differently in the elderly compared with younger patients. Studies in patients with renal or hepatic insufficiency should be conducted, although often studies involving the young suffice, and separate studies in the elderly may not be needed. Pharmacodynamic dose-response studies usually do not have to be conducted except for sedative/hypnotic agents and other psychoactive drugs, or where phase II/III studies suggest age-associated issues. Drug–drug interaction studies should be done when appropriate and do not necessarily have to be limited to the elderly.

FDA Guidance and Geriatric Rule

In 1997, the FDA (62 FR 45313) established the "Geriatric Use" section in drug labeling, which was phased in over time. In October 2001, the FDA issued guidance on this rule (see www.fda.gov). It reviews the requirements for geriatric information in the various sections of approved labeling, such as "Indications and Usage" and "Clinical Pharmacology, Warnings, Precautions". Regarding safety specifically, the FDA states that the labeling should include the following: "A statement describing a specific hazard with use of the drug in the elderly that references appropriate sections (e.g., 'Contraindications, Warnings, Precautions') in the labeling for more detailed discussion."

The FDA also issued a document aimed at consumers entitled "Medicines and You: A Guide for Older Adults", which summarizes some of the issues in geriatric use of medications. There are several "Medicines and You" articles in this series.

Reporting requirements for AEs that occur in the elderly are the same as those for other age groups. Data on particular issues for a drug in the elderly should be included in the product labeling.

The elderly present a different picture from that seen with children. There are generally more data available about drugs in the elderly and about conditions more commonly seen in the elderly, such as renal or hepatic insufficiency, diabetes, and alcohol use. It is, in general, easier to study drugs in the elderly than in children, since with children there are often issues of informed consent. Informed consent issues may also be a concern in the elderly, who may have experienced a decline in mental acuity. Thus, if there are not actual data from studies in the elderly, there are often data on these conditions that allow the healthcare professional to alter doses, change duration of therapy, order special tests, and so on to suit the elderly patient in question with some degree of medical science and data behind the decision. Drug–drug interactions pose a particular risk in the elderly, and much has been written about this partial vacuum.[4]

The FDA developed a plan for drug evaluation in seniors starting as a workshop in 2021. A review of this workshop and several articles can be found at Roadmap to 2030 for Drug Evaluation in Older Adults. Clin Pharmacol Ther. 2022 Aug;112(2):210-223. doi: 10.1002/cpt.2452. Epub 2021 Nov 8. The goal is to have more seniors enrolled in clinical trials and develop better safety and efficacy data.

EMA

The EMA issued a special report on medicines in the elderly. The conclusions include recommendations to define elderly, frailty, and adequate age cutoff points for drugs, to continue adding a specific section on elderly in the Committee for Medicinal Products for Human Use (CHMP) guidelines and to update these where necessary, to emphasize in discussions with sponsors the need to recruit an adequate number of elderly subjects of various ages in the studies, and to systematically require the appraisal of elderly exposure for drug approval. See also the "Medicines for the Elderly" section at the EMA website (www.ema.europa.eu).[5]

In deliberating drug safety considerations for the elderly, the CHMP considers PRAC conclusions in the context of benefit. They must determine how to bring together available evidence, which is not necessarily constrained or limited to technical and regulatory requirements. Also, CHMP considers various stakeholders (e.g., drug developers in industry and academia; quality assessors in regulatory agencies; patients and patient representatives; other medicinal product experts in industry and regulatory agencies). In addition, use of the term "older patient/people/population" versus "the elderly" versus "the geriatric population" may provide confusingly categorized data.

There is also an EU Geriatric Expert Group (GEG), formed according to Doc. Ref. EMA/CHMP/137793/2011, that provides scientific advice on topics related to the elderly to the Committee for Medicinal Products for Human Use (CHMP) and the European Medicines Agency. The GEG considers topics such as the frailty of elderly (physical frailty, comorbidity status, and mental frailty) and also provides advice on:

- Geriatrics guidelines;
- Geriatric aspects regarding development, assessment and safety monitoring;
- Meetings to provide geriatrics expertise; and

[4] Bressler, Bahl, *Mayo Clin Proc*, 2003; 78: 1564–1577; see also the editorial and the multiple references in the *Archives of Internal Medicine*. Polypharmacy: a new paradigm for quality drug therapy in the elderly? *Arch Intern Med*, 2004; 164: 1957–1959.

[5] EMA/CHMP/137793/2011, EMA geriatric medicines strategy.

- Providing advice on the geriatric implementation plan (GIP).

Despite these efforts, the number of clinical trials specifically dedicated to the elderly remains limited, and the elderly included are often not representative of the population of the same age in terms of co-morbidity and co-prescriptions, which limits the external validity of the obtained results. Furthermore, the chosen outcomes in these trials are sometimes less appropriate for this population, in which it is preferable to assess functional outcomes (feelings of autonomy, levels of psychological, social, and physical functioning) rather than more conventionally assessed outcomes such as overall survival.[6]

Other Special Groups

It is now generally recognized that there is significant biodiversity among humans. There are probably many reasons for this. One major cause relates to drug metabolism pathways. The cytochrome P450 system, which plays a major role in drug metabolism, is well known to exhibit enormous diversity (genetic polymorphism), producing major differences in metabolism of drugs from individual to individual.[7]

Because of the differences in how drugs are absorbed, metabolized, distributed, and excreted by groups and by individuals, a more rational and tailored use of drugs will allow the maximization of effectiveness and the minimization of AEs. For more product-specific details on the role of cytochromes in drug metabolism and interactions, see the extensive series of reference tables curated and hosted by the Department of Medicine at Indiana University (search for "Flockhart drug interaction tables.")

Two further examples of special groups (women and African Americans) follow. If pharmacogenetics fulfills its potential and allows subgroups (and perhaps even individuals) to be identified in terms of who will be at risk for or safe from particular ADRs. The availability and growing popularity of consumer DNA databases may provide future tools for tailoring safer therapeutic regimens. How pharmacology and medicine will evolve and characterize these differences in the upcoming years is a fascinating and unanswered question.

Women

Women have, in general, a smaller proportion of body water and a greater proportion of body fat than men. Men and women may metabolize drugs differently. For example, men have more alcohol dehydrogenase than women and thus metabolize the same amount of alcohol more rapidly.[8] Women also handle cardiac drugs differently from men in many instances.[9] As might be anticipated, pregnant or lactating women also handle drugs differently.

African Americans

It is well known that different groups in the US have significant differences in their general health. For example, a review by the Centers for Disease Control and Prevention[10] noted that "for many health conditions, non-Hispanic blacks bear a disproportionate burden of disease, injury, death, and disability".

Similarly, African Americans may respond less well to certain drugs, such as anti-hypertensives[11] or may have more AEs, such as angioedema associated with

[6] Ruiter R, Burggraaf J, Rissmann R. Under-representation of elderly in clinical trials: An analysis of the initial approval documents in the Food and Drug Administration database. Br J Clin Pharmacol. 2019 Apr;85(4):838–844. doi: 10.1111/bcp.13876.

Working Group on Functional Outcome Measures for Clinical Trials. Functional outcomes for clinical trials in frail older persons: time to be moving. J Gerontol A Biol Sci Med Sci. 2008 Feb;63(2):160-4. doi: 10.1093/gerona/63.2.160. PMID: 18314451; PMCID: PMC2645663.

[7] See Evans, Relling, Pharmacogenomics: translating functional genomics into rational therapeutics. *Science* 1999; 286: 487–491; Court, A pharmacogenomics primer. *J Clin Pharmacol* 2007; 47: 1087–1103; and Nakamura, Pharmacogenomics and drug toxicity [editorial]. *N Engl J Med* 2008; 359: 856–858.

[8] Frezza, di Padova, Pozzato, *et al.*, *N Engl J Med* 1990; 322: 95–99.

[9] Jochmann, Stangl, Garbe, *et al.*, *Eur Heart J* 2005; 26: 1585–1595.

[10] *MMWR* 2005; 54(01): 1–3.

[11] Levy, ed., *Ethnic and Racial Differences in Response to Medicines: Preserving Individualized Therapy in Managed Pharmaceutical Programs*, National Pharmaceutical Council, Reston, VA, 1993.

angiotensin-converting enzyme inhibitors.[12] From these and other data, additional studies of the effects of drugs in various ethnic or racial groups are desirable. See an excellent commentary on the need for greater diversity in clinical trials by Professor Kenneth Davis of the University of Cincinnati in "African American Health. Clinical Trial Diversity: The Need and the Challenge".

Another example occurs when African Americans have more adverse events during treatment producing poorer outcomes. See Reactions to drugs results in poorer outcomes for African American breast cancer patients, Indiana University genetics research revealed outcome differences http://news.medicine.iu.edu/releases/2017/10/breast-cancer-drug-outcomes.shtml.

There are many refereed references on ethnicity and differences in drug metabolism.[13]

The collection and analysis of data based on ethnicity is quite tricky, however. The FDA issued a guidance on the collection of ethnicity data in clinical trials in 2005. The guidance offers practical guidelines on how to collect race and ethnicity data in clinical trials and how to present the data in INDs, NDAs, and BLAs.

However, there is limited guidance on whether an investigator (or in many cases, a prescriber of a marketed drug) should make his or her assignment or whether this should be self-designation by a study subject. Should the investigator ask? Further, the categories are based on antiquated US census designations that are not globally applicable. When the topic of race/ethnicity was discussed at ICH in relation to safety reporting, it was decided by consensus, that no clear definitions could be applied. But how ethnicity and the data are to be interpreted in people or groups with mixed ethnic backgrounds is unknown. We await pharmacogenomics. Over time, it would be expected to encounter less genetic diversity on a global basis. So, we await future developments that may impact patient safety.

In 2022 the FDA initiated a project to increase diversity in clinical trials. This was summarized in a press release entitled: "FDA Takes Important Steps to Increase Racial and Ethnic Diversity in Clinical Trials". Although aimed primarily at increasing diversity in clinical trials, safety is not specifically addressed, it is likely that additional safety (and efficacy) data will be collected, however imprecise. A search within the FDA on Clinical Trial Diversity will lead you to the agencies current thinking and recommendations on this topic.

[12] Kalow, *Trends Pharmacol Sci* 1991; 12(3): 102–107.

[13] For example, see Phan, Moore, McLachlan, *et al.*, Ethnic differences in drug metabolism and toxicity from chemotherapy. *Expert Opin Drug Metab Toxicol* 2009; 5(3): 243–257.

CHAPTER

37

Acute and Chronic (Late Occurring) Adverse Events, Adverse Events That Disappear

Introduction

Adverse events (AEs) seen shortly after starting or stopping drugs are common and relatively easy to recognize (though if it were that easy, there would be little need for this book). There is usually a high index of suspicion, a close temporal relationship, and often biologic and pharmacologic plausibility.

This is not the case for adverse events (AEs) that occur weeks, months, or even years after stopping the drug ("long-latency period"). There may be no medical record available, the patient's memory of using the product may be hazy, the index of suspicion is low or non-existent, and there may be no logical, biologic, or pharmacologic reason for this AE to be associated with the liver, brain, or other target organ(s).

It is now increasingly recognized that drug therapy, particularly advanced therapeutic products (e.g., immunomodulators) as well as other therapies (radiation therapy, neutraceuticals, OTCs, etc.) can produce late-emerging AEs. Usually, it takes an insightful clinician or a good epidemiologic study to show that a particular drug caused (or is associated with) a particular AE years later. Such a finding is often first met with disbelief and even ridicule. However, public health and good science demand that all contingencies be kept in mind and examined when appropriate. A high index of suspicion is key. Perhaps the most difficult situation occurs with a cancer that develops years after drug exposure. Other areas with possible late appearing adverse events are seen in dermatology though the same issues of determining clear causality remain.

From empirical observations, the latency period from starting or stopping of a drug to the onset of the AE is variable. AEs can be seen immediately after starting a drug, shortly thereafter, or even after weeks or months of taking the drug with no other obvious problems. AEs can also be seen long after stopping the drug. Examples that follow are of AEs seen long after starting or stopping a drug.

Bendectin®: A False Alert

Market Removal

Bendectin® was a fixed combination of three active ingredients used for treating nausea and vomiting during pregnancy:

1. Doxylamine, an H1 anti-histamine that acts as an anti-nausea and anti-vomiting agent;
2. Pyridoxine, vitamin B6;
3. Dicycloverine, removed from the product shortly before market withdrawal of Bendectin.

This product was incorrectly suspected of causing congenital abnormalities. In 1977 a lawsuit was filed that claimed that Bendectin® resulted in a birth defect called Poland syndrome (a deficit in the pectoralis muscle). Then, in 1979 an article appeared in the National Enquirer that linked Bendectin® to birth defects and this triggered great public concern. The FDA issued a statement for prescribers and patients that stated, "... the current physicians labelling for the drug reflects the FDA's evaluation that there is no adequate evidence linking Bendectin with an increased risk of birth defects."

Several case-control studies were performed, and their results confirmed that there was no measurable teratogenic effect. These data formed the basis for the exoneration of this product. It had been on the market for about 27 years and was taken by some 33 million pregnant women in the US, representing 20–40% of all pregnant women. It was voluntarily withdrawn from the US market and never returned even after its exoneration. The product remains available in other countries under various names (see below).[1]

Return to the Market in Canada and Europe

A laboratory was authorized to sell a product containing doxylamine and pyridoxine under the name of Diclectin®. To reduce the remaining suspicions held by obstetricians, it was specified in the product labeling that the therapeutic category for which this combination was approved was "anti-nausea agent for the nausea and vomiting of pregnancy". A group of Canadian experts published a statement on August 11, 1989, affirming that this fixed association was safe. The British authorities had also expressed the same opinion. The Canadian government had, thus, maintained a marketing authorization for this product for a Canadian manufacturer.[2] An epidemiologic study in 2003 compared the rate of birth defects in the United States in the years 1970 to 1992 and found no change in the rate of birth defects after the cessation of Bendectin® in the 1980–1984 period.[3]

There is an enormous literature on Bendectin, and it is maintained by some workers that this is the most studied drug in pregnancy ever. There are several books and hundreds of references available.

Various organizations of physicians, governments and academia have considered Bendectin® and Diclegis® to be first line treatment for morning sickness though an unpublished study has suggested that the efficacy may be less clear. See "medicine and pregnancy" on FDA WebSite or Guidelines on the exposure to medicinal products during pregnancy on the EMA WebSite.

Adriamycin®

Examples of drugs producing late AEs include Adriamycin (doxorubicin HCl), which may produce cardiac problems years after therapy has ended.

Myocardial toxicity manifested in its most severe form by potentially fatal congestive heart failure may occur either during therapy or months to years after termination of therapy. The probability of developing impaired myocardial function, based on a combined index of signs, symptoms, and decline in left

[1] Fleming, *BMJ* 1981; 283: 99; CSM/MCA, *Curr Problems Pharmacovigilance* 1981; 6; *Lancet* 1984; 2: 205; *BMJ* 1985; 271: 918.

[2] CSM/MCA, *Curr Problems Pharmacovigilance* 1981; 6; *Lancet* 1984; 2: 205; Medico-Legal Committee Opinion, *J Soc Obstet Gynaecol Can* 1995;17: 162; Koren, *Can J Clin Pharmacol* 1995; 2: 38.

[3] Kutcher JS, Engle A, Firth J, Lamm SH, Bendectin and birth defects II: Ecological analyses, *Birth Defects Res A: Clin Mol Teratol* 67(2): 88–97.

ventricular ejection fraction (LVEF) is estimated to be 1–2% at a total cumulative dose of 300 mg/m^2 of doxorubicin, 3–5% at a dose of 400 mg/m^2, 5–8% at a dose of 450 mg/m^2, and 6–20% at a dose of 500 mg/m^2, given in a schedule of a bolus injection once every 3 weeks. In a retrospective review, the probability of developing congestive heart failure was reported to be 5/168 (3%) at a cumulative dose of 430 mg/m^2 of doxorubicin, 8/110 (7%) at 575 mg/m^2, and 3/14 (21%) at 728 mg/m^2.

This toxicity may occur at lower cumulative doses in patients with prior mediastinal irradiation or on concurrent cyclophosphamide therapy or with pre-existing heart disease (Package Insert for Adriamycin, Pharmacia/Pfizer, 2010).

■ Gene Therapy

The FDA issued a Guidance for Industry entitled: *Gene Therapy Clinical Trials—Observing Subjects for Delayed Adverse Events* in November 2006 and updated in 2017. They state:

> "Study subjects exposed to gene transfer technology may be at risk of delayed adverse events as a consequence of persistent biological activity of the genetic material or other components of the products used to carry the genetic material."

■ Anti-retroviral Drugs

It is now well recognized that many human immunodeficiency virus drugs can produce late toxicity. The FDA has issued guidance noting that long-term follow-up should be done in clinical trials:

> "Because multiple adverse events have been observed with chronic administration of anti-retroviral therapy, mechanisms should be used for systematically evaluating adverse events over prolonged periods following traditional approval. Controlled comparisons and prospectively evaluated cohorts may be helpful in characterizing and defining drug associations for late-occurring adverse events. Therefore, after traditional approval, the Division strongly encourages sponsors to continue to collect safety data in key randomized studies or other treatment cohorts for prolonged periods (3–5 years)." (*Guidance for Industry, Antiretroviral Drugs Using Plasma HIV RNA Measurements — Clinical Considerations for Accelerated and Traditional Approval,* Center for Drug Evaluation and Research, October 2002).

See also The National Center for Biological Information (NCBI) Anti-retroviral Therapy (ART) for HIV Infection in Infants and Children: Towards Universal Access: Recommendations for a Public Health Approach: 2010 Revision.

Drug-related adverse reactions while on ART can occur immediately (soon after a drug has been administered), early (within the first days or weeks of treatment) or late (after months or more of treatment). See https://www.ncbi.nlm.nih.gov/books/NBK138571/.

■ Diethylstilbestrol (DES)

Perhaps the most interesting and striking example of delayed-onset AEs is that of vaginal cancer in the offspring of women who took DES. This has been examined in detail.

DES is an estrogen first synthesized in 1938. In 1941, DES was approved by the FDA for human use. In 1947, the agency approved the use during pregnancy for the treatment or prevention of spontaneous abortion (miscarriage) based largely on the work of Harvard researchers George and Olive Smith, work that eventually proved to be wrong; the drug did not prevent miscarriages.

The suspicion of a problem arose in 1970, when clinicians observed a rare vaginal cancer occurring in women aged 14–22 years. This cancer, clear cell adenocarcinoma (CCA), was classically seen only in women in their seventies. No explanation seemed apparent until the mother of one of the young cancer patients mentioned that she had taken DES to prevent a miscarriage. Questioning of the other mothers revealed that they too had taken DES, and Arthur Herbst and collaborators confirmed the association between DES and CCA in a case-control study in 1971.

Delayed Onset of Malignancy (Long Latency)

The delay in the appearance of the adverse drug reaction after the last dose (the latency period) of DES is among the longest ever seen. The delay in detection has several logical explanations:

- The AE did not occur in the women who took DES but in their female offspring exposed during the critical window of vaginogenesis.
- The AE was not visible in the female offspring at birth.
- The AE was not evident until after puberty during a gynecologic examination.
- Obstetric problems appeared only when a pregnancy occurred.

The spontaneous reporting consisted of a publication of the first series of cases and a case-control study. The reported risk of developing CCA in DES-exposed women is approximately 1 in 1,000 from birth to 34 years of age. The risk increases rapidly from the onset of puberty until the late teens and early twenties. Subsequently, the risk drops dramatically, although a few cases have been reported in women in their forties. Other less serious but more frequent obstetric and gynecologic problems in the DES-exposed progeny have also been commented on in the medical literature:

- Vaginal adenosis, cervical ectropion (normal, albeit misplaced, columnar epithelium);
- Structural anomalies, such as cervical hoods, hypoplastic, and T-shaped uterus;
- Functional problems, such as decreased fertility, ectopic pregnancy, spontaneous abortions (relative risk, 92:1), and pre-term births (relative risk, 5:1);
- Possible abnormalities in children of daughters whose mothers received DES (i.e., third generation);
- Benign malformations, such as small testicles and epididymal cysts in males exposed in utero.

Actions Taken

In 1971, the FDA banned the use of DES in pregnant women (FDA Drug Bulletin 1971). In the same year, a registry was established at the University of Chicago with Arthur Herbst as the chairperson. In 1978, the national cooperative Diethylstilbestrol-Adenosis (DESAD) Project was developed to identify and study DES-exposed women with adenosis. In 1973, the US National Institutes of Health notified medical schools and gynecologic oncologists about increased cancer risk. In 1977, France withdrew the obstetric indication. A movement known as DES Action was created in the United States, Canada, France, the United Kingdom, and elsewhere. See its website.

In 1999, the US Congress directed the National Cancer Institute to fund a 3-year DES National Educational Campaign housed at the Centers for Disease Control and Prevention (CDC).[4] The third generation (offspring of DES sons and daughters) are now being followed for possible health issues related to DES use by grandmothers. CDC maintains a complete website with multiple links https://www.cdc.gov/des/index.html.

There are other examples of long-latency AEs, though rarely as long or as dramatic as DES. Using the Yellow Card system in the UK, it was reported that practolol, a beta-blocker withdrawn from the UK market in 1975, was associated with sclerosing peritonitis, which did not appear until an average of 201 weeks after the drug start date (range 0.5–11.5 years).[5]

■ Future for Long-Latency AEs

The US Institute of Medicine addressed long-latency AEs seen after vaccinations in "Research Strategies for Assessing Adverse Events Associated with Vaccines: A Workshop Summary" (1994); however, no particular new strategy was identified to better find such AEs.

---

[4] Herbst, *N Engl J Med* 1971; 284; 878–881; Wilcox, *N Engl J Med* 1995; 332: 1411; Giusti, *Ann Intern Med* 1995; 122: 778; DES Action VOICE, Summer 2000 (section adapted from Cobert and Biron, *Pharmacovigilance from A to Z*).

[5] See Mann RD, Sclerosing peritonitis due to practolol, *Pharmacoepidemiol Drug Safety* 2007; 16(11): 1211–1216.

The best and only real strategy as of now is to do long-term follow-up of patients at risk for long-latency AEs using pharmacoepidemiologic techniques.

■ Frequently Asked Question

Q: This seems to put the practitioner in an impossible position. How can one even begin to make a rational attempt to determine whether a particular sign, symptom, or AE is due to a drug (or drugs) taken weeks, months, or even years ago? The patient may not even remember or know precisely what he or she was taking. And how can we even approach AEs due to the drugs a parent took a generation ago?

A: A valid point. The practitioner really can't make such a determination. The finding of very long-term or skipped-generation AEs remains primarily in the domain of epidemiology and observational studies. There is a tendency to run the safety arm of clinical trials for longer periods of time after the acute study is over. However, even that will not pick up the rare AE due to the small number of patients involved and the difficulties of long-term observational studies of safety. If subjects are followed long enough, all will have AEs (and will eventually die). That is, there are confounding and coincidental events that make interpretation of the long-term results very difficult. It may well be that when large populations have electronic health records, a more formal health authority-driven-review of large databases in an ongoing manner will have more sensitivity in discovering long latency, low frequency AEs.

Spontaneous reporting by astute clinicians remains the best current approach based on the examples seen to date. Perhaps pharmacoepidemiology and genomics will provide more answers. From the practitioner's point of view, a high level of suspicion must be maintained. The patient should be quizzed on both recent and remote drug history, including over-the-counter medications. Beyond that, we must await better techniques and methodology for tracking drugs taken and resulting AEs.

It is possible that new techniques coming from AI will aid in diagnosis of late occurring AEs. But as of now this is only a hypothesis.

CHAPTER

38

Pregnancy and Lactation

Testing pregnant animals is done as part of the usual preclinical development of new drugs, but a drug that is not teratogenic (leading to congenital malformations) in some or all animal species tested may sometimes, unfortunately, still be noxious in pregnant women. For increasingly controversial[1] ethical reasons, clinical testing is almost never done in pregnant women during the development of new drugs unless the drug is developed expressly for use in pregnancy. Thus, the safety and efficacy of drugs in pregnant women are largely unknown at the time of marketing, and only a little additional information is gained from spontaneous reporting of adverse events (AEs).

■ Introduction

Two tragic stories highlight the risk for the baby when the mother takes a drug during pregnancy:

- **Thalidomide:** In the early 1960s, thalidomide was used as an antiemetic to treat morning sickness in pregnant women. It was found to damage the development of unborn babies, when taken during the first weeks of pregnancy. The drug mainly led to phocomelia (atrophy of the limbs, with the feet

[1] Payne P. Including Pregnant Women in Clinical Research: Practical Guidance for Institutional Review Boards. Ethics Hum Res. 2019 Nov;41(6):35–40. doi:10.1002/eahr.500036.

Check on the EMA WebSite : "Benefit-risk of medicines used during pregnancy and breastfeeding"

and hands implanted directly on the trunk). More than 10,000 babies were affected around the world, particularly in Europe.

- **Diethylstilbestrol (DES):** From the 1940s to the early 1970s, DES was given to pregnant women because it was thought it would prevent miscarriages. In 1971, DES was shown to cause clear cell carcinoma, a rare vaginal tumor, in girls and women when they reach puberty who had been exposed to this drug in utero; recent studies have demonstrated deleterious effects on granddaughters and grandsons as well.

These two stories justified the implementation of more non-clinical testing before marketing and robust PV systems to warn patients about risks during pregnancy. In addition, these new systems were intended to ensure a rapid and accurate safety signal detection; they are the cornerstone of the current regulations.

Some drugs are used and, to some degree, tested in pregnancy, usually in situations in which treatment is obligatory for either the mother or unborn child (e.g., hypertension, asthma, rheumatoid arthritis, epilepsy). These studies are usually not blinded and are prospective or retrospective observational or surveillance studies.

Pregnancy registries are now required for manufacturers and Marketing Authorization/New Drug Application holders for most marketed drugs. That is, every use of the drug that the company becomes aware of in a pregnant woman or by a pregnant woman's partner is recorded and, with consent, is followed to outcome (birth, miscarriage, etc.)

Situation in the United States

According to one report,[2] there are more than six million pregnancies in the US each year and 50% of pregnant women in the US take at least one prescription medicine during pregnancy. Further, use of four or more medications in the first trimester has tripled (9.9–27.6%) from 1976 to 2008. Healthcare practitioners and patients need information on medicines that is relevant for decision-making during pregnancy (and lactation).

One approach adopted by the US FDA in 1979 was letter categories to "differentiate" products with data available regarding product use in pregnancy (see 21CFR201; 44FR37434, June 26, 1979, and subsequent updates). However, these letter categories were not considered adequate to provide prescribers with enough relevant information for critical decision-making when treating pregnant or lactating women.

Thus, a December 2014 final rule (79 Fed Reg 72064; December 4, 2014) required removal of the letter categories from labeling in favor of more complete statements of known risks, based on the available data and medical/disease factors, as well as non-clinical data placed in the context of human data. The final rule provides an enhanced framework for communicating information on benefits and risks of using a drug during pregnancy and lactation to help with prescribing decisions. The final rule also includes a subsection on females and males of reproductive potential after or during attempts at pregnancy.

Before discussing the 2014 final rule, it is of interest to review the five former letter categories:

- **Category A:** Adequate and well-controlled studies have failed to demonstrate a risk to the fetus in the first trimester of pregnancy (and there is no evidence of risk in later trimesters) (see § 201.57(k)(6){i}).
- **Category B:** Animal reproduction studies have failed to demonstrate a risk to the fetus and there are no adequate and well-controlled studies in pregnant women (see § 201.57(f)()(ii)).
- **Category C:** Animal reproduction studies have shown an adverse effect on the fetus and there are no adequate and well-controlled studies in humans, but potential benefits may warrant use of the drug in pregnant women despite potential risks (see § 201.57({)(6)(iii)).
- **Category D:** There is positive evidence of human fetal risk based on adverse reaction data from

[2] Mitchell AA, Gilboa SM, Werler MM, *et al.*, Medication use during pregnancy, with particular focus on prescription drugs: 1976–2008. *Am J Obstet Gynecol.* 2011; 205(1): 51.e1–8.

investigational or marketing experience or studies in humans, but potential benefits may warrant use of the drug in pregnant women despite potential risks (see § 201.57{](6)(iv)).

- **Category X:** Studies in animals or humans have demonstrated fetal abnormalities and/or there is positive evidence of human fetal risk based on adverse reaction data from investigational or marketing experience, and the risks involved in use of the drug in pregnant women clearly outweigh potential benefits (see § 201.57(fl(63(v)).

The letter categories were considered too simplistic and were sometimes misinterpreted as a grading system. And they did not adequately communicate risk information for clinical decision-making. Thus, FDA changed the labeling rules for pregnancy and lactation and all letter categories were removed by June 29, 2018. The final rule replaces the letter categories with three new narrative sections, illustrated in Figure 1. Note that the affected products have had the letter categories removed, but elimination of the standard statements that previously followed the letters was not required.

The A, B, C, D and X risk categories, in use since 1979, are now replaced with narrative sections and subsections to include:

1. Pregnancy (includes Labor and Delivery):
   a. Pregnancy Exposure Registry
   b. Risk Summary
   c. Clinical Considerations
   d. Data
2. Lactation (includes Nursing Mothers)
   a. Risk Summary
   b. Clinical Considerations
   c. Data
3. Females and Males of Reproductive Potential
   a. Pregnancy Testing
   b. Contraception
   c. Infertility

Pregnancy

There is now a single subsection (8.1) for "Pregnancy", including labor and delivery. If there is a scientifically acceptable pregnancy exposure registry for the drug, the "Pregnancy" subsection must contain a specified statement about the existence of the registry, followed by contact information needed to enroll or to obtain information about the registry.

Next is a summary of the risks of using a drug during pregnancy. If data demonstrate that a drug is not absorbed systemically, this must be stated. If the drug is absorbed, risk statements must be included that are based on data from all relevant sources (whether human or non-clinical), that describe, for the drug, the risk of adverse developmental outcomes.

The labeling must also contain relevant information, if it is available, to help health care providers make prescribing decisions and counsel women about the use of the drug during pregnancy; this could include information on disease-associated maternal and/or embryo/fetal risk, dose adjustments during pregnancy and the postpartum period, maternal adverse reactions, fetal/neonatal adverse reactions, and/or the effect of the drug on labor or delivery.

A good source for further information can be found at the FDA Office of Women's Health website.

Also of note is that The FDA and the Substance Abuse and Mental Health Administration of the US government strongly advise against the use of cannabidiol (CBD), tetrahydrocannabinol (THC), and marijuana in any form during pregnancy or while breastfeeding.

Lactation

This subsection (8.2) must contain a summary of the risks of using a drug during lactation. If data demonstrate that the drug is not absorbed systemically, there must be a statement to this effect. If data demonstrate that the drug is absorbed systemically by the mother, this summary must include, to the extent it is available, relevant information on the presence of the drug in human milk, effects of the drug on a child fed breast milk, and effects of the drug on milk production. For drugs absorbed systemically, a risk and benefit statement must appear at the end of the summary of risks, unless breastfeeding is contraindicated during drug therapy.

The "Lactation" subsection must also include, to the extent information is available, relevant information concerning ways to minimize drug exposure in the breast-fed child in certain situations, e.g., timing of dosing relative to feeding. If available, information that describes available interventions for monitoring or mitigating the adverse reactions presented elsewhere in the labeling.

Females and Males of Reproductive Potential

The "Females and Males of Reproductive Potential" subsection (8.3) includes relevant information when pregnancy testing or contraception is required or recommended before, during, or after drug therapy or when there are human or non-clinical data that suggest the possibility of drug-associated effects on fertility.

The final rule ("Content and Format of Labeling for Human Prescription Drug and Biological Products; Requirements for Pregnancy and Lactation Labeling" is available at https://federalregister.gov/a/2014-28241.

FDA also issued draft guidance to assist manufacturers in preparing this section of the labeling ("Pregnancy, Lactation, and Reproductive Potential: Labeling for Human Prescription Drug and Biological Products — Content and Format Guidance for Industry", December 2014).

In July 2020 a draft guidance entitled: "Pregnancy, Lactation, and Reproductive Potential: Labeling for Human Prescription Drug and Biological Products-Content and Format" was issued by FDA and should be reviewed as it is gives detailed information on how the labeling should be prepared. Although not finalized as of early 2024, it is, in general, a good idea to follow FDA draft guidances where this is feasible.

The FDA has also required pregnancy registries to be maintained by the industry. That is, whenever the sponsor is aware of a pregnancy it must be recorded and, with consent, the pregnancy should be followed to term. These cases are reported in PADERs and/or PSURs/PBRERs.

■ FDA Guidance on Pregnancy Registries — 2002

In August 2002, the FDA issued guidance for industry on Establishing Pregnancy Exposure Registries. The 2020 draft guidance noted in the previous section should also be reviewed as it covers pregnancy registries also.

In this guidance, the FDA gives a specific definition of a birth registry to differentiate it from a teratology registry:

> "A pregnancy exposure registry is a prospective observational study that actively collects information on medical product exposure during pregnancy and associated pregnancy outcomes."

This type of registry is not a pregnancy prevention program.

Note: The FDA did not recommend a registry for all drugs in this document though now it is expected that all pregnancies seen during marketing will be followed to outcome and reported in the periodic reports. These may not be formal registries as defined in this document but the data must be tracked and kept:

- "We recommend that a pregnancy exposure registry be seriously considered when it is likely that the medical product will be used during pregnancy as therapy for a new or chronic condition."
- "A medical product may also be a good candidate for a pregnancy exposure registry when one of the following conditions exists:
  - Inadvertent exposures to the medical product in pregnancy are or are expected to be common such as when products have a high likelihood of use by women of childbearing age.
  - The medical product presents special circumstances, such as the potential for infection of mother and fetus by administration of live, attenuated vaccines."
- "Pregnancy exposure registries are unlikely to be warranted in the following situations: (1) there is

no systemic exposure to the medical product, or (2) the product is not, or rarely, used by women of childbearing age."

A registry can be established at any time during the life of a drug. The applicant or the FDA may initiate the request. The design of the registry is a function of the objective. The design may range from an open-ended surveillance tool to testing of a specific hypothesis.

As of 2023, there were 171 pregnancy registries being followed by FDA.

Good Epidemiologic Practices

The guidance then details critical elements of a registry, including objectives, exposure, sample size, eligibility requirements, data source and content, fetal anomalies sought, use of an independent data monitoring committee, an investigational review board, and informed consent. The reader is referred to the guidance for these epidemiologic details.

A few points of note from the guidance:

> "When estimating the number of exposed pregnancies to be enrolled prospectively, it is important to be aware that approximately 62 percent of clinically recognized pregnancies will result in a live birth, 22 percent will end in elective termination, and 16 percent will result in fetal loss (i.e., spontaneous abortions and fetal death/stillbirth)."[3]

Birth defects occur "spontaneously" in a high number of women. The March of Dimes Birth Defect Foundation, Fact Sheet 2001, reported the following rates for various pregnancy outcomes and fetal abnormalities:

- Spontaneous abortions/miscarriage (loss before 20 weeks): 1 in 7 known pregnancies;
- Low birth weight (<2,500 g): 1 in 12 live births;
- Fetal death/stillbirth (loss after 20 weeks): 1 in 200 known pregnancies;
- Any major birth defect: 1 in 25 live births;
- Heart and circulation defects: 1 in 115 live births;
- Genital and urinary tract defects: 1 in 135 live births;
- Nervous system and eye defects: 1 in 235 live births;
- Club foot: 1 in 735 live births; and
- Cleft lip with or without cleft palate: 1 in 930 live births.

The guidance also notes that other types of studies, such as case-control studies, may be useful to evaluate rare adverse birth outcomes and to identify whether the drug in question is an associated risk factor. They are useful when long-term follow-up is needed. They can be nested within other existing pregnancy registries.

Automated database studies (e.g., health maintenance organizations, Medicaid) may be useful also.

Regulatory Reporting Requirements

Registries are considered solicited information and, thus, must be evaluated and reported as if they were clinical trial AEs: the cases must be serious, unexpected, and have a reasonable possibility that the product caused the AE. See 21CFR310.305(c)(1), 314.80(c)(2)(iii) and (e), and 600.80(c) (1), (c)(2)(iii) and (e)). Congenital anomalies are considered serious AEs (21CFR314.80(a) and 600.80(a)). Registries that are run independently of applicants holding New Drug Applications are not subject to post-marketing reporting requirements. However, such registries frequently supply annual reports to applicants and, once aware, the NDA holder is subject to regulatory reporting.

The applicant must also submit an annual status report to the FDA on any registry being run. A registry may be discontinued if:

- It has accumulated sufficient data to meet the registry objectives;
  - The feasibility of collecting sufficient information diminishes to unacceptable levels due to

[3] Ventura, Mosher, Curtin, *et al.*, *Vital Health Stat* 2000; 21: 56.

low exposure, poor enrollment, or unacceptable loss to follow-up;
- Better methods are developed to address the objectives of the registry;
- Termination criteria should be listed in the original protocol.

In conclusion, sponsors or applicants who are studying or marketing drugs that may pose a pregnancy/teratology threat must give careful and early consideration to adequate data gathering to determine whether a safety problem exists. If it is already known to exist, a registry might be established to quantify and track safety problems. The obvious aim is risk minimization using the various means available.

See also FDA's web page on Women's Health and pregnancy registries

https://www.fda.gov/ScienceResearch/SpecialTopics/WomensHealthResearch/ucm251314.htm.

Situation in the European Union

Good Vigilance Practice Module VI addresses pregnancy and lactation (GVP VI, B.6.1). The Marketing Authorization holder (MAH) should follow-up all reports from healthcare practitioners of drug use in pregnancy; the same rule applies to consumer reports. If an adverse event (AE) or an abnormal pregnancy outcome occurs, this should be an expedited report. This includes congenital anomalies, fetal death or spontaneous abortion, and serious adverse reactions. The health authority may require exposure data (even without ill effects) for certain products, such as those with high teratogenic potential or those where pregnant women would be exposed. An example of the latter is pregnant women who are or become infected with HIV.

The MAH is encouraged to collect complete data and report even normal outcomes in periodic reports, as this is useful information (reports without an outcome must be kept but should not be considered as ICSRs). This is, in effect, a pregnancy registry and such reports should be included in the PSURs/PBRERs along with aggregate data on exposure and outcomes. Formal prospective pregnancy registries should also be included.

Further details are available in the European Union Guideline on the Exposure to Medicinal Products during Pregnancy. This document notes the issues to be addressed in Risk Management Plans, data sources, and types of studies (e.g., case series from spontaneous reports, record linkage, pregnancy registries, birth-defect registries, clinical and observational studies, and non-governmental sources of data). It "aims at providing criteria to select medicinal products for which active surveillance for collecting post-authorization data in pregnancy is necessary. It provides guidance on how to monitor accidental or intended exposure to medicinal products during pregnancy and specific requirements for reporting data and adverse outcomes of pregnancy exposure. The guideline also includes detailed recommendations regarding presentation of data collected on exposure in pregnant women." There is also a discussion of data quality and data standardization. This excellent overall review of drugs and pregnancy is worth reading.

Details on Pregnancy Prevention Programs are provided in the guidance in GVP Module VI (Section B.6.1); this is applicable to products known or suspected to be teratogenic.

Labeling in the European Union (the SmPC) should include the following, as per the 2008 European Union Guideline (Guideline on risk assessment of medicinal products on human reproduction and lactation: from data to labeling):

- Clinical data from human experience in pregnancy with the frequency when appropriate;
- Conclusions from developmental studies that are relevant for assessing risk associated with exposure during pregnancy. Only malformative, fetotoxic, and neonatal effects should be mentioned in this paragraph;
- Recommendations on the use of the medicinal product during the different periods of gestation, including a sentence on the reasons for these recommendations;
- Recommendations for managing exposure during pregnancy when appropriate (including relevant specific monitoring, such as fetal ultrasound and specific biological or clinical surveillance of the neonate).

This 2008 guideline includes a table combining available non-clinical and human data which helps categorize the risk. A decision tree is also provided to help in prescribing a drug. Finally, standard wording, depending on the known/available non-clinical and human data, is proposed for inclusion in the Product Information.

Lactation

In general, no breast-feeding infant should be exposed to products the mother takes. In practice, it is not always feasible for the mother to stop certain critical drugs. Fortunately, contrary to pregnancy studies, lactation studies are relatively easy to do and can be done in the study of new drugs; however, robust data on new drugs are quite limited as very limited studies are conducted.

Recommendations for Drugs in the 11th WHO Model List of Essential Drugs": "There are very few kinds of treatment during which breastfeeding is absolutely contraindicated. However, there are some drugs which a mother may need to take which sometimes cause side effects in the baby." This publication gives specifics for many drugs, with specific recommendations such as "compatible with breastfeeding", "avoid if possible", "avoid breastfeeding", and "no data available". The Sainte Justine Hospital (Canada, Quebec) has provided robust advice and references for drug use (article in French) during lactation.

In the European Union, the 2005 guideline about lactation briefly noted:

> If available, clinical data should be mentioned, including studies on the transfer of the active substance or its metabolite(s) into human milk. Information on AEs in nursing neonates should be included if available. Recommendations should be given to stop or continue breast-feeding or to stop or continue treatment. Data on animal studies should be given only if no human data are available.

Note: The FDA and EMA issued guidances

- — FDA: see FDA WebSite: Clinical Lactation Studies: Considerations for Study Design Guidance for Industry (2019)
- — EMA: see EMA WebSite: Guideline on good pharmacovigilance practices (GVP) 3 Product- or Population-Specific Considerations III: Pregnant and 4 breastfeeding women (2019)

AEs in Pregnant Partners of Males Taking a Drug

This is an area with little information. Reproductive studies in animals are done to determine the effects of new drugs on the testes and sperm. Thus, there are often animal data in regard to whether a drug is toxic to the male reproductive system. The major known issues in this area relate to decreases, often temporary, in fertility in males. There are few data, however, on toxicity in the female and the fetus due to transfer of the drug into the female from the male's semen or other body fluids. In general, advice is given to avoid use. This includes cannabis. An example:

PegIntron and Ribavirin is an antiviral used in combination with interferon-alpha used for treating hepatitis C and which should clearly not be used in pregnant women, women who may become pregnant, and male partners of women who are pregnant. The FDA-approved Package Insert notes as follows:

> "PegIntron Monotherapy: Pregnancy Category C: Nonpegylated interferon alfa-2b has been shown to have abortifacient effects in Macaca mulatta (rhesus monkeys) at 15 and 30 million IU/kg (estimated human equivalent of 5 and 10 million IU/kg, based on body surface area adjustment for a 60-kg adult). PegIntron should be assumed to also have abortifacient potential. There are no adequate and well-controlled studies in pregnant women. PegIntron therapy is to be used during pregnancy only if the potential benefit justifies the potential risk to the fetus. Therefore, PegIntron is recommended for use in fertile women only when they are using effective contraception during the treatment period."
>
> "Use with Ribavirin: Pregnancy Category X: Significant teratogenic and/or embryocidal effects have been demonstrated in all animal species exposed to ribavirin. REBETOL therapy is contraindicated in women who are pregnant and in the male partners of women who are pregnant [see Contraindications (4) and the REBETOL Package Insert]."

> "A Ribavirin Pregnancy Registry has been established to monitor maternal-fetal outcomes of pregnancies in female patients and female partners of male patients exposed to ribavirin during treatment and for 6 months following cessation of treatment. Physicians and patients are encouraged to report such cases by calling 1-xxx-xxx-xxxx" (Package Insert for PegIntron)."

The area of female exposure to drugs or teratogenic effects from male partners taking the drugs requires significant additional study. However, the methodology for such work is and will remain exceedingly difficult.

■ Other Resources

From a practical point of view, the critical issue for healthcare practitioners, consumers, and health authorities is to determine what drugs may be safely taken before and during pregnancy (including the weeks after conception and before diagnosing the pregnancy) and lactation.

perinatology.com

perinatology.com is an excellent website. This site has multiple links as well as information on specific drugs, their effects in the various trimesters (if known), lactation information, neonatal AEs, and a literature search.

Teratology Registries and Organizations

Given the scarcity of information, it is now recognized that tracking the pregnancy and its outcome in women who have taken products either accidentally (not knowing they were pregnant) or knowingly is an important way to understand the potential toxicity (and efficacy) of drug products.

- OTIS — The Organization of Teratology Information Specialists (OTIS) is the professional scientific society made up of the experts that provide the MotherToBaby service and the researchers that conduct MotherToBaby Pregnancy Studies. OTIS was established in 1987 as a way of connecting experts in the field of birth defects research to the general public. OTIS has a call routing system so that anyone in the United States and Canada can be routed to an affiliated service to speak with an expert. They have "MotherToBaby Fact Sheets" which summarize the available scientific information to determine whether or not parents and their developing babies are at risk because of an exposure in their environment. See: https://mothertobaby.org/about-otis/
- A European counterpart is the European Network of Teratology Information Services (ENTIS — https://www.entis-org.eu/.
- EUROCAT (https://eu-rd-platform.jrc.ec.europa.eu/eurocat_en) is a large European network of population-based registries grouped geographically for the epidemiologic surveillance of congenital anomalies; Full, Associate, and Affiliate Members contribute data with various levels of granularity. As of 2023 multiple registries in 21 countries survey nearly 1.5 million births a year (25% of EU births)/. One center of particular interest is the Swedish Medical Birth Registry, at, which is a part of the Centre for Epidemiology at the National Board of Health and Welfare in Sweden. What makes this center of unique interest is that it aims to collect prospective gestation and pregnancy data on almost all births in Sweden — between 86,000 and 120,000 per year. Data collected include information on previous gestation, smoking habits, medication, family situation, hospital, length of gestation, type of delivery, diagnoses of mother and child, operations, type of analgesia, sex, weight, length, size of head, birth conditions, place of residence, nationality, and outcome, delivery, and infant information. There are also various teratology and mutagenicity societies around the world in the pharmaceutical and chemical industries, among others.

As regards lactation, the LactMed web site is well designed and easy to use (https://www.ncbi.nlm.nih.gov/books/NBK501922/. To this end, many health agencies around the world now urge or require pharmaceutical companies, hospitals, and so on to track all known pregnancies.

Finally, the extraordinary and tragic situation with DES deserves mention here. The possibility that ingestion of a drug during pregnancy could produce an AE years later in the patient or even the offspring is a challenge to medical research that does not seem solvable with the existing state of the art.

■ Frequently Asked Questions

Q: What about the more complex areas of drug–drug, drug–food, or drug–alcohol interactions in the pregnant and lactating woman?

A: This is really an unknown area. Because gold-standard, prospective, blinded studies are rare to impossible with pregnant women, data are difficult to obtain even in the "simpler" situations of a single drug taken by a pregnant woman. The complexities of interactions, particularly with agents known to be toxic (e.g., alcohol) are not able to be studied adequately (if at all) at this time. The critical issue is the inability to test hypotheses other than those suggested by epidemiologic studies. That is the state of the art today.

Q: Is there not a paradox of sorts here? If a drug that is known to be harmful to the mother or fetus but the registry still shows some women taking the drug, doesn't that show the failure of the warning and the risk management program?

A: Indeed, a successful risk management program, or REMS/RMP, to avoid pregnancies with a known teratogen will theoretically make the registry unnecessary and undoable. It is one of the tragedies in medicine today that women who are pregnant knowingly or unknowingly take drugs that are clearly known to be teratogens. Much more attention is now being paid to risk management programs to prevent pregnancies in women taking these drugs. Whether this will be successful remains to be seen. This is an area of public health that also requires "good pregnancy behavior" by the mother (and father) in terms of smoking, alcohol, eating, medications, and drugs (both licit and illicit).

Q: Can we quantify the risk when a drug has been taken by a woman during her pregnancy?

A: When a drug is identified as "teratogenic", it fortunately does not mean the risk of harm is 100%. The percentages vary across time since conception, drugs, dose period of exposure, and other environmental factors. As an example, a "major" risk with thalidomide means 20–25%. For each pregnant woman, a decision is to be taken depending on the indication, the drug, the dose, the period of exposure, etc.

Q: Which textbooks are the best references on drug exposure during pregnancy and lactation?

A: Many ... but try the three edited by Briggs, Schaefer and Ste Justine for pregnancy and Hale for lactation. Keep in mind however, that there is often a lag between the writing of a textbook and its publication (including this Manual!). Textbooks also go out of date as new information is amassed. So, one should also refer to online resources in addition to published (paper) textbooks.

Q: It seems there is a dearth of evidence-based information to support decision-making in this area. What is the direction of research?

A: We are in an exciting age where science is evolving and new medical technologies continue to emerge. Some of these that may be important in generating new information for women's health include nanotechnology, pharmacogenomics, novel imaging technologies and methods, 3D printing, and developments in regenerative medicine. Incremental progress in these areas should spawn new methods and tools for evaluating sex and gender factors related to the use of medicines. Indeed, advancing research should support development of innovative products and technologies for better management of medicines used in the healthcare of women.

CHAPTER 39

Product Quality Issues

Adverse events are not the only issues of concern when it comes to monitoring the safety of a product. Product issues due to manufacturing, quality control, challenges with the packaging or labeling, storage, tampering, counterfeiting, sterility, impurities, contamination, and so on, can also lead to risks associated with product use. The public health implications of poor quality control of product in all stages of manufacturing lend to the important of understanding the critical link between functions such as Quality, Manufacturing, Labeling, etc. and Safety & Pharmacovigilance. This chapter summarizes briefly issues that revolve around quality and manufacturing as it relates to concepts within pharmacovigilance.

■ Introduction

Issues in addition to bad reactions to the active chemical entity in the product play a significant role in drug safety and pharmacovigilance because of the realization that a safety issue may be related to more than just the active ingredient (active moiety). Excipients, residues from the manufacturing process, quality control (or lack thereof), the container and packaging, storage issues in the pharmacy or home, tampering, counterfeiting, and other misadventures that occur before and after the product has left the factory can produce bad effects. So, an adverse event (AE) can be more than just a bad reaction to the active chemical entity.

How did we get here? In 1955, more than 200,000 children received a polio vaccine in which the process of inactivation of live virus proved to be defective. Within several months, about 40,000 cases of polio had occurred; 200 children had various degrees of paralysis and 10 died from poliomyelitis.[1] Fortunately, most of the frequently seen product quality issues do not generate such serious safety concerns.

Basics

What is a product quality issue? What is a Product Quality Complaint? What is a Medication Error? There are a few definitions available for reference in regional regulations and ICH, however in general a Product Quality Complaint (PQC) is any written, electronic or verbal communication regarding the failure of, or defect, in a drug product (either real or perceived) to meet any of its specifications or standards of quality, purity, identity, safety or potency. Similarly, there are medication errors which are any preventable events that may cause of lead to inappropriate medication use or patient harm while the medication is in the control of a Health Care Professional, patient, or consumer. Medication Errors (MEs) can include incorrect route/formulation, improper dosage (including overdose/underdose), incorrect dosing schedule or frequency, an incorrect medicinal product administration, such a mix-up of drug names or accidental administering a contraindicated subgroup such as to children, and accidental/unintended exposures to the product.

The FDA defines a Drug Product Complaints as "... involving the possible *failure of a drug product to meet any of its specifications* and for such drug products, a determination as to the need for an investigation in accordance with 211.192" (21 CFR 211.198). Additionally, 21 CFR 211.192 incorporate further guidance regarding the Product Complaint Review, stating "All drug production and control records, *including those for packaging and labeling*, shall be reviewed and approved by the Quality Control Unit to determine compliance with all established, approved written procedures before a batch is released or distributed". When a drug product or its packaging fails its specifications at a clinical site or by an investigator, then it should be considered a complaint.

Below are some examples of PQCs. It is important that a company establishes their own list of PQCs specific to the product type and known or anticipated/potential complaints, concerns, or failures. These, as stated above and as per regulations, should be described in SOPs and provided in regular training materials to employees.

1. Package Integrity (Container broken, stopper/seal not intact, stopper difficult to penetrate, etc.)
2. Suspected counterfeit/falsified product
3. Label/Labeling missing or errors
4. Discolored product
5. Patient preference (color, small, funny/odd taste, bad taste, metalic taste after injection, burns upon injection, etc.)
6. Lack of Efficacy for labelled indication (also should be an AE)
7. Evidence of product tampering
8. Particulate or foreign matter
9. AE associated with a specific batch which was not experienced with other batches (also report as AE)
10. Patient or healthcare professional product complaints can revolve around the following:
    - The drug did not work (lack of efficacy);
    - The drug produced an adverse event (AE) (safety issue);
    - The drug looked, tasted, or smelled funny or different. It was crumbling. There was a powder on the pill and so forth (product manufacturing or quality issue);
    - The drug was a tablet in the past, but this time it was capsules (quality issue in packaging, dispensing, etc.);
    - I want my money back or I am going to sue;
    - I ordered these pills on the Internet from a pharmacy supposedly in Canada (possible counterfeit or quality issue);
    - I saw on the Internet that this pill should....; or
    - Others ("My dog accidentally ate the pills").

[1] The cutter incident: How America's first polio vaccine led to a growing vaccine crisis, *J R Soc Med.* 2006; 99(3): 156.

Frequently, one sees multiple issues with a single phone call: "The pill was the wrong color, and when I took it, I developed chest pain, and I want my money back or I'll sue." Part of the issue here involves getting the correct people within the pharmaceutical company (or health authority or call center if they are the first to receive the call) to act on each of the issues involved: the AE component, the product quality component, and the monetary/legal component. In this chapter, we address product quality issues.

Manufacturing Considerations

Manufacturing is regulated in most countries and regions by a set of regulations, directives, laws, and guidances that go under the general rubric of "Good Manufacturing Practices", or GMP. The International Conference on Harmonization (ICH) has addressed manufacturing issues in a series of "Quality Guidelines", covering such topics as stability, analytical validation, impurities, and so forth. The key document is Q7: Good Manufacturing Practices which has been adopted/implemented in the EU, the USA, Canada, Japan and Switzerland, along with a Q&A that was published on June 10, 2015, which clarified several sections of the Q7 Guideline. Since then, each country or region has enacted its own requirements for GMP. Additional countries beyond the original adopters have now integrated the ICH Q7 Guideline into local requirements.

- In the United States, in the Code of Federal Regulations Part 211 (21CFR211) Current Good Manufacturing Practice for Finished Pharmaceuticals.
- The European Union published its new Directive for pharmaceutical manufacturing sites that has replaced the existing Directive (Directive 2003/94/EC) for human medicines. The new EU GMP Directive, (EU) 2017/1572, was issued on September 15, 2017 and became law by March 31, 2018.

To a large degree, the GMP requirements are quite similar around the world, and one factory will frequently produce products sold in many (or all) global markets, thus meeting all standards.

In the United States, the specific section covering product quality issues is 211.198 Complaint Files:

> "(a) Written procedures describing the handling of all written and oral complaints regarding a drug product shall be established and followed. Such procedures shall include provisions for review by the quality control unit, of any complaint involving the possible failure of a drug product to meet any of its specifications and, for such drug products, a determination as to the need for an investigation in accordance with Sec. 211.192. Such procedures shall include provisions for review to determine whether the complaint represents a serious and unexpected adverse drug experience which is required to be reported to the Food and Drug Administration (21CFR211.198)."

This section obliges the manufacturer to maintain written procedures on the handling of all complaints and specifies that a review must be done for serious and unexpected AEs. The US FDA performed a total of 5,615 GMP inspections of registered drug and device domestic and foreign establishments in 2015 (FDA 2016 Annual Report on Inspections of Establishments in FY 2015). Product quality issues are often cited. An example follows from a Warning Letter to a pharmaceutical company in December 2017. Note that Warning Letters are usually sent to the CEO of the company:

1. "This warning letter summarizes significant violations of current good manufacturing practice (CGMP) regulations for finished pharmaceuticals. See 21CFR, parts 210 and 211.
2. "Because your methods, facilities, or controls for manufacturing, processing, packing, or holding do not conform to CGMP, your drug products are adulterated within the meaning of section 501(a)(2)(B) of the Federal Food, Drug, and Cosmetic Act (FD&C Act), 21 U.S.C. 351(a)(2)(B)."
3. "We reviewed your (date) response in detail."

4. During our inspection, our investigators observed specific violations including, but not limited to, the following.
5. "Your firm failed to thoroughly investigate any unexplained discrepancy or failure of a batch or any of its components to meet any of its specifications, whether or not the batch has already been distributed (21CFR211.192)."
6. "You failed to thoroughly investigate release and stability testing failures concerning two batches of your drug products. These product failures included viscosity and appearance. During stability testing, you also identified packaging defects. You did not initiate investigations for each of these drug quality issues. When you did investigate, you failed to adequately evaluate the manufacturing process and associated records, identify root causes, and implement effective corrective actions and preventive actions (CAPA)."

The responsibility for investigating product complaints generally falls within the competence of one of the quality units in a company. The drug safety department usually becomes involved when there is a product quality complaint (PQC), a medication error, or an AE associated with a PQC. That is, even though there was an issue with the manufacturing or quality of the product, the subject took the product and had an AE. Sometimes, of course, the quality issue is only discovered or noted after the use of the product (e.g., the patient had an AE and went back to look at the package and noted the tablets smelled funny and were off-color a quality issue).

Within the pharmaceutical company, this is a "double issue", with an evaluation of the AE by the drug safety group and an evaluation of the product complaint by the quality unit and the manufacturing unit concerned. There are several critical operational issues:

- All units (e.g., drug safety, manufacturing, and quality control) must be informed that the other units are involved in the same case if it was received and triaged elsewhere (e.g., in Medical Affairs or Medical Communications). Each unit follows its procedures and does its evaluation, usually simultaneously.
- The units must communicate their findings to each other because one or both will likely be required to submit the findings to the health authorities. A mechanism must be developed to request that the patient who filed the complaint return any unused product to the company for analysis. Some companies do this for all complaints, whereas others set up specific criteria for requests for return of the product. The quality workup may include reviewing batch records, testing the retained sample, and testing the sample returned by the patient.
- The results of this testing must be conveyed to the drug safety unit to include in the report to the FDA and any other concerned health authorities. If this is an expedited report, the quality unit must get the new information to the drug safety unit so that the follow-up to the agencies is done within the required time (often 15 calendar days or less for serious/urgent issues). The quality unit must not delay sending the information to the drug safety group. Similarly, relevant clinical follow-up information (e.g., lot numbers) from the drug safety unit should be forwarded immediately to the quality unit on the case.
- The case may have two or more different identification numbers, one in the drug safety unit and the other in the quality unit. If the computer system(s) cannot handle the two numbers for the same case, then another method of tracking must be developed to ensure that the case does not fall through the cracks. For large companies, the volume of such investigations may be quite high, with many data flowing back and forth between the departments. In addition, a third or even fourth department may be involved if the case involves a refund of money to the patient or a possible legal or police action (e.g., a lawsuit or police investigation for tampering).
- Now that the manufacture of many products is outsourced and sometimes done in more than one factory (e.g., one for raw materials and another for finished product and packaging), coordination and investigation may become complex and require careful and meticulous coordination and tracking.
- AEs and product quality complaints are now considered "two sides of the same coin". That is, if an AE occurs after taking a drug, it is not always

evident that the event is due to the active ingredient. It might be due to an excipient or a problem in manufacturing, storage, or shipping, or perhaps the product is a counterfeit. It is good pharmacovigilance practice for the drug safety group or the pharmacovigilance or risk management group to examine product quality issues on a regular basis to determine whether a clue or suggestion indicates that quality issues have produced AEs. The methodology for this evaluation (the relationship of quality issues to AEs) has not been fully harmonized yet and remains a methodology of "global introspection". Some of the newer transactional safety databases are now able to capture product quality issues for cases in addition to the usual AE data. The analysis should attempt to see whether there are similar cases (AEs and product complaints) seen with that product's lot, batch number, or geographic area. Mail-order pharmacy systems distributing drugs from centralized locations to all parts of the United States now make geographic tracking much harder and less useful. The days when a particular batch of a drug was used in a localized geographic area are disappearing in the United States but less so in smaller countries or regions.

- Many of the AE/product quality issues are often small and non-critical. Examples include the discovery that a part of the packaging (e.g., vials or stoppers) was obtained from a new vendor and looked or acted differently, or late stability testing showed problems. Sometimes it is discovered that a part or procedure was slightly but clearly out of specification. The determination of how far to proceed in terms of analysis and recall of products is often a difficult decision that requires the assistance of multiple departments within the company and the concerned health agencies. Complications can arise if one health agency wants or demands a recall and another does not. A formal written procedure must be developed and used.

Note: In the EU as well as in Japan, reports of infections in patients who used an injectable drug must be considered serious and managed as a safety signal. In the United States, this would be considered a manufacturing issue.

Product Recall

Significant and severe product quality issues, in particular those that risk patient health or produce serious AEs or suggest tampering, must be acted on immediately. The pharmaceutical company must have a mechanism in place to recognize such issues, investigate them, and bring the information to the responsible levels of the company and the health agencies in a timely fashion. If necessary, a product may need to be withdrawn immediately, public and internet/social media announcements made, protocols stopped, and so forth. The company should have a procedure whereby the team that would need to perform these actions is easily mobilizable for action. It is also a PV role to identify safety signals due to quality defects.

The definitions of recalls and withdrawals in the United States are as follows:

- **Class I recall:** This is a situation in which there is a reasonable probability that the use of or exposure to a violative product will cause serious adverse health consequences or death.
- **Class II recall:** This is a situation in which use of or exposure to a violative product may cause temporary or medically reversible adverse health consequences or where the probability of serious adverse health consequences is remote.
- **Class III recall:** This is a situation in which use of or exposure to a violative product is not likely to cause adverse health consequences.
- **Market withdrawal:** This occurs when a product has a minor violation that would not be subject to FDA legal action. The firm removes the product from the market or corrects the violation. For example, a product removed from the market due to tampering, without evidence of manufacturing or distribution problems, would be a market withdrawal.
- **Medical device safety alert:** This is issued in situations in which a medical device may present an unreasonable risk of substantial harm. In some cases, these situations are considered recalls. Examples of recalls, withdrawals, and safety alerts can be seen at the FDA's website.

Recent examples are provided as follows:

- Cracked glass at the rim surface of the vials;
- Product mix-up;
- Potential microbial contamination which compromises sterility or lack of sterility assurance;
- Potential serious side effects;
- Mislabeling;
- Presence of particulate matter;
- Presence of glass particles;
- Violations of current good manufacturing practice regulations;
- Contains dexamethasone instead of hydrocortisone;
- Unapproved drug;
- Potential for product to be below specification; or
- Missing expiry/lot information.

Generally, most countries have mechanisms for emergency recalls or withdrawals from the market of products that have severe or dangerous or high-risk quality problems. This may be for the entire drug or only for certain formulations, lots, or other subgroups. These may be handled as expedited, reports or "rapid alerts" using the Rapid Alert Procedure in the European Union. Although the safety group may be closely involved, the operational issues of the withdrawal or alert will involve multiple groups, including manufacturing, regulatory, legal, and communications (if the public has to be contacted).

Counterfeiting & Falsified Products

Counterfeit, fake, specious products are now a major concern. This is especially true for certain high-margin, highly desired drugs on the market (e.g., erectile dysfunction drugs, narcotics). Many companies and health agencies are confronting this issue. Warnings are issued almost weekly by health agencies to consumers and medical personnel regarding fake products that can be harmful to patients.

In 2011, FDA issued a guidance on mechanisms companies can implement to identify counterfeit products: *Incorporation of Physical-Chemical Identifiers into Solid Oral Dosage Form Drug Products for Anticounterfeiting*. This was followed by another FDA guidance document in 2016 titled, *Drug Supply Chain Security Act Implementation: Identification of Suspect Product and Notification Guidance for Industry*.

See also the World Health Organization's information on drug counterfeiting.

In the European Union, "falsified medicines" are not the same as "counterfeit medicines". A counterfeit medicine is a medicine made by someone other than the genuine manufacturer, by copying or imitating an original product without authority or rights. Counterfeit medicines infringe trademark law. In contrast, a falsified medicine is a fake medicine that is designed to mimic a real medicine. Falsified medicines do not pass through the usual evaluation of quality, safety and efficacy that is required for an EU authorization procedure.

Every company marketing or distributing a product should have an SOP dealing with counterfeit or suspected counterfeit products. It should set up procedures for drug safety, corporate quality/manufacturing, legal, and regulatory to deal with matters in their domains. The manufacturing/quality groups should determine that the product is fake, ideally by requesting that it be sent to the company (in a postage-free mailer) for evaluation and testing.

Unfortunately for drug safety, the case usually arrives as a "normal" SAE or non-serious AE and must be handled as such even if it is suspected to be from a counterfeit medication. Such suspicions should be noted in the narrative of the initial report, if present, and a note made that follow-up verification is being pursued. The physical product should be requested immediately, including the packaging, and forwarded to manufacturing/quality for testing upon receipt. Obviously, all communications and receipt must be well documented in the database.

If a case turns out to be due to a counterfeit and not due to the company's product, this should be notified in a follow-up to all concerned health authorities. How it is handled in the database in periodic reports (PSURs) is tricky and not standardized. As a rule, the case should not be included (necessarily) in the tables, listings, and analyses of the company's product, but rather addressed in a separate section of the report. It may be difficult to handle this within the safety database. Drug safety may want to work with the legal and regulatory departments as well as manufacturing to set up a coordinated system to handle this. Some companies are now setting up security departments just to deal with counterfeits. Safety databases should be updated to manage such AE reports from suspected/confirmed/disproved counterfeit (or falsified) products. This issue actually increases dramatically in many countries (Africa, Asia among others).

General Remarks

This chapter is not the end of the discussion regarding PQCs, MEs, counterfeiting, falsified products and other GMP/GVP concerns. This should just be the beginning. Companies should have the appropriate qualified staff in place who can have enough foresight to ensure processes are in place to handle these situations even if their occurrence in some instances is remote. It is also important for employees in pharmacovigilance, quality, manufacturing and labeling to be trained in GMP regulations and fully understand the human/public health implications should some of these events occur and go on unaddressed and uncorrected. Ask yourself these questions:

1. Do you have these events defined within your organization?
2. Are you able to collect and report on these types of events? Is there a database or a means to collect and store, then analyze and report on these events?
3. Do you have procedures in place to cover these topic areas?
4. Is your company able or equipped to handle a product recall in reaction to a PC/PQC or other manufacturing issues?
5. Is there training available in your company regarding these topics?

If you can't answer these questions, hire an external consultant who can help setup these processes and assist in evaluating the established system for quality and compliance purposes.

Frequently Asked Question

Q: This doesn't seem fair. Why should a company have to report and waste time and resources on tracking down safety matters concerning counterfeit drugs?

A: Well, of course, life is not fair. But this is still an important public health issue and the company will serve both the public health and its own interest (to protect its products) by pursuing and resolving issues around counterfeits. In practice, it is not always clear whether a drug is or is not a counterfeit, especially if the original packaging is no longer available. A counterfeit may present a health threat and, thus, possibly cast a negative shadow on the true product. Preventing a legitimate product from being tarnished by such an assault should be a priority for the company.

CHAPTER

40

Safety Data Volume, Archival, Record Retention, and Good Documentation Procedures

This chapter focuses on post-marketing case reports. The quantity of adverse events (AEs) received by the FDA on CDER-regulated, marketed products continues to increase year after year.

■ Introduction

The number of AEs received by companies and health authorities is rising dramatically. In this post-covid era, there is a measurable and general increased public awareness of terms such as "safety and efficacy". After COVID-19, there was an influx in publication and public training on what was considered "Safe" and "effective" and were encouraged to report these things called "side effects" to their health care professional. We saw educational programs and media posts regarding what to look for and how to report to the agencies. In fact, COVID probably helped shed some much-needed light on the world of drug safety and pharmacovigilance. But with that added attention, we are seeing a more educated public who is more apt and willing to report events as they see them. This is likely due to several reasons:

- An increased awareness by healthcare practitioners that reporting AEs to the health authorities (and companies) is critical for public health and better communications.
- An increased awareness among patients and consumers of the importance of reporting AEs, at least in the United States, Europe, and Canada, where these reports are encouraged.
- Expansion of ICH membership and awareness of the importance of PV elsewhere, e.g., to Russia, China, Brazil, India, etc., and broader adoption of ICH consensus PV guidelines.
- More clinical trials producing more AEs.
- Increasing prescribing of drugs by physicians and the increasing use of drugs by the general population

(both prescription and over-the-counter, OTC) producing more AEs.

- An increase in the number, design, and creativity of customer engagement programs with the opportunity for two-way communication between patients and drug manufacturers (e.g., disease management programs and patient support programs, etc.).
- More toxic (and more efficacious) drugs being produced, treating diseases that, 20 years ago, were badly treated or untreatable by drugs (e.g., AIDS, certain malignancies, Crohn's disease, rheumatoid arthritis).
- More drug use by the elderly, more polypharmacy, more drug interactions, and AEs.
- The explosion of eHealth coupled with improved technology, better communications, and easier methods of AE reporting (online, e-mail, EDC, automatic "pulling" of AEs from databases, manufacturer and patient advocacy websites, etc.).
- Better training in pharmacy, nursing, and medical schools as well as increased awareness in hospitals and other healthcare facilities of quality programs and the need to report AEs.
- Increasing life expectancy.
- Larger visibility of PV, thanks to media attention on safety issues (Fen-Phen, cerivastatin, rofecoxib, benfluorex, etc.).
- The spread and use of PV systems to health agencies in resource-constrained countries that either did not have such systems in place or did not pay much attention to them.
- An increase in health agency reporting requirements and increasing audits and inspections of PV departments with significant penalties for failure to handle safety adequately.

Databases

Access to the most recent statistics and volume of reports received can be accessed at any regional public database, such as the FDA public dashboard for the FAERS AE Database.

For historical perspective, prior to 2015, when electronic reporting of structured data in ICSRs became mandatory, FDA did not enter all non-serious case reports into their database. This accounts for discrepancies in the FDA data, for example in 2000 FDA received a total of 266,866 reports, but only 75% ($n = 199{,}632$) of the total was entered into the database.

The European Union also has a central database for individual case reports. The database, which is housed by the EMA, contains both post-marketing reports and expedited reports from clinical trials.

Launched in 2001, the EudraVigilance database recorded 1,238,000 case reports in 2016. Out of them, 27% ($n = 339{,}000$) were from the European Economic Area (EEA) and 73% ($n = 899{,}000$) were from non-EEA countries. Until November 2017, case reports were sent by manufacturers to regulators in Member States and, in turn, reports were forwarded to the EudraVigilance database by the national authorities. Beginning in November 2017, EMA is receiving ICSRs from marketing authorization holders and is forwarding the reports to the concerned EU national competent authorities. A good reference for the activites related to EudraVigilance would be to conduct a search for the EMAs "Annual Report on EudraVigilance", which is publised typically in June for the previous year.

Such numbers of AE reports must be interpreted and/or compared between regions/countries or between years, with caution. It should be kept in mind that prior to 2015 certain non-United States non-serious AEs and non-United States serious-labeled AEs did not have to be reported to the FDA by companies.

In the EU, patient/consumer reports have only been recorded since 2010. Prior to 2010, certain EEA countries required healthcare provider confirmation of consumer reports; this is no longer required. So, the numbers cited above are less than the total AEs captured. As another potential bias, a safety crisis can generate "over-reporting" (e.g., Levothyrox® in France in 2017 with a dramatic increase of patient/consumer reports). This is known as a "secular effect".

These large and increasing numbers of AEs were reported every year to Health Authorities:

- Highlight the relevance of the work done over the last 20 years to improve case report collection and transmission, i.e., using E2B to structure data in case reports and using MedDRA® as a single, global dictionary to code AEs (and other relevant data elements).

- Justify the increasing interest of ongoing big data analysis for signal detection, since the older isolated qualitative approach used by health agencies and companies is insufficient.
- Highlight the need for better trained PV employees and improved processes and tools with increased automation in data handling.
- Promote continuing research on how artificial intelligence can facilitate screening digital data for safety signals, as well as handling and analyzing large numbers of case reports (both valid and not valid).

The FDA expects that manufacturer-submitted case report forms will be complete and of high quality. In its document *Enforcement of the Postmarketing Adverse Drug Experience Reporting Regulations*, September 30, 1999, as well as in other SOPs, the FDA instructs its inspectors as follow:

Verify the completeness and accuracy of the selected reports against other information in the firm's files as follows:

1. Was information on the form available at the time of submission?
2. Was all relevant information included on the form?
3. Was the initial receiving date supplied to the agency the same date as the initial receipt of information by the manufacturer?
4. Was new information obtained by the firm during the follow-up investigation and was this information submitted to the agency?
5. Where feasible, particularly when hospitalization, permanent disability, or death occurred, did the firm obtain important follow-up information to enable complete medical evaluation of the report?

In addition, the document further instructs the auditor as follows:

Document deviations from the ADE regulations. Clear deviations such as, failure to submit ADE reports, failure to promptly investigate an ADE event, inaccurate information, incomplete disclosure of available information, lack of written procedures or failing to adhere to reporting requirements, should be cited.

These violations are cited in a "483" form addressed to the company, ordinarily at the close of an inspection. More severe violations may produce a "Warning Letter" or an "Untitled Letter", usually addressed to the chief executive of the company:

The following violations are considered significant to warrant issuance of a Warning Letter:

- Failure to submit ADE reports for serious and unexpected adverse drug experience events (21CFR 314.80(c)(1) and 310.305(c)).
- 15-day alert reports that are submitted as part of a periodic report and which were not otherwise submitted under separate cover as 15-day alert reports. This applies to foreign and domestic ADE information from scientific literature and post-marketing studies as well as spontaneous reports (21CFR 314.80(c)(1) and 310.305(c)).
- 15-day alert reports that are inaccurate and/or not complete.
- 15-day alert reports that are not submitted on time.
- The repeated or deliberate failure to maintain or submit periodic reports in accordance with the reporting requirements (21CFR314.80(c)(2)).
- Failure to conduct a prompt and adequate follow-up investigation of the outcome of ADEs that are serious and unexpected (21CFR 314.80(c)(1) and 310.305(c)(3).
- Failure to maintain ADE records for marketed prescription drugs or to have written procedures for investigating ADEs for marketed prescription drugs without approved applications (21CFR 314.80(i) and 211.198).
- Failure to submit 15-day reports derived from a post-marketing study where there is a reasonable possibility that the drug caused the adverse drug experience.

In other words, the auditors/inspectors will cite lack of standard operating procedures as well as late, incomplete, inadequately followed-up, or unsent

15-day reports. It thus behooves the company to be sure that quality and compliance procedures are in place to ensure the following:

- All cases are received in the appropriate department in the company. For example, sales representatives and other company personnel, if told about an AE, must report these cases to the drug safety department for the appropriate handling. This must be documented in standard operating procedures, with training provided and documented and violations noted and corrected.
- Cases must be rapidly triaged in the drug safety unit (or elsewhere if appropriate) to ensure that they are handled in the appropriate time frame. This applies most markedly to cases that may be 15-day post-marketing expedited reports (and, of course, those clinical trial cases that may be 7- or 15-day expedited reports). In practice, this means that all serious AEs should reach the drug safety group within 1–2 (working) days after receipt anywhere in the company.
- Serious AEs should be promptly entered into the database and medically reviewed, and those valid cases that are 15-day expedited reports promptly sent to the health agencies. Follow-up should be requested in those cases where there is incomplete information. It is highly unusual for a case to be complete with the initial report, and, in practice, all serious AEs will have follow-up performed.
- Data should be reviewed against the source documents for completeness and accuracy.
- Data should also be reviewed by a physician for medical content.

Audits and inspections performed by the EMA or other European Union health authorities are similar in their fundamental nature but have certain European Union twists that are different from those in the United States In any case, all the points noted above would apply to a European Union audit as well.

Similarly, the European Union national authorities, MHRA, and other agencies stress the importance of quality, timelines, consistency, analysis relevance, and the appropriateness of the training and skill set of the individuals handling particular functions.

Archiving

Over the years, with the vast majority of product development work being conducted electronically and no longer on physical paper case files, the activity of archiving has actually become a lot easier to handle. Regardless, the drug safety department must maintain an archive for each case whether serious, whether submitted to the health agencies, whether it fully meets validity criteria, and whether considered important. These records should be kept in a secure (physical or electronic) and protected (from intrusion, fire, water, bugs, rodents, etc.) file room if on paper and in HIPAA and other data security and privacy compliant computer systems whether in the cloud or on individual machines. In more recent years, a different threat of cyber security and data breaches must be taken into account when protecting product development data from piracy and other types of cyber threats.

For systems still utilizing paper cases for processing, access to the file room or electronic storage should be limited, and files that leave the file room physically to be worked on by the staff or examined by someone else should be formally signed out and tracked. Electronic files should have full audit trails or be kept in a system that is capable of tracking and creating version control. The files should be treated the way a library treats rare and expensive books.

Old cases may be archived off-site either on paper, electronically, or both, in a similarly protected environment, but they must be available for an audit within one working day or less. Hence, the filing, indexing, and retrieval system must be clearly worked out and efficient.

Source documents and cases from outside the country, especially those not in English, may be kept at the source (e.g., the company's subsidiaries or affiliates or business partners), but must be available within a day at most for an inspection or other safety review. Similarly, if images are stored electronically, the IT systems must be protected and readily available.

All paperwork, including scrap paper, jotted notes, and telephone logs, must be kept in the permanent files of the company. Some companies scan all documents and retain only the electronic files. If stored as paper, these documents, where appropriate, should be kept in the paper folders for each individual case safety report and be easily retrievable during an inspection or audit by internal auditors or health authorities. Pencils, erasers, and whiteout should also be banned from the drug safety department. All notes should be in pen. Sticky notes should also be avoided because they may fall off or disappear and may contain important data. Data corrections or changes should be done by putting a single line through the incorrect value (leaving it still readable) with the new value written nearby and dated and initialed or signed.

The best form and format of archiving should be left to professional archivists and IT experts. Paper retention produces enormous volumes of files, especially if a company or health authority is receiving tens or hundreds of thousands of cases and hence hundreds of thousands to millions of pieces of paper per year. Thus, non-paper archiving is now, in practicality, obligatory. Most validated software used for safety data processing will have an automated audit trail function. However, a problem in adopting an IT solution is the rapid pace of change in technology that creates obsolescence of the electronic storage systems.

Historical data stored on "floppy disks", zip drives, etc. are now useless because the diskettes themselves may no longer be readable if stored badly and because there are few computers that still have disk drives that can read such disks, therefore larger and longer-standing entities should ideally be making efforts to re-catalogue, save, and archive material previously saved on outdated technology.

Any decision made in regard to archiving should be discussed with the appropriate experts (archivists, regulatory, legal, IT) in the institution and reviewed periodically to see whether the methods and procedures in use are still appropriate but also to check whether the needed software is maintained.

Record Retention Times

There are various time limits that have been established, usually by the legal department or by the records retention department of a company, for all documents. While retention times are specified in various regulations, companies have various time frames for keeping records, allowing their destruction after certain dates, such as 25 years, 3 years after the NDA or MA is closed, 2 or 3 years (depending on product life span) after the last product is sold, meets the expiration date, or is no longer used in a clinical trial, and so on.

In practice, safety records should be kept forever. One never knows when one might need the records either for health authority issues, litigation, or licensing arrangements. Keep in mind that diethylstilbestrol produced AEs in the offspring (and even in granddaughters) decades after the original patients took diethylstilbestrol. One of the authors is aware of a lawsuit in which a third party audit of the safety department was subpoenaed over a decade after the audit.

Good Documentation Practices

Finally, some additional comments on good documentation practices are as follows:

- All safety information received must be handled and recorded.
- If it is not written down or stored electronically, it does not exist and did not happen.
- Documents must be detailed, accurate, and timely.
- Documentation should be contemporaneous; that is, it should be written down at the time it occurs and not at a later date.
- Page numbers, dates, and versions must be tracked.
- No documents should ever be backdated.
- Eschew obfuscation (= avoid lack of clarity)!
- Documents should be written in a business-like manner, with correct tone, grammar, vocabulary, and syntax.
- Documents should be written so that they are understandable to people whose first language is not that of the document. Such practices have been codified by some agencies mainly under good manufacturing regulations.

CHAPTER

41

PV Quality System

United States, European Union, and other health authority regulations require that companies have written Quality Documents (QDs), i.e., Standard Operating Procedures (SOPs), working practices, decision trees and process charts, etc., to handle drug safety and pharmacovigilance (PV). These are documents that describe the general or specific steps to be done in a process, job, or function to ensure that the result is obtained in a complete, reproducible fashion and delivers what is sought.

■ Introduction

The practical goals of a Pharmacovigilance (PV) Quality System are to

- Have Quality Documents (QDs) (Standard Operating Procedures (SOPs), working procedures, questionnaires, manuals, forms, quick reference guides, decision trees, flow charts, manuals, etc.) in place and periodically updated;
- Provide up to date and accurate training for everyone involved in PV and Drug Safety (employees, contractors, etc.);
- Ensure a periodic/ongoing compliance check (metrics/KPIs) to identify deviations; and
- Maintain a clear governance to implement sustainable corrective and preventive measures.

The ultimate goals are to support the PV system in order to:

- Detect and manage safety signals and/or changes to the risk-benefit balance of the medicinal products;
- Prevent harm from adverse reactions;
- Promote safe and effective use of medicinal products;
- Be fully compliant with current regulations.

The following is from the US Food and Drug Administration's (FDA's) document for inspectors conducting adverse event (AE) audits: Post-marketing Surveillance and Epidemiology: Human Drugs, Enforcement of the Post-marketing Adverse Drug Experience Reporting Regulations, September 30, 1999 revised 2012, Field Reporting Requirements.) https://www.fda.gov/downloads/drugs/guidancecomplianceregulatoryinformation/ucm332013.pdf.

The US regulations (21CFR211.198) require that manufacturers have written procedures for complaint files including provisions for determining whether a complaint represents a serious and unexpected ADE. The regulations (21CFR211.25) also require that qualified personnel investigate and evaluate ADEs. If serious deficiencies are found during the inspection, obtain copies of the procedures, and determine personnel qualifications and staffing, especially if the firm utilizes computerized reporting. Any person subject to the ADE Reporting regulations, including those that do not have approved applications, shall develop written procedures for the surveillance, receipt, evaluation, and reporting of post-marketing adverse drug experiences to FDA (21CFR314.80(b) and 21CFR310.305(a)).

In the EU, Good Vigilance Practice (GVP), Module I (Pharmacovigilance systems and their quality systems — EMA/541760/2011) specifies that written procedures exist and goes on to list those that are required (at a minimum).

Note: Printing out and filing all agencies' regulations to have in a specific folder does not make sense as this risks having staff work with outdated versions if the newest version has not been added. It is best to keep them electronically and clearly identify the latest version in use. For any question on regulations, the best is to frequently check and search on the Agencies websites (FDA, EMA, etc.).

An essential element of any PV Quality System is that there are clear, written procedures in place. Care should be taken to ensure that quality control and review are appropriately addressed in the various processes and reflected in the relevant procedures. See the table below for a listing of the basic requirements. There may be other requirements in specific situations. One should customize the Quality System so that it is "fit for purpose". Here is a high level listing of what should be checked. It should be customized for each function and company:

Table 1. High Level Overview of Pharmacovigilance Quality System Requirements.

Theme	Topics to be Addressed in the Quality System

PV Organization/ Function	■ PV Policy;
	■ EU-specific:
	  ■ QPPV Roles & Responsibilities (including back-up procedure to apply in their absence);
	  ■ PV System Master File (PSMF);
	■ Organizational chart, job descriptions;
	■ Safety agreements with partners;

Case Report Management	■ Reports of different types:
	  ■ Organized data collection schemes (solicited, unsolicited, clinical trials, literature review)
	  ■ Process should ensure that reports from all the different sources are captured:
	    ■ AEs in clinical research, including investigator-initiated trials as well as phase I–IV studies, AEs from marketing and sales, legal, telephone operators, webmasters, and the mailroom, spontaneous reports, consumer reports, social media controlled by the company;

Table 1. (*Continued*)

Theme	Topics to be Addressed in the Quality System
Case Report Management	■ EEA and third countries, other Marketing Authorization Holder personnel, licensing partners; ■ Competent Authorities; ■ Collection, processing (including data entry and data management), quality control, coding (MedDRA® coding conventions and versioning), classification, narrative preparation, medical review, quality review and reporting of ICSRs; ■ Detection of duplicate ICSRs; ■ ICSR reporting: ■ Breaking the blind independent of study team (SUSARs from clinical trials); ■ Handling of 7-day expedited reports (Death or life-threatening SUSARs from clinical trials); ■ Handling of 15-day expedited reports (clinical trials & post-marketing surveillance); ■ E2B electronic case reporting; ■ ICSR data exchange when trading partner is not E2B-enabled; ■ Follow-up of reports for missing information and for information on the progress and outcome of the case(s); ■ Handling of reports sent to business partners and internal clients; ■ Reporting requirements for employees not normally involved in safety, specifying that all AEs must be sent to drug safety within certain time frames (i.e., if an accounting department employee hears from a neighbor over the weekend that one of the company's products made him sick, that AE must be reported to drug safety); ■ Handling of AEs in animals associated with medicinal products intended for human use ■ Medical literature cases; ■ Archiving and retrieval of cases;
Aggregate Reports	Preparation, processing, quality control, review (including medical review) and reporting for: ■ PSUR/PBRER, DSUR, PADER; ■ Investigational New Drug Application annual reports; ■ Annual Safety Reports; ■ New Drug Application periodic reports; ■ And other aggregate reports;
Safety Signals & Benefit-Risk Assessment	Global PV activities applying to all authorized, approved or marketed medicinal products: ■ Signal detection, validation, analysis & prioritization, assessment, recommendation for action, exchange of information; ■ Benefit-Risk assessment; ■ Senior Pharmacovigilance Committee (members, organization, roles and responsibilities, deliverables, escalation for dispute resolution, etc.); ■ Handling of urgent safety restrictions and safety variations; ■ Interaction between safety issues and product defects; ■ Life cycle risk management and preparation of risk documents (e.g., REMs and RMPs) including assessment of risk-minimization effectiveness; ■ Program Safety Analysis Plan, including Safety Assessment Committee (overall Clinical Development program per product); ■ Medication error handling; ■ Product quality handling;
Quality Assurance	■ QA Policy (objectives, organization, means, PV System performance & effectiveness measurement, etc.); ■ Quality Document preparation and maintenance;
	■ Training (training matrix, plans & records — PV and non-PV employees, CROs, partners and other third parties); ■ Audit, inspection, self-audit; ■ Filing, archival, and retrieval; ■ Pharmacovigilance QA governance;

(*Continued*)

Table 1. *(Continued)*

Theme	Topics to be Addressed in the Quality System
Health Authority Exchanges/ Compliance	■ Responses to requests for information from regulatory authorities; ■ Meeting commitments to Competent Authorities in relation to a Marketing Authorization; ■ Contacts with government agencies; ■ Reporting and communication notifying HA and HCP of changes to the benefit–risk balance of products;

Other	■ Record/Document management:
	  ■ Record management and data retention policy;
	  ■ Management, access and use of databases or other recording or analysis systems;
	■ DMC/DSMB (initiation, scope specifications, member selection, operating, etc.);
	■ Crisis management and disaster recovery;
	■ Pharmacovigilance due diligence processes;
	■ Pharmacovigilance outsourcing policy and governance;
	■ Litigation.

The scope of a pharmacovigilance system and its quality system should not be limited to PV employees; many PV partners need to be involved (non-clinical, clinical development, regulatory affairs, medical affairs, legal, marketing/sales, communication, complaints written to senior management directly, etc.). This must be considered both in the development and updating of QDs, but also in training.

A list and copies of the global and EEA procedures should be available within 24 hours on request by the Health Authorities. Any additional local procedures should be developed and available to respond to specific requests.

One of the first requests that an inspector from the FDA, the Medicines and Healthcare Products Regulatory Agency (MHRA), or European Medicines Agency (EMA) will make at the beginning of a drug safety inspection is for an organization chart and copies of the drug safety SOPs and related documents (such as guidelines, working documents, manuals, etc.). Usually, the company has an index or listing of these documents that is given to the inspector, who then chooses which ones to examine.

Companies then must expect that the government inspectors, corporate auditors, vendors doing due diligence, and others will read the SOPs in detail and expect those people in the company governed by the SOPs to follow them scrupulously. Auditors will also look at working documents, manuals and guidelines, and other documents (see below) that groups prepare to aid in their work in addition to SOPs. The auditors expect the staff to adhere to these guidelines too, especially if they are approved by some formal or semiformal company mechanism.

Note that putting a process or requirement in a "working document" rather than in the SOP does not free the staff from adhering to the requirement. Thus, it is not a good strategy to relegate certain requirements to a working document or guideline in the hope that the inspector will not examine them or hold the staff responsible for these requirements, too. All procedural documents are "fair game" in an audit or inspection.

Companies or health agencies may create multiple levels of procedures. For a large company, there may be a very high-level ("global" or "corporate") SOP that states the scope, mission, and broad outlines of the safety policy. Then, each division within the scope may develop its own localized policy, and subdivisions may then develop theirs. Usually, two to three layers are the practical limit of this hierarchy. For example, for a large multi-national company, one way to approach this is to create three levels of SOPs:

1. **High-level corporate policy that applies to all divisions of the company:** This is the corporate policy to have the highest level of compliance to laws, regulations and ethical behavior. This demonstrates the company intent to collect, analyze, and report to the appropriate health authorities and internal and external clients all AEs, product quality complaints, and medication errors that the company learns about regarding its products.

2. **Division level:** Each division of the company then prepares a more detailed version of the high-level policy that applies only to that division:
   - Human products division: Creates a broad policy to put the high-level policy into effect. This would cover all research and marketing in the home country and abroad (directly or via subsidiaries or affiliates) and directs them to prepare their own local SOPs (in their local language with a translation into English for review by the quality group).
3. **Subdivision level:** Each section (e.g., the French affiliate) within a division then creates its own SOPs to put the policies noted above into place in their local language. There may be multiple policies needed to accomplish this, and they should specifically cover such things as responsibility by job title (e.g., the medical monitor is responsible for ...), timing (e.g., all SAEs from investigational sites will be sent to the company within 24 hours of occurrence by electronic transmission, fax, e-mail, etc.), and so on.

For example, the following units could create one or more SOPs to cover the following:

- The drug safety unit SOPs would cover the specific details of the handling of spontaneous AEs (serious and non-serious, reports from healthcare professionals as well as from consumers), literature AEs, clinical trial AEs from phase I–IV studies, clinical trial AEs from investigator-initiated trials, AEs from business partners periodic reporting, signal detection, and so forth;
- The clinical research unit SOPs would cover instructions to investigators and monitor what and when to send AEs using a particular written form, or how to handle the case in the electronic case report form (EDC system);
- The animal toxicology/pharmacology unit(s) should have SOPs covering how and when animal findings regarding safety and toxicity should be reported and to whom, because in many jurisdictions, animal findings that may result in safety issues in humans must be reported as expedited reports within 15 calendar days.

Other QDs at any level can also be created. At any point, a unit may create documents to assist staff in doing their daily jobs. These documents might be manuals (e.g., a data entry manual explaining screen by screen how to enter AE cases into the safety database), guidelines, guidances, "cheat sheets" (e.g., a table of all AEs listed in a drug's Package Insert to aid in the rapid determination of whether an AE is labeled), process guides, and various other work aids. These should be done somewhat formally with version control and verified to be correct and consistent from person to person within a group.

QDs must be kept in tight control because they represent the "bible" and contain instructions to the employees that must be followed. Only the latest versions should be used and available to all employees. Keeping only the latest versions online should ensure that employees do not use older, outdated versions. However, in practice, especially if there are many QDs, employees print out copies rather than looking online every time they have a question (e.g., they might have to log out of a case they are entering into the database to look up an SOP question). This tends to defeat the purpose of QDs but is probably unavoidable. In that case, the printed version should contain a statement to the effect: "This printed copy does not necessarily represent the latest in-force version of this SOP. The current in-force copy may be found online at [give link or URL]." Alternatively, the QA group may issue to every employee covered printed copies of the QDs that are numbered, dated, and version controlled. When a new version of a QD is published, a member of the QA group should update each binder, replacing the old version with the new version.

Clearly, very tight version control must be maintained. This should be spelled out in the SOP that governs QDs creation and maintenance. It should cover how and by whom it is determined that a QD is needed and its creation, review, approval, and updating. A system of version control and numbering should be described. It should also mandate training appropriate employees on the new procedures.

Copies of older, outdated QDs should be retained, as a health agency inspector may wish to see the QD in force at the time when a case that is months or even years old is examined. The company may avoid a citation by showing that a particular SOP requirement that is in place now was not in place when the case was actually received and processed.

Training on QDs is obligatory and must be done before the QD goes into effect. Training should not be simply distribution of the QDs and having each person read them. Efforts should be made using professional, dedicated trainers (e.g., employees who have some skills in teaching and training) to develop a methodology to ensure that training is effective. This includes setting up training and retraining schedules and curricula and using effective technology (interesting presentations, video, web-based training, etc.).

Many companies will conduct testing after the training to ensure that the content was absorbed. This is somewhat controversial, though most companies will test manual data entry, as this critical function must be done correctly. Many companies have training departments that "certify" trainers ("train the trainers") within divisions of the company. The trainers themselves may not train on all QDs but may enlist subject-matter experts to do the actual training. The trainers may review and approve the training materials. In addition, detailed records of training must be kept! They should be at the employee level and at the group level so that it can be easily demonstrated (with written records) to an auditor that every employee was successfully trained. Copies of the training materials (such as PowerPoint decks) must also be retained. See Chapter 34 for further details.

It is not sufficient to write and publish QDs. They must be followed. The Quality Assurance department should review (audit) QDs on several levels:

- Do the QDs meet the mission and standards they set? For example, if a safety SOP requires adherence to US and European Union expedited reporting requirements, the SOP should be audited against the US and European Union regulations, laws, and guidelines. This is often a difficult job for an auditor, because it requires that he or she must be familiar with these laws and regulations. Historically, the groups doing pharmacovigilance audits also did clinical research audits as well as, in some cases, financial, Good Laboratory Practice, and Good Manufacturing Practice audits. This would often mean that the auditors had only a superficial knowledge of safety requirements and best practices.
- The trend now is for developing specialized drug safety auditing units that have employees with detailed knowledge of PV — often former case processors or staff from the drug safety unit who wish to move out of the "firing line". Thus, the auditor is able to make a learned judgment on whether the SOP meets the appropriate regulatory requirements and is best (or at least acceptable!) practice.
- The second level of review is the more common and, in general, easier level to audit: Are employees adhering to the requirements of the SOP? If the SOP is clear and prescriptive, the auditor is easily able to verify whether the procedures are done appropriately. For example, if the SOP requires that each AE report coming into the safety department is manually or electronically date-stamped immediately on receipt and then entered into the database within 2 working days, it is relatively straightforward for the auditor to check the date stamp and compare it with the date of data entry.
- Another level of review is internal consistency.
  - If each subsidiary in the countries where a multi-national company sells the drug has a safety SOP, these SOPs should be reviewed for consistency with the higher-level SOP and, if desired and appropriate, with each other. This is one reason to have a high-fidelity translation of the SOP into the official company language (usually English).
  - For every new or updated QD, a consistency check is to be conducted against the other applicable QDs.

Although CIOMS and ICH have done much work to harmonize safety requirements and regulations, there are still significant differences between and among each country's requirements, particularly in clinical trials, where there is less harmonization than in the marketed drug arena. These differences, on the working level, can be substantial and difficult for companies to work out in a manner satisfactory to all parties.

In our age of globalization, it is now common for companies to work with many other companies (either pharma/biotech companies or CROs) in co-development, co-marketing, and other joint arrangements. Some of these can involve multiple companies throughout the world. Such situations require that some level of coordination and agreement is reached on how SOPs and processes will be handled.

The specific requirements of SOPs may also present problems in such situations. If one company uses only E2B case submission and the other company uses paper forms, there will be issues to resolve. Or, if two companies agree to exchange with each other completed CIOMS I forms for all SAEs and one company bases its procedure on completing the forms by calendar day 7 and the other by calendar day 11, there may be significant timing and process issues, forcing one of the companies to alter its procedure to accommodate a shortened preparation schedule. One company may require a legal review of each case and the other may not. At some point, most companies harmonize as much as they can and "agree to disagree" on the remainder of the issues. Generally, the larger the company, the less flexible it is.

Although it would be ideal to have only one set of QDs in place for a study or drug on the market, it is often the case that each company uses its own QDs. Differences in case handling, processing, medical review, and so forth, must be ironed out before the study is begun or the drug marketed. There is no one correct or ideal way to do this. Each situation is usually customized, and compromise may be required by one or all parties. This can be difficult for large companies with rigid systems in place that do not wish to make exceptions or "one-offs". Sometimes companies may not permit their (highly proprietary) QDs to leave their building. The other company may see them but only by physically visiting the site where the first company keeps the QDs. This can make harmonization of QDs between the companies rather difficult.

The list of proposed QDs in this chapter is not exhaustive and will be tailored by each organization. Some organizations will be "lumpers" and others will be "splitters", creating fewer or more QDs. Some companies develop "end-to-end" SOPs; the purpose is to consider one single process across departments rather than one SOP per department/function.

For example, the management of clinical trial SAEs from the initial information to HA reporting may require numerous persons and departments to be involved depending on the company organization. This might include the CRAs, Data Entry Persons, PV physicians, Regulatory Affairs Managers, etc. One single SOP is then developed and applicable to all personnel involved in the process. Such an approach is appealing but can be complex to develop, implement and keep up to date.

All SOPs, working documents, manuals, and such should be reviewed periodically (at least yearly and more frequently, if appropriate, for example, when a regulation changes) to be sure they are still applicable and up to date. They should, in particular, be compared with regulations and requirements in force, best practices, and what is really happening in the organization they apply to. It may surprise that what is written in the SOP may not be what is really happening "in the trenches". Adjustments in process and SOP should be made. All changes in the documents should be carefully documented and noted in the "changes in the new version" section of the document. Training should be performed as necessary. For a good review of SOPs in the pharma industry.[1]

New PV requirements that Health Authorities continue to put forth have not usually produced many surprises Most of the "new" regulations will have been developed in consensus forums, in which the company will have had an opportunity to participate, either in the expert working group, a feeder group, or during the public consultation. An experienced person dedicated to keeping abreast or even influencing evolution of new pharmacovigilance requirements in the external environment must be identified (usually within the regulatory affairs function).

Metrics and "Key Performance Indicators" (KPIs) should also be set up; the purpose is to get an objective and periodic view on both the compliance, performance

[1] See Gough, Hamrell, Standard operating procedures (SOPs): How to write them to be effective tools, *DrugInfJ* 2010; 44: 463–468.

and efficiency of the PV System; metrics and KPIs can also be developed to get an objective view on volume, workload, actual resources, etc. Following table provides some examples of KPIs that a company can follow:

Table 2. Examples of Pharmacovigilance Performance Metrics.

Key Performance Indicators (KPIs)	
Metric/KPI	**Topic**
Percentage of expedited case reports submitted by the due date to HAs	Compliance
Percentage of PSURs/PBRERs submitted by the due date to HAs	Compliance
Number of questions raised about PSURs/PBRERs by the HA assessor after their review	Medical Assessment Quality
Number of identified safety signals and possibly "missed" (e.g., raised by the HA assessor)	Medical Assessment Quality
Number of confirmed safety signals leading to a change or corrective action (e.g., labeling update, time from detection to labeling update at the corporate level, time for labeling update in each country, etc.)	Efficiency in Patient Protection
REMS/RMP commitments (1) achieved (2) by the due date	Compliance & Efficiency
Cost per case report (stratify by clinical trial versus spontaneous serious)	Efficiency
Number of case reports (valid versus invalid)	Volume/ Workload
Number of case reports managed per headcount	Performance
Other	

Similar metrics/KPIs are developed by all companies on compliance of obligatory submissions to HAs; for other topics, metrics/KPIs are company-dependent. It is fruitful to have metrics/KPIs comparing periods (weekly, monthly, quarterly, yearly, etc.). The number of useful metrics/KPIs does not have limit. If an activity can be measured, it can be improved. Select KPIs that are most useful for continuous improvement.

A specific PV team or person must be responsible for governance of the quality system. Metrics and KPIs must be periodically communicated to appropriate employees and to the Pharmacovigilance Quality Governance team. At pre-defined intervals, the Pharmacovigilance Quality Governance team should meet and address all identified deviations in order to define and design CAPAs (process updates, re-training, etc.). An *ad hoc* dashboard to manage all open/closed CAPAs is strongly recommended and all meeting topics and decisions must be minuted.

CHAPTER 42

Training

Two broad and related areas are addressed here: (1) training of the drug safety staff and (2) training of the other employees in the organization who need to know something about drug safety but are not in a drug safety or pharmacovigilance (PV) group.

Introduction

The first thing that must be emphasized is that no one should start doing his or her job without training. A governmental inspector or auditors will look at the training records of individuals to be sure that they were appropriately trained on the functions they are doing and that this training was done BEFORE the person actually started doing the job. Although this seems obvious (no one wants to fly in a plane where the pilot was not trained on that plane), it is not always honored. Failure to do this can result in findings in an audit or inspection.

In any organization, there are two broad areas of training required. The first includes the corporate/organizational requirements and includes such things as policy on obeying laws and regulations, using the computer systems, corporate ethics, behavior and mission, equality in the workplace, getting along with coworkers, safety in the workplace, filling out needed forms for payroll and benefits and other corporate level matters that everyone in the organization needs to know. These programs are usually taught to all employees by the corporate-level training group. These are not addressed further here.

The other area of training, discussed in detail in this chapter, involves job-specific drug safety training. Nearly all companies now have a training function, and many groups now have full-time dedicated trainers whose job it is to handle all the aspects of training and instruction. Some drug safety and pharmacovigilance

(PV) groups in large companies have their own dedicated trainers. Smaller companies do not usually have this "luxury".

This group sets up a training system with tailored curricula, depending on the personnel being trained and jobs being performed. Usually, a fair amount of customization is required to train the right people on the right things. This may include back-up personnel. If the training group is at the corporate level and has the function of doing drug safety training, then they usually have the drug safety and PV personnel act as subject-matter experts (SMEs) and prepare the curriculum and training material. Sometimes the experts do the training themselves; sometimes the training group uses the material and does the training. The trend now is to develop computerized self-training courses using automated self-training. Course design may simply be "read and apply" or, for more critical functions, may have metrics to measure understanding and retention.

For live training, the training group sets up schedules for training and makeup sessions for those who missed the first session. Although they may do much of the training themselves, especially on high-level or more general subjects, the training group will usually create a roster of SMEs who will be called on to train in highly specialized or technical areas that the trainers are not able to teach. The training group works with the quality and compliance groups, as well as with the drug safety group, to determine which employees should be trained in which areas. They determine which training can be "one shot" and which requires updating or refresher training. Some groups with high turnover require frequent training sessions for new employees (e.g., the sales force), whereas others are often more stable and do not require training sessions as frequently. Obviously if SOPs or laws and regulations change, then retraining is usually required. In some instances, annual training is required for all employees, e.g., on safety reporting obligations and how to triage an adverse event to the safety group.

The training job may require significant travel if training is done at various sites around the home country or the world. This is particularly true for multinational organizations and those that have employees working at home or off-site. The levels of training for full-time employees versus consultants should also be taken into account. Vendors, third parties, consultants, part-timers, interim employees, and other non-full-time employees still need training for their jobs. This may require significant effort for far-away companies, vendors, remote employees, etc. Turnover of personnel, particularly among vendors, will need to be monitored for training needs of new hires. Issues of training of non-English-speaking employees also need to be addressed. Although English is often the international language in companies and institutions, training in local languages may also be required. A global company may have one language as the "official" company language for safety and other records, local governments may require transactions in the local language. Training on how social media safety issues (e.g., Tweets or Facebook comments on drug safety issues) needs to be covered.

Much training now is being done as "distance learning", using electronic resources such as live or recorded webinars, teleconferences, smartphone and training apps, and software that allows personal study at the time and pace that the trainee desires. There are now many vendors who will take on the training for a company using very sophisticated technology. The training group should have a good understanding of these newer technologies and how training records are stored and their access. The use of consulting and outsourcing in the appropriate circumstances should be considered as business globalizes and multiple partnerships are set up in the pharmaceutical world under various business arrangements.

The training group should set up a record-keeping system, both for the training department to document globally who was trained and for employee-specific training files, which usually remain within each employee's human resources or departmental dossier. Copies of the training materials (e.g., PowerPoint slides, training apps) should also be retained in the master file. Many organizations now have cloud-based training document and data storage obviating the need for multiple and sometimes duplicative paper folders.

During an inspection by the health agency, the training group can demonstrate that training of a particular function (e.g., handling 7-day expedited reports) was completed for the appropriate groups (e.g., drug safety, clinical research, regulatory affairs), with the training documentation used or given to the students (slides, handouts) on file. In addition, the training group can go to each employee's (paper or electronic) file and show the record, indicating that the employee was trained on this function on this particular date. All of this documentation must be readily available. What is the plan for training records if a vendor is replaced?

The training group should work with the departments to be trained as well as with drug safety to prepare a "Training Matrix" of which employees (by title or function) need which training modules and at what frequency. They should determine which employees, consultants, vendors etc. need refresher training even if the standard operating procedures (SOPs) and processes have not changed.

Companies should have a general corporate policy that requires all employees and agents of the company (including consultants and temporary employees) to report AEs to the drug safety group or safety CRO if they hear about them during and outside of work. This usually refers to marketed drugs and covers such items as when a neighbor or relative casually notes that he or she took your company's drug XX and had a bad reaction. The policy requires the employee to report the AE to the drug safety group or safety CRO by the next business day with sufficient contact information to allow drug safety to follow-up on the report and to get the details of the case. This should be routinely done (with periodic reminders) in all companies with marketed products with an e-mail blast, memo, or company newsletter. The sales force comes in regular contact with healthcare workers, who may comment on adverse events. The primary role of these colleagues is not drug safety, so they may need more frequent reminders of their obligations.

On drug safety issues, it is necessary to train several groups ("feeder groups") within the company on their duties regarding sending AEs to drug safety and then the handling and distribution of the cases. Groups that require training include the marketing and sales groups, the legal department, the mailroom staff, the telephone operators, senior corporate management and their administrative staff (who often receive complaint letters and email or social media addressed to the Chief Executive Officer or President), all clinical research and support groups, medical affairs, the product complaint department, the quality and compliance groups, regulatory affairs, medical information/services, the new business development group, the library, IT and webmasters, and any other groups identified as being involved with AE or safety reports.

Outside groups needing training include vendors, partners and clinical or contract research organizations doing work with or for the company as well as all other contractors and outsourcers (e.g., hired sales forces, such as rent-a-reps), investigators doing clinical research who need to report AEs to the company, outside legal counsel, and other business partners who, by contract, need to adhere to the company's SOPs. This includes vendors and others engaged in patient support programs. It may sometimes be difficult to determine which groups need training and at what level.

As the training needs of the organization increase because of new hires, expansion, and changes in regulations and requirements, it is unlikely that the personnel and travel budget in the training department will increase proportionately. This forces the group to increase productivity and to "work smarter". There are many ways to do this, including web-based training or simply recording a training session as a video and posting it online with required viewing and some level of assurance that the employee actually viewed the information, such as a test of the material. Documentation must be kept.

There is controversy in the training world as to whether actual training needs to be done with either live training sessions or electronic training versus having the person read and review the appropriate SOPs — this is called "read and understood" training. It basically involves giving the appropriate SOPs and other procedural documents to the person and having him or her read and "understand" them. There is often (but not always) someone assigned who can answer the reader's questions. We have seen training files of new hires showing that the employee read as many as 20 SOPs on one day. It is highly unlikely that this will be satisfactory and may be cited in an inspection or audit, particularly if problems are found in the inspection suggestive of training issues.

The issue of testing arises frequently. Some determination of whether the material taught or read has been absorbed is usually required. This can be done by formal testing at the end of training or by having another person observe the trainees functioning on the job (e.g., watching the employee enter a case into the safety database). The testing may be anonymous, or the results made known only to the person being tested and not the trainer or supervisor. Retraining and retesting for people who fail may be required. In all cases, good pedagogic techniques must be followed, such as "praise publicly, reproach privately". The training group typically prepares modules covering each section or sub-section listed below and can thus pick out which modules should be used to train which employees as a function of the employee's job and experience. For example, internal hires may need less training than new hires.

Considering the development and evolution of PV training, *ad hoc* training sessions might be a possibility to ensure that the PV group is up to date regarding current PV standards. As an example, for those working within a company without a pharmacoepidemiology (PE) group, at least one or two PV members must have knowledge about PE basics: when requesting external PE support, this will help their ability to challenge the consultant's proposal and avoid whatever is proposed. Additional training sessions may also be needed, depending on the employee education and experience levels. In addition, there may be a need to consider the company's products, because specific business training sessions may also be needed that cover such topics as: various disease states, PK, PD, clinical development, etc.).

For non-native speakers of English, continued English training may be quite useful to help avoid mistranslation in case reports, aggregate reports, white papers, meetings, etc.

A training plan and a training record must be maintained for every PV employee and everyone trained in any PV or PE or related areas.

Organizational Structure and Site Information

Training should cover the following:

- New employee orientation (usually done by human resources);
- Introduction to staff and organization;
- Review of training curriculum;
- Site information, including "other" sites;
- Telephone, password, voice mail, email, other computer and web functions, databases needed;
- Smartphone/mobile and social media policies, apps used; use of personal or non-company approved apps;
- Safety department overview — structure and functions, teams, support staff;
- Subsidiary, affiliate, and country operation;
- Duties and responsibilities of the position;
- Performance objectives and measures; goal setting;
- Support groups;
- Training from other divisions (e.g., as provided by clinical research, legal, regulatory affairs, informatics);
- Emergency and disaster recovery procedures if the site is not accessible or the computers are down; and
- Data privacy and protection.

Computer, Forms, Electronic, and Print Resources

- Computer and internet accounts and password, applications;
- Help desk;
- E-mail policies, smartphone, and social media use;
- Corporate website and portals;
- Services accessible online: library, benefits, forms;
- Logging on from off-site; and
- Policies regarding "off limit" websites.

What is Pharmacovigilance?

- Mission of drug safety;
- Governing US, European Union, and other country or region regulations, laws, guidelines, directives (may be needed for business arrangements, even if the company has no direct business in a given jurisdiction);
- SOPs, manuals, job aids, guidelines, work instructions (WIs), and how to access them;
- Terminology;
- Functioning and duties of the health agencies (competent authorities) governing the company's products: US FDA, European Union EMA, MHRA, and so forth;

- Who should contact government authorities and under what conditions;
- Labeling — Summary of Product Characteristics (SmPC), Package Insert, Investigator Brochure, Company Core Safety Information and Data Sheet; and
- High level concepts including expedited and periodic reporting.

Corporate and Drug Safety SOPs, Working Documents, Guidelines, and Manuals

- High-level corporate SOPs;
- Divisional SOPs;
- Drug safety SOPs;
- Other departments' SOPs that touch on drug safety, e.g., product defects;
- International Organization for Standards (ISO) or the European Committee for Standardization (CEN) requirements if applicable.

Medical Dictionary for Regulatory Activities (MedDRA®) and Other Dictionaries

- Introduction to MedDRA;
- The MedDRA browser;
- Coding AEs and other data: Maintenance and support service organization and FDA and other conventions;
- Requesting new codes and periodic updates;
- Drug dictionary; and
- Other dictionaries, code lists, abbreviations, and conventions.

Safety Database

- Access to the database: IDs, passwords, inactivity time-outs, changing passwords, retiring IDs;
- Screen-by-screen training on data entry;
- Pregnancy cases, mother–child cases, and other special situations;
- Data privacy;
- Laboratory data;
- Source documents and scanning;
- Archiving and deleting cases;
- Clock start date, time zone, and other date issues;
- Duplicates;
- Transmission of expedited reports to the FDA or other regulatory agencies by paper or electronically;
- Transmission of cases to business partners;
- Workflow;
- Quality checks (QA and QC);
- Requesting follow-up information from the reporter/investigator;
- Preparing reports, cover letters, investigator letters;
- *Ad hoc* queries, structured query language, query by example;
- Device, combination product, vaccine, biologics, blood product issues; and
- E2B & other import and export mechanisms.

Workflow

- Handling 7-day clinical trial expedited reports;
- Handling 15-day clinical trial (IND) expedited reports;
- Handling 15-day expedited reports (post-marketing and clinical trial);
- Global expedited reports;
- Electronic data capture (EDC) safety handling in clinical trials;
- E2B and non-E2B report submission (including backwards forwards conversion with different versions);
- EU — EudraVigilance submission;
- Non-expedited serious reports;
- Non-serious reports;
- Pregnancy cases;
- Literature reports;
- Stimulated reports and reports from investigator-initiated studies;
- Medication errors;
- Product quality reports, including transmission of infectious agents in a product;
- Medical (physician) review;
- Quality checks;

- Aggregate reports: PSURs/PBRERs, Annual Safety Reports (if still used), IND annual reports, NDA periodic reports (PADERs), DSURs;
- Interactions with other departments (e.g., clinical research, regulatory); and
- Breaking the blind in clinical trials: individual cases and at the end of the trial for all cases.

Partner and CRO Interactions

Signaling and Pharmacovigilance

- Signal generation, handling, workup, and management over time;
- Risk management and preparation of REMs and RMPs;
- Crisis management and urgent safety notifications;
- Drug withdrawal, protocol changes, stopping studies, tampering/counterfeits, and other urgent issues;
- Label changes; and
- Media training.

Academic Training

Many universities and academic institutions are now offering courses or programs that teach drug safety, PV, risk management, and signaling. Some cover DS as part of larger programs in "pharmaceutical medicine." This is a rapidly evolving area and we expect that some institutions will offer formal training programs (with "certifications") that will get people jobs. We're not quite there yet, however.

Other External Training

There are now many organizations (both profit-making and non-profit) around the world that now offer training in drug safety and PV.

There are many conferences done around the world often lasting one to 4 days. Some government organizations offer training (EMA and MHRA). There are many region-specific training conferences.

They are of variable quality and depth. ("Apply for Drug Safety and Pharmacovigilance Certification Training. Get ready for a lucrative career in Drug Safety and PV in 3–4 months.") Be very careful of what is being offered. If "a certificate" or "certification" is offered be very wary of what that actually means. The authors are not aware of any certification programs that are officially or widely recognized by companies of governments to train people for drug safety employment.

Some are quite useful and accurate. Others are incomplete, contain incorrect information or are high on opinion and low on fact. As regulations change, they may not be updated. They are usually quite expensive, and the buyer should be wary (caveat emptor).

CHAPTER

43

Audits and Inspections

The US Food and Drug (FDA), the European Medicines Agency (EMA), the United Kingdom's Medicines and Healthcare Products Regulatory Agency (MHRA), Health Canada, and many other national health authorities are permitted or required by law to perform inspections of companies to ensure that they comply with all safety reporting regulations.

■ The Basics

Although the terms often used interchangeably, audit and inspection are not quite the same. An inspection in the drug safety context generally refers to an inquiry, examination, and verification of processes, data, records, regulatory compliance and databases, etc., by a government or official authority. An audit is the same but, in contrast, is done by a non-governmental entity, such as one's own company, or a partner, vendor, supplier, client, and so forth. Note: In this chapter, unless otherwise specified, the terms will be used interchangeably.

Another term frequently heard now in the context of inspections and audits is "gap analysis". This is an audit/inspection in which the primary aim is to find the gaps in the system, i.e., any difference between the requirements and actuality. This approach can differ somewhat from an audit or inspection in the sense that a government or third party audit/inspection is essentially an "adversarial procedure". The auditors are there to find gaps, but may do so in a not very friendly manner. Tension tends to run high. A gap analysis is usually done in a non-adversarial way to help the company (auditee) understand the gaps and problems and ways to fix them. The auditor may actually coach or give advice during the audit in a "friendly" manner that an auditor in an adversarial setting would not.

Government inspections are largely done to protect the public health: to verify compliance to the regulations, to monitor the industry, as part of normal business (e.g., a routine every 2- to 3-year inspection) or "for cause" to investigate a problem. Audits are done primarily for business reasons: compliance to regulations; due diligence of a new or ongoing vendor, partner, client, supplier; investigation of a problem; routine as part of a quality management system, and so forth.

Such audits and inspections may be periodic and routine (e.g., yearly) covering one or more products, general or specific (e.g., look at a newly installed IT system) or they may be non-periodic for cause, looking at a specific problem or issue. "Targets" of the audit include the pharma company (headquarters, regional or national offices, clinical research, monitors, legal, the CEO's office, telephone operators, websites and webmasters, regulatory, legal, sales, marketing, ad agencies, data entry, IT department, training department, medical writing, aggregate reporting group (DSUR, PSURs/PBRERs, NDA Periodic Reports, etc.), licensing group, compliance/quality group, manufacturing, product quality partners, distributors, co-developers, licensees and licensors, vendors, contractors, CROs, data storage facilities, archiving, investigator sites, and anyone in the safety "chain". It may cover clinical research and unapproved drugs or marketed products or both.

Most agencies now are doing inspections on a risk basis. That is, they classify and inspect on a priority basis those companies perceived to be at higher risk of having issues and problems with their safety system. The agencies use either a formal risk rating system or a more informal ranking (companies that just merged, have safety problems, launch a major new or toxic drug, company's first product on the market, etc.) to prioritize their inspections.

For inspections in the European Union, a very detailed document must be supplied some 6 to 8 weeks before the inspection. This document is called the EU Pharmacovigilance System Master File (PSMF) by the EMA. It must be prepared and be available before an inspection. It may run, with appendices, hundreds of pages, and, when supplied, it is usually on a CD, thumb drive or DVD or some other electronic means.

Scope of the Audit

Anything and anyone involved in AEs and safety are fair game. The audit will cover the processing and handling of safety information from all sources; SOPs; working documents, guidances, manuals; measurable and quantifiable data; follow-up; coding (MedDRA®, drugs); literature review; medical information; queries and questions; expedited reporting (7-and 15-day reports); periodic reporting; signal detection and management, risk management and epidemiology, problem escalation; safety agreements with partners, co-developers, CROs, and so forth; handling of technical and product quality complaints; medication errors; registries; call centers; outsourcing and off-shoring; quality systems; IT; data privacy and security; data backup and archiving; training; off-hour and weekend/holiday coverage; business continuity plans and crisis management; safety information communication; safety labeling, and governance.

The auditors will likely ask for the following documents:

- **General**
  - Organizational charts to ascertain the personnel involved in handling AEs, complaints, and safety data;
  - All procedural safety documents including standard operating procedures (SOPs), working documents, guidelines, manuals;
  - All correspondence, meeting minutes, and notes relating to AE handling both internal and external (including health authorities);
  - A list of all products marketed in the country concerned along with their approved current labeling;
  - A list of all collection sites, processing sites, and reporting units that handle cases;
  - Copies of all contracts or safety agreements covering the receipt, handling, evaluation, and reporting of AEs to the health authorities;
  - Job descriptions and training records;
  - The quality system in place;
  - How medical literature is searched (which databases) and handled;

- Compliance governance against regulation and internal commitments (Quality documents, metrics & key performance indicators (KPIs), deviations/violations identification & management, corrective action preventive action (CAPA) plan, meeting minutes, etc.);
- For European Union inspections, all information pertaining to the EU Qualified Person for Pharmacovigilance (QPPV) and his or her duties and function as well as the PV Safety Master File which was probably already supplied.

- **Specific Products**
  - Drugs most likely to have unexpected SAEs;
  - Drugs that could cause serious medical problems if they fail to produce their expected pharmacologic actions;
  - Drugs most likely to have unexpected AEs are those meeting one or more of the following criteria:
    - Approved recently (e.g., last year or two);
    - New additional indication;
    - New molecular entities;
    - Known or suspected bioavailability or bioequivalence problems; or
  - REMS/RMPs, post-marketing safety commitments.
- **Specific Cases**
  - A list of late expedited reports for the last year or two;
  - Serious unlabeled AEs, particularly those involving death or hospitalization;
  - Incomplete, serious, unexpected AEs or reports with unlabeled AEs and no outcome;
  - Incomplete or non-valid cases;
  - "Non-cases" — that is, cases that do not have all four minimum criteria; and
  - Pregnancy listings.

They will examine the cases for completeness and accuracy to ensure that all serious and unexpected spontaneous reports were submitted to the health agency within 15-calendar days:

- Was information on the form available at the time of submission?
- Was all relevant information included on the form?
- Was the initial receiving date supplied to the agency the same date as the initial receipt of information by the manufacturer?
- Was new follow-up information submitted to the agency?
- Where feasible, particularly when hospitalization, permanent disability, or death occurred, did the firm obtain important follow-up information to enable complete evaluation of the report?
- **PSURs/PBRERs/PADERs**
  - Copies of some or all of the reports for the drug(s) for the last year or two;
  - Are all the appropriate reports and listings included?
  - Were the reports submitted in a timely manner?
  - Periodic reports that include unexpected SAEs that should have been submitted as 15-day reports.
- **IT Matters**
  - Validation documents, change control SOP, disaster recovery procedures and results of testing, a system demonstration.
- **Clinical Trial Safety**
  - Study protocol and amendments;
  - IRB approvals, amendments, and yearly re-approval;
  - Informed Consent (including any amendments or translations);
  - Investigator brochure and updates;
  - Investigator meeting presentations;
  - Data Safety Monitoring Board (DSMB)/Data Monitoring Committee (DMC)/Independent Data Monitoring Committee charter and meeting minutes, Drug Safety Boards; and
  - Investigator/IRB/ethics committee notifications for 15-day reports.

The inspectors will request meetings with the appropriate people (both managers and staff) to go through the documents received. The company needs to make preparations (see below) to handle these requests. Questions may include the following:

- Knowledge about both Quality System and Regulations content & expectations?

- How does each type of AE come into the company and how are they handled?
- Are AEs being missed? Are all possible routes of entry into the company covered to ensure that cases are not missed?
- How are cases numbered and tracked?
- Case handling specifics: How are electronic (EDC, E2B), mail, and phone cases triaged and handled? How are AEs or potential AEs and complaints logged in?
- Are medical evaluations performed for each case and by whom and when?
- How and when is follow-up done?
- Who assesses seriousness and labeledness? Is the correct label used? (latest version)
- Who determines whether a case is a 15-day alert report or is to be included in the PSURs/PADERs?
- Who sends the expedited reports and periodic reports to the Health Authorities? Where are these documents stored (paper or electronically) or archived?
- How is labeling handled and how does the company ensure that the labeling reflects the safety status of the drug?
- Is there a consistency check between the Company Core Data Sheet (CCDS) and all local Summary of Product Characteristics (SmPCs)/Patient Information Leaflets (PILs)?
- Are all the databases (commercial or custom-built) used for drug safety functions in compliance regarding validation, change control, data security and privacy, audit trails, and so forth?

In general, the government inspectors can see everything, though in general they do not look at commercial and money issues. The question of whether to supply internal or external audit reports of a company's drug safety system often arises. The companies do not want to provide internal audit reports, arguing that they do not want to be "hanged by their own reports" and will avoid writing down anything problematic to avoid this. The FDA usually has not pressed for these reports, accepting a summary or the CAPA rather than the report itself. The European Union, conversely, requires a summary of these reports in the PSMF.

How an Inspection Flows

There are different methodologies from agency to agency and from company to company. Broadly speaking, inspectors arrive (announced or unannounced; see below) and should be immediately welcomed and brought to a well-equipped workroom. The drug safety group and the "host" (usually someone from the company compliance or auditing group who handles the logistics and flow) decide on the agenda. If governmental, the inspectors may or may not reveal up front all the reasons for the audit (routine, for cause, etc.)

The inspectors will ask for various documents (Quality Documents, EMA line-listings, organization charts, late expedited reports and PSURs/PBRERs, follow-up for RMP/REMS commitments, labeling, IT documents, etc.) either up front or as the inspection unrolls. They may request copies of some to take with them. (Sometimes they will request documents before the inspection.) The company must be able to provide these rapidly, usually within 24 hours, no matter where in the world they are stored. The inspectors will then read the documents, interview personnel, and visit the drug safety group (and others), the server/IT areas (if any), and so forth. Company staff should take copious notes and minutes. Informal or formal summary closeouts may occur at the end of each day. Ideally, inspectors give continual feedback.

On the last day, there is a formal, scheduled closeout meeting, which senior management usually attends. The inspectors sum up their findings and issue a report. Usually, a short, written summary is handed to the company at that meeting and a more formal report issued later on. In situations where very serious problems are found, the mechanisms for escalation within the health agency may be invoked (leading to severe public chastisement and other penalties) and this may be revealed at the closeout meeting. The company must then prepare a CAPA Plan (corrective action, preventive action) and put it into force.

Many agencies, particularly in the European Union, charge the company being examined for the inspection. Fees may be upward of $25,000 and more, depending on the length of the inspection. Travel expenses must also be covered. Inspections usually last a week or so at the minimum and, in egregious cases, may run months.

Findings

There are usually three categories of "findings": (1) critical, (2) major, and (3) minor (other) in EU inspections. The FDA does not call them findings but rather observations and they are not stratified by critical, major, minor:

- FDA
  FDA auditors/inspectors (now called "investigators") use a similar approach for pharmacovigilance and Good Clinical Practice inspections. Investigators look for infractions that impact the validity/usability of data or have a significant subject protection/safety implication. This includes fraud, repeated and deliberate lack of obtaining informed consent, non-reporting of a reportable adverse event. Lesser infractions would not directly impact data usability/validity or patient safety or regulatory compliance, but if repeated consistently, could compromise data or subject/patient safety. Examples of other minor infractions include non-adherence to internal procedures or requirements. All of these "observations" will be described in a written report (with a disclaimer that the cited observations may not be an exhaustive list of all infractions).
- EMA
  - **Critical finding:** A fundamental weakness in one or more pharmacovigilance processes or practices that adversely affects the whole pharmacovigilance system and/or the rights, safety or wellbeing of patients, or that poses a potential risk to public health and/or represents a serious violation of applicable regulatory requirement;
  - **Major finding:** A significant weakness in one or more pharmacovigilance processes or practices, or a fundamental weakness in part of one or more pharmacovigilance processes or practices that is detrimental to the whole process and/or could potentially adversely affect the rights, safety or well-being of patients and/or could potentially pose a risk to public health and/or represents a violation of applicable regulatory requirements which is however not considered serious;
  - **Minor finding:** A weakness in the part of one or more pharmacovigilance processes or practices that is not expected to adversely affect the whole pharmacovigilance system or process and/or the rights, safety or well-being of patients.

Penalties

These vary by country and region. For example, in the United States, several levels of penalties are possible. One or more may be imposed.

- **FDA 483:** A report of deficiencies following an FDA inspection. Requires a response and an action plan for correction of deficiencies.
- **Establishment Inspection Report (EIR):** Prepared by the investigators, giving a very detailed account of the findings.
- **Warning Letter:** A letter to the CEO following repeated, uncorrected violations. Requires an urgent response and plan. An Untitled Letter is similar to a Warning Letter. Both are publicized on FDA's website.
- **Seizure of Product:** Cessation of sales, termination of the NDA.
- **Consent Decree:** A restrictive agreement with FDA before a federal judge on action steps, penalties, and auditing and reporting requirements regarding the observed deficiencies. This is usually effective for 5 years and may be renewed if the desired goals are not met.
- **Criminal Prosecution:** Willful and repeated violations can result in civil or monetary penalties for the company or responsible individuals.

In the EU, necessary measures may be taken by Health Authority "to ensure that a marketing authorization holder is subject to effective, proportionate and dissuasive penalties" (Directive 2001/83/EC):

- CAPA plan review and control;
- Regulatory measures (urgent safety restriction, variation, MA suspension or revocation, registration delay, product recall, etc.) depending on the finding(s);
- Advertising information update;
- Re-inspection to ensure compliance is achieved;
- Warning Letter;
- Publicized list of MAHs found to be seriously or persistently non-compliant;
- Financial penalties (up to 5% of the MAH's Community turnover in the preceding business year); or
- Referral for criminal prosecution with possible imprisonment or fines.

Common Inspection Findings

- Failure to submit (or late) expedited and periodic reports;
- Inaccurate or incomplete reports to agency questions and requests;
- Failure to do follow-up for serious and unexpected AEs;
- Lack of or inadequately written SOPs;
- Failure by the company to follow its own SOPs;
- Database issues, including inadequate validation and security;
- EU QPPV deficiencies (training, coverage, oversight, etc.);
- Technical issues: incorrectly formatted submissions and reports, poor quality;
- Safety signals missed, ignored, or poorly assessed;
- Lack or inadequate metrics and performance measures;
- No or poor quality management system;
- Labeling problems, i.e., Reference Safety Information; and
- Problems and CAPAs from previous inspections not corrected and promises not kept.

The Response to the Inspection or Audit

A written response is required to the findings in most inspections by governments. The response should address each point in the inspectors' report. In most cases, the company agrees with the issues cited and responds with high-level commitments to correct the issues with the promise of more detailed reports as the CAPA is performed. The document must be well thought-out and agreed to fully by the company management as it represents a formal and written commitment to the government(s) in question. In the case of FDA, the written response must ordinarily be provided within 15 days.

If the company chooses to contest some of the findings or not correct them, this should be well thought out and legal counsel obtained from attorneys familiar with FDA or other agency dealings. This can produce a very adversarial situation and FDA can act without prior notification with severe penalties. Rather, if a company disagrees to a degree, they will cite this, along with their reasons, and make an alternate proposal for the CAPA. This can usually be negotiated with FDA and a reasonable resolution can be arrived at.

Responses to findings from non-governmental audits are a business decision, but if the findings are violations of governmental requirements that an agency inspector would cite also, then they should be corrected. The findings should be prioritized, with the critical ones acted on first. The document must be specific and detailed (responding to each point made by the inspectors), with clearly assigned responsibilities, action steps, and time frames for completion. For inspections that have critical or major findings, expect a re-inspection within 6 months to a year.

The Corrective Action Preventive Action Plan (CAPA)

Separate from the initial response letter, a CAPA plan must be set up to deal with the specific findings of an inspection by a health agency. This is an internal company document and usually does not have to be sent to the health authority or auditor though in many cases a high-level summary of the CAPA is sent to the authority. It should specifically be a series of actions to correct and prevent the findings of the inspection or audit. It should be "owned" and tracked by someone in the company.

Action items should be clear and discrete with a specific person named as the responsible party to ensure any CAPA commitment will actually be addressed and solved. Each item should have a due date. In severe cases, a summary or periodic progress report of the CAPA may be sent to the health agency to show good faith and progress. The goal here is for the company to give assurance to the health agency that the problems are recognized and are being corrected in a clear, systematic, and well-documented way.

FDA Safety Inspections

In the United States, the FDA does two types of PV/safety inspections: (1) routine surveillance inspections, and (2) "for cause" or "directed" inspections. The selection criteria include simple routine surveillance, looking at all companies on a periodic basis (e.g., every couple of years), or some sort of trigger at FDA, such as a history of violations (late expedited reports or late periodic reports, significant recalls, etc.) or the recent launch of a major new chemical entity. Inspections may be done in the United States or abroad, and all drugs marketed in the United States are "fair game". If the inspection is for cause, the inspectors have specific information, including case reports or other information that they may or may not reveal to the company under inspection. The FDA investigator may have reviewed previous FDA inspections of the company as well as AE lists from the FDA database (FDA Adverse Event Reporting System, FAERS) and periodic reports.

The investigators (usually one or two per inspection) are ordinarily from the local FDA office and are sometimes accompanied by inspectors with a particular specialty from other offices in the US or the main office. They are guided by an inspection manual that summarizes what the inspectors should examine. Obviously, it behooves the company to review this document and to ensure that the areas scrutinized in an FDA inspection are handled correctly.

The high-level goals of the inspection are to ensure that the company adheres to all appropriate federal regulations regarding safety data collection, analysis, and storage (both paper and electronic), reporting to the FDA, and product labeling, and that drug risks are recognized rapidly and handled in an appropriate manner to protect the public health. Areas inspected include AEs, medical errors, and product-quality complaints.

Inspections are usually unannounced, and the FDA investigator(s) simply arrive at the offices of the company. They present their credentials and documentation for the company to sign, acknowledging their arrival and the review of credentials. Applicants, sponsors, manufacturers, packers, and distributors are subject to inspection of safety process and procedures.

The FDA has global reach and has increased the number of inspections it performs. It is hiring more investigators and other personnel and has established offices outside the United States, in Asia, South America, and elsewhere. A former FDA commissioner has noted that some FDA enforcement efforts have been weak and that this is changing in order to deter other potential violators, communicate the issues to the public, create a level playing field for industry, and increase public confidence in the FDA. Vigilance is expected by companies in regard to how they handle safety problems with their products. They are expected to act quickly and thoroughly to correct problems. Failure to act will produce enforcement and penalties. Warning Letters may be sent in egregious situations. The receipt of a Warning Letter is a very serious matter. It is addressed to senior management (usually the chief executive officer, CEO, of the corporation) and requires a detailed written response within a short time (usually 15 working days), indicating the corrective actions to be taken.

For all inspections and audits, whether FDA, EMA, MHRA, third party etc., a file with all documents must be maintained electronically or on paper (or both in some cases) so that the auditee can rapidly and easily find the documents involved. In particular, if the auditor or inspector has questions or issues months later, the company/auditee must be immediately ready to respond. This means rapid and easy access to the needed documents. Sometimes the person responding may not be someone who participated in the original inspection and not familiar with the documents.

■ Comments on EMA and MHRA Inspections

Inspections by the European Union and other governments around the world usually follow the same general principles noted above. Some differences do apply. European Union inspections are usually announced in advance, and both parties agree on a mutually acceptable date. The inspectors will usually request many documents from the company being inspected covering the PV system, regulatory, quality, etc. as well as most of the documents to be reviewed during the inspection. This may be massive, and the documents are sent on a CD, DVD, thumb drive, uploaded to a secure "vault" in the cloud, or some other secure electronic means many weeks before the inspection. Thus, the inspectors walk in knowing the company's PV situation rather well, as they have reviewed the documents before arriving.

A detailed inspection agenda is provided by inspectors before the inspection or sometimes only upon arrival. The company must then be prepared and any employee who might be interviewed must be informed before the inspection. The inspectors control the agenda and flow of the inspection. Some companies believe that they can take control of the inspection; this is not the case.

In European Union inspections, the Qualified Person for Pharmacovigilance plays a critical role. He or she may be the lead for the drug safety group during the audit and in the response. At the very least, he or she must answer for the entire system, actions, effectiveness, and handling of drug safety for the audit or inspection. As noted above, in the FDA section, an electronic or paper file of the audit must be maintained.

■ Quality Systems and Inspection Preparation in Companies

It is highly recommended that companies set up within their quality or compliance groups a regular schedule for inspections of the company's PV functions, covering pre- and post-marketing situations and paralleling the type of inspection done by the health agencies. PV is now so specialized that dedicated, PV-experienced auditors should be used. These should be done at least yearly, especially if the company's products (new or old) have significant safety issues producing severe or unusual SAEs or toxicity.

Every company, whether selling or doing trials in the European Union, should have an up-to-date Summary/Description of their PV System on file, ready to produce during an inspection or. If a company does not have a quality or compliance group, it should outsource this function but should still ensure that someone in the company has the responsibility for quality and compliance and oversees all outsourced functions.

Every company should have an SOP in place on how to handle outside audits. It should cover the following:

- A procedure should be in place to alert the receptionist at all company sites on what to do when inspectors show up, particularly unannounced FDA inspections. Whom to call (immediately) to greet the inspectors and then who will handle all logistics during the inspection.
- An "escort", "host", or "facilitator" should be designated who will accompany all inspectors at all times. The host handles all the logistics and ensures that meeting rooms and refreshments (usually limited to no more than coffee, tea, water and biscuits) are available, and that the appropriate company representatives are available to meet with the inspectors. If there is more than one inspector (as there usually is), the company should ensure that there are

sufficient hosts to accompany all inspectors should they split up. These are often company representatives from the quality, compliance, or regulatory sections. It is generally not wise to have company attorneys present unless the inspectors also have an attorney present.

- A minute-taker ("scribe") must be present at all meetings to record all issues brought up, to note all promises made by the company, and to ensure that all promised deliverables are delivered in the timeframe promised. The minute-taker should write up the minutes of the meeting (including listing all documents requested and delivered) at the end of each day's audit.
- A document summarizing the rules to follow and behavior to adopt can be provided to all interviewees.

A system to have copies made of documents that are requested by the inspectors must be in place. Copies should be done on special paper marked (or watermarked) "confidential" or the equivalent. Duplicates of everything handed to the inspectors should be retained in the company's inspection files. If copies are made available electronically, a system to ensure that the documents are securely uploaded and copies kept in the electronic file maintained for the inspection.

The meeting/interview room should be separate from the drug safety section. It is generally not wise to have the auditor wandering around the section being inspected unless this is arranged in advance or officially requested. Obviously, the drug safety section should ensure that all documents are in their appropriate places and that the staff is aware the inspectors are present.

Never lie. Always tell the truth. Directly answer the questions posed. Do not volunteer information. Do not guess. If the answer is "Yes" or "No" answer "Yes" or "No" and wait for the next question. Never be afraid of a silence. If you do not know the answer to a question, say so. Try to find (with the help of the facilitator) someone who can answer it. If you do not understand a question, ask for it to be repeated or clarified.

Key Documents

The URLs for the location of these documents seem to change frequently. We suggest you google them on the website of the FDA or EMA.

- US FDA
  - 7353.001 (Compliance Program Guidance Manual) Chapter 53 — Post-marketing Surveillance and Epidemiology: Enforcement of the post-marketing adverse drug experience reporting regulations;
  - Regulatory Procedures Manual
  - Office of Regulatory Affairs, Compliance References (usually reviewed and updated annually, as indicated);
  - Guidance for Industry Good Pharmacovigilance Practices and Pharmacoepidemiologic Assessment,
- EMA
  - REGULATION (EU) No. 1235/2010 OF THE EUROPEAN PARLIAMENT AND OF THE COUNCIL
  - DIRECTIVE 2010/84/EU OF THE EUROPEAN PARLIAMENT AND OF THE COUNCIL
  - Guideline on good pharmacovigilance practices (GVP) Module III: Pharmacovigilance Inspections;
  - Guideline on good pharmacovigilance practices (GVP) Module IV: Pharmacovigilance Audits;
  - REGULATION (EU) No. 536/2014 OF THE EUROPEAN PARLIAMENT AND OF THE COUNCIL of 16 April 2014 on clinical trials on medicinal products for human use, and repealing Directive 2001/20/EC;
  - COMMISSION REGULATION (EU) No. 488/2012 amending Regulation (EC) No. 658/2007 concerning financial penalties for infringement of certain obligations in connection with marketing authorizations granted under Regulation (EC) No. 726/2004 of the European Parliament and of the Council.

■ Summary and Comments

Audits and inspections are now a requisite fact of life in the pharmaceutical industry, and drug safety is no exception. High quality work must be done, it must be monitored through formal systems, and all must be documented. The health authorities are now inspecting companies (pharma companies, vendors, licensors, IT companies, etc.), and the ability to "withstand and survive" such inspections is obligatory. Internal PV audits must be done and must become a routine part of life.

Many issues remain to be resolved as more countries are starting to do inspections and are getting tougher and better at it. One can easily envision the day when dozens of countries do inspections, producing "an audit a week", as one health authority arrives as soon as the last one leaves. Obviously, international coordination to avoid duplicative efforts will likely occur. The concept of mutual recognition of inspections, wherein one government recognizes the inspection capabilities and inspection results of another agency, is now becoming more frequent and may make the overall inspection process more efficient and improve compliance. However, as inspections seem to be either revenue-neutral or actual profit centers for health agencies, it may be difficult for the agencies to give up such lucrative sources of income. How this plays out remains to be seen.

CHAPTER

44

Ethical Issues and Conflicts of Interest

The ethical issues of business and medicine have become complex and difficult. Years ago, before medicine was thought of as "big business," as it is now, the ethics of medicine were somewhat cleaner (at least on paper). Physicians adhered to the Hippocratic Oath, which says, regarding drugs, "I will neither give a deadly drug to anybody who asks for it, nor will I make a suggestion to this effect." It is not so simple now that we know almost all drugs can be "deadly" or at least produce significant adverse reactions and harm. See *The Hippocratic Oath Today: Meaningless Relic or Invaluable Moral Guide*? (https://www.thepublicdiscourse.com/2016/03/16447/)

■ Introduction

The physician's obligation for most of the years since Hippocrates was primarily to the individual patient. Other than clinical acumen, the physician had little in his or her armamentarium that was effective in diagnosis or treatment. Diagnosis, for the most part, relied on the physician's brain without laboratory tests or other investigations. Real medications were few, and often useless, adulterated, impure, or even toxic. Clinical research dates only to the 18th century and serious use of clinical research to the 19th century. Surgery was, at least until anesthesia was developed, also in the 19th century, crude and painful at best and fatal at worst. The physician comforted and predicted and often did little else.

How that has changed! Physicians (plus nurses, physician assistants, nurse practitioners, midwives, and many other healthcare providers) now have an extraordinary array of diagnostic and therapeutic choices available. There are far more choices than the practitioner is able to keep up with and to use appropriately.

But the cost of this great improvement in diagnosis and therapeutics has been the introduction of complexity and conflicting agendas, as healthcare professionals now have obligations to society, employers, governments, insurance companies, partners, and hospitals. The days when the patient paid his or her $5 cash for an office visit (and $8 for a home visit) in developed countries are long gone. The world of big business and corporations has now caught up with big medicine. Costs of physician and other healthcare provider services, procedures, surgeries, laboratory tests, medications, and devices have skyrocketed, all with an eye on potential litigation for "defective" or misused products. The entire dynamics of medicine and healthcare have changed. The next frontier will be how to handle the rationing that will occur (it's here already, in fact) as the population of baby boomers, millennials and GenZ's ages and resources are unable to keep up with the demand for healthcare services such as very costly drugs and biologics.

The question of what is a pharmaceutical company's responsibility should be addressed. There are, broadly speaking, two schools of thought on corporate responsibility. The first is the one of "fiduciary responsibility", which states, roughly, that a company's role is to maximize profitability and shareholder/stockholder value while staying within the law. The second view holds that companies have additional moral obligations to their "stakeholders" above and beyond simply making as much money as possible for the stockholders (owners) of the company. The stakeholders include the patients and their families, healthcare personnel, employees, the communities where the company is located, the public at large, vendors the environment. America and other parts of the world have shifted somewhat from the first view toward the second one or some combination thereof. There is currently a major and ongoing debate on corporate ethics and responsibilities, with one side saying that "corporate ethics" is a contradiction in terms, or an oxymoron, and the other that we are moving to a new view of corporate behavior. This debate then tempers the view one takes regarding the behavior of companies and their individual employees, regulators, customers, bystanders, and others. The debate is not unique to the pharma world and has been seen with BP and the Gulf of Mexico oil spill, Union Carbide and Bhopal, and many other tragedies. Business ethics is now a hot topic in business schools.

Accompanying the changes in the structure of medicine have been changes in the roles and obligations of physicians and other healthcare providers. For example, the physician's role in clinical research is ambiguous. By doing clinical research, the physician is experimenting on participants (either patients or normal subjects) with new medications that may not help the individual patient. However, the results may help humankind (if the new product represents a breakthrough) and definitely will help the drug company involved. This is a concept not envisioned in Hippocrates' time. An excellent review of the issues appears in the Stanford (University) Encyclopedia of Philosophy entitled The Ethics of Clinical Research. (See Stanford Encyclopedia of Philosophy, The Ethics of Clinical Research, First published Fri Jan 30, 2009; substantive revision Wed Jun 23, 2021)

The multiple views and conflicts are discussed relating to a basic philosophical question: "Clinical research poses a very practical and practically vital example of one of the most fundamental concerns in moral theory. When is it acceptable to expose some to risks of harm for the benefit of others?"

The specific ethical obligations and considerations in regard to the pharmaceutical industry is a topic of lively discussion, and many websites offer opinions.

For an excellent review of the ethical issues in the pharmaceutical world, see M. D. B. Stephens's superb section entitled, "Ethical Issues in Drug Safety".[1] This article covers clinical trials, the use of placebo, ethics committees, conflicts of interest, informed consent, patient protection, publications, symposia, advertising and promotion, labeling, and relations with government.

[1] Stephens MDB, Ethical issues in drug safety, *Detection of New Adverse Drug Reactions*, 5th edition (Wiley, Hoboken, NJ, 2004), pp. 591–648.

Companies are set up, as noted above, to make money. They do so by selling various drug/device/biologic products that have known faults or defects listed in the labeling as adverse events (AEs) or suspected adverse drug reactions (ADRs), warnings, and precautions. The main thesis of this manual is that the full and complete safety profile for a product can never fully be known. One always approaches a more complete understanding of the safety profile over time, but one never arrives at "complete" and "final" knowledge.

For all new products, a more comprehensive risk profile is not completely known until well after marketing begins and exposure to much larger and heterogeneous populations than during clinical trials occurs.

For just about all drugs, the safety of use in pregnancy has not been studied (as for children as well). The company has invested enormous amounts of money in the development and then promotion of the products that have a finite (financial) life span due to patent expiration and new and better products coming along. When a drug is approved, it is judged by health authorities to have a benefit profile greater than its risk profile, translated by the public into the shorthand of "safe and effective", although it really means "relatively safe and relatively effective and hopefully more of the latter than the former when used as directed".

Companies will do everything within reason to promote and protect their products. The drug safety group (along with the product quality department, if separate) is the department that receives only bad news about product use. This department must determine, in very short-time frames, whether the serious or fatal problems reported are likely due to the drug. Some of the cases must be reported to the government within a week or two and others tallied up in summary reports as signals for internal corporate review and, sometimes, submission to the health authorities.

The primary duty of the drug safety group is to protect the public health. A secondary duty is to protect the company's products only insofar as this does not conflict with the primary protection of the public health. It is always interesting to read the introduction to the corporate standard operating procedure or mission statement for the drug safety group to see whether this distinction is respected. It usually is, at least on paper.

It is interesting to note that universities in the United States, for the past 20-plus years, have had the right to patent and make profit from pharmaceutical discoveries from their labs. This has led to some phenomenal successes, with hundreds of millions of dollars of royalties from drug sales coming into the university treasuries. Not surprisingly, the universities are reacting just like for-profit pharmaceutical companies when their monetary stream is threatened or interrupted. They sue one another and drug companies to protect their interests.

The following sections address some of the areas of controversy that touch drug safety.

Dynamics in Play Regarding Drug Safety and Companies

- Corporations are rarely run by physicians or clinicians and more often by non-medically trained marketers, sales personnel, lawyers, and accountants. Such managers, who work their way up the corporate ladder, usually do not do a rotation in the drug safety department. It is, thus, understandable that the senior corporate view on drug safety is sometimes vague and often ill-defined.
- The rules governing drug safety are arcane, highly technical, and very difficult to understand (even for those in the business). Management rarely wants details but rather prefers "executive summaries" of data that may not capture the nuances of the clinical judgment involved in drug safety decisions. In addition, there is legal discouragement about writing down real or potential "bad things" about the drug products in e-mail or memos. Management may work on the MEGO ("my eyes glaze over") or MITIN ("more information than I need") principles regarding drug safety.
- The drug safety group is a "cost center" and not a profit center. Pharmacovigilance professionals often argue that their approach saves the company money and shame by preventing safety concerns from becoming safety crises, resulting in crisis management procedures, patient harm, litigation, restrictions on use, or even product withdrawal from the market. This argument, of theoretical future dollars

saved by the safety department, usually carries little weight.

- The drug safety function is not glamorous and usually not well funded — at least not as well funded as the clinical research and commercial organizations. The same often holds true in drug regulatory authorities: there is more staff studying dossiers for approval of new products than studying adverse drug reaction reports. And in most medical schools, pharmacovigilance is not even part of the curriculum. As the saying goes, drug safety is the "poor stepchild". This may be changing somewhat, as various "scandals" and the public awareness that drug safety really does matter may increase funding and resources available; moreover, the anti-Covid mass-vaccination process highlighted the needs for an accurate safety surveillance. New drug regulations are often generated in response to safety concerns.
- In many multi-national companies, the drug safety group is often scattered at several sites around the world and frequently away from the main campus or headquarters of the company ("out of sight, out of mind"). This distributed model, coupled with a good technology infrastructure, can facilitate load-sharing of safety obligations. An ever increasing trend is the outsourcing of drug safety to third parties (CROs) often in far-away lands. Sometimes there is a different CRO for each continent.
- The use of artificial intelligence in drug safety is now being studied and tested and will introduce real changes sooner rather than later.
- Delivering bad news up the corporate ladder is, in the best of times, accepted but not welcomed. In the worst of times, it is actively discouraged and punished. It is hard to "speak truth to power". The messengers are, indeed, sometimes "killed". The mechanism of reporting on signals that could drastically reduce sales, if confirmed or made known, is often convoluted, requiring the safety message to work its way up the corporate chain before it reaches someone with decision-making power.
- Delivering bad news is generally not as well paid as delivering good news (completing clinical trials, selling more drug, etc.) in companies. No one is awarded extra compensation for sending in additional 15-day alert reports.
- Rightly or wrongly, the reputation for honesty of drug companies (including their drug safety groups) is not high in the eyes of health authorities, regulators, consumer groups, and the public. This tends to produce a defensive mentality within the companies of "circling the wagons". Companies, again rightly or wrongly, put little trust or credence into AE reports from certain groups such as consumer groups, disease groups, social media, and attorneys, and often react defensively.
- The drug safety group ("the sales prevention department") is usually grudgingly accepted as a "necessary evil" by other groups in the company.
- The group handling business negotiations for in-licensing new products often do not think of drug safety or bring it into play at the very last minute.
- It is often very difficult to convince sales and marketing departments of the need to train both new and current salespeople on AE reporting ("The job of the sales force is to sell"). Training is often relegated to giving out reading material, or if an actual physical presentation is permitted, it is often done at 4:30 p.m. on a Friday afternoon.
- Drug safety often reports into the medical research department. Less commonly, it reports into the legal or regulatory departments. It should never report to a marketing or sales function. The drug safety organization may report to a non-empowered, low-level, relatively junior employee with little organizational voice or influence and thus, drug safety has no internal "champion".
- There are few ways for management to measure drug safety performance. Clearly, measuring the on-time reporting performance for 15-day case reports, PSURs/PBRERs, DSURs, New Drug Application periodic reports, and Investigational New Drug Application annual reports is the most common metric used, but this simply captures mechanical performance and not the medical protection and risk management aspects of pharmacovigilance. Softer measures such as "the health authority's satisfaction with our performance" are nearly impossible to measure. Most often feedback comes after a regulatory inspection or company audit. Usually, this type of feedback requires corrective action.
- It has been proposed that an indirect way to measure the Drug Safety performance could be to check

a ratio of the number of signals identified by regulators vs the number of new signals identified by the company. Such a Key Performance Indicator (KPI) being as close as possible to zero would be of interest. Unfortunately, there is no reference or standard for this. But a company should look carefully at why a signal was first picked up by the health agency and not by the company.

- Pharmaceutical companies are asked to present statistically significant efficacy data from clinical trials to prove that a drug should be approved by the health authorities to market a product. Thus, many in senior management assume that safety data work in the same way. Drug safety does not.
- Management often takes the view that a serious safety issue must be proven with hard data. There must be clear causality associated with the drug and no alternate explanations for the safety problem. Thus, some managers will not accept drug safety physicians' views that a particular serious and severe medical problem is probably or possibly due to the drug and that a change in the product labeling is warranted. "Clear proof" in several or many patients is demanded.
- Alternative explanations are often presumed to be the cause of the problem: "This patient smokes, drinks, is hypertensive and both parents have heart disease. How can you say our drug caused this patient's heart attack?" Sometimes the drug truly is the cause of the problem even though there are other possible causes.
- The problem may be reduced to a simpler question: is the drug innocent until proven guilty of a safety problem or is the drug guilty of a safety problem until proven innocent? In the past, the "innocent until proven guilty" view predominated. Now, the pendulum is swinging toward early notification of the public of potential safety issues and signals even if events are not clearly due to the drug. Whether this will prove to be good for the public health (moving people off dangerous drugs) or bad for the public health (moving people to other more toxic or less effective or costly alternatives) remains to be seen. People feel better about warning the public and medical providers of possible issues ("virtue signaling"). Whether this improves health outcomes has not been shown.
- The "level playing field" argument is often made by non-medical personnel regarding reporting and acting on safety issues. The argument for this runs roughly as follows: "If we, as a company, have to report that our drug X seems to be causing ventricular fibrillation, then our competitors' products, which also cause ventricular fibrillation (as evidenced by Freedom of Information Act or medical literature reports), should also be obliged to change their labeling." This then puts pressure on the drug safety department either to not report or to minimize such events until they are "proven". Companies thus sometimes try to make deals with the agencies ("We'll change our label if you make our competitors also change theirs", or "This should be class labeling"). This approach rarely works.
- Interestingly, physicians are now found more and more commonly in marketing departments, where they tend to take on the coloration of marketers and lose the (hopefully) objective mindset of physicians. They then may take on an adversarial ("devil's advocate") role in relation to the drug safety physicians.
- In a similar vein, physicians working in the medical research department (phases II and III) often become quite "protective and possessive" about the drugs they are studying and may take a doubting view that "their" drug could produce such serious AEs and, thus, that these serious AEs are "unrelated" to the study drug. This is one reason the final determination of causality, labeling, and reportability should rest with the drug safety group.
- Physicians and, to a lesser degree, other healthcare professionals working in industry (including drug safety) are/were often looked down on by physicians and healthcare workers "out in the real world". Some consider pharmaceutical professionals to have "sold out".
- There are few formal training programs for drug safety personnel either in medical, nursing, or pharmacy schools. There are courses on drug safety lasting from a day to a week or two (usually by non-academic institutions), and there is a scarcity of textbooks. Training tends to be similar to an apprenticeship and occurs only after a person is hired into the industry ("on the job training"). Hopefully, medical academia will discover drug

safety and pharmacovigilance. This seems to be happening with Translational Medicine.

- Company drug safety officers, unless they previously worked for health agencies, really do not have a good feel for how the drug safety agency works (and vice versa). Although there are contacts between industry and the agencies through consensus organizations, such as the International Council for Harmonization, the Council for International Organizations of Medical Sciences, the Drug Information Association, and others, such contact is usually at a distance and defensive because of perceived conflicts of interest, secrecy requirements and different "agendas".
- Drug safety personnel, as with any other company personnel, receive performance bonuses and may own stock or stock options. Hence, pay is tied to company performance as well as to the individual's work. Sometimes the drug safety group will work incredibly hard during a safety crisis but the outcome for the company may still be negative with a new warning in the label, a product restriction, or even product withdrawal from the market. The drug safety group will rarely be "rewarded" for their hard work. This can be quite discouraging to those personnel.
- Drug safety units are under continued scrutiny by the health agencies (particularly in the form of inspections) and internal auditors.
- There are significant pressures on drug safety personnel regarding work volume and time allocated to complete tasks (especially those time frames regulated by law), difficulty in finding experienced safety officers, and difficulty in training safety officers.
- Outsourcing and off-shoring are moving many drug safety jobs out of Europe and North America, forcing a larger pool of workers in these venues to compete for fewer and fewer jobs.
- The upward corporate career mobility for personnel in drug safety groups is limited usually to drug safety or related functions such as epidemiology and safety signaling. Rarely do employees move high up in the corporate hierarchy unless they leave the drug safety unit.

Data Safety Management Boards and Ethics Committees/Institutional Review Boards

Another interesting area is Data Safety Management Boards (DSMBs), which are composed of experts generally hired and paid by pharmaceutical companies to independently and objectively review safety data in a single ongoing clinical trial. The US FDA requires comprehensive safety assessments to be done at the "program" level (see section on Safety Assessment Committees). Board members, usually external physicians and drug safety experts (including statisticians), must make medically correct and honest judgments on patient safety and trial integrity independent of the company. A trial sponsor is ordinarily not strictly obligated to heed the recommendation(s) of a DSMB, but if they do not follow this advice, they need to be able to carefully explain why they did not. When one single group is set up to handle both safety and efficacy data, we do not refer to DSMBs but IDMCs (Independent Data Monitoring Committees). In the EU and the US, such external committees are more and more "recommended", mainly during early development phases.

In February 2024, the FDA issued clear guidance regarding the implementation of DSMBs during clinical trials and how to appropriately select members and deal with conflicts of interest. The inherent conflicts here are clear: board members are paid by the company but must make decisions that may adversely affect the company (and the board members' income if the trials end early). Nevertheless, DSMB and Ethics Committees/Institutional Review Board (EC/IRB) members usually do not work full time for one single DSMB or EC/IRB; therefore, their opinion and advice are easier to deliver since, most often, such opinions do not impact their daily activities and incomes.

Similarly, EC/IRB members are usually paid to provide expert advice on scientific and ethical aspects of protocols before a study starts and periodically monitor safety in ongoing trials. Some ECs or IRBs are "for-profit" companies, and even non-profit university ECs/IRBs may bring in a stream of income for the institution. For more detailed information on DMCs, please refer to that chapter in this Manual.

Safety Assessment Committee

In December 2015, FDA issued a Draft Guidance on Safety Assessment for IND safety reporting. In addition, FDA has a proposal (not yet a requirement) for the sponsor to have access to a Safety Assessment Committee (SAC) that periodically evaluates overall safety in a clinical development program, i.e., across all studies. The SAC may be composed of company employees or non-employees but must operate independently of those engaged with day-to-day conduct of the clinical program. The SAC provides advice to the sponsor, who has the sole responsibility for informing FDA of safety issues. The same concerns for the potential for the appearance of a conflict of interest apply to all of these groups.

Dynamics in Play Regarding Drug Safety and Health Agencies

- Personnel in government health and drug safety agencies are not involved in the monetary aspects of profit-making companies. Their job is more clearly that of protecting the health of the public, though they are no freer from outside political, financial, and other influences than are pharma company personnel.
- In the United States, the Food and Drug Administration and the personnel in the FDA have multiple masters to answer to (either formally in the organizational structure or informally), including the senior management of the FDA, the cabinet department to which they report (Health and Human Services), the president, Congress, and various other watchdogs, including the Justice Department and the Public Health Service. Funding is not always dispersed at a level perceived to be necessary for adequate functioning. Similar multiple masters may be seen in other countries, although in many instances the reporting line is much cleaner when the safety function reports through the Ministry of Health only.
- The health agencies are heavily scrutinized by the media and on-line (at least in the United States and the EU), more so than safety departments in pharmaceutical companies. Scrutiny in social media has elevated this to a much higher level as some news or accusations can go viral in an instant.
- In the past, employees at the agencies tended to make less money with fewer benefits than corresponding personnel in pharmaceutical companies. This is now changing significantly and is no longer true everywhere.
- The agencies tend to be underfunded and understaffed compared with the resources in pharmaceutical companies if one looks at the number of AEs received and the drugs under scrutiny. Some multinational companies' drug safety departments are bigger than the small country health agency safety staffs. This may not always be the case, however, in countries that have large and powerful agencies (e.g., US, UK, France, Germany, etc.).
- The perception is that the agency is not expected or "allowed" to make mistakes. Bad outcomes, serious outcomes, and patient deaths are not supposed to occur in drugs approved by the health agency. Others feel, however, that the agencies (especially FDA, where a 6-month review period is now the norm), approve drugs "too quickly or too slowly", according to one's point of view.
- The FDA and other agencies often go through a turbulent period (short-term leadership, loss of experienced personnel, reorganizations, criticism from the outside, drug withdrawals, etc.) following an election. Indeed, an entire change in the name, structure, and even functions of the agency may occur. This happened in the EU for the EMA when it moved from London to Amsterdam after Brexit but also in France in the last decade after some scandals.

- Many agencies have been accused of being in bed with the industry, and critics point to the large number of people who move from health agency to industry jobs and occasionally vice versa. The claim here is that an agency person will not be tough on industry if he or she hopes to get a job in industry in the next couple of years.
- Duplicative and, in a sense, competitive pharmacovigilance is done by other major health authorities around the world. If a drug is removed from the market or the labeling is changed in one country or region, particularly a "major" one like the United States or the European Union, the other agencies often feel obliged to follow suit. Many drug regulatory agencies operate under formal information-sharing agreements (Memoranda of Understanding) that permit exchange of data, such as ongoing analyses and internal discussions, non-public decisions, and documents, etc. The major agencies have personnel exchange programs, whereby an employee of one agency is embedded in another agency for a set period of time, e.g., 1 year.
- Health agency workers often feel they are doing "God's work", and are "purer" than those folks in industry who are just interested in making money.
- Many agencies have limited regulatory powers. For example, there is limited regulatory power to force label changes and regulate neutraceuticals and healthstore products. However, FDA has the authority to unilaterally make changes in safety labeling if an applicant refuses to do so within a set timeframe. It is also difficult and time consuming to change regulations.
- Government safety officers, unless they previously worked in industry, often do not have a good feel for how corporate decisions and governance occur.
- Similarly, company employees do not always have an understanding of how government agencies function (though many will say they do, having fought battles to get a driving license or resolve a tax dispute). Some government jobs, usually at the senior or ministerial level, are political appointees and may change when the government changes.
- It is not clear how the lower-level safety officers are able to get their views brought up the line in health agencies. Whistle-blowing is a dangerous action.

Dynamics in Play in Regard to Drug Safety and Academic and Non-academic Healthcare Facilities

- In the United States, and to a lesser degree in Canada, the role of universities and medical, nursing, and pharmacy schools in drug safety training, surveillance, and research is minimal. These schools train healthcare practitioners but offer minimal training in drug safety, interactions, and so forth. Courses tend to focus on the concepts of pharmacology and the clinical use of medications. In recent years, some pharmaceutical companies have joined medical schools to design elective programs in drug development or drug safety for medical students and house staff. In the EU, more and more academic pharmacology departments are offering pharmacovigilance training.
- Occasionally, industry physicians hold academic positions at medical schools, often in the clinical research or pharmacology units and occasionally in the clinics (seeing patients, though malpractice insurance issues tend to prevent this in the United States). But there is little "cross-fertilization" among colleagues. Similarly, medical personnel in health agencies rarely hold academic positions at medical institutions, also minimizing cross-fertilization. In contrast, France, for example, has a very tight relationship between the regulatory agency and the regional university hospitals in handling drug safety (31 regional PV centers report to the French Agency).
- Academics perform heavily paid consultation and clinical research for the pharmaceutical industry. Physicians and other scientists in academia perform clinical trials and post-marketing studies, give lectures in speakers' bureaus funded by the industry, and so on. They are sometimes referred to as "key opinion leaders (KOLs)". They may own stock in pharmaceutical companies. This has produced a wave of scandals in the United States and elsewhere, as it is revealed that some academics have created for-profit companies to develop, research,

and market products or receive hundreds of thousands or even millions of dollars from pharma companies. Although this is not forbidden in most cases, these ventures and endeavors were not declared to the universities as required in their rules. This has changed a bit in the US with the passage of the so-called "Sunshine Act" where payments from industry to physicians are posted on a website. See the section in this manual for further details. Many pharmaceutical companies also publish payments on the company website.

When an applicant submits a marketing application for a drug, biological product, or medical device to FDA, e.g., a New Drug Application, Biological License Application, etc, the applicant must comply with the Financial Disclosure by Clinical Investigators regulation (21 CFR part 54). This regulation requires applicants to certify and submit certain information concerning the compensation to, and financial interests and arrangements of, any clinical investigator conducting clinical studies covered by the regulation.

- In the EU, any expert or committee member working for a national agency or for the EMA must produce a declaration of interest which is made public on the agency website. "Members of the Management Board, members of the committees, rapporteurs and experts shall not have financial or other interests in the pharmaceutical industry which could affect their impartiality. They shall undertake to act in the public interest and in an independent manner and shall make an annual declaration of their financial interests. All indirect interests which could relate to this industry shall be entered in a register held by the Agency, which is accessible to the public, on request, at the Agency's offices" (Regulation EC 726/2004, Article 63).
- Likewise, FDA employees (and their spouse and minor children) are prohibited from having a financial interest in any FDA "significantly regulated organization". This must be declared on a confidential financial disclosure form (Office of Government Ethics form 450) prior to employment (or within 30 days) and every year thereafter. Based upon an exceptional circumstance, however, a written exception may be granted. An example of possible justification of an exception might be a pension from a regulated organization if the holding does not conflict with the employee's official duties. The government maintains a list of prohibited financial interests. An FDA employee who acquires any prohibited financial interest (or a revised list captures an employee's existing holding) must complete and submit a report on HHS form 717-2 within 30 days of acquiring the financial interest. The agency monitors disclosures and will guide the employee as to divestiture.
- Academics sit on health agency advisory committees in the United States, Europe, Canada, and elsewhere, where they play key roles. Ideally, they should have no conflicts of interest or the appearance thereof. If any exist, they must be declared. It is sometimes hard to find an expert in a drug or disease who has not, at some point in his or her career, worked with the industry to study new products or new uses. No one is "pure".
- Academics may sit on hospital formulary committees and have a major say in which products are used (and sold) in that institution, even when they have been paid to study these products.
- Some academic research units and "transitional medicine" units receive some funding from industry, and clinical trials in academic units usually charge industry significant "university overhead" to allow the trials to be done at their institutions. Thus, industry becomes a significant source of academic funding at some institutions. In addition, some institutions in the United States now make significant money from drug sales for which they hold patents and receive royalties. There are virtually no medical or pharmacy faculties that do not receive direct or indirect grants, awards, scholarships, speakers' fees, unrestricted educational grants, continuing medical education (CME) grants, expenses, professorships (chairs), and so forth, from industry. Some companies go so far as to install a pharmaceutical research center or an endowed chair on the campus of prestigious medical faculties. This entire situation is now being questioned but given that governments seem to have less money and companies more money, it is not clear how this will evolve.

Dynamics in Play Regarding Drug Safety and Consumer Groups, Disease Groups, and the Internet (Blogs, Websites, Social Media, etc.)

- These groups are usually non-profit organizations created by patients with common diseases or medication use.
- There are organizations or sites set up with other goals in mind. They alert their readers about dangerous drugs and may refer the person to an attorney if appropriate.
- Also see Worst Pills, Best Pills (www.worstpills.org/), run by the Public Citizen's Health Research Group. This nonprofit group notes that it gives an "expert, independent second opinion for prescription drug information".
- A common view among some patient groups (and even some medical groups) is that the industry is monolithic and "bad". The groups often believe (sometimes quite rightly) that the industry regards them as adversaries. They often believe industry cannot police itself and do not trust industry drug safety conclusions. Of course, the same has been said about banks, stockbrokers, tobacco manufacturers, etc.
- There are now many blogs, websites, Facebook/Meta sites, podcasts, webinars, tweets, and all sorts of other social media sources of "information", often uncurated, on drugs, drug safety, and related issues. Some are polemical and have "aggressive" points of view; others are more "balanced"; some are academic; some are for-profit groups; some are from pharmaceutical companies (though this is not always evident) and more. Social media (Twitter/X, Facebook/Meta, etc.) are now being used for drug safety information both by companies and health agencies and attempts are underway to try to use increased buzz on social media as an early signal for drug safety problems. Artificial intelligence and machine learning are evolving to automate certain aspects of screening these sources for meaningful safety information. As always, a healthy skepticism is necessary when visiting these sites, especially when their provenance and funding are unclear.
- Drug safety issues draw eyes to websites, blogs, and television.
- Such stories do not need to be based on scientific data but may rather rest on accusations or human interest issues. Safe drugs do not make good stories. Dangerous ones or potentially dangerous ones do. "Fake news" occurs.
- There is no obligation to present both sides of a story.
- There is little obligation to correct stories that turn out to be incorrect, fake news or overblown ("A lie can travel halfway around the world while the truth is putting on its boots" — Mark Twain).
- Experienced reporters and television personalities are far more skilled at communicating on television and in the media than drug safety personnel (even those who have had "media training") and can make a non-media-savvy interviewee look quite silly or foolish.
- Data presented in the media may be "precise" but not "accurate". Data may also be presented that are of little clinical meaning or that represent a hypothesis, or a "study" based on a handful of patients ("coffee linked to pancreatic cancer").

Dynamics in Play Regarding Drug Safety and Lawyers/ Litigation

- Few people in the medical profession want to have anything to do with lawyers or litigation. Drug safety personnel in the industry and government are no different and generally do not like to give depositions or testify in court; most try to avoid lawyers and litigation.
- Dealings with lawyers and litigation tend to take enormous amounts of time and offer little in return to the safety personnel involved. Testimony, whether in court or at depositions, is usually highly stressful and time-consuming.
- Law and litigation involve, usually, adversarial procedures and are very different from the collegial, consensual, and scientific approach most safety officers have from medical training, experience, and affinity. There is no obligation to be even-handed or to present both sides of the story.

- There are monetary goals involved in lawsuits in addition to the claimed goals of fairness and justice.

Codes of Conduct

Various groups have put out codes of conduct (usually voluntary) for marketing and detailing drug information to physicians and other healthcare professionals. See, for example, the codes put out by the American pharmaceutical industry association PhRMA at https://phrma.org/ or by the EFPIA in the EU (https://www.efpia.eu/). Furthermore, strict codes putting limits on detailing have been put forth by hospitals, medical centers, and certain US state governments. There is a lively debate ongoing about the best way to convey information on pharmaceuticals to physicians and other healthcare providers as well as patients. Similarly, direct-to-consumer advertising in the United States has elicited strong and sometimes angry discussions. The use of social media and the Internet is now playing a large role in this now rapidly changing area and is often out of the control of government or industry. Most physicians now use handheld devices, e.g., smart phones, to access medical information. Whether this is improving the health of the public is unclear though.

Comments and Summary

The entire field of drug safety is chock full of potential conflicts of interest and personal or institutional agendas, some of which are obvious and some less so. No one owns the truth. Trust but verify. All statements should be questioned, and skepticism is a virtue. Safety profiles of products are incredibly dynamic and change almost daily. What is true today may not be so tomorrow. Beware of statements such as those listed below. They may not all be false, but they should be viewed with skepticism until proven otherwise:

- "Of course I've consulted for XX, Inc., or received a speaker's honorarium or accepted travel funds, but they do not influence my judgment in any way."
- "Of course I see drug reps, but they are not my sole source of information and I make independent judgments."
- "I've never received a dime from industry. (But I own a lot of their stock. Or my wife or children do.)"
- "This drug is (perfectly) safe."
- "This drug has no side effects."
- "Our only interest is the public health."
- "I only do what is right for the patient, not the clinical trial or company."
- "This drug has not been proven to produce atrial fibrillation" (or some other serious AE). "The cases we do have are under investigation and all the patients had risk factors." "The serious AE was due to the patient's lifestyle and risk factors." (This may be true today but it may change tomorrow).
- "We have no reports that this drug caused atrial fibrillation." (But someone else might and we haven't looked.)

But all is not lost, nor does cynicism reign everywhere. The current system, which is made up of multiple competing forces sometimes pulling in different directions and sometimes even in the same direction, has tended to arrive at the truth after all is said and done. It arguably takes too long and some people are hurt and some even die in the course of getting to the "truth".

From the ethical viewpoint, PV people working in the pharma industry must be clear about what is and is not acceptable to them in their daily business. Each person must have clear ideas on which limits are ethically acceptable (patient protection and healthcare professional information) and which ones are not. Unfortunately, most ethical issues are grey, not black and white. Thus, the line between acceptable and not acceptable is not hard and fast. What was acceptable 40 years ago (e.g., placebo controlled trials, trials in prisoners) and what is acceptable now may change. Each person must decide in each tricky case what is acceptable and what is not; and he or she must decide what could justify further actions such as: (1) disagreeing with management (for a proposed labeling update for instance) or (2) even going up the company chain to the chief medical or safety officer, (3) an alert to make public your disagreement within the company, public media information, etc., or (4) as a last resort, resignation. Fortunately, such situations tend to be rare and exceptional within pharma companies, but they do happen.

We have nothing better yet, but many people in the health agencies, the industry, and elsewhere are searching assiduously for better validated methodologies in the world of drug safety. That will probably arrive sooner rather than later as we learn glean insights from the massive volume of accessible data in digital form. The conflicts of interest, however, will likely continue. The history of science suggests we will get better and better, though slowly, asymptotically, and with pain along the way.

CHAPTER

45

Universities and Academic Medical Centers

This chapter was written to give you a sense of how these entities may interact with the safety and pharmacovigilance function. It also provides some historical context so that one may understand how we came to where we are today in terms of the often unique interactions between institutions and the pharmaceutical industry.

Universities and academic medical centers have multiple areas in which they interact with the drug safety world:

- Discovery and licensing;
- Translational medicine;
- Specialized clinical research units (CRUs) that run studies;
- Other clinical divisions that run studies;
- Development of "companion" diagnostics for novel therapeutics;
- Training medical students, pharmacists, nurses, epidemiologists, and other healthcare professionals;
- Ethics Committees/Investigational Review Boards;
- Data safety monitoring committees and adjudication committees;
- Consultation to the industry and regulatory assessment panels;
- Reporting suspected ADRs that occur in the hospital or public health clinics.

The Bayh–Dole Act in the United States

The Bayh–Dole Act, or Patent and Trademark Law Amendments Act, was passed in 1980 (35USC200-21 and 37CFR401). Among other provisions, it gave universities the right to hold patents for discoveries from research that they performed that also had federal funding. Government agencies had been hesitant about letting universities and small businesses obtain or license government-held or government-sponsored patents. This law encouraged universities and small businesses to move discoveries into the marketplace. Examples include the following:

- Professor Jan Vilcek and colleagues at the New York University School of Medicine developed the drug infliximab (Remicade®), from which many millions of dollars in royalties were made. Professor Vilcek donated $105 million to the medical school (*New York Times*, August 12, 2005). NYU made $1 billion in research-related income, primarily from Remicade®. Such arrangements eventually made it possible for NYU medical students to study tuition-free.
- Emory University entered into a royalty agreement for $525 million from the sales of emtricitabine (Emtriva®), a nucleoside reverse transcriptase inhibitor.
- Northwestern University received $1.3 billion in pregabalin (Lyrica®) licensing revenue.
- Columbia University received $790 from the "Axel" DNA splicing patents.
- Cohen–Boyer patents on recombinant DNA technology, which were licensed nonexclusively to over 400 firms, brought in $255 million to Stanford University.

Not all patents from universities are biomedical, however. The University of Florida made $288 million from Gatorade® licenses (an electrolyte-replenishing drink used by many athletes). Many other universities have made significant income from information technology patents.

In the American setting, the development of university-held patents has, of course, produced lawsuits over royalties:

- In 1999, Glaxo Wellcome agreed to pay the University of Minnesota royalties on the company's worldwide sales of abacavir sulfate (Ziagen®), an antiviral AIDS drug, to settle a lawsuit brought by the university over royalties for patents held by a College of Pharmacy professor and subsequently licensed to Glaxo.
- Princeton University and the drug manufacturing company Eli Lilly filed a lawsuit, "... against Barr Laboratories, alleging that Barr was infringing on a University patent covering the active chemical in the cancer drug Alimta.® The suit aims to prevent Barr from manufacturing a generic version of the drug that brought in more than $1 billion in revenue for Lilly last year" *The Daily Princetonian*, May 11, 2009.
- Stanford versus Roche (2011) involved the issue of who was the primary owner of a patent. This case went to the US Supreme Court which held that a patented invention vests first in the inventor and assignments of the patent to a third party (e.g., Roche) are secondary (563 U.S. 776 (2011)).

If universities and medical centers conduct clinical studies, they also have the usual obligations of the investigator to report certain safety information to health authorities, ethics committees, and IRBs, as well as to contractual partners.

In the EU, even if some academic people are developing drugs, devices or other treatments, it remains complex to create an ad-hoc specific private company which will be in charge of developing, submitting and marketing the treatment.

Clinical Research Units/ Academic Study Units

Many universities have established clinical research units (CRUs) in the US, Canada, and elsewhere, including the University of Chicago, University of Buffalo, University of Medicine and Dentistry of New Jersey–New Brunswick (Rutgers), Duke University, University of Miami, University of Pennsylvania, Georgetown, NYU, University of Virginia, State University of New York, University of Arizona, University of Kentucky, McGill University, University of Alberta and many more. In addition, there are units in the United Kingdom, Belgium, Canada, Germany, France, and many other countries.

Duke University in Durham, North Carolina, for example, runs a clinical research organization, which is one of the largest academic clinical research organizations (CROs) in the world. They have over 200 faculty members and do phase I–IV trials in 19 therapeutic areas.

These units may perform both inpatient and outpatient studies in phase I–IV. When functioning as sponsors, the CRU takes on all sponsor responsibilities as outlined in the local laws and regulations (and institutional policies) for the study wherever it runs as if it were a pharmaceutical company or a large consortium running trials (e.g., cancer trials, National Institutes of Health). When it functions as a study site for a pharmaceutical company, its safety functions revolve primarily around sending AEs (particularly serious ones) to the sponsor and notifying the IRB of serious cases. Thus, such units may take on some or all of the safety functions in the trial.

Frequently, individual investigators within universities or medical centers contract with pharma companies, CROs, consortia, the National Institutes of Health, and others to run studies or participate in multi-center clinical trials. These trials are run separately from the CRU (if such a unit exists in the institution). In such a case, the investigator is responsible for complying with all safety obligations under the regulations and local university policies. Many universities now set up offices within the administration that handle such "extramural" research activities. They offer assistance to the investigators and ensure that the university collects the appropriate fees for use of their facilities. Doing clinical trials may serve as a significant source of revenue for academic centers. Some pharma companies encourage their medical staff to remain in contact with medical centers, and physicians in companies often hold appointments in academia. Some controversy has arisen where academic physicians and researchers form for-profit companies that aim to discover, market, or do further research on drugs. Universities in the US and elsewhere are now attempting to create clear "firewalls" between companies and academia even to the point of forbidding company detailers (reps) from coming on site. Some academic centers do not allow their staff to use pens with drug or company logos.

Some countries have much tighter ties between academia and government. The French health authority has a network of over 30 academic medical/Pharmacovigilance centers that collect ADRs, advice and train physicians and other health professionals on drug safety matters. They also are involved in the safety signal detection & risk management processes and provide consultative work for the agency upon request.

■ Translational Medicine

This concept has two definitions:

1. "For many, the term refers to the "bench-to-bedside" enterprise of harnessing knowledge from basic sciences to produce new drugs, devices, and treatment options for patients.
2. For others...translational research refers to translating research into practice; i.e., ensuring that new treatments and research knowledge actually reach the patients or populations for whom they are intended and are implemented correctly."[1]

Translational medicine aims to combine disciplines, resources, expertise and techniques from the benchside, bedside and community to promote enhancements in prevention, diagnosis and therapies. It is interdisciplinary and plays a large role in universities doing clinical trials. For example, at NYU the Translational Medicine Division's goals are as follows:

- To understand the action and metabolism of drugs currently in use;
- To help translate laboratory discoveries into agents for use in clinical care;

[1] From Stephen Wolfe, The meaning of translational research and why it matters, *JAMA* 2008; 299(2), https://web.archive.org/web/20100612200225/http://medqi.bsd.uchicago.edu/documents/TranslationaltheoryT1T2WoolfJAMA1_08.pdf.

- To understand the genetic and metabolic bases for responses to and toxicity of pharmacologically active agents;
- To understand and influence those factors that govern the patient's capacity and willingness to comply with pharmacologic regimens;
- To study the effects of drugs upon human diseases as a means to investigate the underlying pathogenic mechanisms.

Drug Safety Training in Academia

North America

Academia in the United States and Canada plays a growing role in drug research though less so in drug safety and pharmacovigilance. This is unlike the situation in France, the UK, and elsewhere. There are at most a handful of departments of pharmacology, medicine, or epidemiology in North America that play major roles in the drug safety world. Although academics sit on advisory committees for health authorities (FDA, European Union member states, Japan), many more make speeches (often for a fee paid for by the pharmaceutical companies' "speakers bureaus") around the US regarding drug therapy. This is now changing as conflicts of interest are being actively sought out and, in theory, stamped out (if that is possible) or at least minimized. See "Bad Behavior" section.

In addition, many academics perform clinical trials paid for by pharmaceutical companies often as part of academic CROs or Translational Medicine Units, thus removing them as neutral observers or consultants on safety. Pharmacology departments in medical schools have historically played only a minor role in pharmacovigilance. Much of the drug safety interest and research is coming from IT and biostatistical departments in universities looking at pharmacoepidemiology, data mining, electronic health records, drug utilization, and such.

Pharmacovigilance is rarely taught to medical or nursing students in North America. On the positive side, pharmacy schools seem to be incorporating more drug safety concepts into their curricula, and some universities are now developing academic certification and degree (MS, PhD) programs in pharmaceutical medicine.

Some universities and medical centers offer training in pharmacovigilance and pharmacoepidemiology both on site and via distance learning. These include Temple University, Rutgers University, in the US and the University of Hertfordshire, London School of Hygiene and Tropical Medicine, University of London, and the University of Portsmouth. Some offer degrees (usually at the Masters level) and others offer "certificates".

The training that does occur usually involves classical pharmacology and treatment with minimal (if any) discussion of the pharmaceutical industry, the FDA or Health Canada, and the subjects addressed in this book. Similarly, nursing and other allied medical programs also have little emphasis on drug safety. Some pharmacy schools and public health training programs cover drug safety and epidemiology in their curricula and may establish rotations through industry or health agencies during the training of the students. The rudiments of epidemiology (though not pharmacoepidemiology in most cases) are taught to medical students.

Europe

Unlike the US, European academic institutions play a major role in drug safety, often working with the government and health authority. In several western European countries, drug safety teaching seems to be well integrated in those university hospitals where a pharmacovigilance reporting center, a drug information center, a poison control center, or a pharmacoepidemiology or epidemiology department exist.

See the European Programme in Pharmacovigilance and Pharmacoepidemiology (https://www.eu2p.org/about-eu2p/education-programme). This is a consortium of several universities, two regulatory agencies and 15 industry partners. The universities are University of Bordeaux, France; Fundacio Institut Catala de Farmacologia Barcelona, Spain; U of Hertfordshire, UK; Erasmus Univ Medisch Centrum Rotterdam, The Netherlands; Univ Utrecht, The Netherlands; University degli Studi della Campana Luigi Vanvitelli, Italy and associated partners including pharmaceutical companies and a CRO. They offer short courses, certificates, Masters and PhD degrees. Most of the training is on line. Independent Drug Safety Certificates are also available (Lyon, France)

There are other programs offered in Europe and Asia as well as occasional courses in South America and Africa.

Academia in the United States is discovering pharmacovigilance and transitional medicine and the other functions of the industry and incorporate them into training healthcare professionals and others.

Obviously, it is in everyone's interest for drug safety and pharmacovigilance to become topics in which all healthcare professionals are trained and contribute.

Academic Consultation

When academic researchers (physicians primarily) and healthcare workers consult to the pharmaceutical industry, much controversy results. This can include giving (for a fee) opinions on clinical trial programs, protocols, clinical development, and drug safety issues. In particular, a sponsor may ask one or more academic clinicians or pharmacologists to review one or more case reports of AEs reported with the use of a drug. The review would help determine whether the AE is related to the drug.

A google search on "universities partnering with pharmaceutical companies" will reveal many instances of these arrangements. Bad Behavior

Various reports in the news and online have indicated that some physicians involved in clinical trials have been consulting with Wall Street financial analysts (for a fee) and it appears that the analysts wanted some indication of how the particular drug was faring in the clinical trials, usually in matters of safety as the efficacy data were blinded. Trouble can ensue. In one case a physician was charged with leaking insider information on a clinical trial to a hedge fund ("Bail Set for Doctor in Insider-Trading Case", *Wall Street Journal*, November 26, 2010).

Other examples include companies using undue influence (e.g., money) to influence physicians to prescribe their drugs. The Oxycontin story involving Purdue Pharma is another example of harmful interactions between pharma and physicians, pharmacists and others. Books, articles, television shows and other media have documented this situation. Servier is still involved in litigation in France over their product Mediator for appetite suppression in which some 500 people died from heart valve problems. The product remained on sale in France even though the drug was withdrawn years earlier from the US, Italian and Spanish markets.

Consultation also includes giving "scientific marketing talks" (discussions of diseases or particular drugs) to other physicians and healthcare workers on marketed drugs that the sponsor makes. The controversy here revolves around the independence and impartiality of consultants who are also receiving sums of money for scientific marketing activities. Some believe that full disclosure of all financial ties, even remote, permits objectivity. Others believe that objectivity in such a circumstance is never truly possible and that comments on clinical trial efficacy or drug safety are not unbiased. Because this practice is fairly widespread, it has produced, in some cases, difficulties in finding consultants with no industry ties to serve on FDA advisory committees and data safety management boards.

See the important article by Marcia Angell, MD entitled "Drug Companies & Doctors: A Story of Corruption" in the NY Review of Books January 15, 2009. The Pharmaceutical Research Manufacturers of America (PhRMA), the organization of the pharmaceutical companies, has put out several codes and guidances on industry actions and behavior in research, marketing, and sales. It has been signed by some 50 companies and sets certain voluntary standards on drug marketing.

Universities and medical centers are placing more and more limits on what drug company representatives ("reps") can say and do in their institutions. In the United States, many institutions are limiting samples, free lunches, detailing, and other pharma company activities in their centers. In France, limits have been placed on what reps can say and how many free samples are dispensed to physicians, and it is claimed that these requirements are now stricter than those in the United States and Canada.[2]

The Joint Commission standard COP.11.6 requires organizations to monitor the effects of medications on patients. However, the requirement is not explicit on reporting adverse drug reactions (or medication errors) to the FDA, although this is encouraged by the FDA via the MedWatch Program. Thus, hospitals must develop some level of drug safety expertise and local standards of behavior. This is usually via the pharmacy department or the formulary committee (the group that decides which drugs will be kept on formulary and which will not). Requirements outside the United States vary from country to country.

■ The Sunshine Act

Since 1999 there have been financial disclosure rules in the US for Investigators, Industry, and FDA staff. The regulation (21CFR§54) requires applicants who submit a marketing application for a drug, biological product or medical device to file certain information concerning the compensation to, and financial interests and arrangements of, any clinical investigator conducting clinical studies covered by the regulation. The regulation requires applicants to certify the absence of certain financial interests and arrangements of clinical investigators that could affect the reliability of data submitted to FDA. If the applicant does not include certification and/or disclosure, or does not certify that it was unable to obtain the information despite exercising due diligence, the agency may refuse to file the application. The government publishes this (see below). Many companies also disclose all payments to investigators (including fair value of any donated equipment, etc.) on the company website.

In 2010, the US enacted the "Physician Payments Sunshine Act" (also called "Open Payments"). This law requires that drug, biologics, device and medical supplies manufacturers collect and publish all financial relationships with "covered recipients": physicians, dentists, podiatrists, optometrists, chiropractors and teaching hospitals. The law covers companies which provide products to Medicare, Medicaid and the State Children's Health Insurance Program. This essentially covers most of the health companies in the US. It went into effect in 2013.

It covers such things as the cost of meals provided to the covered recipients, payments made for services including advisory boards speakers' programs, consulting as well as other "transfers of value" not in cash such as travel expenses, journal articles, equipment, or subscriptions, etc. It includes indirect payments made by a third party. It also covers research payments. The reporting threshold is about $10.

The goal is to make the financial relationship between the physicians (and other healthcare providers) transparent to expose and lessen conflicts of interest.

See the Centers for Medicare & Medicaid Services website covering open payments: https://www.cms.gov/OpenPayments/

The data is available at https://openpaymentsdata.cms.gov

There is a search tool for the database which is moderately user-friendly. One can find summary payments but also specific physician and hospital payments and how much the company actually paid that physician. The data can also be downloaded. The summary page shows that in 2022 the total money involved was $12.59 billion to 588,514 physicians and 1,200 teaching hospitals.

Unsurprisingly, various organizations have analyzed these data and listed the highest monetary companies and physicians. See for example: https://projects.propublica.org/docdollars/ which has data 3 through 2019.

[2] Silversides, Tight regulation of French drug reps mean French doctors get more balanced information than doctors in the US, *BMJ* 2010; 341: c6964.

This site also allows one to search by doctor or company name is a user-friendly way. The top company was Genentech at $478 million and the top doctor received $29 million in 2018. The top teaching hospital (University of Pennsylvania) received $26 million.

Comment: Has this worked? Is the sunshine helping? The jury is out. Fair compensation for time and talent at market value is reasonable, but high payments continue.

CHAPTER

46

Vaccinovigilance

By Lisa Beth Ferstenberg

Vigilance for vaccine safety is different from vigilance for drugs. At a high level, drugs are frequently used to treat disease, i.e., in individuals who have signs and symptoms of disease, whereas many vaccines are usually designed to prevent disease in otherwise healthy individuals. We will review some of the key differences between vaccinovigilance and pharmacovigilance and illustrate by describing selected initiatives.

Differences between Vaccinovigilance and Pharmacovigilance

Adverse event reporting, whether associated with a drug or a vaccine, captures information on known or suspected reactions to administered substances; however, in the case of a drug, the substance is usually administered as an intervention for an existing illness or condition, and in the case of a vaccine, it is usually given to prevent an illness. This critical difference, between prevention and intervention, affects the entire analysis, interpretation, and implications of vigilance data. Because the target population for vaccines, in general, is ordinarily healthy (and frequently includes young children), the window for an acceptable safety profile is narrow.

In many countries, specific vaccines are mandatory (children's infectious diseases or travelers' diseases for instance). Patients being healthy before vaccine injection, they are most often in a mindset to recognize and report a problem if they develop a vaccine-induced ADR, than patients with possible drug reactions.

Causality versus Attribution

When an illness appears, we want to know why: Why did someone get cancer? Why did someone get an infection? What caused a person to have a heart attack? While our need to know a cause may not alter the medical event, attributing an outcome to a reason seems to give us assurance. Pharmacovigilance, and vaccinovigilance, are clinical sciences that aim to either establish or reject attribution of symptoms to receipt of a treatment or a vaccine. Their methods are, unfortunately, inadequate sciences, since conclusions can only be based on available reported data. Data are often incomplete and sometimes misleading. The two fields differ from each other in significant ways that have major implications for what we attribute, and what we assume, about causality.

The first significant difference between detecting safety signals for vaccines relative to drugs are that people receiving vaccines are usually healthy. In fact, people with immunosuppressive conditions such as cancer, or recent illnesses, are warned not to receive vaccines that contain live infectious agents. The advantage of this situation is that temporal symptoms associated with vaccination, such as fever, swelling, pain and glandular enlargements, are more easily attributable to the vaccine as the causal agent, since no other symptoms or interventions are concurrent. The disadvantage, on the other hand, is that anything that occurs later may be falsely attributed to the vaccine simply because no other causality is suspected.

Temporal Association

The contextual differences between intervention and prevention affect the interpretation of data derived from adverse event reporting. For a drug-related adverse event, the patient presents to the health professional with an array of symptoms. If new symptoms develop following treatment, there is a reasonable likelihood that the provider following the patient will be informed of their occurrence and will be able to assess them in the context of the illness. The association of a drug with a side effect is strengthened if the drug is stopped and the symptoms resolve. If the drug is restarted and the symptoms reappear (rechallenge), this is frequently confirmatory.

Vaccines, on the other hand, are given once (often in a series) or repeated only after a period of several years, in people who have no other reason to see the clinician. Temporal events in a previously asymptomatic person are again, fairly easy to attribute. Delayed events can be problematic, since the patient may have experienced so many other exposures, events and treatments since the time the vaccine was administered.

In general, serious adverse events to vaccines are rare. A majority of reported adverse events are mild and self-limiting and usually involve local reactions, such as pain or itching at the site of administration, or systemic reactions, such as fever or irritability. The rest of reported serious adverse events may include seizures, high fevers, life-threatening illnesses, or death. The notable difference between vaccine-related adverse events, whether serious or non-serious, and those associated with drugs is that vaccine-related adverse events are usually immunologic and are related to immune responsiveness.

Drugs are Metabolized; Vaccines are Processed

Most drugs confer activity by being metabolized and distributed throughout the body; the drug and its metabolites are delivered by the blood stream to target tissues. When adverse events occur, they may indicate that the drug or its metabolites have toxic effects on an end organ, such as liver or kidneys. The pharmacology of drugs, following metabolism, results in their being eliminated from the body in predictable ways. Vaccines, on the other hand, are processed by the immune system and generate a persistent effect, such that an offending foreign agent or antigen (e.g., bacteria or viruses) can be neutralized or removed the next time it is encountered without needing another inoculation. That is what makes vaccines effective over the long-term. Since the vaccine's objective is to elicit an immune response to a target antigen, the emergence of an immunologic or inflammatory response can indicate that the patient is developing a desirable immune response, whereas in drug-related toxicity, the reaction almost invariably indicates an undesirable effect. Vaccines are frequently given in the context of broad public health initiatives, so that little to no information may be captured and recorded about how many doses of the vaccine have been administered in the population, to whom, and with what outcomes.[1] As a result, it can be quite difficult to detect a trend of adverse events to vaccines until a substantial number of cases come to the attention of medical practitioners and Health Authorities.

Incidence and Prevalence of Adverse Event Symptoms

Determination of efficacy can be more difficult when studying a vaccine than when studying a drug. Vaccine trials are usually designed to detect disease prevention, which is generally assessed by a decrease in the expected incidence of new cases of illness, like infections. Drug trials are easier in this regard, in that the disease is already present and you are trying to cure it. Participants in vaccine trials may not have been exposed to the etiologic agent, whether they received the vaccine or not. Some studies are not designed to measure incidence of new cases of the target disease. For example, it is routine to measure antibody titers rather than actual disease prevention when testing annual influenza vaccine preparations. Further, some vaccines are designed as therapeutics, i.e., to treat disease, such as the vaccines to treat rabies, hepatitis, or cancer. See section on "Vaccine Efficacy".

To illustrate the case of preventative vaccines, suppose a company is developing a vaccine for the common cold. They give it to a group of 100 participants with half of them getting a placebo and half get the new vaccine. The study is blinded, so no one knows who gets the vaccine and who gets the placebo until after the study is over. Suppose that 30 people in the placebo group catch a cold during the study period, and 20 people in the vaccine group get a cold. Does this mean that the vaccine prevented 10 additional people from catching a cold? Or were those people just not exposed to a cold virus anyway, just like the other 20 people in the placebo group?

To answer this question, we need to know the expected number of people who would have been expected to catch a cold in that time period. This is the incidence, and to get an accurate number we would need a great number of participants before we had enough to detect a difference between treatment groups. Now suppose that of the 50 participants in each group, 10 participants from each one reported an adverse event of itching at the injection site. The placebo group may have gotten nothing but saline and the new vaccine group got an active substance. So is itching at the injection site an adverse event caused by the vaccine? Clearly, we would be unable to come to that conclusion since the same number of participants who received placebo developed itching as did those who got vaccine. Again, it would take a large number of subjects to determine if subjects who got the vaccine were more likely to develop itching than those who got placebo. If no difference in the incidence of itching occurs even with a large sample of subjects, the conclusion may be that the vaccine itself does not specifically cause itching.

There are two important points from this example. The first is that vaccine trials need to be adequately powered with a sufficient number of participants in each group to clearly identify both the efficacy and the safety of a new vaccine. The second point is that it is easy to assume that a side effect is due to the vaccine. Popular opinion may be that vaccines cause itching, but until a sufficient sample size is studied, and the statistics confirm that, a difference could be found, one should not assume that a side effect is definitely related to the vaccine.

Vaccines have been attributed to the development of many long-term illnesses, including autism, encephalitis, autoimmunity, and others. Data establishing these associations can only be based on the thoroughness of the reports received and analyzed from subjects who develop problems. Unbiased, prospective trials to detect true associations are impractical and unlikely, given the rarity of the events. This discussion does,

[1] Hanslik, Boelle, *Med Sci [Paris]* 2007; 23(4): 391–398.

however, illustrate the caution one must use in coming to conclusions about events that occur in subjects who also received vaccines, versus events that resulted from receiving vaccines.

Vaccine Efficacy

In addition to safety, establishing vaccine efficacy requires knowledge of the epidemiology of the disease to be prevented. Ideally, efficacy is expressed as a reduction in the incidence of the disease in vaccinated subjects as compared with the unvaccinated population. But the epidemiology of the disease includes more than just knowledge of incidence and prevalence. Other factors that can influence when, how frequently and in whom a disease occurs include climate factors, migration of species that may be vectors (carriers) of the disease, exposure patterns that are altered by current events, underlying health issues common in older age, and many other factors. This is why vaccine studies try to limit the population studied to those in whom other factors are not present, but that clearly limits our ability to predict how effective (and safe) the vaccine will be when it is used in the general public.

■ United States Initiative: The Vaccine Adverse Events Reporting System

Given the limitations of even large clinical trials, described above, it is clear that far more is learned about the safety and efficacy of a new vaccine (and a new drug as well) after it has been marketed for use in the general population. However, outside of the strict mandates of clinical trial data gathering, reporting of adverse events by the public is more or less voluntary. Note that reporting of certain suspected reactions is mandatory for healthcare providers in the US (see below). In response to the dire need to understand the safety of vaccines in populations with a large variety of features, the Vaccine Adverse Event Reporting System (VAERS) was established.

VAERS is the post-marketing safety surveillance program created by the Centers for Disease Control and Prevention (CDC) and the US Food and Drug Administration (FDA) for vaccine safety in response to the National Childhood Vaccine Injury Act (NCVIA) of 1986. This law requires health professionals and vaccine manufacturers to report to the Department of Health and Human Services (HHS), of which both CDC and FDA are divisions, specific adverse events that occur following vaccine administration. The objectives of the program are as follows:

- To detect new, unusual, or rare adverse events associated with vaccine administration;
- To monitor increases in the incidence of known adverse events;
- To identify potential patient-associated risk factors that may pre-dispose individuals to vaccine associated adverse events;
- To identify vaccine lots that may be associated with an unusually high rate of adverse events;
- To assess the safety of newly licensed vaccines in large diverse populations once they have been released to market.

Just as with any medical product, anyone can report an adverse event to VAERS, including patients and health professionals. The system is a passive surveillance program, which means that it suffers from several limitations, including the following:

- Underreporting of adverse events;
- Differential reporting, which is a pattern of increased reporting when a vaccine is new that falls off with time;
- Stimulated reporting, which occurs when a new adverse event is first recognized and a flurry of similar or alleged events are then reported (perhaps after media attention);
- Coincidental events, which occurs when an unrelated temporal event is reported as being associated with receipt of a vaccine;
- Poor data quality, with a great deal of missing information and lack of patient follow-up; and

- Lack of denominator data, when information on the number of doses of a vaccine administered in the population is not available.

Nevertheless, approximately 30,000 adverse events are reported to VAERS annually, of which only about 10–15% are serious, i.e., associated with disability, hospitalization, life-threatening illnesses, or death.

GACVS and the European Commission

The Global Advisory Committee on Vaccine Safety (GACVS) was established by the World Health Organization (WHO) to address issues of vaccine safety throughout Europe. They established directives around two general issues regarding Adverse Events Following Immunization (AEFI). The first issue is monitoring vaccine safety. The committee called for prompt data transmission by member countries, assurance of data quality, and the processing and analysis of data for timely signal detection and implementation of action as required.

The second issue focuses on using data collected for detailed examination of pressing questions that affect the efficacy of vaccination programs. This includes an understanding of the safety of excipients, e.g., preservatives and other "inert" ingredients used in manufacturing and formulating vaccines. Excipients also include adjuvants, stabilizers, and residuals, such as formaldehyde, toxins, viral growth media substrates or sub-cellular particles, and vectors.[2]

Preventing loss of confidence in vaccine programs is a major objective of understanding their safety. Lack of immunization and subsequent risk of disease has generally proved to be of far greater risk than risk of toxicity from either the antigenic or the non-antigenic materials in vaccines. If an appropriate proportion of the population is not immunized, there is a risk of losing "herd immunity". Herd immunity is the resistance to spread of an infectious disease in a population. The level of vaccination needed to achieve herd immunity varies by disease and is affected by other factors (vaccines.gov).

GACVS has worked with manufacturers to analyze detailed information concerning complexity of the vaccine formulation and manufacturing processes, storage and handling processes, administration procedures, and host-related factors. Other researchers have also analyzed their institutional databases to identify antigenic and non-antigenic components that could be specifically associated with vaccine-associated adverse events, e.g., risk of anaphylaxis or Guillain–Barré syndrome after influenza immunization.[3] Issues related to specific vaccines have become major subjects of study for GACVS in answer to their mission of vaccine safety and public protection. For example, understanding the association between the genetic characteristics of mumps vaccines and their association with neurovirulence has resulted in the development of more precise and consistent neurovirulence assays.[4]

These maybe particularly important in understanding the potential of specific strains of a vaccine to cause aseptic meningitis. Another example has been identifying specific strains of BCG, the vaccine for tuberculosis (TB), that cause systemic infections, termed BCGosis/BCGitis in young children and infants who are immunocompromised.[5]

The European Commission and the World Health Organization (WHO) have initiated several programs to set standards for immunization programs, their monitoring, and collaboration of concerned stakeholders on various aspects of vaccine safety. For example, The

[2] Lankinin, Pastila, Kilpi, *et al.*, *Bull World Health Organ* 2004; 82(11): 811–890.

[3] Nakayama T, Onoda K, Vaccine events reported in post-marketing study of the Kitisato Institute from 1994–2004, *Vaccine* 2007; 25(3): 570–576.

[4] Rubin SA, Afzal MA, Powell CL, Bentley ML, Auda GR, Taffs RE, Carbone KM, The rat-based neurovirulence safety test for the assessment of mumps virus neurovirulence in humans: an international collaborative study, *J Infect Dis* 2005; 191(7): 1123–1128, doi: 10.1086/428098.

[5] Ying, W, Sun J, Liu D, Hui X, Yu Y, Wang J, Wang X, Clinical characteristics and immunogenetics of BCGosis/BCGitis in Chinese children: A 6 year follow-up study, *PLoS ONE* 2014; 9(4): e94485, https://doi.org/10.1371/journal.pone.0094485.

European Centre for Disease Prevention and Control (ECDC) was established in Solna, Sweden, as an agency of the EU (www.ecdc.europa.eu/). ECDC focuses on three strategic areas: (a) It supports evidence-based decision-making within its remit; (b) It strengthens public health systems; and (c) It supports the response to public health threats. A key activity has been to improve influenza immunizations across the EEA, particularly in sub-populations that are at high risk of complications from influenza. To provide ECDC with reliable data on vaccination coverage in the EEA, a European VAccination COverage Collection System (EVACO) was established. EVACO data are used to assess relevant phenomena that affect vaccination campaigns and to verify correlations with outbreaks of infectious diseases.

The Vaccine European New Integrated Collaboration Effort (VENICE) was formed in 2006 to collect, share, and disseminate knowledge and best practice in the field of vaccination through a network of European experts (venice.cenica.org). This program is funded mostly by the ECDC, partly by the European Commission, and is renewable periodically, e.g., VENICE I (2006–2008), VENICE II (2009–2013), VENICE III (2013–2017). The VENICE network migrated into an official ECDC Vaccine Preventable Diseases network, with experts appointed by the Competent Bodies of each member state. This remains only part of a wider EU network on vaccine safety.

The WHO operates a post-marketing safety database, VigiBase, that includes vaccine case reports. VigiBase is housed and is operated by a WHO Collaborating Center, the Uppsala Monitoring Center, located in Uppsala, Sweden. WHO also coordinates a Vaccine Safety Net and the following provides a link to a list of vaccine safety web sites: http://www.who.int/immunization_safety/safety_quality/approved_vaccine_safety_websites/en/index.html.

These programs extend to special target populations identified for enhanced attention. At the outset, the objective was to evaluate all aspects of immunization programs, including planning, administration, funding, and monitoring. Special populations targeted included immigrants, especially illegal immigrants who easily escape the healthcare system and frequently carry new strains of disease across borders; refugees, who are not covered by legislation; military recruits and staff, who may cross in and out of foreign countries and who routinely receive as many as 18 different immunizations; occupational risk groups, such as prison workers and healthcare professionals; and travelers.

Vaccine Adverse Event Reporting

The value of post-marketing vaccinovigilance as the key to understanding the role of vaccines in protecting individuals from contracting disease and protecting communities from the spread of disease is clear. The differences inherent in studying a vaccine in otherwise healthy patients in clinical trials and learning about vaccines when they are delivered widespread in a population make it imperative that effective vaccinovigilance systems are established and maintained.[6] VAERS and the European MedDRA-based databases are essential for tracking, documenting, and elucidating safety signals in complex settings, but are only as good as the data that enter the system. Through multiple websites, such as FDA, EMA, CDC, UMC, and others, data can be entered by anyone familiar with an adverse event that occurs in association with a vaccine. The following list can be used as a guideline for information that should be gathered before accessing these websites so that information will be as complete and as reliable as possible.

Information Checklist for Vaccine Adverse Event Reporting:

- Case description (case narrative);
- Patient age;
- Patient medical history;
- Time interval from receipt of vaccine to adverse event;
- Trade name of vaccine;
- Lot number of vaccine dose;
- Dosage administered;
- Date of administration;
- Vaccination site/route of administration;
- Concomitant vaccines administered;

[6] Mayans, Robertson, Duclos, *Bull World Health Organ* 2000; 78(9): 1167.

- Concomitant medications taken;
- Rechallenge data if patients have had this or other vaccines before;
- Outcome information.

In the United States, AEs to vaccines should be reported to the FDA. Full reporting information is available on the FDA and CDC websites. Voluntary reports may be submitted online, by email, or by regular mail. Knowingly filing a false report to VAERS is a violation of federal law (18 U.S. Code § 1001) and is punishable by fine or imprisonment or both.

European Union System

It is also useful to recognize what the European system has classified as Adverse Events of Special Interest (AESI), which are believed to be particularly significant as potentially serious adverse events that may be associated with vaccine administration.[7] The AESI include the following:

- Neuritis;
- Convulsions;
- Severe allergic or anaphylactic reactions;
- Syncope;
- Encephalitis;
- Thrombocytopenia;
- Vasculitis;
- Guillain-Barré syndrome;
- Bell's palsy.

Further information concerning vaccine adverse events, data about relatedness of particular adverse events associated with vaccines, and links for reporting adverse events are offered in the following section.

Sources of Additional Information

Useful links can be found at the websites for FDA, CDC, WHO (see above), National Institutes of Health, and HHS. Other useful sources of information include the following:

- Immunization Action Coalition;
- Clinicaltrials.gov: Vaccine Adverse Reactions;
- Institute for Vaccine Safety (Johns Hopkins University School of Public Health);
- National Network for Immunization Information (NNii);
- VAERS.

The last two sites are particularly useful for submitting reports to VAERS.

In the European Union, the EMA's Vaccine Working Party (VWP) was established to provide recommendations to the Committee for Medicinal Products for Human Use (CHMP) on all matters relating directly or indirectly to vaccines.

The VWP's tasks include the following:

- Preparing, reviewing, and updating guidelines to ensure that vaccine-specific issues are fully addressed;
- Supporting dossier evaluation of new Marketing Authorization applications for vaccines and of any post-marketing submission (e.g., variations, follow-up measures);
- Providing to the CHMP and European Commission scientific advice on general and product-specific matters relating to the pharmaceutical and biological aspects of vaccines, as well as the development and clinical use of vaccines in children and adults;
- Liaising with interested parties (e.g., trade organizations, pharmaceutical industry, academia, and patients' organizations);
- European cooperation on vaccine-specific issues;
- International cooperation, for example with the WHO;
- Contributing to and organizing vaccine-related workshops and training;
- On request of the CHMP, constituting a rapid-acting crisis group to take on board-specific issues relating to vaccines, with the objective of exchanging information at the European level and of coordinating responses to the public in a timely manner, for example in relation to an influenza pandemic, vaccines for emerging or reemerging diseases

[7] Greenberg, *et al.*, *New Engl J Med* 2009; 361(25): 2405–2413.

(including against pathogens potentially used for bioterrorism), and other public health issues;

- Supporting the conduct of vaccine-specific epidemiological studies;
- Supporting the implementation of the Vaccine Identification Standards Initiative (VISI) for recording vaccine usage at the European level to ensure effective pharmacovigilance activities and to facilitate epidemiological investigations;
- Monitoring the development of new vaccine technologies (e.g., DNA-based vaccines, cancer vaccines, AIDS vaccines) and the development of new adjuvants;
- Monitoring and providing input for developing new centralized vaccines, with a view to gradually fostering harmonization of immunization schedules in such a way that flexibility is maintained for local, specific public health needs;
- In the United Kingdom, the MHRA monitors vaccine safety as they do drugs. See their website.

In Canada, the Public Health Agency of Canada handles vaccine safety. They have established the Canadian Adverse Events Following Immunization Surveillance System (CAEFISS). See their website for further information on submission of AEFI.

CHAPTER

47

Real-World Issues: Case Studies

Introduction

Many who are not in pharmacovigilance struggle to understand the purpose of the activities described in this textbook. When we, as safety scientists, step back to look at the mission of product development, it almost always includes attempts to ensure patient safety and efficacy without creating additional or undo harm: "Primum Non Nocere". Agencies such as the EMA and FDA continuously evaluate the received data for potential safety concerns. In this chapter we review historical product effects and their influence on the evolution of laws and practices of today.

Ongoing Activities

FDA publishes a new list of potential signals of serious risks/new safety information identified each quarter in accordance with Title IX, Section 921 of the Food and Drug Administration Amendments Act of 2007.

Title IX, Section 921 of the Food and Drug Administration Amendments Act 2007 (FDAAA) (121 Stat. 962) amends the Federal Food, Drug and Cosmetic Act (FDCA) to add a new subsection (k)(5) to section 505 (21 U.S.C. 355). This section in FDAAA, directs FDA to "conduct regular, bi-weekly screening of the Adverse Event Reporting System (now called FAERS) database and post a quarterly report on the Adverse Event Reporting System Web site of any new safety information or potential signal of a serious risk identified by Adverse Event Reporting System within the last quarter." When a potential signal of a serious risk is identified from AERS data, it will be posted in the required report in the quarter in which it is first identified. A potential signal of a serious risk may in some cases constitute new safety information as defined in FDAAA (newly created section 505-1(b)(3) of the FDCA) which includes, among other things, information derived from adverse event reports about a serious risk associated with use of a drug that FDA has become aware of, since the drug was approved or, for drugs that have REMS, since the REMS was required or last assessed. FDA will post each potential signal of a serious risk in the quarter in which it is first identified. If additional new safety information is developed concerning a potential signal that has already been posted, it will be addressed by FDA in new safety communications but will not appear again as a new quarterly posting.

As companies continue to develop and monitor their products in market, it is wise for safety & pharmacovigilance professionals to maintain awareness of the agency's ongoing evaluations and efforts and have a process in place to continuously monitor their own safety data along with them.

Case Studies

Throughout the course of drug development, there are several case studies which illustrate the importance and outcome of pharmacovigilance and the ongoing evaluation of these products once on the market. The cases outlined within are historical examples, it would be wise for those who have interest in learning from historical challenges to find a way to stay abreast of product recalls or withdrawals.

Fialuridine

Fialuridine (FIAU) was a drug used to treat hepatitis B virus (HBV) in the early 1990s. Its use in one clinical trial in particular produced seven cases of severe hepatic toxicity (including five deaths) in 15 patients. This trial produced major fallout in the world of clinical research in the United States. The events are briefly reviewed here, and a few comments are made in regard to the drug safety aspects of the study.

FIAU is a pyrimidine nucleoside analogue that was believed to be a promising treatment for HBV patients. It had previously been studied in a major cancer hospital against other viral infections, including cytomegalovirus (CMV) and various herpes viruses, with some promising results. Animal studies revealed vomiting, diarrhea, mild cardiac toxicity at high doses, and bone marrow toxicity. No liver toxicity was noted in any of the standard animal models (rat, mouse, and monkey).

In 1989, a small pharmaceutical company, together with the National Institutes of Allergy and Infectious Diseases, did a phase I/II dose escalation trial in human immunodeficiency virus (HIV) patients with positive CMV cultures using fiacitabine (FIAU is an active metabolite of fiacitabine). The study of 12 patients did not show an effect on CMV. Adverse events (AEs) reported were nausea, fatigue, and an increased creatine phosphokinase in one patient. No subject died during the study. However, follow-up revealed four deaths, including one subject who had hepatitis B about 6 months after the end of the study. His death was believed to be due to the underlying hepatitis and other hepatotoxic medications he was taking.

In 1990, a short-term treatment (2 weeks) study of FIAU was done on HIV patients. During the study, it became clear that there was a potential, possibly significant effect on HBV, but probably little CMV efficacy. The protocol was amended to allow HBV patients to be enrolled. Investigators at the National Institutes of Health (NIH) joined the study team. Significant decreases in HBV DNA were noted. Some patients also developed doubling or tripling of serum transaminase levels. It was unclear whether the transaminase elevations were AEs due to the drug or due to the so-called flare phenomenon of elevated transaminases seen when HBV viremia drops with other drug treatment (e.g., interferon).

In 1991, the positive results from this trial led to a trial of 4 weeks of FIAU therapy in HBV-positive patients. The trial showed excellent results in groups receiving the highest dosages, with major reductions in HBV DNA. No AEs producing dropout or dose modification occurred. "Flares" and HBV DNA rebound were noted in several subjects, but three of nine subjects had continued suppression of HBV DNA, normal liver tests, and were HBV-antigen negative. One subject developed abdominal pain (but with normal liver and pancreas tests) that resolved 4 months after the trial. One subject was diagnosed with cholelithiasis, and another had an episode of peripheral neuropathy. One subject died. He had chronic hepatitis B and had a good result with FIAU in the trial as judged by his HBV DNA level. He had nausea and fatigue during the trial. One month after the last dose of FIAU, his transaminase was noted to be four times normal, and he complained of nausea, fatigue, and abdominal pain. A non-study physician recommended cholecystectomy, which was done under general anesthesia. Liver biopsy revealed chronic active hepatitis and steatosis. He deteriorated after surgery and died a few months later. An autopsy revealed steatosis. At the time, his death was attributed primarily to the anesthesia drugs administered.

On the basis of these results, the NIH and Eli Lilly (now developing the drug) began a study in 1993 of carefully selected hepatitis B subjects with a planned treatment period of 6 months of FIAU. Within the first few weeks of the study start, some subjects complained of fatigue, nausea, cramps, and diarrhea. Some subjects had dose interruption. No abnormal laboratory tests were noted. However, all subjects had decreases in HBV DNA, and 6 of 10 became HBV DNA negative. The data were reviewed at about 6 weeks into the trial, and because of the encouraging results, the investigators opted to continue.

A few days later, one subject, who had discontinued the drug two weeks previously, presented to an emergency room with nausea, weakness, and hypotension. The transaminases were normal, but the bilirubin and lactic acid levels were elevated. The subject went on to develop liver and renal failure and died, despite liver transplantation. The autopsy revealed pancreatitis, glomerulonephritis, esophageal varices, and pneumonia. The liver showed micro- and macro-vascular steatosis, cholestasis, and chronic active hepatitis.

Within 2 or 3 days of the subject's first showing up at the emergency room, the study was stopped, and all subjects still on FIAU were told to stop the drug. All subjects (n = 15) were admitted to the NIH Clinical Center for observation. Despite stopping the drug, seven subjects developed hepatic failure, pancreatitis, neuropathy, and myopathy and were to have liver transplantation. Five died (some after transplantation) and two survived. Eight of the 15 subjects had no AEs.

As a result of this disaster, several inquiries were set up. The US Food and Drug Administration (FDA) established an internal task force and issued a report in November 1993. It was believed that there were many episodes of "missed toxicity" and that the AEs were inappropriately attributed to the disease under study rather than to the investigational drug. The task force also felt that the informed consents and the study monitoring and oversight were not adequate. The FDA issued warning letters to the investigators charging, among other things, failure to immediately report serious AEs to the sponsor and institutional review boards, failure to reduce or terminate dosing in subjects with moderate toxicity, failure to describe all foreseeable risks in the informed consent, failure to follow-up on serious AEs, failure to include complete and accurate safety data in the investigator brochure, and failure to adequately monitor by not ensuring that all AEs were reported in the case report forms.

Subsequently, the NIH did its own investigation and concluded that the rationale for the studies was strong, especially in light of the lack of other (oral) therapy for the disease in question. The NIH sent in an inspection team. They concluded that the protocols were "meticulously" prepared and implemented and that fatal outcomes could not have been predicted from the AEs. They also determined that the AEs were adequately reported. Thus, NIH and the FDA investigations reached opposite conclusions!

Next, an investigation was done by the Institute of Medicine (IOM) at the request of the Secretary of Health and Human Services, the US government agency that has direct oversight of FDA. The IOM, a private, non-profit, non-governmental organization, is part of the US National Academy of Sciences. Its review largely agreed with that of the NIH. It concluded that excellent attention was paid to safety monitoring and that there were no significant violations of study conduct or informed consent. They concluded that rapid action to stop the study actually saved lives and prevented an even worse tragedy.

These events were extensively discussed and criticized. Press coverage was vivid and lurid, and a congressional investigation in 1994 occurred with strong charges thrown about. Further work revealed that the FIAU toxicity was due to mitochondrial damage by the drug.

Much has occurred since then in regard to tightening and harmonizing regulations and clinical trial oversight. It is not the intent here to review the issues in clinical trial regulation, oversight and monitoring, or politics. Instead, the drug safety implications are discussed.

- Serious and non-serious AEs due to (study or marketed) drugs may occur that mimic the disease being treated. The implications of this are important.

  It is not adequate to attribute serious AEs to the disease or condition being treated, background medical conditions, intercurrent problems, or other non-drug causes without a careful consideration of a possible drug-related etiology. A very high level of suspicion that the drug produced the serious AE must be maintained at all times when evaluating whether a drug has produced a particular AE. The drug is not "innocent until proven guilty".
- Clinical trial safety oversight by the sponsor (company) and the investigator must be "meticulous". All regulatory requirements (protocol design, investigator qualification, AE collection, reporting and review, consent forms, institutional review board oversight, safety data review committees, etc.) must be followed strictly and completely.
- A data safety plan (risk management) must be drawn up and in place before the study starts. This concept is embodied in the US FDA's IND reporting regulation and associated guidance documents.
- Pre-study signals (from animal data or other clinical trials or class drugs) must be considered and addressed carefully.
- Investigator (and sponsor and monitor) training must be done before the study starts and during the study if new personnel become involved. The training should be of high quality, customized to the study, and done by a training specialist (not simply printed material).
- A sponsor physician must be designated as clearly in charge of the ongoing safety review. Qualified institutional review boards with high-quality experienced personnel who have sufficient time to review safety data must be used. Sponsors and investigators must supply the institutional review boards with easily reviewable data sent at frequent periods, as agreed by the boards.
- Companies and institutions doing clinical trials must have a crisis management plan in place to do a preliminary investigation and to take appropriate actions on critical safety issues within a few hours.
- Larger political and governmental solutions should also be considered (presumably they are), including full-time dedicated national safety monitoring committees, a separate safety organization within the federal government, involvement of academia in ongoing safety monitoring (as in France), limitation of proprietary secrets, an AE reporting system in a federal database for clinical trial AEs combining the safety efforts put into case report form safety reporting with those for regulatory serious AE reporting (this refers to duplication of reporting in clinical trials: to the drug safety group and in the case report form), continued research into trend analysis and early signaling, and so on.[1]

Fen–Phen

What is now called the "fen–phen" issue refers to the combination of fenfluramine and phentermine used for weight control. Both products had long been approved as single agents (in 1973 and 1959, respectively) by the US Food and Drug Administration (FDA) as appetite suppressants.

Reports in the literature of pulmonary hypertension and fenfluramine appeared in the 1980s and 1990s. Reports of headache, insomnia, nervousness, irritability, palpitations, tachycardia, and elevations in blood pressure were seen with phentermine. Few long-term data were available for the use of these drugs at the time.

The combination of fenfluramine and phentermine was never approved by the FDA, and their use in combination was "off-label". However, millions of prescriptions for their use were written.[2]

After this increased use, reports of toxicity started to appear. One report cited the death of a 29-year-old

[1] See an excellent review on the FIAU safety issues: Nickas J, Clinical trial safety surveillance in the new regulatory and harmonization environment: lessons learned from the "Fialuridine crisis", *Drug Inform J* 1997; 31: 63–70. An excellent review of the situation is available: Saag M, A review of the FIAU tragedy and its effect on clinical research. *J Clin Res Practice*. 1999; 1: 21–32. Also see the IOM report: Manning FJ, Swartz M, eds. *Review of the Fialuridine (FIAU) Clinical Trials. Committee to Review the Fialuridine (FIAU/FIAC) Clinical Trials.* Division of Health Sciences Policy, Institute of Medicine. Washington, DC: National Academy Press, 1995.

[2] Diet pills redux [editorial]. *N Engl J Med*. 1997; 337: 629–630.

woman after only 23 days of the combination.[3] Also in 1997, the Mayo Clinic reported 24 women who developed valvular heart disease (mitral, aortic, and tricuspid, sometimes more than one valve) after a mean of 12 months of combination therapy (with one woman using the drugs for only 1 month). One third had pulmonary hypertension, and several required valve surgery.[4] Valvular disease with only fenfluramine or only dexfenfluramine was also reported.

By November 1997, the Centers for Disease Control and Prevention reported 144 spontaneous cases of fenfluramine or dexfenfluramine with or without phentermine producing valvular disease. Reports of abnormal echocardiograms in fen-phen or dexfenphen patients were received by the FDA. They noted 30% abnormal echocardiograms in 291 asymptomatic screened patients, primarily with aortic regurgitation. Many of the patients were women.

Fenfluramine and dexfenfluramine were withdrawn from the market in late 1997. Phentermine was not withdrawn because no cases were reported to the FDA with this drug alone (as of September 1997).

The FDA noted in its Q&A of September 1997 that because valve disease is not usually associated with drug use, it was not screened for in patients and no cases were detected in 500 patients in a 1-year clinical trial. It noted that the link between symptoms and drug use was not "obvious". In addition, there were few animal data to suggest this toxicity, and early on most patients and physicians did not give too much thought to pulmonary or pulmonary toxicity with these drugs.

After this publicity, not surprisingly, many new cases were noted and lawsuits were filed. In October 1999, the manufacturer agreed to a class action settlement of up to $4.75 billion. A trust was established by the manufacturer by order of the US District Court to administer the claims and payments of benefits to registered class members, providing for benefits including refunds for the costs of Pondimin and Redux, medical monitoring and some medical treatment or payment for monitoring and treatment, and compensation for specifically defined valvular heart conditions. Several safety lessons were learned:

- Untested combinations of approved products may be quite dangerous even if the individual products are not — and especially if the individual products have a safety concern or even of a hint of one.
- Old products are not always "well known" or completely studied.
- Old safety lessons or safety clues may be minimized or forgotten.
- Unintended consequences (AEs) may occur at any time in an unexpected organ system or patient.
- Dose matters. But sometimes it does not.
- "Absence of evidence is not evidence of absence". That is, just because there is no finding of a particular AE or disease in clinical trials or patients treated with a drug does not mean that it was sought. And if it was sought, it might not have been sought in the right patients at the right time with the proper diagnostic tools, tests, or case definition.
- Companies, physicians, and regulators should be very careful about off-label use, and better ways to monitor their effects need to be developed. There are many valid medical reasons for certain off-label uses, especially in oncology, but extreme care must be exercised, particularly when there is no clear clinical or scientific basis for such use.
- Intelligent and clever clinicians can still discover serious drug-related AEs in the course of their daily practice. Such serious AEs should indeed be reported to the health authority or company.
- Drug usage, when popular and extrapolated to the populations of North America, Europe, Japan, and elsewhere, can produce enormous benefits to individuals, healthcare practitioners, and society. It can also produce major disasters.

Nomifensine

Nomifensine (Merital®) was first used as an antidepressant in Germany in 1976, in the United Kingdom in 1977, and in the United States in 1985. From 1978 to 1985, some 165,000 to 251,000 prescriptions were

[3] Mark, Patalas, Chang, *et al.*, *N Engl J Med* 1997; 337: 602–606.
[4] Connolly, Crary, McGoon, *et al.*, *N Engl J Med* 1997; 337: 635.

written each year. Between 1978 and 1979, the manufacturer received four reports of hemolytic anemia. A case report was published in the medical literature in 1979. From 1981 to 1982, three more cases in the United Kingdom were reported. From 1979 to 1980, the company did immunologic studies of some 300 patients. In 1981, the United Kingdom labeling was changed to indicate that rare cases of hemolytic anemia were reported.

At that time, the labeling also stated that rare cases of liver enzyme elevation were noted. In the 1980s, the use of nomifensine increased, and by 1986, 296 AE reports were received by the manufacturer, including 16 positive Coombs tests and 45 hemolytic anemias, as well as 27 jaundice reports, 12 abnormal liver function tests, six hepatitis reports, and one hepatic necrosis report. The first United Kingdom fatalities were reported in 1985. Further case reports were published from 1980 to 1985, noting hemolytic anemia (with and without renal failure), thrombocytopenia, hepatitis, fatal alveolitis (a systemic lupus erythematosus-like fatal reaction), and fatal immune hemolysis. By June 1985, the estimated incidence of hemolytic anemia was one in 20,000. Further reports were received, and by November, the estimated rate was one in 4,000.

"Dear Doctor" letters were sent out in 1985 in the United Kingdom, and the drug was withdrawn from all worldwide markets in January 1986.[5]

During this time (late 1970s to the 1980s), the state of drug safety and pharmacovigilance reporting was markedly different from today. The ICH, European Medicines Agency, and MedWatch were not yet in existence, and many countries had disparate or non-rigorous AE reporting systems.

The drug was approved by the US FDA in 1984 (after some 6 years reviewing the dossier), and marketing began in the United States in July 1985. Up to 10,000,000 patients were exposed to the drug by then. The drug was withdrawn from all markets (including the United States) in January 1986.

In the United States, the question then arose regarding how the FDA could have approved the product and then permitted marketing while the crescendo of cases was building up, especially in 1984–1985. Hearings in the US House of Representatives (Congress) were held in early 1986, and the FDA launched an investigation in August 1986.

A summary report was issued by the FDA (Kurtzweil, FDA Consumer, September 1991, p. 42). The FDA investigation revealed that two deaths, an Italian in 1980 and a French woman in 1984 (before the approval in the United States), were known to the company but not reported to the FDA until 1986, months after the drug was withdrawn from the market. Nine other deaths, including three in the United States, also occurred. As the FDA notes in its report: "The investigation, which lasted a year and a half, was lengthy because officials of the US company refused to allow personnel who had been directly involved in analyzing and reporting adverse drug reactions to speak to FDA investigators. In addition, months often passed before they provided written answers to investigators' questions."

The FDA was able to gather evidence showing that the company, Hoechst AG in Germany, and a former medical director of the clinical research division "had been aware of the deaths of the two European women shortly after they had occurred but had failed to report them to FDA as required." The FDA found no evidence that the US division of the company (Hoechst-Roussel) had withheld information from the FDA. In December 1990, the US federal attorney in New Jersey charged Hoechst AG and the medical director by name with failing to report the two European deaths. No charges were filed against Hoechst-Roussel. In April 1991, Hoechst AG and the medical director pleaded guilty to the charges and were fined the maximum amount allowed by law. Nomifensine became something of a worldwide cause *célèbre*.

Several safety lessons were underscored:

- Always do the right thing;
- Do not withhold safety data from the FDA and other health authorities;
- The company should speak with one voice and say the same (correct) thing to all health authorities at the same time;
- Report all data in a proper and timely manner and document it with meticulously kept records;

---

[5] Stonier, *Pharmacoepidemiology Drug Safety* 2002; 1: 177–185; Stonier, Edwards, Nomifensine and haemolytic anemia, *Pharmacovigilance* (Wiley, Hoboken, NJ, 2002).

- Proper written procedures must be in place to ensure that all safety data are reported to all branches of the company (especially multinational companies) that need these data. The company should perform periodic internal audits to ensure that this is happening. Any deficiencies should be remedied immediately, and data that should have been reported must be reported to the health authorities as soon as the issue is discovered (painful though this may be);
- Cooperate fully with all health authority investigations;
- The senior officers of the company must understand the significance of the drug safety function and put their full weight, support, and resources into ensuring that safety is done correctly;
- Maintain a high index of suspicion that AEs may be due to the drug and not to other causes;
- Physicians and those in positions of senior responsibility in the company should be aware that they may be held personally liable (criminally and civilly) if they do not do their safety duties; and
- Ensure that safety information is reported to the health authorities as required before, during, and after Marketing Authorization submission and approval.

TGN-1412/TAB08

TGN-1412 is a monoclonal antibody that is a strong agonist for the CD 28 receptor expressed by T cells. It was originally developed in a German university. It was felt that it might be useful in preferentially activating "regulatory T cells" to act as an immunomodulator for treatment of autoimmune diseases. A company was created and they developed a "humanized" antibody for use in clinical trials. It was tested in cynomologus monkeys, which have a CD 28 receptor homologous to the human receptor. Testing in monkeys showed no serious AEs. The question of whether TGN-1412 was specific to the CD 28 receptor and whether it might also stimulate other T cells producing unexpected consequences was unclear.

In March 2006, six healthy male volunteers received the TGN-1412 antibody and two healthy male volunteers received placebo in a clinical research unit in the UK. Within an hour of the infusion, several of the TGN-1412 treated subjects complained of nausea, headache and severe lumbar (back) pain. Over the next several hours, hypotension, tachycardia, fever, lymphopenia and monocytopenia occurred in the TGN subjects. Shortly thereafter multi-organ failure, including lungs and kidneys, occurred. They were hospitalized. Neither of the placebo subjects became ill. It was not totally clear how these subjects should be treated. Nevertheless, all of the 6 men survived though there were permanent disabilities including necrotic fingers and toes that required some amputations. The reaction was determined to be a "cytokine storm" — the release of pro-inflammatory cytokines. Evidently, TGN-1412 was not as specific as originally thought. The early results were published in a *New England Journal of Medicine* article. See http://www.nejm.org/doi/full/10.1056/NEJMoa063842#t=article.

A UK government-established commission investigated and found that all regulatory requirements were met. Others noted, though, that not all of the preclinical data was made available to the health authorities and that clinical trials with similar antibodies did activate T cells leading to cytokine storm.

The starting dose was also analyzed. It was found that the chosen starting dose, though hundreds of times lower than the "safe" dose in the monkeys, was still high enough to cause about 90% of all CD 28 receptors in man to be occupied by TNG-1412 antibodies which can lead to a cytokine storm. It also seems that studies of other antibodies by other companies used a starting dose that allows for a receptor occupancy of no more than 10% — much lower than in this study. So, using this criterion, the starting dose was much too high. Other researchers also discovered that monkeys, unlike humans, can lose their CD 28 receptors in certain conditions, thus, preventing the activation of these T cells. So the monkeys' T cells could not be activated but the humans' could be and, indeed, were activated. Many other publications followed summarizing the subsequent work. See, for example, https://www.ncbi.nlm.nih.gov/pmc/articles/PMC2964774/.

This was indeed a phase one disaster that involved drug safety. However, TGN-1412 was not finished in spite of the tragedy that occurred. In 2006 a Russian investor acquired the rights to TGN-1412 and renamed it TAB08. A Russian company continued the development of the drug. Further lab research on the drug elsewhere resulted in the development of an *in vitro* test to determine the effect of TAB08 on T cells. This, plus the work that showed that human CD4+ effector memory T cells retain their CD 28 receptors (unlike the monkeys which lose them), allowed more precise evaluation of TAB08 for use in clinical trials. This information was not available during the original study.

A new clinical trial was started in Russia in healthy human volunteers. A much lower starting dose was used which would bind only 1% of the CD 28 receptors (unlike the 90% binding in the first study). Dose elevation was also done with smaller increments and the subjects were very closely monitored. No serious AEs were noted and the study results were published which showed that these low doses selectively activated regulatory T cells but not the inflammation producing T cells — exactly the result desired. See https://www.ncbi.nlm.nih.gov/pubmed/24374661 and https://www.clinexprheumatol.org/article.asp?a=10866.

Additional studies were designed. A phase I PK and tolerability study was done without evident safety issues. A multi-center phase II trial in rheumatoid arthritis patients in whom methotrexate was not effective, as well as studies in psoriasis vulgaris, solid neoplasms, and systemic lupus erythematosis (SLE) were conducted.

An editorial summarizing the TGN1412/TAB08 story as of 2015 was published in the *British Journal of Clinical Pharmacology*.[6] The return of the prodigal son and the extraordinary development route of antibody TGN1412 — lessons for drug development and clinical pharmacology.) See https://www.ncbi.nlm.nih.gov/pmc/articles/PMC4386939/.

So what lessons can be drawn from this?

Well, the first is fairly obvious. Testing new drugs, particularly the first in humans, is a risky business. Detailed preparatory work before going into humans must be done. This includes animal, *in vitro*, and clinical pharmacology work.

The first dose and doses of the new drug must be done under tight, carefully monitored conditions — ideally as an "in-patient" where safety, rather than efficacy, is the primary concern.

The second lesson is for the drug safety personnel both in the phase I unit and in the Drug Safety unit. Careful attention must be paid to both serious and non-serious AEs in all subjects.

FDA has stated that in phase I studies (normal volunteers) the likelihood of a serious AE happening by chance or due to other causes than the drug is highly unlikely. Thus, one should strongly consider that any serious AE in this setting is possibly due to the drug. This view should be emphasized for all phase I studies, i.e., all serious AEs should be handled as expedited reports (15-day reports) as the default unless there is clearly another cause for the serious AE. The threshold for concern about safety matters in phase I studies and trials should be very low. Be conservative, particularly regarding new and potentially impactful safety information early in product development.

[6] *Br J Clin Pharmacol* 2015; 79(4): 545–754, doi: 10.1111/bcp.12605.

CHAPTER

48

Medical Marijuana and Pharmacovigilance

■ Overview

There is one drug that has a unique pharmacovigilance picture in the United States: Marijuana. This section will primarily summarize the status in the US (2023) and discuss the nascent approach to pharmacovigilance for medical marijuana and touch upon recreational marijuana. The situations in a few other jurisdictions are also summarized to illustrate the lack of a harmonized approach to pharmacovigilance in this area.

Marijuana has been known and used since antiquity with reports of use dating back to 5000 BCE. It is the most commonly used illicit drug in the US with reports that roughly 1/2 of all Americans have tried it at least once (see news.gallup.com/poll/353645/nearly-half-adults-tried-marijuana.aspx

Usage is extensive in the US with reports of some 55 million Americans currently using marijuana. In addition, marijuana use during the pandemic increased in states where it is legal and in states where it is illegal. Legality varies from state to state.

Marijuana, also known as MJ, Mary Jane, bud, hash, roach, toke, weed, hashish, hemp, grass and more, is a preparation from the *Cannabis sativa* plant.

Marijuana contains about 400 chemicals of which 70 are "cannabinoids" (a chemical class that acts on cannabinoid receptors in the brain). The most notable marketed cannabinoid is tetrahydrocannabinol (THC). Cannabidiol (CBD) is another cannabinoid on the market and is reported to have fewer psychoactive effects. In the US, the Congress passed the Agriculture Improvement Act in 2018, which removed CBD from the controlled substances list (if made from hemp). However, not all states have followed suit.

Marijuana is made using leaves, flowers, stems and/or seeds. It can be used as is or as an extract of these parts of the *C. sativa*. It is used by smoking, vaporization, food, capsules, lozenges, patches sprays, etc. The potency of marijuana varies by strain, by preparation and by changes made by manufacturers and sellers.

The onset of action is nearly immediate if smoked, 30–60 minutes if eaten. Effects last 2–6 hours, it is lipid soluble and after it is metabolized can be found in blood, urine, hair, oral fluid, and sweat. A good starting reference on marijuana pharmacology can be found at https://www.ncbi.nlm.nih.gov/pmc/articles/PMC5312634/.

Concentrations of THC in flower products in the US are not standardized and vary from 1% to over 22%. Some fractions and distillates are often in the range of 50–90% THC. The products available on the market today are much more potent than those sold 10 or 20 years ago, as different hybridized cultivars varietals are now being grown, imported (legally and illegally) and sold. In the Netherlands, there actually is a standardized strain with 22% THC that has been available for over 20 years.

The quality of marijuana production is currently not standardized across the US and elsewhere. The US Pharmacopeia states: However, the lack of consistency in the quality of cannabis for medical use makes it difficult for regulators, prescribers, manufacturers, distributors, and patients/consumers to maintain confidence in the products on the market. One potentially serious health risk is the cannabis plant's ability to absorb heavy metals, many of which are known human carcinogens. A lack of consistent quality assurance can expose patients to the risk of substandard, super-potent, contaminated, or adulterated cannabis products. In many parts of the US, cannabis is available for medical use under state law. Prescribers, manufacturers and distributors — not to mention patients — are all concerned about the safety and quality of cannabis for medical use. States have adopted different approaches to oversight, but the lack of consistency may leave patients at risk. See: https://www.usp.org/dietary-supplements-herbal-medicines/cannabis

Please note that the websites listed here are up to date as of this writing but since this field is rapidly changing some may change or disappear. Please use google to find the correct URL.

■ US Federal Regulatory Action

Medical cannabis, being used as a therapy to treat medical conditions, has garnered more national attention in recent years. There are complexities associated with the use of cannabis as treatment including its administration, packaging and dispensing. Limited clinical data associated with its use, adverse health outcomes, and potential associated deaths from marijuana intoxication have contributed to challenges with its development as an approved clinical product. From a safety point of view there is no national (federal) requirement for AE/safety reporting. Some states do have requirements, but it is not clear how the states handle any AEs reported. There is no national database collecting safety data so most safety information is obtained from published journal articles, social media and such.

In the US, the regulatory status is unlike that of any other drug. Marijuana is a Schedule 1 drug (note that it is clearly defined as a drug). Schedule 1 includes "Drugs with no currently accepted medical use and a high potential for abuse. They are the most dangerous drugs of all the drug schedules with potentially severe psychological or physical dependence." Other drugs in this category include heroin, LSD, ecstasy, peyote and others. Many in and out of the medical community feel that this is not the appropriate category for marijuana. Several petitions to the Drug Enforcement Agency requesting a move of marijuana to one of the less dangerous schedules have been rejected by DEA. It may require an act of Congress to get this changed.

Marijuana use is illegal in the US and possession is a federal offense as of this writing (late 20230. Physicians cannot legally prescribe it. The US Supreme Court has held that Congress may outlaw cannabis and patients may be prosecuted even if it is legal in a specific state. The federal government has said it doesn't "target sick & dying people" but some prosecutions have occurred.

In 2013, the US Department of Justice issued a memorandum (known as the "Cole Memorandum") which basically stated that the federal government would largely take a "hands off" approach to marijuana use in states that have legalized it and "set up a strong and effective regulatory and enforcement system…for prevention of distribution of marijuana to minors, revenue from flowing to criminal enterprises, the use of marijuana activity as a front for other illegal acts, and violence or threats to public safety." In early 2018, the Cole Memorandum was rescinded by the US Department of

Justice. In late 2023, the President indicated that prior offenses for marijuana possession should be pardoned as well as requesting the Department of Health and Human Services and Attorney General to look further into changing the Category 1 DEA schedule. There has been a proposal in Congress to change this to Category 3. This has been proposed before without success. We shall see.

In 2023, additional protections were put in place to protect states, patients and other entities in states where cannabis is legal from being prosecuted by the Department of Justice (Rohrabacher-Farr Amendment). See also the FDA webpage on cannabis: https://www.fda.gov/news-events/public-health-focus/fda-regulation-cannabis-and-cannabis-derived-products-including-cannabidiol-cbd#relatedinfo.

The reason this is so important is that as of 2023 some 38 states have legalized medical marijuana and 24 have legalized recreational marijuana. Many states that have legalized medical marijuana and some that have not legalized it do allow products with CBD but not THC. Some 20 states have decriminalized marijuana.

The FDA has stated over the years that as marijuana products are not approved drugs, they cannot regulate it. The FDA has stated: "The FDA has not approved any product containing or derived from botanical marijuana for any indication. This means that the FDA has not found any such product to be safe or effective for the treatment of any disease or condition. The agency has received reports of adverse events in patients using marijuana to treat medical conditions... CBD products are also being marketed for pets and other animals. The FDA has not approved CBD for any use in animals and the concerns regarding CBD products with unproven medical claims and of unknown quality equally apply to CBD products marketed for animals. (See https://www.fda.gov/newsevents/publichealthfocus/ucm421168.htm# notapproved.) However, statements by the FDA Commissioner have indicated that FDA may take a further look at this.

Although FDA does not regulate cannabis, if adverse events are received, they are examined and entered into the FDA post-marketing safety database, FAERS. A search of that database revealed over 7500 AEs, 7200 serious and approximately 300 deaths reported as of December 31, 2022. Many of the deaths were complicated cases with potential involvement of multiple drugs.

The FDA is looking into regulation of various products that they have not previously regulated. They issued a draft guidance in June 2023 on Psychedelic Drugs: Considerations for Clinical Investigation noting that clinical trials done under an IND must meet all the safety reporting requirements plus An evaluation of psychedelic responses that occur during clinical studies should be obtained through the inclusion of validated subjective scales and through monitoring abuse-related AEs, such as euphoria, hallucinations, stimulation, and emotional lability. Abuse-related AEs are monitored and reported as a safety concern even if they are hypothesized to be associated with the therapeutic response. FDA has issued warnings to companies for illegally selling CBD products. The FDA concluded in January 2023 that the existing regulatory frameworks for foods and supplements are not appropriate for cannabidiol and will work with Congress on a new way forward.

FDA approved two synthetic THC products (Marinol (tm) and Casamet (tm) which have been on the market for several years and are approved for the nausea and vomiting seen in cancer chemotherapy and for weight loss treatment in AIDS. They are Schedule 2 drugs. In 2018, FDA approved Epidiolex (tm) which is made from cannabidiol (CBD) for two rare and serious forms of epilepsy, Lennox-Gastaut syndrome and Dravet syndrome.

The situation with CBD is also complex. Hemp-based CBD which is federally legal everywhere. However, some states of made its use conditionally legal and a few states still consider all cannabis products illegal.

The regulation of cannabis, lacking any FDA regulation, is thus left to each state. Many states, but interestingly, not all, have set up state level regulations through commissions or divisions of the state government. In some states medical use of cannabis is not regulated at all. In some states there are also local regulations at the city or county level.

Many states have set up their own systems to register growers, vendors, and manufacturers. Since physicians and other medical practitioners cannot legally prescribe marijuana, systems have been set up in each state to register medical personnel to recommend cannabis. Each state does it differently with medical "recommenders" registering, usually online. They are then permitted to recommend medical cannabis online or sometimes in writing. The systems, in many states are not in place yet or are not yet operational.

Few states have addressed the concept of adverse event reporting. Most states have addressed quality issues and problems seen with the cultivation of marijuana but have not set up systems that require the reporting of adverse events to the state, FDA or anyone else. Few states require documentation of adverse events by growers, middlemen or dispensaries.

There are thousands of dispensaries in the US though not all are registered or "legal". Some dispensaries sell only medical marijuana, some sell recreational marijuana and some sell both. Whether, after registration, a dispensary may sell both remains to be seen and will differ from state to state.

This field is dynamic and changes are occurring daily.

■ Efficacy

As noted, it is not the intent of this chapter to review efficacy. Briefly, from the National Academies of Science report referenced above, the efficacy can be briefly summarized as follows.

The data are complex and sometimes contradictory. Data are variable. For some diseases there are data from "real life use and/or clinical trials", other data are only statistical associations of efficacy without real life or trial data. The results can be briefly summarized as follows:

- *Conclusive evidence of effectiveness*: multiple sclerosis spasticity, chronic pain in adults, anti-nausea & vomiting in chemotherapy;
- *Moderate evidence*: Short-term sleep improvement with sleep apnea, fibromyalgia, chronic pain, multiple sclerosis;
- *Limited evidence*: Weight loss in AIDS/HIV, Tourette Syndrome, Anxiety disorders, Post-traumatic Stress Disorders, Dementia, Glaucoma, Depression with chronic pain or MS.

A more recent review has noted cannabis has some evidence of efficacy in neuropathic pain, cancer pain, nausea and vomiting, appetite stimulation, anxiety, spasticity (e.g. in multiple sclerosis). Conditions where evidence does not support its use include acute pain, tremor in MS, Huntington's disease, glaucoma, schizophrenia and depression. See: https://www.google.com/url?client=internal-element-cse&cx=012222452693656877933:myuumbqxnzu&q=https://doh.dc.gov/sites/default/files/dc/sites/doh/publication/attachments/Medical%2520Cannabis%2520Clinical%2520Efficacy%2520V2.pdf&sa=U&ved=2ahUKEwjAlqyimq__AhVtkmoFHRa3APcQFnoECAgQAQ&usg=AOvVaw3xt8GiP_fvgMuXUzBuEUxQ

There are multiple other disorders with no evidence one way or the other. There is evidence that cannabidiol (CBD) is effective in seizure disorders in children. There are many claims, especially in the social media world, of efficacy for many other diseases. There is, though, little clinical evidence to support this beyond anecdotal reports. There is much work going on, including clinical trials, throughout the world though less so in the US because of the Schedule 1 category for cannabis.

■ Safety

As with efficacy, there is limited data on cannabis safety. Again, from the above-cited consensus report, following are the safety data results in brief:

- Substantial evidence: Being male and smoking cigarettes are risk factors for progression to problem marijuana use, starting marijuana at an early age is a risk factor for development of problem marijuana use.
- Moderate evidence: Being male, use of alcohol, tobacco, and other illicit drugs, during adolescence the frequency of cannabis use, oppositional behaviors, a younger age of first alcohol use, nicotine use, parental substance use, poor school performance, anti-social behaviors, and childhood sexual abuse are risk factors.

- Substantial statistical evidence: Increased risk of car crashes, increased risk of overdose, lower birth weight in offspring of users, development of schizophrenia and other psychoses especially with frequent users.
- Limited statistical evidence but no clear clinical evidence: Increased risk of cancer or leukemia, triggering a stroke or myocardial infarct, worsening of respiratory symptoms, pregnancy complications, impairment of learning, increased risk of depression, suicide attempts, anxiety disorders, increased severity of post-traumatic stress disorder, impaired operation of machinery.

Marijuana crosses the placental barrier and gets into the fetus. It is also found in breast milk. There is weak data suggesting that the babies of users were twice as likely to end up in the neonatal ICU, have smaller heads and lower birth weight and later problems of cognition, memory and behavior.

A report in the *New England Journal of Medicine* (N Engl J Med 2014; 370(23): 2219–2227, doi:10.1056/NEJMra1402309.) noted that there is a real risk for addiction particularly in adolescents (9–16%). There is also a withdrawal syndrome of irritability, sleeping difficulty, dysphoria, craving, and anxiety. They also noted several similar safety issues cited above in the National Academies of Sciences report cited above. The authors concluded: "As policy shifts toward legalization of marijuana, it is reasonable and probably prudent to hypothesize that its use will increase and that, by extension, so will the number of persons for whom there will be negative health consequences."

As use of cannabis increases and as more attention is paid by the medical community, new safety issues are being noted. For example, recently there have been reports of severe cyclic nausea and vomiting in heavy users that abates upon cessation. See https://www.ncbi.nlm.nih.gov/pmc/articles/PMC5360975/.

The latest safety labeling for the two FDA approved synthetic THC products include: Asthenia, palpitations, tachycardia, vasodilation, abdominal pain, nausea, vomiting, amnesia, anxiety, nervousness, ataxia, confusion, depersonalization, dizziness, euphoria, hallucinations, paranoid reactions, somnolence and abnormal thinking & (rarer): low blood pressure, diarrhea, fecal incontinence, myalgia, depression, nightmares, speech problems, tinnitus, flushing, conjunctivitis, drug interactions.

There are warnings and precautions about use in patients with seizures, heart problems, psychiatric drugs.

From the public health point of view there are data supporting increased incidences of marijuana-related traffic deaths (http://www.factcheck.org/2016/08/unpacking-pots-impact-in-colorado/), emergency room visits for marijuana related-problems and increased ER visits for children and babies who consume edible marijuana products http://www.denverpost.com/2016/07/25/colorado-kids-emergency-room-visits-marijuana-increased/). There are reports of tainted marijuana products. See https://www.ncbi.nlm.nih.gov/pmc/articles/PMC3568288/.

There have been reports of contamination of marijuana products with arsenic, lead and the mold Aspergillus producing serious illness. Cannabis is a type of plant known as a "hyperaccumulator" or "accumulator" which means it absorbs and accumulates from the soil such things as heavy metals (cadmium, nickel, and lead), fertilizers, pesticides and other harmful products. See: https://ehp.niehs.nih.gov/doi/10.1289/EHP12074.

Reports and studies have been published suggesting problems in pregnancy with gestational use including low birth weights, birth lengths and gestational age at birth independent of or synergistic with smoking tobacco.

Drug Interactions: This is an area that has been explored to some degree. The pharmacology is known: THC and cannabinoids are metabolized by cytochrome P450 (CYP)3A4; THC is also metabolized by CYP2C. It has been found that the use of ketoconazole (a CYP3A4 inhibitor) can double the THC and cannabidiol concentrations. CYP2C9 inhibitors would be expected to increase THC exposure also. Cannabadiol inhibits CYP2C19 increasing levels of clobazam. Reports of elevated INR levels and bleeding have been reported with marijuana and warfarin. See the review in the Canadian Medical Association Journal CMAJ v.192(9); 2020 Mar 2.

The best FDA site for the status and news of marijuana is: https://www.fda.gov/news-events/public-health-focus/fda-regulation-cannabis-and-cannabis-derived-products-including-cannabidiol-cbd#relatedinfo

Canada

Medical and recreational cannabis is now legal in all of Canada. Similar issues as reported in the US have been seen in cannabis used in Canada. See https://www.canada.ca/en/health-canada/services/drugs-medication/cannabis/personal-use/reduce-risk-choose-legal.html

Europe

In Europe, the situation is complex and fluid. There is no harmonization on cannabis yet. In most countries, recreational use is forbidden but many have decriminalized its possession. In several European countries medical use is legal including Croatia, Cyprus, Czech Republic, Denmark, Finland, Germany, Greece, Ireland, Italy Luxembourg, Malta, The Netherlands, Poland, Portugal, Spain, Switzerland, UK. Others may follow (trials are ongoing in France among others).

See the websites below on the legal status of possession, salc, transport and cultivation country by country. See http://www.emcdda.europa.eu/publications/adhoc/ and https://en.wikipedia.org/wiki/Legality_of_cannabis_by_country. A summary report from the European Centre for Drugs and Drug Addiction addresses the legislation concerning cannabis possession and use in Europe. See http://www.emcdda.europa.eu/system/files/publica-tions/4135/TD0217210ENN.pdf/.

Comments

Clearly medical and recreational cannabis use is an idea that is spreading rapidly in the US, Canada, Europe and elsewhere. The authors cannot remember any similar situation where a Schedule 1 drug that was universally illegal (and still is at the US federal level) has been approved for medical and recreational use at the local level. Perhaps the prohibition of alcohol in the US from 1917 to 1933 is the closest example.

Since this is an unprecedented situation, we do not have any real precedents to look towards for guidance. Nonetheless, several points can be made, some of which are self-evident and some are less so:

- **Cannabis is a drug:** Cannabis in all forms should be considered a pharmacologically-active drug no matter what the delivery system. Some have said that when cannabis is delivered in food it should be considered a food and not a drug. We feel this is not correct and the reality is that this is a drug packaged in a food delivery system.
- **Chain of Control is not assured:** The chain of control for both recreational and medical cannabis products is not as tight as the chain of control for commercial drug products. That is, consumers and patients have a strong assurance that a drug product purchased in a licensed pharmacy or an over-the-counter setting is the correct, unaltered, and unadulterated product. The product leaving the production plant will be the same as the one the patient picks up in the pharmacy.

  This is not clearly the case with cannabis. If a firm is vertically integrated (the producer is also the retailer), then there should be good assurance that thc product is as intended and expected. If, however, the cannabis is to be baked into food, have other flavorings or ingredients added or even tampered with, then any assurance of a pure and unchanged product is lost.

  There are reports of anti-coagulants, fentanyl, glass and many other substances being added illicitly to cannabis products producing severe toxicity in users requiring hospitalization. In addition, some patients may use a mix of various cannabis preparations, illicit and/or licit, making the identification of the responsible product impossible.

  See also the National Institute on Drug Abuse webpages: https://www.drugabuse.gov/drugs-abuse/marijuana.
- **Regulations are not harmonized:** The laws and regulations regarding safety (amongst other things) are not standardized in the US or the EU for

cannabis. Some states allow it; some do not. There is no FDA oversight of cannabis. Users, producers, middlemen, and vendors must look at state and local laws which are inconsistent with each other and are often even non-existent. In addition, the black market of illegally produced and sold marijuana continues to flourish. The advent of legal marijuana does not mean these illegal sources will disappear. Often the illegal marijuana is cheaper than the legal marijuana.

- **Quality:** Not all manufacturing or use follows the predicate rules of Good Manufacturing Practice (GMP), Good Clinical Practice (GCP), and Good Pharmacovigilance Practice (GVP).
- **Indications for use:** These have either not been defined well or have been defined very broadly for indications for which there is little or no data. For example, at the time of this text, Pennsylvania has approved cannabis use for these conditions (https:// www.pa.gov/guides/pennsylvania-medical-marijuana-program/#17MedicalConditions):
  - Amyotrophic lateral sclerosis
  - Anxiety disorders
  - Autism
  - Cancer, including remission therapy
  - Chronic Hepatitis C
  - Crohn's disease
  - Damage to the nervous tissue of the central nervous system (brain-spinal cord) with objective neurological indication of intractable spasticity, and other associated neuropathies
  - Dyskinetic and spastic movement disorders
  - Epilepsy
  - Glaucoma
  - HIV/AIDS
  - Huntington's disease
  - Inflammatory bowel disease
  - Intractable seizures
  - Multiple sclerosis
  - Neurodegenerative diseases
  - Neuropathies
  - Opioid use disorder for which conventional therapeutic interventions are contraindicated or ineffective, or for which adjunctive therapy is indicated in combination with primary therapeutic interventions.
  - Parkinson's disease
  - Post-traumatic stress disorder
  - Severe chronic or intractable pain of neuropathic origin or severe chronic or intractable pain
  - Sickle cell anemia
  - Terminal illness
- **Dosing:** Dosing for medical use has not been well-established or established at all nor has potency been standardized.
- **Labeling:** The labeling for cannabis products is also not standardized and may be minimal or non-existent. Often it is wrong! A 2017 study from the University of Pennsylvania found that nearly 70% of cannabidiol extracts sold online were mislabeled (see https://www.pennmedicine.org/news/news-releases/2017/november/penn-study-shows-nearly-70-percent-of-cannabidiol-extracts-sold-online-are-mislabeled).
- **SAEs and death:** Adverse events and deaths are not being collected or reported consistently or, in many cases, at all. Most states do not require the collection by producers or vendors or reporting to health authorities of SAEs and deaths.

It is not clear how recreational and medical marijuana will interact. Will patients go through the effort and cost to see a health care provider, register and obtain medical marijuana or will they simply go in and buy some recreational marijuana right away. Will more easily obtained recreational marijuana drive out medical marijuana?

Bottom Line

At this point there really is minimal pharmacovigilance in place for cannabis. Adverse events and deaths are often not reported or not reported consistently and problem products may be left on the market. To complicate matters, individual cases often involve multiple pharmacologically-active agents at doses that are unknown. Signaling cannot be done adequately. Causality and potential interactions are difficult to assess. There is clearly a strong need for a consistent and national or regional (e.g., EU) control of cannabis and its use and safety. There will also be non-medical interested parties involved such as business people, investors, stockbrokers and others who will affect the way the cannabis story plays out.

Marijuana use, both recreationally and medically, may well become a major public health problem. It is highly likely that regulations will tighten up particularly if a major health disaster occurs with cannabis use.

Abbreviations

ACK Electronic Acknowledgement
ADE Adverse Drug Experience or Event
ADR Adverse Drug Reaction
AE Adverse Event
AEFI Adverse Event Following Immunization
AEMPS Spanish Medicines and Healthcare Products Agency, Agencia Espanola de Medicamentosy Productos Sanitarios, www.aemps.gob.es/
AESI Adverse Event of Special Interest
AIFA Italian Ministry of Health (Agenzie per i Farmaci)
AMP Authorised/Authorized Medicinal Product
ANM Romanian National Medicines Agency (Agentia Nationola a Medicamentului), http://www.anm.ro/en/home.html
ANSM French National Agency of Safety of Medicines and Products of Health (Agence National de Sécurité des Médicaments et Produits de santé), formerly Afssaps, http://ansm.sante.fr/
API Active Pharmaceutical Ingredient (sometimes Application Programming Interface)
AR Adverse Reaction, sometimes Assessment Report (EU)
ATC Anatomical-Therapeutic-Chemical classification
ATMP Advanced Therapy Medicinal Product (EU)
BCP Business Continuity Plan
BCPNN Baysian Confidence Propagation Neural Network

BfArM	German Federal Institute for Drugs and Medical Devices, Bundesinstitut für Arzneimittel und Medizinproducte, http://www.bfarm.de/EN/Home/home_node.html, also see PEI for vaccines and therapeutic biologics
BLA	Biologic License Application, formerly Product License Application (US)
BMI	Body Mass Index
BDA	Bulgarian Drug Agency
BPI	Association of the German Pharmaceutical Industry, www.bpi.de
B-R	Benefit-Risk, sometimes BR or Risk-Benefit
BTC	Behind the counter (as opposed to Over The Counter, OTC)
CA	Competent Authority, see NCA
CAEFISS	Canadian Adverse Events Following Immunization Surveillance System
CAP	Centralised Authorisation Procedure (EU), sometimes College of American Pathologists
CBER	Center for Biologics Evaluation and Research at FDA (US)
CCSI	Company Core Safety Information, part of CCDs, see CSI
CCDS	Company Core Data Sheet for marketed products, see CDS
CDC	Centers for Disease Control (US), www.cdc.gov/
CDER	Center for Drug Evaluation and Research at FDA (US), http://www.fda.gov/Drugs/default.htm
CDRH	Center for Devices and Radiological Health at FDA (US), www.fda.gov/medicaldevices/default.htm
CDS	Core Data Sheet, see CCDS; sometimes Clinical Diagnostic Scale
CEM	Cohort Event Monitoring
CEN	Centre Européen Normalisation (the European Committee for Standardization), www.cen.eu/
CI	Continuous Improvement
CIOMS	Council for International Organisations of Medical Sciences, www.cioms.ch
CONSORT	Consolidated Standards of Reporting Trials
CPMP	Committee for Proprietary Medicinal Products, replaced by CHMP (EU)
CFR	Code of Federal Regulations (US)
CHMP	Committee for Medicinal Products for Human Use, formerly CPMP (EU)
CIOMS	Council for Organisations of Medical Sciences
CNA	Competent National Authority, see NCA
CMDh	Coordination Group for Mutual Recognition and Decentralized Procedures (human) (EU), sometimes CMD(h)
CMS	Concerned Member State (EU)
COSTART	Coding Symbols for Thesaurus of Adverse Reaction Terms (US), largely superseded by MedDRA
CPRD	Clinical Practice Research Datalink (UK), http://www.cprd.com/home/ also see GPRD
CRF	Case Report Form
CRO	Contract Research Organization/ Clinical Research Organization
CSI	Core Safety Information
CSP	Core Safety Profile (RSI for work sharing PSUR assessment in the EEA)
CSR	Clinical Study Report
CT	Clinical Trial
CTA	Clinical Trial Authorization, sometimes refers to Clinical Trial Agreement
CTASR	Clinical Trial Annual Safety Report, see ASR (EU), replaced by DSUR
CTC	Clinical Toxicity Criteria, sometimes refers to Clinical Trial Certificate, see CTCAE
CTCAE	Common Terminology Criteria for Adverse Events

CTD	EU Clinical Trials Directive, or EU CTD, see CTDir; mostoften CTD refers to ICH M4 Common Technical Document and the electronic format to eCTD
CTEP	Cancer Therapy Evaluation Program (US), ctep.cancer.gov/
CTM	EudraVigilance Clinical Trials Module, see EVCTM
CTX	Clinical Trials Exemption Certificate, now incorporated into the CTA
CV	Curriculum Vitae, sometimes cardiovascular or other terms
DCSI	Development Core Safety Information
DD	Due Diligence
DDD	Defined Daily Dose
DDL	Dear Doctor Letter, see DHPC
DHHS	Department of Health and Human Services, often HHS (US), www.hhs.gov/
DHPC	Direct Healthcare Professional Communication, see DDL
DIA	Drug Information Association, or simply DIA, www.diahome.org
DIBD	Development International Birth Date, sometimes D-IBD
DILI	Drug-Induced Liver Injury
DKMA	Danish Medicines Agency, Laegemiddel Styrelsen
DLP	Data Lock Point
DMC	Data Monitoring Committee
DMEC	Data Monitoring and Ethics Committee
DMP	Development Medicinal Product
DOI	Digital Object Identifier
dQP	Deputy Qualified Person, see QPPV
DSMB	Data Safety Monitoring Board
DSRU	Drug Safety Research Unit, University of Southampton (UK)
DSUR	Development Safety Update Report, see E2F and CIOMS VII Report
DTC	Direct To Consumer
DTD	Document Type Definition (specification used in electronic transactions)
DTP	Direct To Patient
DUI	Drug Utilization Information (Japan)
DUS	Drug Utilization Study
E2A	ICH guideline on definitions and terminology for key aspects of clinical trial safety reporting titled, "Clinical Safety Data Management: Definitions and Standards for Expedited Reporting"
E2B	ICH guideline on standard data elements for the transmission of ICSRs titled, "Clinical Safety Data Management: Data Elements for Transmission of Individual Case Safety Reports"
E2B(R3)	ICH revision standard data elements for the transmission of ICSRs
E2C	ICH guideline on the content and format for Periodic Safety Update Reports for marketed products, see E2C(R1) and Addendum to E2C(R1)
E2C(R1)	ICH guideline on Periodic Safety Update Reports titled, "Clinical Safety Data Management: Periodic Safety Update Reports for Marketed Drugs," which incorporates the E2C(R1) Addendum as of November 2005
E2C(R1) Addendum	Addendum to ICH E2C guideline on Periodic Safety Update Reports titled, "Addendum to E2C: Periodic Safety Update Reports for Marketed Drugs," which has been incorporated into ICH E2C(R1); sometimes referred to as Addendum to E2C or Addendum to E2C(R1)
E2D	ICH definitions and standards for post-marketing expedited safety reporting titled, "Post-Approval Safety Data Management: Definitions and Standards for Expedited Reporting"

E2E	ICH guideline on pharmacovigilance planning (risk management) titled, "Pharmacovigilance Planning"
E2F	ICH guideline on pre-authorization safety reporting or Development Safety Update Report (DSUR) titled, "Development Safety Update Report," in development
E6	ICH guideline on good clinical practices titled, "Good Clinical Practice: Consolidated Guideline," sometimes E6
EACPT	European Association for Clinical Pharmacology and Therapeutics, www.eacpt.org/
EBD	European Birth Date (date product first authorized for marketing in the EU)
EBGM	Empirical Bayes Geometric Mean
EC	Ethics Committee (EU), sometimes European Commission or Council of the European Union of the European Council or European Community, see IRB
ECDC	European Centre for disease Prevention and Control
EDI	Electronic Data Interchange
eCTD	Electronic Common Technical Document
EDC	Electronic Data Capture
EEA	European Economic Area
EFPIA	European Federation of Pharmaceutical Industries and Associations, www.efpia.org
EFTA	European Free Trade Area
EGA	European Generic Medicines Association, www.egagenerics.com
EHR	Electronic Health Record, see EMR
ELA	Establishment License Application (US)
EMA	European Medicines Agency, formerly EMEA, www.ema.europa.eu/
EMEA	European Medicines Agency, now EMA
EMR	Electronic Medical Record
ENCePP	European Network of Centres for Pharmacoepidemiology and Pharmacovigilance, www.encepp.eu/
ENS	Early Notification System
ENTIS	European Network of Teratology Information Services
EOF	Greek regulator, National Organization for Medicines
EORTC	European Organization for Research and Treatment of Cancer, www.eortc.be
EPAR	European Public Assessment Report
EPITT	European Pharmacovigilance Issue Tracking Tool
EPPV	Early Postmarketing Pharmacovigilance (Japan)
ePSUR	Periodic Safety Update Report in structured electronic format
ESCOP	European Scientific Cooperative on Phytotherapy, www.escop.com/
ESMO	European Society for Medical Oncology, www.esmo.org
ESTRI	Electronic Standards for the Transfer of Regulatory Information (ICH M2 topic)
ETASU	Element to Assure Safe Use (of the drug)
EU	European Union
Eu2P	European Programme in Pharmacovigilance and Pharmacoepidemiology
EU-HBD	European Harmonised Birth Date for marketed medicinal products (related to PSUR within the EEA), see EBD and IBD
EudraCT	European Union Drug Regulating Authorities Clinical Trials
EURD	European Union Reference Date
EuropaBio	European Association for BioIndustries, www.europabio.org
EU TCT	European Union Telematics Controlled Terms
EV	EudraVigilance, European database of ICSRs, eudravigilance.ema.europa.eu/

EVACO	European Vaccination Coverage Collection System
EVCTM	EudraVigilance Clinical Trials Module, see CTM
EVDBMS	EudraVigilance Database Management System, see DBMS
EVMPD	EudraVigilance Medicinal Products Dictionary, sometimes MPD, also see XEVMPD
EVPM	EudraVigilance Post-Authorization Module, sometimes PM
EVWEB	EudraVigilance web interface
EWG	Expert Working Group
FAERS	Federal Adverse Event Reporting System (US FDA)
FAQ	Frequently asked questions
FDA	Food and Drug Administration (US and several other countries), www.fda.gov
FDA 3500	Form FDA-3500 (MedWatch form for voluntary reporting of Individual Case Safety Reports to FDA)
FDA 3500A	Form FDA-3500A (MedWatch form for mandatory reporting of Individual Case Safety Reports to FDA)
FDAAA	Food and Drug Administration Amendments Act (FDA)
FDARA	Food and Drug Administration Reauthorization Act (FDA)
FIC	Family of International Classifications (WHO)
FIMEA	Finnish Medicines Agency, http://www.fimea.fi/
FMQ	FDA MedDRA Query
FOI	Freedom Of Information (primarily US)
FTP	File Transfer Protocol
GACVS	Global Advisory Committee on Vaccine Safety (WHO)
GCP	Good Clinical Practice(s), see ICH E6 guideline
GLP(s)	Good Laboratory Practice(s)
GMP(s)	Good Manufacturing Practice(s)
GPMSP	Good Postmarketing Study Practices (Japan)
GPP	Guidelines for Good Pharmacoepidemiology Practices (ISPE)
GPRD	General Practice Research Database (UK), www.gprd.com/
GPvP	Good Pharmacovigilance Practice(s), see also GVP
GRAS	Generally Recognized As Safe (US)
GVP	Good Pharmacovigilance Practices, sometimes Good Vigilance Practices (distinct guidelines for EU, JP, etc.)
GXP	Sometimes GxP, an all-inclusive reference to GCPs, GLPs, and GMPs
HA	Health Authority
HC	Health Canada, www.hc-sc.gc.ca
HCP	Healthcare Provider, sometimes Healthcare Professional, sometimes HcP
hERG	Human ether-à-go-go related gene, (encodes the potassium ion channel responsible for IKr)
HHS	Department of Health and Human Services, www.hhs.gov/
HL7	Health Level Seven, a Standards Development Organization, www.hl7.org
HLGT	High Level Group Term (in MedDRA hierarchy)
HLT	High Level Term (in MedDRA hierarchy)
HMA	Heads of Medicines Agencies (EU Competent Authorities) see HoA, www.hma.eu
HoA	Heads of Agencies (EU Competent Authorities), see HMA
HPFB	Health Products and Food Branch of Health Canada
HSA	Health Sciences Authority (Singapore), www.hsa.gov.sg/
HTA	Health Technology Assessment
IB	Investigator Brochure
IBD	International Birth Date

ICF	Informed Consent Form, sometimes Information Component (when used in BCPNN)
ICD-9	International Classification of Diseases, ninth revision (see MEDIS)
ICD-9CM	International Classification of Diseases, ninth revision, with Clinical Modification
ICD-11	International Classification of Diseases, eleventh revision
ICH	The International Conference on Harmonization of Technical Requirements for Registration of Pharmaceuticals for Human Use, see www.ich.org
ICSR	Individual Case Safety Report
ICT	Interventional Clinical Trial
IDMP	Identification of Medicinal Products (ISO, formerly ICH M5)
IFPMA	International Federation of Pharmaceutical Manufacturers Associations, www.ifpma.org
IG	Implementation Guide
IIR	Investigator Initiated Research
IIS	Investigator Initiated Study
IIT	Investigator Initiated Trial
IKr	Rapidly-active delayed rectifier potassium ion channel (cardiac)
Iks	Slowly-active delayed rectifier potassium ion channel (cardiac)
IMB	Irish Medicines Board, www.imb.ie/
IMCA	Icelandic Medicines Control Agency (Lyfjastofnun), www.imca.is/
IME	Important Medical Event
IMI	Innovative Medicines Initiative (EU)
IMMP	The Intensive Medicines Monitoring Programme (New Zealand)
IMP	Investigational Medicinal Product (EU)
IMPD	Investigational Medicinal Product Dossier
IMS	IMS Health (a source of healthcare statistics), sometimes Information Management System Now a part of IQVIA www.iqvia.com
IND	Investigational New Drug (US)
INFARMED	Portuguese National Institute of Pharmacy and Medicine, Instituto Nacional da Farmacia e do Medicamento, www.infarmed.pt/
INN	International Non-proprietary Name
IRB	Institutional Review Board (North America), see EC
IRBR	Incremental Risk-Benefit Ratio
ISMP	Institute for Safe Medical Practices
ISO	International Organization for Standardization, www.iso.org
ISoP	International Society of Pharmacovigilance, see www.isoponline.org
ISPE	International Society for Pharmacoepidemiology, see www.pharmacoepi.org
IST	Investigator Sponsored Trial
IT	Information Technology
J-ART	Japanese adaptation of WHO-ART, see WHO-ART
J-MedDRA	Japanese language version of MedDRA® (also MedDRA/J)
JMO	Japanese Management Organization (for MedDRA/J)
JPMA	Japanese Pharmaceutical Manufacturers' Association, http://www.jpma.or.jp/english/
KOL	Key Opinion Leader
KPI	Key Performance Indicator
LAREB	Landelijke Registratie en Evaluatie van Bijwerkingen (Netherlands Pharmacovigilance Foundation), www.lareb.nl/
LEEM	Les Entreprises du Médicament (Association of the French Pharmaceutical Industry), www.leem.org
LFT	Liver Function Test(s)
LLT	Lowest Level Term (in MedDRA hierarchy)
LOINC	Logical Observations: Identifiers, Names, Codes (for lab data), loinc.org/
LPD	Local Product Document
LSSS	Large simple safety studies

M1	ICH topic on international medical terminology, e.g., Points to Consider, see MedDRA
M2	ICH guidelines on electronic standards for the transfer of regulatory information
M5	ICH guideline on the identification of medicinal products
MA	Marketing Authorization
MAA	Marketing Authorization Application
MAH	Marketing Authorization Holder
MAUDE	Manufacturer and User Facility Device Experience database at FDA (CDRH)
MCA	Medicines Control Agency (UK), replaced by MHRA
MDN	Electronic Message Disposition Notification
MDR	Medical Device Reporting program database at FDA (CDRH), historical data, see DEN
MEB	Dutch Medicines Evaluation Board (and the MEB Agency), www.cbg-meb.nl
MedDRA®	Medical Dictionary for Regulatory Activities terminology (ICH Topic M1), see www.meddramsso.com
MedDRA/J	Japanese language version of MedDRA®, sometimes J-MedDRA
MEDIS	Japanese adaptation of ICD-9
MedSun	Medical Product Surveillance Network for medical devices (US)
MedWatch	FDA medical products safety reporting program (see FDA 3500 and FDA 3500A), www.fda.gov/Safety/MedWatch/default.htm
MGPS	Multi-Item Gamma Poisson Shrinker
MHLW	Ministry of Health, Labour and Welfare or Koseirodosho (Japan), www.mhlw.go.jp
MHRA	Medicines and Healthcare products Regulatory Agency (UK), formerly MCA, www.mhra.gov.uk/
MIHARI	Medical Information for Risk Assessment Initiative (Japan)
MLM	Medical Literature Monitoring
MPA	Swedish Medical Products Agency, Läkemedelsverket, www.lakemedelsverket.se/english/
MPD	Medicinal Products Dictionary (EU), frequently EVMPD or EV MPD, also see XEVMPD
MPR	Medicinal Product Report (EU)
MRC	Medical Research Council (UK), www.mrc.ac.uk
MRP	Mutual Recognition Procedure, see DCP (EU)
MS	Member State (EU)
MSF	Médecins Sans Frontières/Doctors without Borders
MSSO	Maintenance and Support Services Organization (for MedDRA), see www.meddramsso.com
NAP	National Authorization Procedure
NB	Net Benefit
NCA	National Competent Authority, see CNA
NCE	New Chemical Entity
NCS	Not Clinically Significant
NCVIA	National Childhood Vaccine Injury Act
NDA	New Drug Application (US), see MAA
NDF-RT	National Drug File Reference Terminology (US)
NDS	New Drug Submission (Canada), see BLA, NDA, and MAA
NEC	Not Elsewhere Classified (in MedDRA terminology)
NGO	Non-Governmental Organization
NICE	National Institute for Health and Care Excellence (UK)
NIMP	Non-Investigational Medicinal Product (EU)
NLM	National Library of Medicine (US), www.nlm.nih.gov
NME	New Molecular Entity

NNH	Number Needed to Harm
NNT	Number Needed to Treat
NoMA	Norwegian Medicines Agency, Statens legemiddelverk or SLV
NOS	Not Otherwise Specified (in MedDRA terminology)
NUI	Non-Urgent Information
OGYI	Hungarian regulatory agency, National Institute of Pharmacy, Országos Gyógyszerészeti Intézet, www.topra.org
OMOP	Observational Medical Outcomes Partnership (US), http://omop.fnih.org
OMS	World Health Organization, also WHO, www.who.int
OND	Office of New Drugs at CDER
OPDP	Office of Prescription Drug Promotion at FDA, formerly DDMAC (US)
OSE	Office of Surveillance and Epidemiology (FDA/CDER), formerly Office of Drug Safety
OTC	Over The Counter
OTIS	Organization of Teratology Information Services
PAC	Patient Alert Card (EU)
PAES	Post-Authorization Efficacy Study (EU)
PAFSC	Pharmaceutical Affairs and Food Sanitation Council (Japan)
PAHO	Pan American Health Organization (WHO), www.paho.org
PAL	Pharmaceutical Affairs Law (Japan)
PAR	Public Assessment Report, see EPAR (EU)
PAS	Post-Authorization Study (EU)
PASS	Post-Authorization Safety Study (EU)
PBRER	Periodic Benefit-Risk Evaluation Report, see PSUR and ICH E2C(R2) guideline
PCC	Poison Control Center
PCORI	Patient-Centered Outcomes Research Institute (US)
PD	Pharmacodynamics
PDUFA	Prescription Drug User Fee Act (FDA)
PEI	German Federal Agency for Sera and Vaccines, Paul-Ehrlich-Institut Bundesamt für Sera und Impfstoffe, see BfArM
PEM	Prescription Event Monitoring
PFSB	Pharmaceutical and Food Safety Bureau (Japan)
PhPID	Pharmaceutical Identification of Medicinal Products
PhRMA	Pharmaceutical Research and Manufacturers Association, www.phrma.org/
PhVIWG	Pharmacovigilance Inspectors Working Group (at EMA)
PhVWP	Pharmacovigilance Working Party, replaced by the PRAC (EU)
PIL	Patient Information Leaflet (EU)
PIM	Product Information Management system (EU)
PIP	Paediatric/Pediatric Investigation Plan (EU)
PIS	Patient Information Sheets
PK	Pharmacokinetics
PK/PD	Pharmacokinetics/pharmacodynamics
PL	Package Leaflet
PLA	Product License Application, superseded by BLA (US)
PLR	Physicians Labelling Rule (US)
PM	EudraVigilance Post-Authorization Module (EU), sometimes Post-Marketing (worldwide)
PMA	Pre-Market Approval (US application for medical devices)
PMC	Post-Marketing Commitment
PMDA	Pharmaceuticals and Medical Devices Agency (Japan), www.pmda.go.jp/english/index.html
PMR	Post-Marketing Requirement
PMS	Post-Marketing Surveillance
POM	Prescription Only Medicine
PRAC	Pharmacovigilance Risk Assessment Committee (EU)
PRO	Patient Reported Outcome
PRR	Proportional Reporting Ratio

PSMF Pharmacovigilance System Master File (EU), replaced DDPS
PSUR Periodic Safety Update Report, see E2C
PT Preferred Term (in MedDRA and other terminologies)
PTC Points to Consider, also PtC
PV Pharmacovigilance, sometimes PhV
PVA Pharmacovigilance agreement
PVSMF Pharmacovigilance System Master File
QA Quality Assurance
QALY Quality Adjusted Life Year(s)
QC Quality Control
QD Quality Document
QoL Quality of Life
QP See QPPV
QPPV EU Qualified Person for Pharmacovigilance, sometimes EU QPPV or QP
QRC or QR Quick Response Code
QS Quality System
RA Rapid Alert, sometimes Regulatory Affairs
R-B Risk-Benefit, sometimes RB, see B-R
RCA Root Cause Analysis
RCT Randomized Clinical Trial
REMS Risk Evaluation and Mitigation Strategy (US)
RMP Risk Management Plan
RMS Reference Member State (EU), sometimes Risk Management Strategy
ROW Rest of World
RSI Reference Safety Information
RTF Refusal To File (US)
RWA Real World Analytics
RWD Real World Data
SADR Suspected Adverse Drug Reaction (US, proposed)
SAE Serious Adverse Event
SAR Serious Adverse Reaction
SCDM Society for Clinical Data Management
SDO Standards Development Organization
SESAR Suspected Expected Serious Adverse Reaction
SFDA State Food and Drug Administration (Peoples Republic of China), sometimes Shanghai Food and Drug Administration (Peoples Republic of China) or Saudi Food and Drug Administration (Saudi Arabia)
SGML Standard Generalized/Generalized Markup Language
SI Scientific Information (Japan)
SLV Norwegian Statens legemiddelverk, see NoMA
SME Subject Matter Expert
SmPC Summary of Product Characteristics, see SPC (EU)
SMG Standardized MedDRA Groupings (for labeling)
SMQ Standardized MedDRA Query
Snomed® Systematized Nomenclature of Medicine (registered mark of CAP)
Snomed CT® Snomed Clinical Terms (Snomed RT plus UK NHS Clinical Terms)
Snomed® PL Snomed Problem List (US Veteran's Administration/Kaiser Permanente)
Snomed RT® Snomed Reference Terms
SOC System Organ Class (in MedDRA terminology)
SOP Standard Operating Procedure
SPC Summary of Product Characteristics, see SmPC (EU); also may refer to Supplementary Protection Certificate for intellectual property protection (EU)
SPL Structured Product Labeling (US), see PLR
SPS Summary of Pharmacovigilance System
SSR Special Situation Report
STN Submission Tracking Number (FDA)
SUKL Czech Republic (Státní ústav pro kontrolu léčiv), www.sukl.cz/, or Slovak Republic State Institute for Drug Control (Slovenska verzia),
SUSAR Suspected Unexpected Serious Adverse Reaction

TCT	European Union Telematics Controlled Terms, see EU TCT
TGA	Therapeutic Goods Administration (Australia)
TPD	Therapeutic Products Directorate of Health Canada
UMC	Uppsala Monitoring Centre, see www.who-umc.org
UMLS	Unified Medical Language System metathesaurus (US-based dictionary repository)
USPI	United States Package Insert
USPR	United States Periodic Report
USR	Urgent Safety Restriction (EU)
VAERS	Vaccine Adverse Event Reporting System (FDA/CBER/CDC)
WHO	World Health Organization
WHO-ART	World Health Organization Adverse Reaction Terminology
WHO-CC	World Health Organization Collaborating Centre
WHO-DD	World Health Organization Drug Dictionary
WHO-DDE	World Health Organization Drug Dictionary Enhanced
XEVMPD	Extended EudraVigilance Medicinal Products Dictionary, sometimes xEVMPD
XEVPRM	Extended Eudravigilance Product Report Message
XML	Extensible Markup Language

www.ingramcontent.com/pod-product-compliance
Lightning Source LLC
LaVergne TN
LVHW081947200926
848484LV00009B/2516